Nursing Management
for the Elderly

Contributors

Judith Atwood, R.N., M.N.
Clinical Supervisor, Medicine and Epilepsy,
Harborview Medical Center, Seattle, Washington

Mari Anne Bartol, R.N., M.N.
Geriatric Clinical Specialist, Geriatric Research,
Education and Clinical Center, Seattle/American
Lake Veterans Administration Hospitals,
Tacoma, Washington

James Bennett, D.M.D.
Director, Hospital Dental Residents,
Health Sciences Center,
University of Oregon,
Portland, Oregon

Suzanne Bither, R.N., M.N.
Coordinator, Pulmonary Rehabilitation Program,
Portland Adventist Medical Center,
Portland, Oregon

Carole Blainey, R.N., M.N.
Associate Professor, Department of Physiological Nursing,
Diabetic Nurse Clinician, Diabetes Research Center,
University of Washington,
Seattle, Washington

Gretchen G. Boyer, R.N., B.S.N.
Former Ophthalmology Nurse Clinician,
Graduate Student, Gerontology,
University of Washington,
Seattle, Washington

Pauline Bruno, R.N., D.N.Sc.
Associate Professor, Department of Physiological Nursing,
University of Washington,
Seattle, Washington

Doris L. Carnevali, R.N., M.N.
Associate Professor, Community Health Care Systems,
University of Washington,
Seattle, Washington

Ann Cordes, R.N.
Nurse Clinician, Iowa Veterans Home,
Marshalltown, Iowa

Dorothy Crowley, R.N., Ph.D.
Professor, Department of Physiological Nursing,
Associate Dean, Graduate Programs,
School of Nursing, University of Washington,
Seattle, Washington

Ralph Goldman, M.D.
Assistant Chief Medical Director for Extended Care,
Veterans Administration, Department of Medicine
and Surgery, Washington, D.C.

Robert Greifinger, M.D.
Medical Director, Community Health Plan of
Suffolk, Inc., Health Sciences Center,
State University of New York at Stony Brook,
Stony Brook, New York

Richard Grossman
Director, Center for Health in Medicine,
Montefiore Hospital and Medical Center,
Bronx, New York

M. Edith Heinemann, R.N., M.A.
Professor, Department of Psychosocial Medicine,
Director, Alcohol and Drug Abuse Nursing,
University of Washington, Seattle, Washington

Margaret Heitkemper, R.N., M.N.
Doctoral Student, Department of Physiology,
University of Illinois, Chicago.
Former Research Associate, Department of
Physiological Nursing, University of Washington,
Seattle, Washington

Tom Hickey, D.P.H.
Associate Professor, Health Gerontology,
Department of Community Health Programs,
School of Public Health, University of Michigan,
Ann Arbor, Michigan

Marianne Ivey, B.S.
Associate Professor, Director of Continuing
Pharmacy Education, Pharmacy Practice,
School of Pharmacy, University of Washington,
Seattle, Washington

George L. Larson, Ph.D.
Chief, Speech Pathology, Veterans Administration
Hospital, Seattle, Washington

Maria Linde, R.N.
Stroke Nurse Clinician, Virginia Mason Hospital,
Seattle, Washington

Doris M. Molbo, R.N., M.A.
Assistant Professor, Department of Physiological Nursing,
University of Washington, Seattle, Washington

Maxine Patrick, R.N., Dr.P.H.
Chairman, Department of Physiological Nursing,
School of Nursing, University of Washington,
Seattle

Caroline E. Preston, M.A.
Associate Professor, Department of Psychiatry and
Behavioral Sciences, School of Medicine,
University of Washington, Seattle, Washington

Nancy J. Roben, R.N., B.S.N.
Nurse Practitioner, Medical Comprehensive Care Unit,
Veterans Administration Hospital, Seattle, Washington

Kathleen Smith-Di Julio, R.N., M.A.
Instructor, Department of Psychosocial Nursing,
Alcohol and Drug Abuse Nursing,
University of Washington, Seattle, Washington

Janet Specht, R.N., B.S.N.
Director of Nursing Service, Iowa Veterans Home,
Marshalltown, Iowa

Lynne Talley, R.N., M.N.
Conference Coordinator, Continuing Nursing Education,
School of Nursing, University of Washington,
Seattle, Washington

Helen Wolff, R.N., M.S.
Assistant Professor, School of Nursing, University of
Portland, Portland, Oregon

Bonnie Worthington, Ph.D.
Associate Professor and Nutrition Chief,
Home Economics and Child Development
Mental Retardation Center—Clinical Training Unit,
University of Washington, Seattle, Washington

Nursing Management for the Elderly

Edited by

Doris L. Carnevali, R.N., M.N.
Associate Professor, Community Health Care Systems

Maxine Patrick, R.N., Dr.P.H.
Chairman, Department of Physiological Nursing

School of Nursing
University of Washington, Seattle

J. B. Lippincott Company | Philadelphia New York Toronto

ISBN 0-397-54229-1
Library of Congress Catalog Card Number 79-4461

Printed in the United States of America

1   3   5   7   9   8   6   4   2

Library of Congress Cataloging in Publication Data

Main entry under title:

Nursing management for the elderly.

   Includes bibliographies and index.
   1. Geriatric nursing. I. Carnevali, Doris L.
II. Patrick, Maxine. [DNLM: 1. Geriatric nursing.
2. Nursing, Supervisory. WY152 N979]
RC954.N89   610.73′65   79-4461
ISBN 0-397-54229-1

To our parents

Signe and Ernest Lambrecht
and
Hannah and Helmer Scholin

Their skill and zest in living their later years as fruitfully as their younger ones, despite age-related changes and eventual chronic disease, inspired us to try to contribute professionally to the health and well being of other old people.

Maxine Lambrecht Patrick
Doris Scholin Carnevali

Preface

Nursing is consistently involved with elderly persons when they seek help with their health care. This is true whether the nurse functions in ambulatory, acute, long term, or home care facilities or agencies. Very often nurses are *major* care providers in the older age group, with other disciplines serving more as consultants. Thus, geriatric nurse clinicians and nurses whose case loads include some elderly need a knowledge base to guide their assessments and management in treating these people effectively.

For the purposes of this book, we are concerning ourselves with individuals in the over-70 age bracket (and their families). It is not that 70 is a magical age when something suddenly changes, but by that time the physiologic decrements associated with aging become more obvious for everyone, even those who age slowly. These changes are, or should be, an increasing factor in health care management.

The perspective of this book is shaped not only by limiting the patient population involved but also by the editors' definition of nursing. We believe that nursing's area of primary accountability is oriented to achieving a *workable* and *satisfying balance* between the demands of daily living, given the patient's preferred or usual lifestyle on the one hand, and his functional abilities, resources, and support systems as they are affected by aging and disease on the other. One of the characteristics of the over-70 age group is that this balancing tends to become increasingly precarious. Increased incidence of disease and life stresses place new or greater demands while abilities as well as internal and external resources tend to wane. This growing risk of imbalance suggests an important area for nursing involvement on either an episodic or long term basis with individuals in varying degrees of independence-dependence.

No health care discipline functions in isolation these days. Nursing is no exception. Since nurses are, with increasing frequency, an early health care contact, as well as an ongoing one, they need some basic knowledge and assessment skills in diagnoses of related disciplines. They need to know when to safely retain management of the patient, when to consult others, and when to refer a patient for contact with another health care provider. Thus, the book incorporates the orientation of other relevant health care areas, as they apply to nursing management—drug, diet, dental.

This book is written for practicing registered nurses and students who care for older people as part or all of their case load. We expect our readers to have a variety of educational and experiential backgrounds. To this end the areas are presented with sufficient depth to encourage more than a superficial approach to nursing management. However, some nurses may wish a more extensive treatment of a subject; this need is met by bibliographies at the end of each chapter. With the growing interdisciplinary approach in health care, members of other disciplines may also find this book helpful in gaining insight into nursing's approach to health care management and areas of expertise. Consultation and referral should be a two-way street.

The field of gerontology-geriatrics is vast. Even if the subject were limited to nursing aspects, it would be possible to write volumes, or at least a heavy tome. This, obviously, is not that kind of book. We have tried to create a compact reference that will be useful to practicing nurses and students. We have opted for a selective, high risk approach to some conditions and situations that practicing nurses encounter regularly in their patients. The situations, diseases, conditions, and phenomena covered are those a nurse sees frequently. *They are common, but complex, in their nursing management.*

One word about the terminology used in this book. You will find the individual who seeks health care services from a nurse identified in the traditional term of *patient*. This is not meant to construe that the person is expected to be in a "sick" role, or in an automatically dependent relationship to the nurse. It is meant to indicate the recipient of nursing care—no more, no less. For the sake of convenience, throughout this book *he* has been used in the generic sense to include both men and women, and *she* has been used to refer to nurses, both male and female. These pronouns have no other significance.

In sequence, the book moves from normal to abnormal. The initial section gives perspective on the normal changes occurring in the elderly in areas significant to nursing management. The remainder of the book addresses high risk health situations in older persons, together with the conceptual basis for assessment and nursing management. Certain omissions occur because of the approach chosen.

One area where we hope for productive consistency is in the format. Nursing is increasingly involved with the branching logic needed to arrive at discriminating diagnoses and effective nursing management. We hope that the organization in this book will make more efficient the data gathering, the differential diagnosis, and rational management. Whenever possible you will find at least the diagnostic concepts organized in the following fashion:

DESCRIPTION	*General description of the phenomenon.*
ETIOLOGIC FACTORS	*Cause of phenomenon, including antecedent and current events, current environment, and changes in coping abilities or support system.*
HIGH RISK POPULATIONS OR SITUATIONS	*Prediction of individuals, groups, ages, or situations in which the nurse should consider this diagnosis.*
DYNAMICS	*Underlying functions and mechanisms of the phenomenon, life situations in the presenting situation, and associated relationships.*
SIGNS AND SYMPTOMS	*Subjective and objective data to be observed for and used in deciding that the phenomenon being observed fits within this concept.*
DIFFERENTIAL DIAGNOSIS	*Criteria for differentiating this phenomenon from similar ones.*
COMPLICATIONS	*Intervening factors or undesired side effects.*
PROGNOSIS	*Predicted direction, duration, and possible-probable outcomes.*
PREVENTION AND MANAGEMENT	*Rationale and guidelines on how the nurse handles care of patients with the phenomenon and how to reduce occurrence.*
EVALUATION	*Criteria of effectiveness of the management and resolution or continuation of the presenting situation.*

Chapters that deal with high risk areas begin with a Quick Review. The aim of this is what the heading says: to aid the reader in finding what he wants to know in a hurry, and then filling in the details by reading the chapter. As a means of locating the Quick Reviews, black tabs have been placed in the upper right hand corners of pages containing Quick Reviews. Chapters with Quick Reviews have also been marked with an asterisk (*) on the Contents pages.

Contents

---

* Chapter begins with a Quick Review or Quick Reviews. See page viii for explanation of Quick Reviews.

I Would Pick More Daisies

If I had my life to live over, I'd dare to make more mistakes next time.

I'd relax. I'd limber up. I would be sillier than I've been this trip.

I would take fewer things seriously, take more chances, take more trips.

I'd climb more mountains, and swim more rivers.

I would eat more ice cream and less beans.

I would, perhaps, have more actual troubles, but I'd have fewer imaginary ones.

You see, I'm one of those people who lived seriously, sanely, hour after hour, day after day.

Oh, I've had my moments, and if I had it to do over again, I'd have more of them.

In fact, I'd try to have nothing else, just moments, one after another—instead of living so many years ahead of each day.

I've been one of those persons who never goes anywhere without a thermometer, hot water bottle, a rain coat and a parachute.

If I had to do it again, I would travel lighter this trip.

If I had my life to live over, I would start going barefoot earlier in the spring, and stay that way later into fall.

I would go to more dances. I would ride more merry-go-rounds.

I would pick more daisies.

Anonymous

Nursing Management
for the Elderly

Part 1

Nursing's Focus in Providing Health Care for the Elderly

Introduction to Part 1

Part 1 is devoted to the focus of nursing in its delivery of health care to the elderly. As such, Part 1 becomes the perspective for the use of the remaining parts of the book.

Chapter 1 deals with the evolution of nursing's territory from the myriad of shared or delegated tasks that have characterized nursing practice. It also suggests a model that may help the reader to translate the definition of nursing into the focus of care.

The second chapter explores values—societal, professional, and personal—and their impact on the nurse and nursing practice. It suggests that these values exert their influence both overtly or covertly, but pervasively, on all facets of the delivery of care by nurses.

Chapter 3 returns to the nursing model of care and differentiates its focus from that of the medical model. The latter is an area where the nurse must also practice skillfully if good health care is to be provided to the over-70 age group.

The fourth chapter applies the nursing model to the focus of the nursing data base. It suggests the core areas of data that are needed regardless of the presenting situation.

The essence of these first chapters should be kept in mind as subsequent parts dealing with normal aspects of aging and high risk problems are considered. It offers a particular frame of reference for determining how the knowledge data and options for management are applied to nursing care of the elderly.

1

Health Care for the Elderly:
Nursing's Area of Accountability

Doris Carnevali and Maxine Patrick

Nurses have been involved as major providers of health care for older people for a long time. They still are involved, but there has been an important and growing change. Without this change, this book would not have come into being.

The geriatric patient population has been a nursing responsibility primarily by default. Nursing has been given this area of health care, but it has neither appreciated it nor assumed accountability for provision of high quality professional management. The fact is that geriatrics has been viewed as a dumping ground—for both clientele and providers.

In this rapidly changing technologic age, many segments of our society have become youth oriented, productivity oriented, and, in relationship to health, cure oriented. It stands to reason that high status would be given and costly health care providers and priorities in health dollars would be directed toward curing individuals who are predicted to have productive years ahead of them. Therefore, older persons, the chronically ill, and, most particularly, those who are both chronically ill and elderly have received lower priority. Even among the elderly, those who have potential for improvement are more eligible for therapy and skilled care than those who must work to maintain what they have or those whose health is declining. Personnel in skilled care nursing homes report utter frustration at admitting individuals with potential for self-care and a better way of

Illustrations in this chapter were executed by George McNeal.

life. The personnel work hard with these individuals to provide the environment and support systems that enable them to function at their highest level. However, as soon as these individuals reach this level of functioning, they are no longer eligible for skilled levels of care and must return to facilities that do not have the level of funding to provide staff and environment to maintain the gains. Within weeks or at best months, without the support systems, the residents regress. It is like a revolving door. Support systems for maintenance do not have the priority of cure systems.

Given this situation of low status and meager financing, it is not surprising that the widely available nursing personnel who do not have the salary scales of many other professional provider groups have been used as health care providers in institutions whose care goal is maintenance, or even custodial warehousing.

The nursing profession itself has not been immune to the cure orientation. For a long time the higher status in nursing has gone to nurses who help to cure people, particularly when they do it in acute, high-risk situations such as in cardiac care units, intensive care units, and emergency rooms. A corollary of this was the assumption that there must be something missing in nurses who directed their careers to health care for the older population, the chronically ill, and those who died, slowly. Only recently a young nurse who had been functioning in an emergency room told her medical and nursing colleagues that she was planning to change her focus and work in a geriatric facility. "But you're a good nurse," they told her, "why would you want to go work in a place like that?" Even within the intensive care settings, nurses have observed and remarked on the distancing maneuvers they engage in with both patient and family when the prognosis changes from recovery to predicted failure to recover. It is as if curing, or at least improving the patient's physical condition is the better part of nursing, while helping individuals to live with persisting conditions can be delegated to those in the profession who couldn't make it among the "curers."

CHANGES IN THE GERIATRICS SCENE

Fortunately several changes are occurring. Some of these changes are in general society, some in the health professions, and some specifically in the nursing profession.

Changes in Society

The numerical distribution of age groups in society is shifting perceptibly because more people are living longer. The older segment of the population is growing. Not only are older people becoming more numerous but they also are becoming increasingly vocal. Communications via the media have made health care consumers of all ages aware of the nature of health care that could be available, and so expectations are higher. Health insurance plans enable older individuals to purchase more health care than they formerly could. In terms of future legislation for health care benefits, they are lobbying and making their voices heard among politicians and legislators. Then, too, in this litigious age in which courts are used to call attention to grievances, lack of health care for a large segment of a population can be seen as discriminatory. There are many forces directing society to attend to at least the illness needs, if not the health needs, of the older population.

Changes in the Health Professions

There are changes within the health professions as well. Special organizations that concern themselves with health care for the chronically ill, elderly, and dying are springing up or gaining popularity and status. Special journals are devoted entirely to each of these areas. There is an increasing amount of research into aging and chronic disease as well as into the process of living while one is dying. Where once there were only pediatricians, pedodontists, and pediatric nurse specialists for particular age groups, now there is seen a need for geriatricians, gerodontologists, and geriatric nurse specialists who are prepared and skilled in addressing themselves to the health care needs of the oldest segment of the population.

Changes in Nursing

In nursing those who have an interest in caring for older persons have banded together in special interest groups, both within the professional nursing organizations and within other organizations. Nor has this been a lackluster group. The geriatric nursing group was the first in the American Nurses' Association to develop specialized standards of care in 1970. Not content with this first, it was also among the first to certify clinicians who showed demonstrable excellence within the speciality in 1974. The field is attracting increasing numbers of enthusiastic, talented new clinicians—nurses prepared to administer nursing services in both community and institutional settings as well as nurse practitioners and doctorally-prepared nurse researchers. Mature nurses who have long practiced in the field are engaged in actively upgrading their knowledge and skills in geriatrics and gerontology through continuing education and independent study. Colleges and universities are offering advanced work in the field.

Part of this turnabout in nursing relative to the care of older individuals must be related to societal changes. But at least an equal part derives from a change in nursing itself. It is coming of age as a profession in its own right with an identifiable area of expertise and accountability.

NURSING'S EXPERTISE AND HEALTH CARE FOR THE ELDERLY

Nurses have been experiencing a growing awareness of the nature and importance of the particular expertise they bring in providing health care in addition to, or as a modification of, the delegated functions they carry out for other disciplines. This conscious definition of practice has created an important change in nursing's orientation to providing health care for the elderly. Look at this definition of nursing and then at the health status and needs of the older population to see the logic of matching nursing providers with health care for older persons. The reason for nursing's natural importance to the health and illness care for this age group becomes apparent.

Nursing Orientation in Health Care

Nursing's *primary* focus and area of accountability* in providing health care is that of *helping the individual and his family to manage the activities and demands of daily living as these affect and are affected by health and illness, at the same time taking into account the individual's lifestyle.* (A basic assumption is made that consumers will seek outside help only when they are dissatisfied or ineffective in managing these activities themselves and that they will continue to use these services only as long as they see them as being needed.) The definition of nursing suggests that nurses' concern is with *balancing the Activities of Daily Living and Demands of Daily Living* (ADL, DDL) on the one hand and *Coping Resources* (CR) and *Support Systems* (SS) on the other (Fig. 1-1), since each of these aspects is influenced by health, illness, and associated experiences. (See Glossary for definitions.)

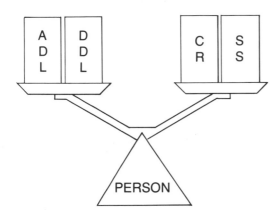

FIGURE 1-1. Nursing model for diagnosis and management.

---

* Primary accountability of a discipline for an area of health care does not mean that the health care provider must personally carry out all of the related activities. It does mean that he is accountable to the patient to know that adequate and valid assessment, diagnosis, and management has been undertaken by someone prepared to assume this responsibility. Nurse surrogates may be physicians, family members, LPN/LVNs, social workers, physical therapists, pharmacists, or any number of individuals on the health care scene.

The individual's and family's lifestyle will be a force on both sides, contributing to the nature of perceived demands and actual activities of daily living as well as to the coping resources and *useable* (as differentiated from available) support systems.

Health Needs of Older Persons and the Nursing Model

For older persons, particularly those over 70, the balancing between activities of daily living, demands of daily living, and the increasingly fragile

---

GLOSSARY

ADL **Activities of Daily Living:** The usual events and behaviors engaged in by the individual during the course of the 24-hour day.

DDL **Demands of Daily Living:** The person's *perception* of expectations he holds for himself or those he perceives others to hold for him that determine his priorities, choices, routines, and pace. They may suggest areas of discomfort if disruption occurs, *the explicit or implicit personal "shoulds."* This includes expectations of compliance with medical or health care regimens prescribed.

CR **Coping Resources:** Personal capabilities (e.g., strength, endurance, knowledge, desire, sensory capability, courage, creativity, problem solving ability, past coping patterns). These are the intrapersonal resources that enable the individual to manage to some degree the present and future challenges to his lifestyle (Little and Carnevali, 1976).

SS **Support Systems:** External environmental and personal forces that sustain and maintain the individual in a preferred or required lifestyle, such as family and important others, equipment, architecture, supplies, housing, neighborhood, stores, finances, transportation, ecologic environment, and laws.

LS **Lifestyle:** The totality of an individual's approach to living, often evidenced by preferences, pattern, and pace in daily living and use of resources or support systems. It incorporates such characteristics as preferences for independence/dependence, high/low stress levels, spontaneity and change/structure and regularity, extroversion/introversion, rapid/slow pace, and high/low physical activity. These preferences are translated into observable behaviors in approaching routine as well as unusual events.

coping resources and support systems tends to become more precarious with the years (Fig. 1-2). True, some activities and demands of daily living seem to be reduced, by necessity or choice, but many continue. And some new demands are added. (See Chapter 5, concerning developmental tasks of later years).

On the other end of the balance, some resources and support systems may diminish. Many basic physiologic functional capacities decrease. (See Chapter 6, Aging Changes in Structure and Function.) Age mates, so integral to satisfying support systems, die off while younger folk become involved in their own very busy lives. Income tends to stabilize, usually at a lower level, while cost of living has tended to escalate. Status decreases for many and so do opportunities for meaningful work. Forms of transportation may become less accessible or useable. Even one's credibility can become diminished. How many professional students are taught that "Older people are notably poor historians in reporting their medical history and current symptoms." (For a more detailed review of other losses, see Losses of Aging, Chapter 26.)

Beyond the losses which diminish personal resources and coping abilities as well as support systems, there is a tendency to settle into the patterns of one's lifestyle in both activities of daily living and preferred coping styles as well as in using support systems that are most comfortable. Changes require more of an adjustment or are uncomfortable; therefore they require more expenditure of physical or emotional energy than older persons may be willing or able to give. The balancing of demands and resources becomes more difficult to manage, even without the additional risk or incidence of illness or trauma.

The Ailing Older Adult

When pathology is added to normal aging, either an imbalance between demands and resources occurs or an increasingly uneasy balance is restored, often at a lower level of activities and with a changed lifestyle (Fig. 1-3). For example, the normally independent person may have to rely on family, friends, or homemakers to do the shopping and maintain the environment. Another have to give up driving, or gardening, or living in his own home. Some who have lived in semi-independent retirement housing may have to shift to nursing home care. The shift to equilibrium at a lower level may take many forms, gross or subtle. The problem is not only the amount of change but also the impact these changes have on the person and the family.

Illness, whether it is acute or chronic tends to reduce physical and psychologic *coping resources*—strength, endurance, ability to maintain a normal sensory environment, even the desire to participate in health care management or life. Over a period of time, illness drains financial resources and personal as well as institutional support systems.

At the same time that coping capabilities are being reduced, more weight is being added on the *demands* side. The ailing older person faces demands to adjust to:

- new signs and symptoms
- diagnostic tests and preparations for them
- self-concepts modified by new diagnostic labels assigned to them
- compliance with treatments for diagnosed and undiagnosed problems
- effects and side effects of those treatments

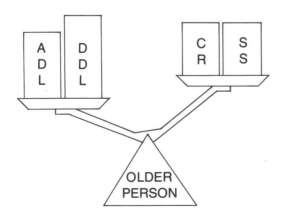

FIGURE 1-2. Risks of imbalance with old age.

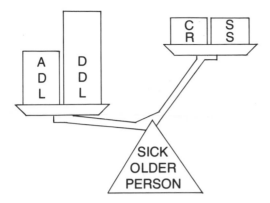

FIGURE 1-3.   Risks of imbalance with illness and age.

- modified relationships with mates, children, friends, and health care providers
- changed living environments
- dietary changes
- forms to be completed
- privacy invasions
- waiting lines to be tolerated
- new knowledge needed, new skills
- more demands on one's courage to face all these changes

Activities that were carried out with minimal thought or energy tend to require more effort, concentration, and rest periods or pacing. Yet, despite these imbalancing forces, most people and their families, including the elderly, accommodate and manage to retain sufficient balance to continue. *Support* systems that formerly worked may be strained and waver but other forms of support often can be located and either added or substituted. These may not be what the individual would prefer, but the result is some form of balance.

Lifestyle as a Factor in Health Care Management

Most older adults have evolved reasonably strong, preferred lifestyles long before they reach their seventies. This lifestyle not only shapes the pattern and tenor of their daily lives but also, importantly for health care providers' planning, influences the kind of changes they will accept and the support services they will use.

"Compliance" is a term used rather routinely by health professionals to indicate the patient's consistency in carrying out correctly a prescribed regi-men. For many older adults involved in self-care for chronic illness or health maintenance, compliance depends on the degree of congruence of the prescribed regimen with their usual lifestyle and goals. Where there is marked deviance, one may predict a high risk of noncompliance in self-care.

Similarly, the use of support systems is strongly associated with lifestyle. The triangle on the left side of Figure 1-4 illustrates the way in which a lifestyle that blocks entrance of additional resources and support systems can lead to difficulties in maintaining a balance between the demand side and the coping side. An extreme example of this is the "loner" who prefers maintaining solitude and privacy to receiving needed health care that will also bring intrusion and loss of control. These individuals often must become desperately ill, to the point where they lose the opportunity for choice, before they will allow others to enter their lives. Another example is the person who "does not believe in pills" and who may or may not fill a prescription and most likely does not comply with the prescribed drug therapy.

The right half of the diagram in Figure 1-4 illustrates balance retained or regained because the person's lifestyle permitted introduction of needed outside additions to his coping and usual support systems. Again, this is not usually a carte blanche situation. Some forms of help are more desirable or tolerable than others.

Finally the reader is asked to add a third version, one with which each is familiar. In this figure the deficits in coping resources and support systems are great. There is a wide opening for all kinds of services and, in addition, a virtual vacuum-type force that creates a voracious demand for health care and support services.

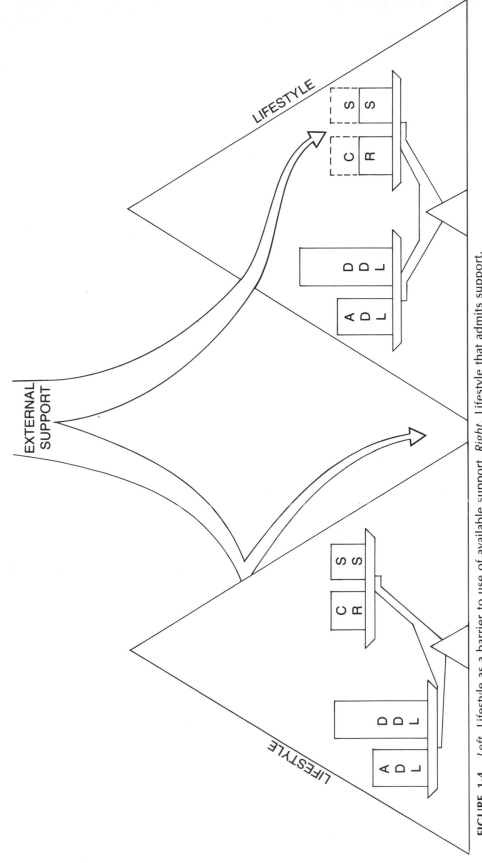

FIGURE 1-4. *Left,* Lifestyle as a barrier to use of available support. *Right,* Lifestyle that admits support.

The Articulation of Illness in Aging and Nursing Management

The older-aged-patient group is one for whom maintenance of both lifestyle and health is becoming increasingly insecure and for whom unfamiliar demands cause difficulty in adjusting to change. Also, there is a predictable shrinking of resources and attenuation of support systems. These factors suggest a group of people who may well work with nurses in a collaborative partnership to search for ways to achieve personally effective patterns of daily living in areas affected by health and illness.

This is not to suggest that only nurses, patients, and their families should be involved in this alliance but that nursing's particular expertise and contribution are significant and crucial. Nurses are and should be involved in health and illness care for the elderly—not just because they are inexpensive or available, nor even because they have been the traditional care providers. Nurses should hold themselves responsible and accountable for a major block of health and illness care for the elderly because the component of care they are prepared to provide helps in managing daily living as it is affected by health and illness and makes a productive fit with the ongoing health-illness needs of older people. This is true whether the older persons are living independently in their own apartments and homes or are in more dependent circumstances.

What is equally important is that others, consumers and providers, recognize and appropriately consult and refer patients for expert nursing management. Nursing has a long way to go in terms of achieving adequate recognition of its contribution. Gerontology and geriatrics is one field in which advances can be made rapidly.

2

The Nurse's Philosophy of Aging and the Aged: Its Impact on Nursing Practice

Doris Carnevali and Maxine Patrick

The individual nurse's practice is shaped not only by the focus of the diagnostic-management model or by the knowledge and skill utilized in applying the model to patient care, as important as these are. In a very basic way the care of the elderly is influenced by the beliefs and values* the nurse holds about the elderly clientele for whom she provides health care services.

Beliefs and values are a strong influence on all aspects of nursing diagnosis and management—the data one notices, the words used to describe what is noticed, the priorities set, the decisions made, the formulation of diagnostic statements, the care prescribed, the way care is delivered, and the criteria set for evaluation. At times, values and beliefs form a conscious basis for behavior. For example, the belief that "Honesty is the best policy" may be a very conscious thought that precedes the return of change to a store clerk who has made an error in the shopper's favor. More often the values and beliefs are subtle, pervasive influences. In other words, beliefs and values shape the nurse's behavior whether or not she is aware of it. This is a particularly important insight for those who, as Farson puts it, have the "arrogance" to be in the "helping professions" (1975). Here, the risk of inflicting one's own beliefs and values on those who are dependent becomes very great. In the case of nurses involved in the care of the dependent elderly, often with ongoing day-to-day contact, one can see the extensiveness of opportunity and the risks of the situation. It becomes very easy and comfortable to incorporate one's own value and belief system in every step of the nursing process and in the accompanying interpersonal interaction, unless purposeful thought is addressed to what is happening.

Given this risk of requiring others to comply with provider's values, it becomes important for the nurse who is working with the elderly to know the *working* values and beliefs that are influencing the nursing care being given. It is important to see the relationship between these beliefs and values and the diagnosis and management evolving from them, including the style in which care is given.

SOCIETAL FACTORS AND THE STATUS OF THE AGED

Since nurses are socialized first by their families and then by professionals, all of whom are a part of a larger culture, it is reasonable to assume that the values a society holds regarding a group of its members will influence the attitudes, values, and beliefs its members are taught to hold toward that group. Subgroups within a society may be identified in a variety of ways. *Age* is one of them. So it is that differing cultures have varying values associated with identifiable age groups—children, adults, and the aged.

---

* *Beliefs* are ideas or opinions which a person or group hold to be true. Beliefs are not always rational. *Values* are preferences for or esteeming of certain activities, ideas, objects, kinds of persons, goals, and so forth.

The status of the elderly within a society has been hypothesized to be related to several forces that are impinging on the entire society:

1. Extent of available resources in relationship to the needs of the population.
2. Availability of written communication for transmission of knowledge, cultural patterns, and skills.
3. Rate of change.
4. Proportion of the society that falls within the group.

Societal Resources, Personal Productivity, and Status

It has been suggested that the status of the elderly is related to their productive capacity to carry their own weight and contribute to the society's product or, alternatively, to the resources available to the society to support nonproductive members. In more primitive societies, which were dependent upon an environment with limited resources, the aged who survived their productive capability were left behind or sent out of the community. The group could not afford to value them as continuing members since they endangered the survival of the group. One reads of nomadic tribes who left behind members who could not keep up. In fact, for some tribes, the religious belief regarding life after death supported early death by holding that dead persons retained throughout eternity the body-age-beauty and functional capacity they had at the time of death. Such beliefs made abandonment of parent or cherished tribal member easier (Simmons, 1960).

In agrarian societies, including rural life in modern societies, the aged often have been able to contribute in ways that relased younger stronger members to participate more actively in producing resources needed. Therefore, the aged were able to retain status and were valued as contributors to family and society.

Modern industrial society's decree of mandatory nonproductivity in the form of formal retirement from the work force places its elder members in a situation where loss of status is a high risk. They are not valued—they are not wanted. The current concern those in the present work force have regarding funding pensions for an increasing number of members who no longer contribute, as well as concern for their own pensions later, is a manifestation of the risk

to status faced by the elderly. Not only do the elderly not produce but also they place an increasing drain on others. This drain may take the form of money, as in pensions, but it may also involve time and physical and emotional energy. In a personal sense, when family members not only cannot provide for themselves but also become a burden on others, they are valued less and status decreases, even though love and affection for them continue.

Transmission of Cultural Patterns and Status

Cultures that had no written language depended upon the elders to teach succeeding generations the history, skills, and traditions of the society. Those with written and other advanced symbolic forms of communication seem to have less need of the wise and skilled elders.

The current resurgence of interest and pride in one's cultural heritage has enhanced the status of many older persons who are the only sources of knowledge about the history, recipes, crafts, stories, arts, music, dances, and religion of the group. Once these are written, the songs recorded for posterity, the dances filmed and recorded, one wonders if again the elders will revert to a devalued state.

Rate of Cultural Change

The status of older persons has also been influenced by the rate of societal change. Slow rates of change have been associated with higher status for older members. The logic of this hypothesis is that when a culture is changing rapidly, the older generations lose their value as they become too out-of-tune with changing times to be useful to younger generations except as a baseline for measuring change. They are seen as knowing only how things were, not how they are.

We have to go no further than our own nursing profession to see the truth in the latter. How much value do currently competent young nurses place on a nurse who decides to return to the field after having been away from it for five years? The langauge is new, the technology has changed, the systems have been reorganized, the role and role relationships have been modified. Even currently-practicing professionals struggle to keep up with change—witness the movement toward mandatory continuing education.

In a society afflicted with the condition of "future shock," the contributions of older people tend to lose value. And with it, unless other sources of value are seen, the people themselves are valued less.

Proportion of Elderly and Status

Another factor seen as leading to loss of status for older persons in a society is the size of the group in relation to the rest of the population. The rare rather than the commonplace is valued. In cultures in which most die young, survivers are revered. Where increasing numbers live long, being an elder member of the society becomes mundane, less valued. The elderly may even be devalued as depriving young people of jobs, housing, and resources.

An example of this may be seen in the changes occurring in the nursing profession. The career patterns of women in the nursing profession are changing from that of short careers with retirement to homemaking and family activities to long nursing careers combined with other activities. The result is that young nurses entering the field are having increasing difficulty locating the job opportunities they prefer. How much value do eager, aspiring young graduates place on a large group of older nurses whose seniority deprives them of career opportunities?

Summary

If we look at just these factors and apply them to our current industrialized society (the older persons who consume more than they currently produce, who are becoming a growing proportion of the group to be supported by fewer young people) and if we add the widespread use of communication (the written word, other audiovisual media, computerization and advanced technology) as well as the rate of societal change and rapid human technologic obsolescence, one sees that there is great risk that older persons will be less valued. This societal attitude of decreased valuing can, in turn, subtly or overtly influence the values and beliefs which nurses, as products of this society, bring to bear as they provide health care services to the older age group. It is important that nurses be aware of this influence.

SPECIFIC BELIEFS AND IMPLICATIONS FOR NURSING CARE

Nurses maturing within any society undoubtedly assimilate the general societal attitudes and those of their more immediate family. These attitudes, plus the process of professional socialization through training and clinical role models in practice, lead to adoption of specific beliefs and values that affect nursing care given to older adults. Some of these beliefs, commonly heard among nurses, are listed in the box on page 16. Potential nursing behaviors that could result from these beliefs are also noted.

The stereotypes and beliefs in the first box are of a negative nature. While it is true that some of these beliefs would hold true for selected older adults, the beliefs are inappropriate if applied without validation across the board to all aged persons. Ideas for a bill of rights which might be created for the older clientele are given in a second box. Examine the ideas and discover the beliefs you hold. Explore the ways in which you currently implement them through the way in which you nurse your older patients.

The boxed material is a sample and is not to be considered as a full exploration. The reader no doubt will think of a variety of other values and stereotypes that influence the health care given to the elderly.

STRATEGIES FOR IDENTIFYING VALUES IMPINGING ON HEALTH CARE

Determining the values at work for an individual or group of health care providers can be done in two ways. The values thought to be held can be identified explicitly—then the behavioral implications in terms of choices, priorities, and style can be considered. Or the approach can be reversed—actions, failure to act, observations made, language used, priorities set, and so forth can be noticed, and the values that tend to generate such behaviors could be hypothesized. The most thorough approach employs both strategies. The first tends to address the ideal; the second addresses the *real working* values.

Not only the value is of concern but also the extenuating factors—all the conditionals—the ifs and buts. Few values are absolute. Each value tends to be tempered by constraints. It is important to know what the constraints are for the individual nurse as well as any group of care providers.

A realistic appraisal of working values (not platitudes) can be a very useful personal exercise or staff development activity; it can pay off in greater self-awareness and more effective care.

If you believe:	You may tend to:
Older people can't learn ("You can't teach an old dog new tricks")	Minimize teaching older adults about health, disease, coping behaviors. (e.g., aged mastectomy patients received less teaching about arm exercises and coping with changed musculature than younger patients)
Intelligence decreases with age	Use simpler words and ideas than you do with younger people without checking to see if it is appropriate.
Older people prefer to live in the past	Encourage reminiscing to the exclusion of including current ideas, future planning, and activities.
	or
	Negate the value of reminiscing.
Older people tend to have "mental" problems	View behavior as reflecting age-related deviances with some skepticism.
Kindness to older people means protecting them from being upset or stressed	Conceal information from them or modify the truth in terms of what you think is good for them.
All older people end up in hospitals with illness	Emphasize illness care rather than prevention, maintenance, and self-care.
Spunky patients are difficult patients	Avoid assertive patients and/or punish them.
Interest in sex is inappropriate among the elderly, particularly among single elderly	Joke about sexual overtures or activities among older persons. Neglect to obtain data on interest in sexual activity and take this into account when prescribing and administering treatments. Fail to consult them in decision-making process when decisions will affect their sexual activity patterns. Make no provision for protected privacy as a norm in in the institutional setting.
Older persons are not credible historians in reporting signs, symptoms, or health history data	Behave as if they don't really know what they are talking about when they report to you. Patronize them, but don't take the reports seriously. Check the data out with younger adults who are more reliable.
Adult children should assume parenting or executor roles with aged parents	Talk over important decisions with children rather than the parent. Help the parent to make the decision already made by the children. Relate to the children as if they were in the parenting role and the parent as if he were in the child role.
Body image is not important when one is older	Minimize the importance of grooming services and attractive clothing. Fail to give information or budget for prosthetic devices and rehabilitative teaching. Fail to help make the older person feel attractive.
Competence decreases with old age, therefore they must be protected from risk	Require people to prove competence before trusting them to perform (e.g., not allow them control of their own money).
Want to be with their own kind (i.e., other older persons)	Structure activities with age mates rather than other generations.
The daily bath is more important than grooming habits of a lifetime.	Equate personal cleanliness and neatness with good nursing care.

If you believe older persons have a right to:	You would tend to:
Make decisions about their own lives	Include them in all decision making in order to maintain this expectation for both providers and consumers of health care services.
Adequate data on which to make informed decisions	Provide information and help the person to explore options.
Have their decisions accepted	Accept their decisions and assist in interpreting them and implementing them to and with the system and family members.
Time and attention of providers and family	Schedule time to be with them. Genuinely attend to them in any encounter rather than engaging in distancing maneuvers, professional busyness, or superficiality.
Access to health care	Locate care where it is convenient to clusters of elderly. Facilitate transportation. Engage in architectural planning and furnishing to give access and provide appropriate support during waiting periods for those with limited mobility or endurance.
Therapy including prevention, maintenance, and restoration	Chronologic age would not automatically rule out certain forms of care.
Make decisions regarding health care with their finances in mind	Know their resources and attitude toward health expenditures. Act in accordance with their wishes where possible.
Live alone if they so choose and maintain their preferred style of living as long as possible	Seek services that would enable the person to remain in preferred environment.
Participate in decisions regarding change of lifestyle if and when this becomes necessary	Explore pros and cons of each option and predict and discuss transition problems. Acknowledge the difficulty of changing lifestyle. Support coping patterns of dealing with change. Allow time for transition when this is possible. Explain signs and symptoms of stress in making change to family/staff.
Maintain independence in areas and ways as long as possible	Seek areas and ways to foster and support independence on a daily basis, in little as well as larger areas, rather than doing for them.
Maintain a personal environment with own cherished belongings	Sacrifice neatness and uniformity if needed to provide a home environment.
Maintain privacy	Where privacy must be violated, help them to understand rationale.
Feel cared about	Seek ways to communicate personal interest in the individual. Find aspects or characteristics to genuinely enjoy.
Talk about or avoid talking about dying	Take time to listen when the individual indicates an interest and need to discuss dying. Listen without judgment or engaging in distancing maneuvers.
Be assertive in coping with the environment	Develop patterns of interaction that value and understand assertive responses rather than dampen it.

SUGGESTED READING

Farson, R.: Problems as Invisible Dilemmas: Myths and Paradoxes in Education. Speech to Western Council on Higher Education for Nursing Conference, Seattle, Wash., 1975.

Little, D., and Carnevali, D.: Values that affect nursing care planning. In Nursing Care Planning, ed. 2. Philadelphia: J. B. Lippincott, 1976, pp. 22–52.

Simmons, L. W.: Aging in preindustrial societies (1945). In Tibbitts, C. (ed.): Handbook of Social Gerontology, Societal Aspects of Aging. Chicago: University of Chicago Press, 1960, pp. 62–91.

3

Models of Diagnosis and Management

Doris Carnevali and Maxine Patrick

At one time health care was considered synonomous with medical care. Now there is a trend to see health-illness care as an area that often benefits from multiple perspectives and management skills. This broader perspective is particularly appropriate for the aged individual whose health problems tend to have multiple ramifications.

Nurses are accustomed to a multidisciplinary approach in giving care. They have a long history of being the most constant health care providers in many settings. Thus, nurses have been carrying out the *tasks* of other disciplines when others were either off duty or working elsewhere. Tasks however, are only one dimension of the service those professionals have been prepared to provide.

In the field of geriatrics and gerontology, nurses will undoubtedly continue to play a multidisciplinary role, particularly in home care and long term care settings. Given this likelihood, it becomes important, if older folks are not to get second class care, that nurses alter their vision of their surrogate roles from the tasks to focus on the perspective, the basic knowledge and basic skills of those disciplines. Nurses need to see themselves functioning in lieu of that other professional, seeing the patient and family through that discipline's eyes. They need to know how that discipline gathers its data base and what its orientation is to the management of patient problems that fall within their domain. Further, nurses need to be aware of *what they know* and *what they don't know* about these other disciplines and to use this

awareness as a basis for making decisions as to when to consult, when to refer, and when to retain management of a patient's care.

By the same token the reverse is also important. Nurses need to hold persons in other disciplines accountable for the quality of nursing care that they deliver when they function in lieu of the nurse. Other disciplines should feel responsible for knowing nursing's contribution to care, nursing's techniques of gathering information for the nursing data base, and the basic knowledge and approach used in management of a patient's/family's problems in the nursing domain. Professionals in other disciplines must be aware of what they know and don't know about nursing so that they too will make astute decisions and appropriately use nursing consultation and referral.

A model may help to clarify these territories and relationships. Figure 3-1 shows a petal-type arrangement of patient and professional contributions on a treatment team. Solid lines and shaded areas are used to suggest areas of discipline expertise and accountability that can't be easily shared or delegated to others, while intermittent lines denote blurring and sharing of responsibility, knowledge, perspective, and care. This particular diagram has six petals; however, it should be imagined as changeable with fewer or greater numbers of components as the presenting treatment team requires. The comparable size of wedges is not meant to indicate area of responsibility in any one situation, only a designated territory of personal or discipline expertise and accountability.

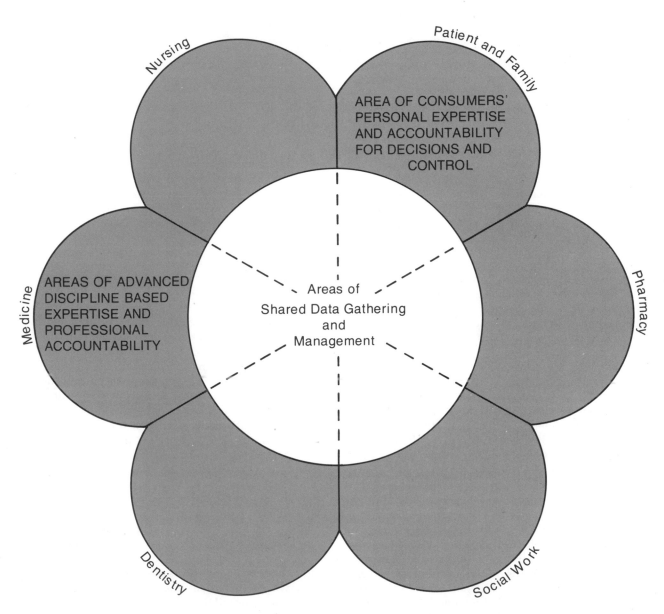

FIGURE 3-1. Model of patient and professional expertise and shared contributions on a treatment team.

This diagram suggests several general ideas and relationships:

1. The patient/family and any disciplines involved in providing care bring a personal or discipline-based perspective and expertise as well as accountability to the situation.
2. At *basic* levels both data gathering and management are shared, usually being assumed by whatever professional (or lay person) the patient selects to encounter or is already encountering.
3. When involved in a health care situation, each one has an area of accountability for the quality of this component of care, whether direct assessment and care is personally given or is performed by a person from another discipline territory.
4. The provider or participant from each component has a degree of specialized knowledge and expertise that goes beyond that normally expected of individuals not so professionally trained. Therefore, consultation or referral are appropriate whenever patient problems require more than the basic knowledge and skills available from current providers.*
5. The patient and family have expertise and skills that are significant and valuable. The consultation and referral process applies to them as validly as to the professionals.

This model has been presented initially in a very general approach. Petals have been labeled merely to demonstrate the disciplines commonly involved in health care for the elderly who might be involved in a presenting situation; other disciplines or groups could as easily be substituted. Quality of care for the geriatric patient is best achieved through this shared/colleagial approach.

To illustrate behaviors in which one profession functions in lieu of another in the shared level of assessment and management, a comparison will be made of the two petals where nurses most commonly practice—nursing and medicine. The basic focus of each discipline, the direction of diagnosis and patterns of management, will be examined.

There is no question that practitioners in each of these fields regularly practice in the mode and area of the other. Nor is there any intent to suggest that this should not be so. It is cost effective and humane for it to continue to occur. The purpose of delineating the territories is to show that differences in perspective do exist, differences in the data base should exist, and differences in diagnosis and management must exist if patients are to receive health-illness care appropriate to their needs.

COMPARISON OF NURSING AND MEDICAL DIAGNOSIS AND MANAGEMENT

It is only in recent years that nurses have accepted the notion that they diagnose and manage medical problems. The truth is that nurses have done this to some degree all along. Many persons would have died earlier or lived in much poorer health if nurses had not been reasonably active and astute in making medical diagnoses. Many persons would be presently suffering unnecessarily if nurses failed to make medical types of judgments in the absence of physicians. The acceptance by nurses of the reality of this aspect of their role means that they openly acknowledge accountability for having some skill in providing health care within the medical model. Thus, when nurses function *in lieu of physicians*, they are accountable for:

1. gathering data the physician would, using the pattern and system—following the *medical* path of branching logic in moving from one sign or symptom to the search for others.
2. arriving at the most valid *medical* diagnosis their knowledge permits.
3. making a plan of *medical* management that safely treats the problem (with or without medical protocols or consultation) *or* making a referral if the knowledge and skill of the nurse is not sufficient. (It is important to know limitations as well as capabilities.)
4. implementing the treatment plan with the patient.
5. using *medical* criteria appropriate to the diagnosis to evaluate the patient's response to management.

Assessment and Diagnosis in the Medical Orientation

According to Foley (1973), physicians observe the following sequence of steps in arriving at a medical diagnosis:

---

* A problem here is that nurses have been trained to consult and refer but not to expect to be consulted or receive referrals when nursing problems exist that require advanced nursing expertise.

1. make a phenomenologic diagnosis (collect data on signs, symptoms, antecedent events, etc.)
2. make a physiologic diagnosis (determine which physiologic functions are primarily involved).
3. make an anatomic diagnosis (determine which target organs are primarily involved).
4. make a pathophysiologic diagnosis (determine the pathologic process that is occurring (e.g., inflammation, neoplastic phenomena, ischemia, atrophy).

Failure to follow these steps in this sequence, taking short cuts, or carrying them out with lack of prerequisite skill and knowledge results in inadequate medical care. Thus, any person taking on this medical assessment-diagnostic function would be expected to follow this pattern in a disciplined, skilled fashion if good medical care is to be initiated. Obviously, this requires a sound body of basic medical diagnostic concepts as well as some degree of skill in medical history taking and physical examination.

To judge by this focus of data gathering, the medical diagnostic taxonomy, and physician behavior, medical diagnosis is concerned primarily with identification of pathophysiology and psychopathology. Medical management is addressed toward curing, stabilizing, palliating, or preventing pathology or trauma. It tends to involve drug therapy, diet therapy, surgery, physical forms of therapy, and psychotherapy. Criteria of evaluation of patient response usually take the form of measurement of return to normal range of findings in body function and structure as well as data on reported well-being and changes in behavioral responses.

If nurses are inadequate or unwilling to respond as physician surrogates when no physician is available, the patient will receive poor medical care. If nurses fail to be responsibly well-prepared in high risk or common areas of medical problems they encounter in their clinical situations, again poor medical care could result.

Diagnosis and Management in the Nursing Model

The primary area in which nurses have accountability for assessing, diagnosing, and managing health care is in their own professional field of expertise—nursing. This should go without saying; however, studies have shown that nurses tend to address a greater proportion of attention to medical management than to nursing management. It is not uncommon to find supposed nursing care plans that have been copies of medical care plans transposed to nursing Kardexes.

If one accepts the premise that the orientation and expertise of nursing are different from that of medicine, it follows that the data and the territory of nursing diagnosis and management are not the same as that of medicine. So, it becomes important that the nurse, or whoever functions in lieu of the nurse be accountable for:

1. collecting an adequate nursing data base and utilizing the nursing pathway of branching logic.
2. arriving at the most accurate and precise nursing diagnosis that can be derived from the data.
3. making a plan of nursing management that will effectively treat the defined problem area.
4. implementing the treatment plan with the patient or family.
5. using nursing criteria appropriate to the diagnosis to evaluate patient's/family's response to nursing management.

If nurses fail to address or cause others to address patient problems requiring nursing perspective and nursing expertise, the patient will receive inadequate nursing care. If others assume the responsibility and nurses fail to maintain accountability for the quality of nursing diagnosis and management, there is also high risk of poor nursing care.

When nurses encounter a patient, they are expected to make a decision as to whether the patient's presenting needs require nursing expertise or that of another discipline. If this decision involves a medical problem and a physician is not available at the time, it is anticipated that the nurse will:

1. determine which needs have priority (obviously medical judgments and treatments come first in some situations, but there are many in which nursing management should have priority).
2. decide whether one or both are needed.
3. be prepared to use either the nursing or medical model for assessment, diagnosis, and management.
4. in situations where both types of care are

needed, determine what management can be undertaken that will treat both medical and nursing problems concurrently.

The nursing model presents a different perspective in diagnosis and management. Where the medical model seeks to pinpoint and define the pathophysiologic or psychopathologic phenomena, the nursing model seeks to specify and define what impact these phenomena and their management have on the activities and demands of daily living for the individual and the family. Or, in the case of prevention, it seeks to determine what effects the individual and family lifestyle have on the maintenance of health. Thus, the nursing model is the one which the nurse, or any person serving in place of the nurse, would be expected to use in order to provide valid nursing diagnosis and adequate nursing management. The nursing model, too, has a certain pattern that is used in arriving at a diagnosis. The nurse gathers data and makes judgments about:

- *Deficits in health-related coping abilities or resources:* Data are collected on signs, symptoms, and antecedent events that indicate the individual/family are not or may not be able to manage daily living effectively in the face of the presenting health-illness situation and/or that present lifestyle may contribute to future health problems.
- *Activities of daily living in which coping deficits will cause disruption:* Data are collected on usual activities and demands of daily living that will be most affected by the lack of coping ability or resources. Consider not only the actual demands and disruption but also the individual's/family's degree of discomfort with it.
- *Altered demands which are being placed upon the individual that cause coping deficits:* Data are collected on current or impending health-related problems that require new or changed coping skills or resources.
- *Extent of the imbalance in terms of severity, direction of change, and duration:* Data are collected (often using medical findings, diagnosis, and prognosis) that predict the severity and duration of disruption, the stress that may be placed on activities and demands of daily living for the patient and family, and other resource and support systems.

As with the medical model, any person taking on the assessment-diagnostic function in the nursing model would be expected to be able to follow the pattern skillfully, have a sound body of nursing diagnostic concepts, and have skills in history taking and utilizing associated objective data from other professionals, the patient, and the environment.

Nursing diagnoses are directed toward identification of specific imbalances between demands of daily living and coping resources in health- and illness-related areas. Nursing management involves mobilizing patient and/or other resources to shore up or replace absent or inadequate coping abilities or support systems. Sometimes these involve provisions of:

- physical assistance
- supplies and equipment
- experiences
- opportunities to practice skill or behaviors
- knowledge or sources of knowledge
- help in applying knowledge to daily living
- assistance or support in planning
- contacts with other resources
- assistance in cutting bureaucratic red tape
- respite from stress to give time to regroup
- modification of the immediate environment
- transportation
- sensory stimulation
- feedback

The forms of nursing therapy and help are wide ranging.

Criteria for evaluation are related to the effectiveness with which the patient and family are able to manage their health problems and daily living but, equally important, they are related to maintaining a satisfying way of life and achieving the patient's/family's own desired outcomes.

APPLICATION OF THE MEDICAL AND NURSING APPROACHES TO THE ASSESSMENT-DIAGNOSTIC PROCESS

When each model is applied to the same presenting situation, the direction of data gathering, branching logic, and differences in diagnoses can be seen. To illustrate this, take an example of an individual who presents with the symptom of *shortness of breath.*

Medical Model

In the medical model the physician (or substituting health care provider) would:

1. *Gather data on signs and symptoms:*
Onset, duration, associated symptoms, antecedent events including psychologic stress, previous history of disease, drug taking, respiratory rate, breathing characteristics, breath sounds, cough, sputum, heart sounds, skin color, signs of respiratory obstruction (flaring nares, depressed sternal notch), history of allergies, intactness of rib cage, neurologic function, breath odor, body temperature, environment (altitude, smog), chest x-rays, blood gases, ECG, blood sugar, blood counts (Hb, WBC).

2. *Determine the physiology that is involved primarily in the disturbance:*
Mechanical movement of air (skeletal integrity, muscle weakness, obstruction of airway), gaseous exchange across alveolar membranes, blood chemistry, metabolic processes, cardiovascular competence, neurologic control systems, psychologic processes (anxiety, hysteria, hyperventilation), drugs acting upon physiologic processes.

3. *Determine primary anatomic target area:*
Lungs, heart, metabolic system (e.g., metabolic acidosis), central nervous system, (organic/psychosomatic), hematologic system, musculoskeletal system.

4. *Determine the pathophysiology:*
Trauma (fractured rib cage, muscle spasms, lung puncture), cerebral vascular accident or trauma, respiratory acidosis, CO_2 retention, inflammation, emphysema, asthma, bronchiectasis, hyaline membrane disease, cystic fibrosis, pulmonary edema, neoplasms, pleurisy, antelectasis, anemia, coronary insufficiency, congestive heart failure, altitude sickness, worry/fear, allergy.

The health care provider, physician or other, could make a diagnosis as to what the phenomenon is and its cause and would institute appropriate management, use consultation with a physician, or make a referral for medical management.

Nursing Model

Using the same presenting situation, in the nursing model a nurse (or substituting health care provider) would use some of the same data but would move in a different direction. The nursing model would require the person to:

1. Gather data (or use data already collected) on signs and symptoms, as in the medical model, but then branch out to *consider how these signs, symptoms, antecedent events, and so forth affect the activities and demands of daily living.* (e.g. Is it an acute situation that demands immediate attention to positioning? Is it an activity that modifies the environment? Does it create problems in communication? What is the status of important others and their reaction to what is happening to the patient?) In the chronic situation, data gathering will move in the direction of the pattern of signs and symptoms in relation to activities of daily living and changes that have been occurring over time—how they affect eating, sleeping, mobility, pace, lifestyle; how the patient and those around are coping with the signs and symptoms or the disease label; what the shortness of breath means to him, how it interferes with his way of life.

2. Determine duration, direction, and imbalancing forces as a basis for diagnosing the nature of the coping challenges the individual must manage: (a) *severity* on the basis of the medical diagnosis determines whether the pathology is likely to cause mild or intense shortness of breath; (b) *duration* determines whether it will be for short or long periods; (c) *direction* determines whether the condition is likely to remain fairly stable, improve, or decline. This, in turn, becomes the basis for assessing the extent of demands the coping resources and support systems must be prepared to meet. Data are collected on what useable coping resources and support systems are available and necessary. Finally, a prediction is made as to whether there is still an imbalance between demands of daily living and capability of meeting them that then requires intervention in the form of nursing management or referral to other agencies as well.

3. *Gather data on target areas in daily living where the person or those around him perceive specific difficulties in carrying out the activities and meeting the demands of daily living* and dissatisfactions associated with required alterations in desired lifestyle caused by shortness of breath. (For example, (a) one woman with shortness of breath whose preferred lifestyle was one of rapid movement and high productivity was continuously distressed at not being able to walk as fast as others when she went shopping. She was also angry and unhappy when she couldn't do the laundry, hang the clothes outside, and do the ironing all on one day, a specific day of the week, as she had for many of her 83 years.

(b) Another person, dependent on oxygen, must adjust a lifestyle to being accompanied by an oxygen tank and tubes.) Pacing of activities and enforced rest poses different problems with different lifestyles and demands of daily living. (One couple experienced total panic and became completely ineffectual when the husband experienced episodes of paroxysmal nocturnal dyspnea.)

4. *Determine the coping and support system deficits* (Fig. 3-2). High risk deficits resulting from shortness of breath include lack of *strength* for ADL, lack of *endurance,* lack of *desire* to alter one's lifestyle to adjust to lower O_2 availability in the tissues, lack of *courage* to face the treatment (as in coronary artery bypass or lung surgery for neoplasms), lack of *support systems* to enable the individual to manage

---

Strength Ability and resources to handle physical, mental, emotional work at a given point in time

Endurance Stamina, staying power with a work load (physical, intellectual, or emotional)

Sensory Input Abilities and resources to maintain an adequate, satisfying sensory environment

Knowledge Status of acquired content in the relevant area to be coped with and level of ability to use that content (e.g., recall, comprehension, application, etc.)

Desire Will or motivation to participate

Courage Risk-taking capacity

Skills Psychomotor, dexterity, communication, interpersonal

FIGURE 3-2. Categories of internal resources. (Reprinted from Little, D., and Carnevali, D.: Nursing Care Planning, ed. 2. Philadelphia: J. B. Lippincott, 1976, p. 168, with permission.)

(e.g., two-flight dyspnea and a fourth floor apartment with no elevator), lack of *knowledge* about phenomena so as to manage it more effectively (e.g., lack of understanding of hemodynamics of paroxysmal nocturnal dyspnea), or lack of *skills* (e.g., the orthopneic person who does not know how to arrange his pillows to minimize risk of falling off during sleep).

From these contrasting examples of utilization of the medical and nursing approaches to assessment and diagnosis it is possible to see the different directions that occur, even when a presenting symptom is the same. It becomes obvious that health care will be incomplete if either approach is neglected or if inappropriate priorities or attention were set between them.

The diagnosing may be done in each discipline area by professionals in that particular discipline or in both areas by one. There is no question that diagnosing at some basic levels is and can be shared responsibility. What cannot be shared is accountability. Thus, whether the physician does the assessment-diagnosis or another does it, *once the patient enters a health care system, the physician is ultimately accountable for medical management.* Similarly, whether a nurse or another does the nursing assessment and diagnosis, once the patient enters the health care system, *the nurse cannot delegate accountability for knowing that nursing diagnosis and management has been done and done adequately.*

IMPLICATIONS OF THESE MODELS FOR NURSES IN GERIATRICS

Within the field of geriatrics there is an unusually high probability that nurses will function in a multidisciplinary approach in providing health care to patient, families, and groups of elderly persons. This suggests certain implications for nursing practice. Nurses who function in situations where they must assume multidisciplinary functions need to:

1. be respected for their expertise as a nurse/in nursing.
2. be or become expert in the diagnosis and management of nursing problems.
3. be well-grounded, as specialists in geriatrics and gerontology, in the knowledge of normal aging and areas of high risk health problems among the elderly.

4. be visible to consumers, colleagues, and administrators in their nursing role.
5. offer consultation and expect consultation and referrals on nursing problems.
6. be aware that nurses' time and energy are finite and that these resources spent in non-nursing pursuits deprive patients of the attention, thought, time, and contribution that should or could be made in addressing and caring for patients' nursing problems.
7. make conscious decisions as to which discipline model to use in a given presenting patient situation and, having done so, move within that model expertly as long as it is appropriate.
8. negotiate for and expect recognition and appropriate renumeration for nursing expertise.

Given the multidisciplinary demands placed upon the majority of nurses who work in geriatric care settings, the remainder of this book assists the nurse in making at least basic assessments in a variety of problems from the perspective of several professional disciplines but with a prevailing sense of the importance of the nursing approach. The hope is that the reader will be a safe basic multidisciplinary practitioner at basic levels but, above all, will be an expert geriatric nurse clinician.

BIBLIOGRAPHY

Foley, J.: Pinpointing organic mental disorders. Med. World News Geriatr., 1973, pp. 26–27.

4

Nursing Assessment in the Elderly

Doris Carnevali and Maxine Patrick

The collection of an adequate data base for nursing management is particularly important and cost-effective with the over-70 age group. This is true for several reasons. First, the health problems encountered tend to be long term, thus impinging on the lifestyle and coping patterns for prolonged periods. Second, the individual's lifestyle and patterns of dealing with health and associated problems are well-established over the years, making change more difficult. Thus, it becomes important for the nurse to know what is usual and important as a basis for predicting any areas of difficulty and planning in such a way as to incorporate the usual lifestyle as much as possible. Finally, most older individuals are managing their health problems in their later years *outside* of hospitals and nursing homes, where they, not the providers, monitor their own well-being and control their day-to-day health care and behavior.

All this suggests that a *compliance model* in which the provider prescribes and the patient obeys may be less effective for many older persons than a *participation model* wherein provider and patient engage in mutually acceptable planning and evaluation of the health care regimen.

The participation model requires a solid nursing data base that identifies activities, perceived demands of daily living, environment and lifestyle, coping resources and patterns, and available/useable support systems. Given this kind of information about the person's style and perspective in living, it becomes easier to present and implement the health care regimen in such a way that it articulates best with what is usual for them. This is true whether the care is given in the home, hospital, nursing home, or clinic. It also helps to predict where the difficulties are going to arise. For example:

The person with shortness of breath who shops at a store two blocks away where he must carry groceries and climb an incline on the way home will have a problem that is more severe than the one who climbs the incline on the way *to* the store when he does not have the extra weight to carry.

The stay-at-home person may experience less life disruption from incontinence than the one with an active outside social life.

The reader, embroiderer, or person whose driver's license is up for renewal will find failing vision more difficult than those whose diversion is braiding rugs or gardening or those who have just passed the licensing test.

Active, fast-paced older persons may have greater difficulty adjusting lifestyle to exertional angina or intermittent claudication than those who have always paced themselves or moved in a leisurely fashion.

The musician may suffer more from hearing loss than the painter, the extrovert more than the introvert.

Persons who value their beauty have been known to find cataract glasses intolerable.

Those who have no faith in Western medicine or in drugs may not use the prescribed medications or may combine them with home remedies.

Persons with a strong fear of cancer or those with a family history of the disease attach different significance and generate different body responses to signs and symptoms from those who do not.

Nursing's primary orientation is the interaction of health and its maintenance and illness and its treatment with the style and activities of daily living. Nursing's area of management is in helping older persons and their families integrate health care practices and daily living more effectively and satisfyingly. This often requires a combination of patient data from the medical history and physical examination, the plan of medical management, and the nursing data base in order to:

1. rule in or rule out problems in living the patient and family will have.
2. develop the plan for nursing management of diagnosed nursing problems consistent with medical problems or other health problems.

This is the orientation, regardless of the setting in which the care is received—hospital, nursing home, clinic/office, or home.

STRUCTURE OF THE NURSING ASSESSMENT

The nursing assessment involves both subjective and objective data. It may take either a comprehensive or presenting problem approach depending on the situation (Little and Carnevali, 1976, 102–104). With either approach, and in any setting, the assessment will incorporate four sections: introduction, body of the assessment, recapitulation, and plans for follow-up. The first section is omitted in subsequent encounters for ongoing data gathering, unless the nurse feels the patient may not have understood or may have forgotten.

Introduction

The introduction is used to help the patient or family understand what the nurse is doing, why she needs to know answers to questions asked, and how the data will be used in the nursing management. Many patients, particularly older ones, have not seen nurses in this role, so its legitimacy should be established, not taken for granted. A short statement on how the medical and nursing plans fit together may also be helpful.

Body

The bulk of the nursing assessment is concerned with gathering subjective and objective data on the patient's situation—functional status, usual lifestyle, activities of daily living, demands of daily living, environment, coping resources, and support systems.

Recapitulation

After gathering the data, the nurse summarizes to the patient what she has heard, noting areas where the patient is coping effectively without assistance and any areas where there seems to be a need for help. The patient is asked to validate or modify the nurse's perceptions. This stage of the assessment requires the nurse to organize the data and also continues to illustrate to the patient what the nurse's role really is in health care management.

Planning Future Interaction

The final section in the initial assessment is used by the nurse and patient to negotiate the role in the health care regimen each will undertake in the interim between visits (or in the nursing home or hospital—the next assessment rounds). This may include patient and nurse activities; guidelines for noting signs, symptoms, feelings, and so forth; phone calls; and what the nurse expects to do in subsequent visits/contacts. It shapes both patient and nurse expectations and commitments.

FOCUS OF THE NURSING ASSESSMENT

The focus of the nursing assessment is on data from both sides of the balance—on the one side the usual or desired lifestyle and on the other the abilities and resources for maintaining it—with the presenting realities of aging, with health or with illness. For comfort it should begin where the patient's current interests and concerns lie and flow from them. However, by the time the assessment is completed in one or more contacts the nurses should have subjective and objective data (at least relevant to the presenting situation) in the following areas (Little and Carnevali, 1976, 128–140):

1. The person's perception of his health status
2. Usual and preferred lifestyle
3. Activities and demands of daily living

4. Functional status
5. Status of support systems

These areas are woven into the nursing assessment in whatever way is appropriate. For example, activities and demands of daily living may be addressed in relationship to areas of functional status that impact upon them or they may be addressed as a separate initial section that is then used as functional capacities are discussed. Both objective and subjective data are collected.

Functional Status

The physician tends to collect data on organs, systems, and their functions in order to determine the pathology. The nurse uses some of the same data in order to determine its effect on daily living. Thus, where a functional deficit is noted, the nurse should collect data on the areas of living (Fig. 4-1) with the presenting situation.

These data are essential to the development of a useable nursing plan, however, asking questions in the same way and same order each time a problem is reported or noted will make for a monotonous interview. Often the person will indicate or give data without being asked. Listen first and then direct conversation or ask as needed to keep the interaction during the assessment natural and interesting for the patient as well as efficient in use of provider time.

Content Areas

Some functional areas are critical in collecting specific data to determine the balance between Ac-

---

Activities or circumstances that trigger the condition or worsen it

Activities engaged in to try to relieve the symptoms or condition

Changes in ADL made or contemplated to adjust to the particular condition of symptoms

Satisfaction with the accommodations he is making

Dissatisfactions with any aspects of the changes he has made, contemplates, or has to make

---

FIGURE 4-1. Data on coping responses to be observed when functional deficits are reported.

tivities and Demands of Daily Living and Coping Resources and Support Systems. Where the nurse has access to the physician's findings on normal or pathologic status, these data may become a foundation to the nursing assessment. However, where the nurse encounters the person first, the nurse's assessment may serve as the initial screening examination.

In Figure 4-2, the categories of functional status are listed in alphabetical order, not necessarily the sequence the nurse would use. Most practicing clinicians or advanced students will have been taught or have developed a particular system or sequence that works for them. Sometimes the presenting situation determines what problems should be addressed first in terms of urgency. What *is* important is that ultimately data are collected and recorded in each area so as to (1) rule out or rule in health-related problems in daily living and (2) define them specifically enough to generate effective plans for nursing management.

The introduction of a *potential problem* area may be done either by the patient or the nurse. The patient may report on signs and/or symptoms, or the nurse may note objective data indicating some dysfunction. For example, the nurse may see that the person has swollen joints and the restricted movement associated with degenerative joint disease, yet the patient may not mention this as a problem. The nurse can approach the problem area with a question such as, "I noticed that you have some swollen joints. Do they give you any trouble?" If the person fails to bring up management areas such as discomfort, analgesia, and impaired activities, the nurse can express an interest in the kinds of adjustment actually being made. The nurse's interest should be explained as not the creation of problems, but the determination of the nature of adjustments the person is making and the attitude toward the situation so that the usual management style can be more effectively used by the health care providers. In the nursing data base it is as important to know health situations in which persons feel they are managing well or are able to ignore deficits as it is to have data on less well-managed problems. Both can be significant in subsequent nursing management.

Where the nurse has data about health problems already under medical treatment (such as diabetes, COPD, alcoholism, CVA), the person's skill and satisfaction in participating in the regimens and managing the disabilities should also be explored. (See specific chapters for guides.)

While much of the data suggested here addresses a lifestyle characterized by self-care and some inde-

Breathing	Shortness of breath, pain on coughing, wheezing, bloody sputum
Circulation	*Heart:* Pain—nature, heaviness, episodes of rapid heart beat, skipped beats, dizziness, blackouts
	Vessels: Varicose veins, cold hands or feet, charley horses, leg pains—walking/at rest
Eating	Appetite, enjoyment of food, diet or dieting, weight, chewing problems
	Cooking: Skill, enjoyment, resources
	Shopping: Transportation, skill, frequency, finances
	Eating Patterns: Meals/day, typical foods
	Locale: Home/restaurant, alone/with others
Elimination	*Bowels:* Frequency, time, concerns, associated problems, medications
	Urine: Frequency, urgency, pain, leaking, up at night
Grooming	Importance to them, capabilities, frustrations
Mobility/Safety	Patterns and location of activities, gait, accidents, balance, weakness, dizziness, stiffness, pain, status of feet/shoes, appropriate clothing available
Senses	Vision, hearing, tactile; sensory stimulation—desired/available—use of glasses/hearing aid
Sleep	Sleep patterns—night/naps, number of pillows, medications, times up at night
Social/Emotional/Cognitive	Memory problems, satisfaction with social life, barriers, use of time, difficult times (See Part 4 for additional guides)

FIGURE 4-2. Categories of functional status areas. (Where a functional deficit is reported or observed, follow the guidelines in Figure 4-1 to determine its impact on daily living and the effectiveness of the individual's coping.)

pendence, they are also important to the nurse assisting the older person to make a transition from self-care to greater dependency in an institutional setting, or the reverse. With older individuals it is extremely important to use the resources and strengths they have as soon as possible so that losses do not occur. The expression, "What you don't use you lose," is particularly significant for the elderly. It is also important for the nurse to document not only the kind of assistance needed but also that which is acceptable to the person. The two may be quite different.

Support Systems

The other component of the nursing data base as suggested by the models in Chapter One is that of the nature of the support systems. For the over-70 age group, both subjective and objective data are crucial. The categories in Figure 4-3 have been found to be useful in nursing care of the elderly. These areas seem to address again the problems of the older person living independently; however, some of them are applicable to care in an institution and discharge planning.

Summary

These, then, are the major areas of nursing assessment with the priorities associated with dealing with an older population. The emphasis is on how patients see the situation as well as the objective reality, how they have been managing to this point, how satisfied or frustrated they are with their adjustments and what they see their needs to be.

The presenting situation with the patient and the style of the nurse will determine which of these areas are initially addressed and what will constitute the total nursing data base for a patient. These areas are suggested as having relevance to the plan of nursing management.

For more detail on issues related to nursing assessment, see Little and Carnevali (Chapter 6, "The

Housing	*Type:* Single family dwelling, yard, apartment, hotel room, retirement center, lighting, risk factors (wires, loose rugs, etc.)
	Neighborhood: Risks, hills, location of stores, transportation, churches, health services, other services
Personal network	Living alone or with spouse/children/housemate/commune
	Relationship and distance from siblings, children, relatives, friends, neighbors
	Club/church contacts, types of contacts (letters, phone, visits)
Communication responses	Phone? Emergency contacts, intercom systems
Transportation	Public transportation availability, personal rides, senior citizen passes
	Barriers to getting in and out of vehicles.
	Own car, status of driver's license
Finances	Adequacy, problem areas, resources, concerns
Need for support	Nature of desired support, useable support, available support
	Ability to maintain support systems (mechanical, personal)

FIGURE 4-3. Nursing data base on support systems.

Client, The Nurse, and the Nursing Assessment Transaction").

MEDICATION HISTORY IN THE NURSING ASSESSMENT

There is an additional area that, in the older person, is wisely handled as a separate component of the assessment. That is the medication history. Nurses have found that with the myriad of drugs that are used by many older persons—prescribed, over-the-counter, and home remedies—it becomes important to address their drug taking patterns, systems, and attitudes as a separate, not integrated, part of the assessment. It is also an assessment that is repeated at intervals appropriate to the drug-taking patterns and skills of the individual as well as changes in his status that affect the taking of medications.

Medication-taking behavior, previous patterns of drug* use, and associated beliefs about medications are an important component of the data base in particular with the older population. While it is true that

---

* The terms "drug," "medicines," and "medications" are used interchangeably in this chapter. However, because of the negative connotation the word "drug" has for some older persons, it is suggested that the terms "medication" or "medicine" be used in talking with them.

in some situations the clinical pharmacists will collect a portion of the data in a drug history, it has been found that nursing's perspective in the area is somewhat different from that of pharmacy.

The pharmacist will focus on the names and kinds of drugs being taken. The nurse will add some different dimensions that include:

1. Previous patterns of utilization of medications.
2. Attitudes toward medications and their effects.
3. Side effects experienced and allergies.
4. Ethnic and/or religious influences on treatment of illness and health maintenance.

The nurse is also interested in any physical or environmental barriers to the safe and effective taking of medications or treatments. So, while it is wise to check the pharmacist's data to avoid duplication, it usually will be necessary for the nurse to gather additional data in order to develop effective nursing management plans for any older patient.

Bringing in the Medications

Nurses who have worked with ambulatory elderly often ask the older person periodically to put all the medications he is using into a sack and bring them to the clinic or office. The person should be told this request refers to all medicines prescribed by all doctors as well as products they get over the counter in drug stores, supermarkets, natural food stores, ethnic shops, and so forth. Give examples of aspirin, vitamins, laxatives, antacids, and medicinal teas. The patient should bring those medicines he takes regularly as well as those he uses on only an occasional basis, including those he has had in the medicine cabinet for some time and those shared with him by his friends, relatives, or neighbors.

The explanation is made to the person that information gained from seeing the medications, the labels, and dates as well as from talking about them with the person will enable the nurse to be more effective in working with him in managing his health care and daily living. Indicate to the patient that many patients require pretty large sacks, since medications are so widely used.

The medication containers and labels offer a concrete point of departure for gaining an understanding of the patient's knowledge about medications and patterns of medication taking. It may also disclose the use of multiple physicians and pharmacists with the increased risk of drug interactions since no one pharmacist will have a complete drug file for discovering drug interaction risks.

Sequence in the Medication Assessment

There is a preferred sequence of topics in assessing the individual's medication-taking behavior. It begins with current prescription drugs and moves on to over-the-counter (OTC) remedies and finally to home remedies. The rationale is that, in sharing information, one discusses areas requiring the least risk —drugs prescribed by the health provider. Here the only risk probably is that of reporting the adjustment of doses, schedules, or noncompliance. The next increment in risk is with the use of OTC products; these are sold by pharmacists or major firms and, therefore, could be seen by the patient as having some modicum of health system/societal approval. The area that may seem riskiest of all for the patient is an honest discussion of the use of home remedies and ethnic practices used in the treatment of illness or in health maintenance. The attitude of the person seeking this information can greatly reduce the risk in discussing ethnic practices.

Data on Current Drug-Taking Practices

Knowledge of Drugs

If the individual brings in his medications, each bottle can be talked about to determine his working knowledge of:

- the name of the drug
- the dosage (mgm./gm. and number of tablets or amount)
- timing of medication
- purpose of the drug and any effects being noted
- side effects: those the individual monitors and those being experienced

For the new patient who does not bring in the drugs and cannot remember drug names, the nurse may ask such questions as:

Do you take any medicines for your heart? for your blood pressure? for your breathing?
Do you take any water pills? vitamins? etc.

Barriers to Safe Medication Taking

Much of the medication assessment is a subjective approach—viewed from the patient's perspective. However, the patient may have some blind spots with regard to some aspects of his capability to follow the medical regimen safely. Therefore, it becomes important that the nurse gather objective data on these areas—from the medical data base and from observations of patient behavior during interactions. Some areas of high risk that predict decreased ability to participate safely and effectively in drug regimens include:

- vision deficits
- hearing deficits (taking in instructions)
- intellectual or memory deficits
- strong aversion to taking any medication
- patterns of drug abuse or addiction
- financial constraints

Perhaps further afield, but still relevant on occasion, is the attitude of family or significant others toward the regimen.

In these and other areas, the nurse needs to note as specifically and precisely as possible the observations made and the inferences drawn regarding the risks to safe medication taking activities. Nursing management of medication taking will be built upon these data.

It is important to know that the risk of errors increases directly and significantly with increases in numbers of medications (Schwartz, 1964, and Neeley and Patrick, 1968).

System for Drug Taking

Another area of data gathering that is particularly important with the elderly is that of learning what system the individual uses to remember and take the right drugs in the right amount at the right time. Herein lies the risk of precarious or ineffective drug taking. The nurse should learn:

> Does he put a day's supply in separated containers so that in the evening that is a check on what has been taken?

For those with vision problems:

> How does he know what pill is in which bottle?

One patient indicated that she recognized pills by the sound as she shook the bottles. (Pharmacists suggest that different sized, colored, or shaped bottles or raised strips of tape on the sides of bottles are safer techniques.)

Schwartz (1964, 109–146) found in the study of medication errors of the elderly that persons who had a system for remembering to take their medicines made fewer errors than those without a system. Almost any predictable daily event can be used as a reminder. One respondent remembered her pills by taking them every time she ate oatmeal. This worked for her because she had once-a-day pills and ate oatmeal once every day.

Timing in Relationship to ADL

Timing of drugs in relationship to meals and sleep and in relationship to other drugs can be important. Three times a day (t.i.d.) or even 9-1-6 can have quite different relationships to meals and sleep for one who eats two meals a day at 11 and 7 and retires at midnight as compared to one who eats 7-12-5 and retires at 9. Further, the way drugs are given in the hospital or nursing home may not be the time they should be taken at home. If something is to be taken "before breakfast," be certain that the person (1) eats breakfast and (2) eats breakfast before noon. Blood levels of certain medications, like antibiotics, need to be maintained for the drug to be effective. This means taking the drug regularly over the 24-hour period; others do not require such regular round-the-clock intervals. Be certain that a round-the-clock regimen is actually required on a medication before subjecting the patient to setting an alarm and being awakened to take a pill at 2 a.m. Also know the person's usual sleep patterns. Often it is possible to schedule the drugs so that they coincide with times the person is normally awake or falls back to sleep readily.

Modifying the regimen

Knowing whether or not older persons adjust their medications in relationship to their signs and symptoms, and how they do it, is also significant. One patient reported to the doctor that his heart beat was "hard as a hammer" on digoxin 0.25 mgm. daily but was fine on half that amount. This same patient has COPD and keeps a supply of tetracycline prescribed by the physician, which he takes when a respiratory infection threatens. He has a known history of being responsible and knowledgeable about recognizing his symptoms and taking drugs. Physicians, however, appreciate a phone call when a patient begins such a self-controlled regimen because then a check can be maintained on the patient. Occasionally a drug change or an office call can prevent the development of a more serious problem.

A less knowledgeable patient was found in a drug history to be taking nitroglycerin and digoxin interchangeably for chest pain. Some patients discontinue antibiotics as soon as symptoms disappear instead of taking the full course prescribed, and then they are hit with relapses. Others staunchly continue to take medications despite side effects.

Some patients are born "savers" and, when money is scarce, many older persons find the expense of medications an almost unsupportable burden. For whatever reason, there are those persons who save medications to use should a condition recur. Others exchange medications with someone who has a "similar condition." These are difficult behaviors to deal with, but they certainly should be delineated and addressed as sensitively and positively as possible since they affect the therapy the older person achieves.

Observing for Response to Medications and Giving Feedback

Because of the increased risk of side effects of drugs in the elderly, another area of data that is important to the nurse is the patient's pattern of observing drug effects:

What is the person aware that he should notice? Will he remember better with written guidelines?

How does he check on his responses? Does he have the *capacity* to notice signs and symptoms?

Does he have the vocabulary to give useable data to the health care provider?

What is his attitude about giving feedback? (e.g., does he tend not to want to bother the doctor or nurse?) Does he tend to ignore symptoms? Does he worry about every twinge?

Does he know the best time to call? Does he have access to a phone?

Does he know when it is important to report symptoms promptly—regardless of the day or hour—and what can wait for office hours?

Flow sheets on which the patient can record data on critical variables may be useful. This technique will control the person who tends to want to report unending minutiae as well as the one who does not know what to report. It also fosters the person's active participation in his own treatment. An example is given in Figure 4-4.

Members of the health team need to be aware of what behaviors they are fostering by their response to patients as they teach them or respond to their calls. Failure to answer simple questions, failure to return calls, condescending attitudes toward data not seen as important to the professional—all can contribute to patterns of inadequate feedback.

Over-the-Counter Products

Patterns in use of OTCs are also important. If the nurse has sensed a reluctance to share information, this section of the assessment can be prefaced by a remark such as, "There are a lot of products available to us in the drug store and supermarkets that help with our health. Do you use any of them?" If the pa-

Bertha Johnson	1/16	1/17	1/18	1/19
Weight	200	201	204	
Episodes of shortness of breath	2	2	4	
Swelling of ankles a.m./p.m.	0/+	+/++	++/+++	
Lasix 1 tab/day	9am	forgot	8:30	

FIGURE 4-4. Medication flow sheet example.

tient's memory seems to require jogging, the nurse can ask about specific types of medicines such as antacids, antidiarrheals, cough and cold remedies, laxatives, vitamins, and ointments.

Another approach is to ask if he has a particular complaint and what he does to relieve it. (e.g., Do you have headaches? What do you do for it?) Include other complaints such as heartburn, gas, indigestion, nausea, diarrhea, constipation, head colds, chest colds, aching joints, and skin problems.

Home Remedies

There is a greater likelihood that the older person has learned family ways of dealing with health problems and complaints. He also may feel, or know from past experience, that health professionals will ridicule these folkways. A means of approaching this subject is to say something like, "My family had some ways of treating colds and aches and pains that worked pretty well. I still use some of them. Did you grow up with some of these too?" If the response is affirmative, the nurse may continue with, "Are there any that you still find useful?"

One form of home remedy is adjustment in diet for particular complaints. For example, in some cultures, persons who feel they have "high blood" (too much blood volume), will restrict red meats and other red foods, while, if the condition is felt to be "low blood," they will increase their consumption of red foods (red meats, beets, red fruits). There are many dietary remedies suggested to prevent or treat arthritis or rheumatism; some people drink lemon juice first thing in the morning.

Home remedies are as effective in some aspects of care as more expensive medications. (e.g., gargles of salt and hot water, cough medicine of honey and hot tea, steam for sinusitis, rice water for diarrhea.) If the health care provider suggests these home remedies and they resolve the problem, the patient will feel the provider's concern for him and his limited funds.

Belief in Medications

Another critical area that may or may not emerge overtly is the credibility that drugs have for the person. Aside from religious groups that overtly disavow reliance on medications, individuals vary markedly in their beliefs about the efficacy of drugs. Some want a pill for any complaint—the more the better. Others will endure major physical dysfunction and discomfort rather than take medications. Most persons fall somewhere between these two extremes but tend to lean toward one or the other. It is important for the nurse to specifically seek data on the preference the person has regarding medications. Even highly educated and sophisticated persons (often health professionals), who do understand the rationale for the medication, may not take the drugs.

Current items in the media—television, radio, newspapers, magazines, and books—can strongly influence attitudes and drug-taking behavior. Therefore, it is important for the nurse to know what is currently in vogue or under attack. She can check whether this input has influenced her patients and their attitudes or behavior in relationship to these drugs.

Summary

The data in the medication assessment is critical to working realistically with an individual in effectively incorporating drug therapy into his life. The data should affect prescription; the way in which drugs, effects, monitoring, and feedback are introduced and supervised; the assistance needed in developing a system for safe and accurate drug taking; and the risks of drug interactions. Understanding of home remedies and patterns will allow for better articulation of prescriptions with the person's and family's usual way of doing things.

The data collected by the nurse should be located in the patient's record in such a way that others who are involved in planning for medications can be aware of the patient's lifestyle in medication taking.

RECORDING THE NURSING DATA BASE

Regardless of the record system being used—traditional or the more recently adopted problem oriented format—the nursing data base, including the medication history, needs to become an easily-locatable component of the permanent legal record. The overall nursing assessment should be recorded on a special form located near the physical examination and medical history forms, so that an integrated composite, interdisciplinary view of the data is easily available. In addition, data collated to SOAP (Subjective, Objective, Analysis, Plan) current presenting problems would reappear on the Progress page or on Nursing Notes, depending on the system.

Further, as the older person moves from one nursing system to another, it seems only fair and cost effective that the nursing data base be carried with him. In some ambulatory care clinics, for instance, patients regularly carry communication to and from nursing home nurses or home health care nurses and the physician-nurse teams in the office or clinic.

REFERENCES

Little, D., and Carnevali, D.: Nursing Care Planning, ed. 2. Philadelphia: J. B. Lippincott, 1976.
Neeley, E., and Patrick, M.: Problem of aged persons taking medications at home. Nursing Research 17: 52–56, 1968.
Schwartz, D., Henley B., and Zutz, L.: The Elderly Ambulatory Patient. New York: Macmillan Co., 1964.

Part 2

Normal Aging

Introduction to Part 2

Part One offered the first cornerstone in the structure for nursing management of the elderly—nursing's focus and area of expertise. Part Two offers the second—the status and processes associated with normal aging. The nurse deals with healthy as well as ill persons over 70. Furthermore, illness in the elderly and its manifestations are affected by age-related changes. Thus, the clinician who wishes to nurse the elderly effectively needs a working knowledge of the nature of age-related changes, their manifestations and implications for daily living, and therapeutic regimens.

Chapter 5 addresses general characteristics of the older age group, including demographic characteristics, theories of social response to aging, and developmental tasks to be achieved.

Chapter 6 explores the anatomic and physiologic changes as the person ages biologically. No nursing implications have been explicitly drawn; however, the reader will no doubt find many she wishes to observe and test with her patients.

The functional changes identified in Chapter 6 are translated into the resultant modification of norms for laboratory values in the elderly. Most laboratory norms are set for younger adults with adjustments for older persons, in most instances, not yet standardized. Chapter 7 reviews the status of ranges of "normal" for the aged compared to younger age groups, as this is available in present literature.

Oral health is so critical to many other aspects of effective living in later years that it has been addressed in a separate chapter. It should be of major concern to the nurse, particularly as attitudes towards oral health and retaining natural teeth are gaining such interest. Chapter 8 explores the anatomic and physiologic changes occurring in the oral cavity, along with a dentist's view of activities to help the person to retain oral health.

Nutrition in the elderly is a critical issue, affecting many aspects of social and physical health of the older person. Normal dietary needs of the elderly and the barriers to meeting these needs as well as resources for overcoming the barriers are all necessary parts of the nurse's knowledge base for effective clinical practice. Chapter 9 treats these areas in depth, building on the biologic aging information of Chapter 6.

Finally, the elderly are a "poly-drug" population, consuming many more drugs than younger age groups and responding to them in much less predictable fashion. Again, building on the knowledge in Chapters 6 and 7, Chapter 10 examines the effect of age related changes on drug-taking behavior and responses.

5

The Elderly
and Their Responses to Aging

Maxine Patrick

Old age is a time of life feared by many. However, the anticipation appears to be worse than the event itself. In a recent survey, for every three people who found life over 65 better than expected, only one found it worse (National Council on Aging, 1975).

It is not unusual to find people who are in their eighties and nineties doing the same things as well as those a decade or two younger, though perhaps a bit more slowly. Too often the sick and institutionalized are seen as the norm of old age. While it is true that the risk of disease and disability increases with age, it is not necessarily incapacitating to many.

Statistics continue to support earlier findings that most older people live independently in the community. Only 5 percent of people over 65 are in institutions on any given day, while an additional 10 percent are housebound (Glick, 1977). This leaves 85 percent who are maintaining themselves in some fashion in the community. Despite these data that continue to demonstrate that the bulk of the older persons live in the community, the greatest amount of health resources and programs are directed to the 15 percent, whose health problems get them into the health care system, rather than toward prevention and support to help persons remain at home.

CHARACTERISTICS

Longevity

Information from vital statistics and biologic studies does not support the common belief that the human life span has increased. Life *expectancy* has increased, but the life span has remained constant (Hayflick, 1976). Treatment of the illnesses of early years has improved, thus allowing more people to survive illnesses to reach the limit of an apparent fixed life span. If the two leading causes of death—heart disease and stroke—were successfully eliminated, approximately 18 years of additional life could be expected. If cancer, the third greatest cause of death were eliminated, two more years would be added to life expectancy (Hayflick, 1976).

MALE AND FEMALE LONGEVITY. It is well known that females outlive males. This is the case for all species. The ratio of men to women decreases with age. At birth there are 120 males to 94.8 females; however, by age 85 there are 100 males to 209.2 females (Brotman, 1977).

Women outlive men by a number of years. For instance, white females born in 1969 to 1971 will live 7.6 years longer than their male counterparts. Nonwhite females will outlive males by nine years. White women aged 65 in those same years will live 3.9 years longer than males, with nonwhite women living 3.1 years longer (Brotman, 1977).

A variety of reasons have been given to try to explain the differences in longevity between women and men. Among those proposed (Waldron and Johnson, 1976) are the following:

- twofold elevation of arteriosclerotic heart disease in males
- high incidence of cigarette smoking and coronary prone behavior in males

41

- male involvement in more hazardous positions
- higher incidence in males of automobile accidents, suicide, and use of guns and alcohol

Women, on the other hand, are thought to have some hormonal protection against aging. Further, progress has been made in decreasing high risk diseases of women such as cancer of the cervix, while there have been few advances in decreasing diseases that take the life of men—cancer of the lung, myocardial infarction, and strokes.

There are some questions as to whether changes in lifestyle will in turn change mortality and morbidity. The work of Lewis and Lewis (1977) supports the view that differences in morbidity and mortality rates are due more to behavioral factors than to biologic ones. Women have had more time at home. They use the health care system more frequently than men. They are the ones from whom children learn health behavior and beliefs. Lewis and Lewis (1977) raise the following questions:

Will sexual equality decrease women's use of health care services?

Will death rates of women increase as they acquire different stresses and greater risks?

Can sexual equality be achieved with individual survival and equal opportunities for personal achievements?

One may speculate as to what could happen with the implementation of equal rights of sexes and acceptance of and by women of roles and behaviors traditionally associated with males. Mortality for women may increase if male roles that women are taking are stressful or involve personal risk. However, if the role changes are unacceptable to men but instead become an added new stressor for them, then the ratio could remain the same or decrease for males.

Proportion of the Population Over 65 Years

The estimate is that from 1976 to the year 2050 the average life expectancy of females will increase from 77 to 81 years, while for males it will rise from 69.1 to 71.8 years (Projection of Population, 1977–2050, 1976). Where in 1977, 10 percent of the population was over 65, the projection is that by the year 2030 between 14 and 22 percent will be in this segment of the population.

Marital Status

There are five times as many widows over 65 as widowers (Glick, 1977). This is due in part to longevity of the female but also to the norms of society. Women usually marry men older than themselves. A woman who marries a younger man, especially one where the age differential is great, e.g., 10 years, is looked at disapprovingly by her peers and relatives. By contrast, a man who selects a bride even 30 years younger may cause comments but is usually accepted.

Men and women over 65 *do* marry or remarry. One percent of all brides and two percent of all grooms in 1965 were in that age category (Glick, 1977).

There are deterrents to marriage between the elderly. One major problem is the attitudes of grown children of either or both potential spouses. If children feel the remarriage of a parent will jeopardize their inheritance, they could stand in the way of the wedding. Children who do not understand the needs and desires of the parent may object to his or her marriage. Older people often give up their own wishes for companionship through marriage in order to please their adult children.

One of the reasons retired persons did not marry in the past was the loss of Social Security income from a spouse. Increasing numbers of couples lived together without going through the legal arrangements of marriage, prior to January 1979, in order to retain an adequate income. The law has now been changed to correct this situation.

Educational Level

SCHOOL ATTENDANCE. Formal education of children in the early 1900s was not highly valued. Many parents were immigrants who went into jobs that did not require formal education. Knowledge of reading and writing was not essential to get a job and earn money. If a family had to make a choice about which of the children should seek higher education, even high school, a boy most likely was chosen over his sister. Girls were expected to marry and raise a family. These roles did not require education in a school. In some cases, the oldest boy in the family had to leave school in order to help support the family. Because of these attitudes it is not surprising that some people 65 and over are functionally illiterate (meaning four years of school or less).

The number of years of school attendance is increasing. A random sample of people in the United States in 1975 (National Council on Aging, 1975, 238) disclosed that only 2 percent of the white people over 65 had no formal schooling. Nineteen percent had one to seven years. This is in contrast to blacks, 12 percent of whom had no schooling and 50 percent of whom had one to seven years. People who lived on rural farms have the least amount of education for whites and nonwhites (Foner, 1968, 112).

IMPLICATIONS. It is well to remember that the number of years of schooling does not reflect an ability to learn nor the intelligence of the learner. Some people who did not have an opportunity to attend many years of school have made and are making major contributions to society. They are in business, skills, and trades. They have learned what they need to know to be effective in a given area.

The number of years of education noted on a health history should not be viewed as a measure of whether or not a person should be taught and/or can learn. Rather, it is a challenge to devise a system so that the patient will learn.

Financial Status

While older people constitute a tenth of the total population, they are 13 percent of the total poor. In 1975, of the 8.2 million families in which the head of the household was over 65, 7 percent had incomes of less than $3000 per year (an average of less than $58 per week). Those older persons who were living alone or with nonrelatives were found to be in the greatest financial difficulty. Of these 6.9 million, almost 390,000 (8 percent) had less than $1500 per year, or an average of less than $29 per week. Forty-two percent of persons living alone had a weekly income under $58 (Brotman, 1977, 24–25). While there are automatic increases in Social Security payments based on rises in the cost of living, these lag behind inflation and older Americans continue to have about half the income of the young.

Social Security legislation initially was passed in 1936. However, the self-employed were not covered by it unless they applied and contributed. The soundness of the program is the concern of old people today; they wonder whether their Social Security checks will keep coming the third of every month.

In April 1978, President Carter signed into law a change in the age of mandatory retirement to 70. Some believe this to be more of an empty gesture than an action which will aid older, low income, disadvantaged workers. Men retiring at a compulsory age

received $3180 (median retirement benefit) compared to $1,640 for those without compensatory retirement. For women the amount was $1940 compared to $890. Whites, professionals, and technical workers are more likely to have a second pension, not just Social Security. Women and minorities are more likely to have only one pension system for retirement (Social Security) and not be in a system with compulsory retirement (Kolobrubetz, 1976). Recent trends have indicated that more people are retiring before age 65. Abolishing mandatory retirement age will be of greatest benefit to a small group of mainly middle and upper middle income workers. Those forced from the labor market with partial disabilities and limited employment opportunities—black, older workers, members of other minority groups, women, and low wage earners—will generally not benefit as much as the others (Kingson, 1978).

There are limitations on the amount of income a person 65 and over can earn before Social Security benefits are reduced. This was $4000 in 1978; the amount will be increased $500 per year until, in 1982, it will be $6000. Then the amount one can earn will automatically increase along with average wage increases. At that time (1982), there will be no limit on earnings of people 70 or older as there is none now for those 72 and older (USDHEW, 1978).

There are two other changes in Social Security which will increase income to those 60 and older. Prior to January 1979, widows/widowers who remarried after age 60 lost their Social Security payments which they received from a deceased spouse. Beginning in January 1979, a divorced wife 62 years or older, married 10 years, can get benefits on her ex-husband's earnings. Before this date a divorced wife had to be married 20 years to collect Social Security from an ex-husband.

Medicare Title 18 began providing financial assistance for sickness care (but not health promotion), in 1965. The advent of Medicare did relieve some of the worry about having money to pay hospital and doctor bills. As of July 1978, Medicare paid for more than 70 percent of the cost of medical insurance (hospital, nursing home, home health) of those who use the health care system (Social Security Administration, 1978). With Medicare, older people are less dependent upon their families or local government agencies for these costs.

IMPLICATIONS. The decrease in available money and the realistic threat of inflation are reflected in the older person's concern for money. It involves many value systems and experiences in earlier life which must be taken into consideration in understanding his perspective in later life.

The nurse should be familiar with and aware of these attitudes of older people towards money. Maybe the patient will not verbalize his concern over the cost of something. Instead of admitting the drug prescribed or the equipment suggested is too costly, he just will not follow the advice. The nurse's awareness of cost is one way of caring. Patients may ask about the cost of items and room charges in an institution. They need an answer with the facts and not a statement of false reassurance, "don't worry."

The work ethic has been a strong factor in many older people's value systems. The belief that one must work and earn a livelihood is basic to their lifestyle. The depression of the 1930s is part of their history. Finding work then and earning enough to live on was difficult if not impossible during the depression because there were few jobs. In the process of seeking work, some families moved around the country, uprooting themselves from the supports they had. This occurred at a critical time in their lives when they were starting families and employment and income should have been stabilized.

When the older people of today became parents, they wanted a better life for their children than they had. Money and education were ways to insure this. These people saved in order to be independent of their children and to be able to care for themselves when they were old or sick. Homeowners felt secure because they had a place in which to live that was paid for. What they did not predict was inflation that had wiped out the value of their hard-earned money. Their homes of decades are being taxed at such a high rate that some are having to move out and others are denying themselves the basics of life, such as food, in order to be able to remain in their cherished homes a little longer.

It is not unknown in this older generation for the parents to deny themselves in order to "leave something for the children." Despite their own precarious financial position, they have a stronger will to be able to give to the children than to receive financial help from them—even where the children might well be able to afford to give assistance.

Health Care Insurance

With the advent of Medicare all persons over 65 are eligible for some basic health insurance. Most people have Part A, (hospital insurance) and do not have to pay for it; they earned it because of credit for work under Social Security. To get Part B (medical insurance), the person must sign up for it; the monthly payments are then deducted from the Social Security check. In addition, many people realize that this insurance does not cover them adequately. They supplement this basic coverage with an additional plan available through most insurance carriers.

However, even though coverage for many is quite effective, few people read and understand the provisions of their health insurance policies. They have not read the policy until after it is needed. Medicare insurance regulations are a good example. The information is difficult to understand. To have to try to understand Medicare coverage when one is still sick or recovering from an illness increases the stress to the patient.

It is important that all health care professionals, particularly nurses, read the Medicare literature. While it is more simply written now than it was originally, it is still difficult to understand. For example, without an understanding of terms like "reasonable charges" or "benefit period," the amount of assistance the nurse can give to patients is limited. The family as well as the patient turn to the nurse for help. Being able to give accurate help with this is part of nursing management in terms of mobilizing adequate financial support systems.

Frequently, the first time a patient has had to apply for benefits from Medicare he is in for a shock at how little of the bills are paid. Some people still think that all hospital and physician bills are covered; this is not true. They do not know that a deductible amount must be paid by the patient on both the doctor and the hospital portion *each calendar year*. Sometimes, after they learn this, or if the nurse helps them to use their coverage wisely, they are able to adjust their health care needs within a calendar year so as to reduce their own costs.

Another area of confusion for patients is the billing system. The entire bill may be sent directly to the patient, or only the portion of the bill the patient is asked to pay after Medicare has paid all they allow. Many old people do not have the money to cover large bills. Frequently, those who have lived a lifetime of paying bills immediately are upset as the bills arrive month after month. Some do not read the overprint that says "This is not a bill." The forms and the numbers look alike. Again this adds to the stress when money is a problem.

Another area of confusion is related to the use of the check that arrives from the third party payor. If the patient does not understand that he is to pay the entire bill when he receives a large check for Medicare, he thinks the check is his to spend. Subsequently, it comes as a shock to continue to receive bills from the doctor and hospital.

The nurse needs to be familiar with these high risk problem areas in insurance as a component of patient care. It is important to help the patient and family to understand his insurance resources and use them most effectively in his planning for health care whenever this is possible.

Old-Aged Children of Old-Aged Parents

As parents live longer, they have children who also are old and who are facing problems in their own lives related to aging. Parents in their eighties could have children in their sixties. Children in their late seventies and early eighties have been known to have parents of 100. Brody (1966) found that 40 percent of elderly applicants to a voluntary home had at least one child who was 60 or older.

Sometimes, in caring for parents, it is difficult to get adult children to participate in their health care management. However, studies have shown that many adult children are and want to be responsible for their parents (Brody, 1977, 43). In a study of health care patterns of elderly in low income residences, the parents were not reluctant to call upon their children in case of illness and 70 percent called upon a member of their nuclear family if they became ill (Carnevali, 1975, 264).

Paths leading to institutional care have shown that this is the last resort for the family and that it is a step which is taken when all alternatives, including personal, social, and economic resources, have been exhausted. This decision is made, even then, with utmost reluctance (Brody, 1966, 1977). The statistics that on any given day only 5 percent of persons over 65 are in institutions seems to bear this out. The implication of this is that when the usual support of old people, their children, is not available, it is not because of lack of interest, but because their resources have already been severely depleted. Alternatives must then be found.

Fears

Young people do not interpret the concerns of older people in the same way as do those who are older. Several years ago, the National Council on Aging Inc., undertook household interviews with both young and old. The interviews with 4254 persons over 65 showed that fear of crime was their "most serious problem"; this was true for people of all incomes. Poor health ranked next, followed by not having enough money to live on, and, fourth, fear from loneliness. The same question was asked of the total public. Table 5-1 shows the contrast in the rankings.

Projecting one's own fears of aging onto those who are aged has considerable likelihood of being inaccurate. Young people at the same income level as the old are far more dissatisfied with their ability to make their income meet financial needs and with poor housing than people over 65. As one lives longer, material needs tend to decrease and the individual learns to expect less.

Some older people, particularly in cities, are living in isolation, afraid to go out of their room or apartment. These people may not be getting adequate food because they are afraid of being attacked or robbed. This is a real problem which has not been addressed in most communities. The old are vulnerable to those who could do them harm and they know it. Some citizens groups have developed and are offering classes on self-defense techniques. Other groups are trying to form buddy systems or offer car pools in order to achieve safety in numbers.

The old are especially affected by the problems of society as a whole. Rape of older women is not uncommon, and prostitutes solicit in rooming houses of old men, especially around the dates that welfare, pension, and Social Security checks arrive. Sexual assault centers or rape relief services are available in many cities to help deal with these problems.

Attitudes

MEDIA. Attitudes of a society are formed in part by television, newspapers, and magazines through

TABLE 5-1. Ranking of fears.

Over-65 Group	General Public
Crime	Not enough money to live on
Poor health	Crime
Not enough money to live on	Poor health
Loneliness	Poor housing
	Not feeling needed

Adapted from Myths and Reality of Aging in America. National Council on the Aging, Inc., April 1975, pp. 130–132.

advertising and editorial policy. The media tend to focus toward the young since they have greater purchasing power than older people. Brooke (1974) looked at the magazines people over 65 read and then reviewed feature articles and ads to see the way older people were portrayed. The respondents to her questionnaires lived at home and indicated that they read magazines regularly. Of 4550 ads reviewed in four magazines only 22 were related to older people. She found that the aged were featured in food, cosmetic, and health ads. Cosmetics were to be used to prevent looking old. Health ads were negative in their showing pain, illness, and soreness. Men were featured as retired. Grandparent and parent roles were shown. She did not find feature articles on positive aspects of aging, how to cope with growing old, and/or retirement. The Gray Panthers are attempting to change the way older people are shown in the media. They also are working to change the way comedians and others stereotype older people in their programs or acts. They feel that presently the media discriminate against the elderly.

Older persons are very much aware that they are seen differently by the young. They know they are patronized or viewed negatively. Some avoid interacting with young people because they fear rejection or are angered at being patronized. This bias takes many forms. When a man of 70 defeats younger men in a sport event it is newsworthy, even though the achievement may not be all that extraordinary. Many older people are as physically fit as the middle aged. This kind of reporting indicates inaccurate stereotyping of the old and a failure to understand the aging process.

HEALTH PROFESSIONALS. Health professionals, including nurses, frequently have negative attitudes toward aging because the older people they see usually are seeking health care. For example, nurses identified more negative characteristics of old age than did psychologists and sociology students (Gibbons, 1963). Most health professionals see old people who are ill; they focus on pathology of age and not normal physiologic age changes. They expect deterioration and disease and do not look for, or are surprised to find, old people physically and mentally equal to other ages.

Negative attitudes of nurses are reflected in their treating hospitalized patients 65 and over differently from younger patients. In one study (Christensen, 1963), registered nurses correctly identified the age range of the person and then altered their behavior in the following ways with older persons:

- raised their voices when speaking
- assisted them with eating without asking if they needed or wanted help, e.g., cut meat, cracked eggs, buttered toast
- provided less privacy while giving care—less attention to pulling screens, closing doors, knocking before entering
- avoided explaining details of diagnostic tests
- taught the family and *not* the older person

Housing

Older people tend to have stable living arrangements. Many have lived in the same place for more than 20 years. They have grown old in the neighborhood. They know the mailman, the druggist, the checker at the grocery store. They like the neighborhood because they have friends there. Frequently these areas do not have many young families.

Often these neighborhoods where older people concentrate become rundown. Their homes are not kept us as well when the owners age and available money decreases. Houses and yards require work for adequate maintenance. Older people lack both the strength and energy to do the work, much as they may want to do it. They do not have the money to hire others to do repairs or maintenance. The result becomes obvious.

This is the kind of area that city planners see as urban blight and tear down without providing for relocation of old people to housing they want or can afford. Cities that have built housing for the low income elderly usually have long waiting lists and cannot keep up with the need.

Many different kinds of housing are needed to meet the diverse living arrangements of older people. Various types are indicated in Table 5-2.

Among people who can live independently, one third of the income is spent on housing. Those with a very limited income spend even more. Some landlords raise the rents every time Social Security payments are increased. Even older people who own their own homes have problems as property taxes and utilities rise with inflation. Many states do provide lower property taxes and utility rates for those over 65 who are below a stated income.

Changing Residence

Any move for an older person is traumatic and even dangerous. Therefore, moves from one living area to another should be planned carefully with full

TABLE 5-2. Kinds of housing for older people.

Type	Benefits
Retirement communities	For people who wish to maintain a high level of activity and interaction. Programs include classes, meetings, and social gatherings. On-site hospitals part of some communities.
Homes for the aged	Usually owned by religious groups. Provide a complete array of services including health care when needed. Residents are active and independent as long as they can be. Infirmary and health care available.
Mobile home parks	Year-round living or seasonal accommodations (e.g., wintering in the South).
Board and care homes	For those who need help with meals and personal care. Health care cannot be provided. These are licensed by most states.
Nursing homes	For people who need some level of nursing care on a regular basis. Licensed by all states.

participation of the person who is moving or being moved. A social worker may visit an older person and decide that he should be moved to a "better place" because he can afford to have a more modern apartment or a more secure neighborhood. Children may want a parent to sell the family home and move to a less demanding type of housing or to another city so he can be closer. A spouse dies and the survivor is advised to move "to get away from memories." All of these are common reasons for moving people. Potentially all can cause problems for the person being moved.

Before a move is made it should be tested on a trial basis with an extended visit. A crisis time is never an appropriate moment to decide to make a major move. Decisions made then frequently are regretted. Moving to please others, or because one can afford better living arrangements, can also be unsuccessful.

Moves into institutions, between institutions, and even within institutions have been found to increase death rates. People with mental illnesses seem to be more vulnerable to moves than those with physical problems. For example, 26 percent of the patients over 65 died within six months following first admission to mental hospitals in one state

(Lowenthal, 1967). In moving patients from one facility to another, the mentally ill had death rates 63 percent higher than other patients. In that study, most deaths occurred in the first three months after the move. In *all* patients the actual death rates were significantly higher than was anticipated, based on the overall condition of the patient (Aldrich and Mendkoff, 1968). It also has been found in studies of people waiting to move into retirement homes that, when the decision is made to move, the person becomes psychologically like those who already live in the facility (Tobin, 1976). The time of decision making as well as the period immediately after a move has been made is one of increased vulnerability for older people.

AGING AND PERSONALITY THEORIES

Considerable research has been done over the years to find out what contributes to successful aging or what is necessary to successfully adapt to old age. The intended outcome was to develop a personality theory for gerontology.

For practical purposes, a personality theory assumes that more can be learned about the actions of a person by knowing something of his past and previous adaptation patterns than by knowing about his immediate actions. Personality theories are better able to explain about continuity than change. They concentrate upon the individual, not on the environment or situations in which he moves. However, a theory which regards how the individual fits into the environment has limitations.

Three developmental theories have been presented: disengagement, activity, and exchange. None of them has been accepted. The disengagement theory has generated the most controversy, mostly by those who have disproven it. Anyone in geriatrics or gerontology should read the original theories before accepting or rejecting them. Look at the characteristics of the people who were studied, where they lived, and how they were selected and tested. Decide whether they are representative of all older people and the group to which you wish to apply the findings.

Disengagement Theory

The disengagement theory is described in the book *Growing Old* (Cummings and Henry, 1955). They see aging as an inevitable, mutual withdrawal or disengagement of the individual from society and society from the individual. This results in decreased interaction between the aging person and others in the social system to which he belongs. This theory states among other things that older people:

- give up roles
- have less social interaction and with fewer people
- disregard task-oriented, goal-directed roles
- are less willing to conform to the norms of society
- seek immediate responses to statements and actions

Women, especially widows who had lived with little interaction, are seen as disengaged and authoritarian. These are just a few of the statements of the theory which could have implications for nursing management.

A theory such as this can assist the nurse in understanding and explaining the behavior of older persons, in developing plans of care, and in evaluating responses and outcomes. For example, behavior of patients who do not conform to the norms of a facility or to instructions given to them by the nurse could be perceived and understood in terms of disengagement theory. Some nurses prefer to care for men rather than women, seeing women as bossy and rigid. Disengagement theory confirms these beliefs, since this theory predicts the behavior. Using this information, expectations and approaches to elderly female patients can be formulated which incorporate an expectation of this kind of behavior into the plan. Hopefully, the outcome is a normal positive relationship.

The nurse and other staff members may have to come to grips with their negative attitudes toward patients who do not conform and toward older women who are rigid and authoritarian. The disengagement theory may be helpful in working this through.

Activity Theory

The activity theory suggests that life satisfaction in older age occurs when the individual is involved in social interaction. According to this theory, people who stay active and maintain the activities of middle age adjust better to old age.

Some facilities that provide services to the elderly seem to support the activity theory. This means keeping people busy in groups, interacting, engaged in activities such as arts and crafts. A philosophy or policy that espouses activity as a successful way to age influences the attitudes and behavior of the staff toward the residents. *All* persons are expected to attend and enjoy programs as essential and therapeutic. There is the risk that residents who do not like to participate can be made to feel "less good" than those who do. Residents are aware of staff attitude.

While these programs serve many purposes, it should be pointed out that the activity programs may not be appropriate for all. An activity history obtained from all persons will help the staff. It will also help the resident determine the kinds of activities in which he would like to participate, the amount of time he wishes to be involved, the present activities he wishes to continue, the new activities he might like to learn, and his general attitude toward this lifestyle. For the person who has difficulty in recalling what he does, ask him to record all his activities for several days.

Nurses who function in situations where the activity theory is the frame of reference for the lifestyle need to be aware that therapeutic or recreational activities must be at an appropriate level and type or they will not be accepted. Men who are used to hard physical labor are more likely to participate in activities which require these skills than they are in making ceramics. Conversely, knitting and needlepoint may be appropriate for other men.

Activities must have a purpose and the person should know what it is. One patient viewed activities as a punishment. He had been sent to occupational therapy without explanation. His view was that he was sent there to see severely deformed people and to learn to appreciate that he was less disadvantaged than others. To make articles without purpose is contradictory to the work ethic of many people born in the early 1900s. Projects that can be sold with the money returning to the person or facility may meet this criterion. Other persons may want to be able to make items for their own use or to give as gifts to family and friends.

Activities also need to be viewed from the perspective of physical capability. Lack of willingness to participate in activities could be due to a physical problem. For example, if a person has a problem with urinary frequency, he may refuse to go to an activity that is of undefined length of time or one where he does not know the location of the bathroom. Such a person is taking a chance to go to this activity. A trip or an outing that does not state the amount of walking or extent of sitting may deter some older people from going when they really wish to go.

Exchange Theory

The activity and disengagement theories state that there is a decrease in social interaction in old age. Patterns of interaction exist among individuals and groups because they are rewarding. However, in seeking rewards there are costs. Profits derived from social exchange are equal to reward minus cost (Dowd, 1975). The social-psychologic theory of exchange postulates that interaction between individuals and groups continues as long as both profit from the interaction. Power is derived when there is an imbalance in social exchange. For example, if one party cannot reciprocate a rewarding behavior, the one who commands the services that another needs attains power over the other. This is done by making the satisfaction of the latter party's needs contingent upon its compliance.

With old people the decrease in social interaction is the result of a series of exchange relationships in which power of the aged is gradually diminished. This is inevitable because of loss of health, friends, and decreased income. When all power resources are gone, all the older person can do is comply with the young or society. This produces an unbalanced exchange relationship. The one who is dependent and less powerful attempts to rebalance the relationship by withdrawal, extension of power network, emergence of status, or coalition formation (Dowd, 1975, 589). None of these have been very successful. What has happened instead is that the imbalance becomes the norm, expected in the situation.

Implications of this theory for nursing include helping older people increase their power resources in the social networks in which they operate. This can be done by encouraging continued involvement in society, in groups, or joining new organizations and remaining socially and politically active. Developing new roles, although difficult, is another way of achieving power. These include volunteer work for nonprofit organizations, foster grandparenting, teaching classes in senior centers, finding new causes (e.g., NOW) and protecting neighborhoods.

In social interaction between young staff and older people, the staff should be aware of the "power" they have and how they use it. The patient is in the truly dependent position.

One function of patient advocates is to protect the dependent person from those in power. Some older people think that adequate or favorable treatment from health care providers requires gifts. Some old people give gifts to staff as a way of insuring adequate or favorable treatment.

The Gray Panthers organization is an example of a coalition of old and young joined together to form a power group to change society. In terms of exchange theory the purpose would be to rebalance the dependent old with the young.

ENVIRONMENT

The individual is a product of the environment in which he lived in the past and in which he lives currently. Social, political, economic, and technologic events that have occurred since 1900 should be listed along with critical times in the life cycle (in World War I, a teenager; the 1929–32 depression, in the work force or raising a family, etc.). This kind of information will aid in understanding and anticipating behavior of people 70 and older.

Values and standards of the Victorian years carried over into the early 1900s. Conservative political attitudes and the Protestant ethic were typical. Children were to be quiet and obedient to elders. All family members were expected to work in order to eat.

Since 1900 there have been four wars. These occurred at critical times in the lives of today's older population. World War I in 1914 to 1918 was fought when they were teenagers; World War II in 1941 to 1945 occurred at a time when they were established in careers and married, raising families. The Korean conflict in 1950 disrupted families for both fathers (50) and sons. The Vietnam War, which began in 1963, involved grandsons.

The technologic advances of the past 70 years have been numerous and diverse. They have included the automobile, the airplane, and space flights. Landing on the moon in 1969, sending equipment into space to Mars. Home life was changed by electric lights and appliances, telephone, television, radio, and microwave ovens to mention just a few. Development and deployment of atom bombs, hydrogen bombs, and neutron bombs have become means for the potential destruction of civilization.

The changes in the economy over the past 70 years include inflation, depression, unemployment, high employment, high wages, and recession. Frequently these changes occurred at critical times in the life span—a depression during the early years of marriage (1929 to 1933) when beginning a family, and retiring at a time of high inflation when money saved had reduced purchasing power (1965 to 1970). The economy is tied to the weather for energy and food production. In the 1930s there was severe draught in the farm belt. Crops that survived sun and drought were eaten by grasshoppers. During these years, in order to survive, many adults moved away from family and relatives to find work in other parts of the country.

National leaders and their personalities and philosophies have been an influence. For the over-70 generation, they include Theodore and Franklin Roosevelt, Wilson, Hoover, Hitler, Stalin, DeGaulle, Adenauer, Gandhi, Churchill, Kennedy, and Nixon.

The roles of women born in the early 1900s were those of wife and mother. They learned from their mothers how to sew, cook, can, and take care of children, frequently their own siblings. This turned out to be useful knowledge when they married during a depression when money had to be stretched and stretched. When men were at war, many women took jobs in defense factories; some remained employed after the war. The money they earned contributed to raising the standard of living of the family. Others returned to their families full time. There were many emotional drains on women of that era: being alone with small children; worrying about loved ones in wars (husbands, brothers, sons, grandsons); widowhood and inadequate finances which forced them into the work field with few skills.

LIFE CYCLE

There are certain general characteristics of each age group in the life cycle (Table 5-3). In the middle years the environment supports risk taking, but the individual has energies to take advantage

TABLE 5-3. Life cycle from the middle years through the very old.

Age	Value Theme	Developmental Task/Life Cycle Women	Men	Supports
Middle Years (45–60)	Dignity Control	Menopause Grandmother	Climacterian Grandfather	Spouse Friends Colleagues
		Children married Children leave home		Peers Parents Children
		Enter job market Volunteer	Major job success Second career	
		Parents die		
Preretirement and retirement (60–70)	Meaningful integration Autonomy	Retire Part-time jobs Widow		Spouse Children Friends Siblings
Old age (70–85)	Survival Acceptance of death	Life review Siblings die Diminished energy Adjustment to chronic illness Widower		Long time friends Neighbors Family Relatives
Very old (85+)		Death of children and friends		Remaining friends Remaining relatives Health care professionals

of the opportunities. People either achieve greatest successes in their careers during this time, or must face the realism that they cannot meet personal and financial goals they had established when they were young. The middle years are reflective, a time to review past accomplishments. They also are a turning point with a beginning awareness of approaching retirement.

The years in the 60s are more complex and dangerous. The individual begins to conform to the demands of the outer world and is less able to change the world in line with his own wishes. The way of coping with these changes is to become more interested in self and to attend to the control and satisfaction of personal needs.

Numerous studies have found that anticipation of retirement is stressful. However, once retired, people adjust to it better than they had expected. Preretirement planning has been helpful to some; others have started second careers. Retirement of a husband can be difficult for the wife. The wife had developed a life based upon being alone, doing what she wanted with friends. When her husband is home all day, she may feel obligated to change and do things with and for him. This can lead to problems.

The premise of this book is that old age is 70 and older. Many people of this age are far from old physiologically, socially, or psychologically. The fastest-growing group are those 75 and older. The average age of people in nursing homes is 82 (U.S. Senate, 1974, 16). Many people are living to be 90 and older. These people are special because they have outlived their peers.

Perkins (1976) interviewed some people 90 and older in her search for common factors that possibly contributed to their long life. She found that they all came from families that had lived to be 80 to 100 years. Although they had outlived friends and family, these people actively sought and made new friends. They had had major health problems but had recovered from them. They considered developing religious attitudes and maintaining beliefs more important than the actual practice of religion or religious activity. All had had stressful periods during their lifetime but they had coped with them. Death was not viewed as a stress. It was the opinion of this group that what happened to them was up to them, not others. The church, exercise, being busy, moderation, and good stock were the reasons they gave for their long life.

SUMMARY

The responses of old people to many commonly occurring events can be understood if one knows the life and times through which they have lived to reach that age. Their concerns and fears are real and can be prevented or allayed using this same information. Most older people live outside institutions yet, as a whole, they are viewed as dependent. To be healthy and wealthy makes life good at any age; unfortunately, that is not the case for many people who are old. When people reach a given age, whether it is 12, 40, or 70, they do not become a "group." Heterogeneity exists at all ages; those working with older people should not need to be reminded of this.

BIBLIOGRAPHY

Aldrich, C. K., and Mendkoff, E.: Relocation of the aged and disabled. In Neugarten, B. (ed.): Middle Age and Aging. Chicago: University of Chicago Press, pp. 401–408, 1968.

Binstock, R., and Shanas, E.: Handbook of Aging and the Social Sciences. New York: Van Nostrand Reinhold Co., 1976.

Birren, J., and Schaie, K. W.: Handbook of the Psychology of Aging. New York: Van Nostrand Reinhold Co., 1977.

Brody, E.: Long Term Care of Older People. New York: Human Sciences Press, 1977.

Brody, E.: The aging family. Gerontologist 6: 201–206, 1966.

Brooke, V.: "Gray Power in Black and White: The Roles and Visibility of the Aged in Four Popular Magazines. Unpublished Masters Thesis, School of Nursing, University of Washington, Seattle, 1974.

Brotman, H.: Income and poverty in the older population. Gerontologist 17: 23–26, 1977.

Carnevali, D., and Little, D.: Nursing Care Planning, ed. 2. Philadelphia: J. B. Lippincott Co., 1975.

Christensen, J.: The Development of a Tool to Guide Observations of the Behavior of Nurses Giving Care to Patients Over 65. Unpublished Maters Thesis, School of Nursing, University of Washington, Seattle, 1963.

Cook, F., et al.: Criminal victimization of the elderly. Gerontologist 18:338–349, 1978.

Cummings, E., and Henry W. E.: Growing Old. New York: Basic Books, 1955.

Dowd, J. J.: Aging as exchange: a preface to theory. J. Gerontol. 30:584–594, 1975.

Gibbons, M.: Development of a Tool to Determine the Attitudes of Nurses Toward Older Patients. Unpublished Masters Thesis, School of Nursing, University of Washington, Seattle, 1963.

Glick, P. C.: A Demographer Looks at the Family. Paper

presented at Gerontological Society's 30th Annual Scientific Meeting, San Francisco, November, 1977.

Havighurst, R. J., Neugarten, B. L., and Tobin, S. S.: Disengagement and patterns of aging. In Neugarten, B. (ed.): Middle Age and Aging. Chicago: University of Chicago Press, pp. 161–171, 1968.

Hayflick, L.: The cell biology of human aging. N. Engl. J. Med. 295:1302–1308, 1976.

Kingson, E.: Mandatory retirement reform—revolutionary change or empty gesture," Generations, 6–7, Winter 1978.

Kolodrubetz, W. W.: Characteristics of workers with pension coverage on the longest job. In Reaching Retirement Age. U.S. Social Security Administration, U.S. Government Printing Office, Washington D.C., 1976.

Lewis, C. E., and Lewis, M. A.: The potential impact of sexual equality on health. N. Engl. J. Med. 297:863—869, 1977.

Lowenthal, M., and Berkman, P.: Aging and Mental Disorders in San Francisco. San Francisco: Jossey-Bass, 1967.

National Council on the Aging, Myths and Reality of Aging in America, April, 1975.

Perkins, A.: The Elite Aged. Unpublished Masters Thesis, School of Nursing, University of Washington, 1976.

Projection of Population 1977–2050, Superintendent of Documents, U.S. Government Printing Service, Series P-25, No. 704, 1976.

Riley, M. W., and Foner, A.: Aging and Society. Vol. 1. New York: Russell Sage Foundation, 1968.

Tobin, S. S., and Negarten, B. L.: Life satisfaction and social interaction in aging. J. Gerontology, 16:344–346, 1961.

Tobin, S. S., and Lieberman, M.: Last Home for the Aged. San Francisco: Jossey-Bass, 1976, pp. 304.

U.S. Department of Health, Education, and Welfare, Recent Changes in Social Security. Social Security Administration, DHEW Publication No. (SSA), 78-10388, March 1978.

United States Senate, Subcommittee on Long Term Care, Nursing Home Care in the United States, Washington, D.C.: Superintendent of Documents, U.S. Government Printing, Supporting Paper No. 1, December 1974, 162 pp.

Waldron, I., and Johnson, S.: Why do women live longer than men? J. Human Stress. Vol. 2, March 1976, pp. 2–13; Vol. 2, June 1976, pp. 19–31.

6

Aging Changes in Structure and Function

Ralph Goldman

From birth until maturity the sum total of biologic change is incremental; from maturity onward the totality shifts and becomes decremental. During the first half of the present century, interest focused on growth and development, and there was the tacit assumption that change after maturity was pathologic in origin. However, when mortality was dramatically reduced during the developmental period, there was a shift in interest to chronic diseases of older individuals. During the past quarter century an increasing body of information has accumulated that indicates that aging is a specific process inherent in the organism and probably independent of, although influenced by, the environment. It is upon these changes, both incremental and decremental, that the processes of injury and disease interact. It is necessary to know and understand these changes in order to achieve the optimal results in the management of patients at all ages.

GENERAL CHANGES WITH AGE

One of the major problems, and perhaps the most perplexing, of gerontology is to identify the changes that are due to age alone, and to distinguish them from specific processes. Strehler (1977) has proposed that aging has four characteristics: it is universal, it is progressive, it is decremental, and it is intrinsic. Just as growth and development, although variable in their manifestations, are universal biologic phenomena, so must aging be if it is a

normal process. It is the component of universality that removes aging from the realm of pathologic processes and identifies it as a normal phenomenon. There is, however, growing evidence that some of the pathologic processes which become manifest may be due to specific individual vulnerabilities. That aging changes are decremental and progressive follows almost by definition. The evidence for the intrinsic origin of the structural and functional changes with age are developed in the course of this chapter.

Cellular Changes

There is a gradual loss of cells as the individual ages. This has been documented by changes in organ weights and total cell counts and by determinations of changes in the amount of potassium, DNA, intracellular water, and nitrogen in the aged compared to the young organism. The somatic cells of the body can be characterized as those capable of reproduction (known as mitotic cells) and those, primarily nerve and muscle cells, incapable of reproduction (known as post-mitotic cells). The post-mitotic cells, when lost, for whatever reason, are not replaced and their number decreases with age. Those cells that remain show age-related changes. The most characteristic change is the accumulation of a pigment within the storage granules of the cytoplasm. There is also electron microscopic evidence of changes in the other cellular organelles such as distortion in structure and reduction in number of mitochondria

53

and fragmentation of chromosomes. Recently, Hayflick (1965) has shown that contrary to the previous belief that mitotic cells are immortal, these cells have a finite capacity for reproduction and, thus, for replacement. Human embryonal cells in tissue culture are capable of approximately fifty divisions; the rate of replacement decreases as the cell line ages, and eventually the line dies. The number of residual generations is inversely related to the age of the individual supplying the cells. The same phenomenon is seen in all vertebrates studied, and the potential number of cell generations is directly correlated with the life span of the species.

The remaining cells, on histologic examination, tend to be larger and the structural pattern of the tissues is increasingly irregular. As a result, while the total number of cells may decrease 30 percent between youth and old age, the cellular mass decreases by a somewhat smaller amount. The decrease in metabolically active cells is paralleled by a decrease in intracellular water, although the extracellular water and plasma volume remain constant (Fig. 6-1). There is an increase in body fat with age which equals or exceeds the decrease in cell mass and may obscure this change in compositional distribution.

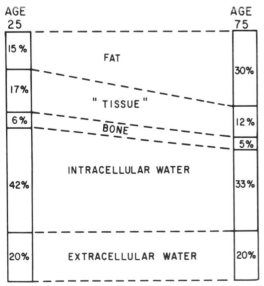

FIGURE 6-1. Distribution of major body components with age. (From Goldman, R.: J. Am. Geriat. Soc. 18: 765, 1970, with permission)

Extracellular Matrices

A fairly uniform series of age-related changes is found in the extracellular matrices of the connective tissue. Most important are changes occurring in collagen, which is a relatively inert long-chain macromolecule produced by the fibroblasts. There is little evidence that once formed, collagen fibers are either altered or reabsorbed. New fibers are produced which form bundles with the earlier fibers and cross-link chemically. The increased density of this widespread tissue component undoubtedly affects diffusion of nutrients and wastes and impairs function, as by reducing pulmonary compliance and vascular elasticity. It is this increase in collagen that affects the tenderness of an old laying hen as compared to a fryer, mutton as to lamb, and beef as to veal. Elastin, another component of the connective tissue matrix, becomes fragmented and calcified with age, also reducing tissue elasticity. The matrix of cartilage becomes brittle, more easily disrupted, and, as a result, contributes to the progressive increase in arthritis. Changes in bone are significant but cannot be so directly related to specific changes in the matrix. Bone changes are discussed in more detail later.

Extracellular Fluid and Solutes

Although the decrease in intracellular water reflects the changes in cell mass, there is no associated change in the extracellular water (see Fig. 6-1). In addition, there are few changes in the solute content of the extracellular fluid and these are so small as to be evident only on statistical analysis. There is a progressive decrease in the serum albumin and an increase in the globulin, with the total protein remaining relatively constant. The serum cholesterol increases slowly until about age 65; then it stabilizes or decreases slightly. The fasting blood glucose is unchanged, but the levels following a glucose challenge increase progressively and significantly with age. The other routine determinations show little age-related change.

PROBLEMS IN RESEARCH ON AGING

There are many problems inherent in research on aging which must be recognized in evaluating the data. Figure 6-2 shows the reduction in total body

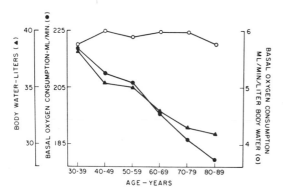

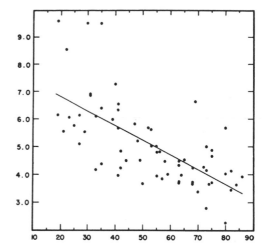

FIGURE 6-2. Relationship of age to total body water (antipyrine space), basal oxygen consumption, and basal oxygen consumption per unit of body water. Drawn from data presented by Shock et al., 1963. (From Gregerman, R. L.: In Gitman, L. (ed.): Endocrines and Aging. Springfield, Ill.: Charles C Thomas, 1967 with permission)

FIGURE 6-3. The relationship between resting cardiac output and age in 67 males without circulatory disorders. The line represents the linear regression on age. (From Brandfonbrener, M., Landowne, M., and Shock, N. W.: Circulation 12:557, 1955, with permission)

water and oxygen consumption at rest with age. When body water is equated to cell mass, there is no change in relative oxygen consumption, implying that there is no alteration in the function of the tissues that remain. It is necessary to examine further to determine if the metabolic process has been altered and, especially, if the functional reserve has been impaired.

Another problem is manifest in Figure 6-3, which shows the decrease in the resting cardiac output with age. It can be seen that some values in the eighth decade are higher than some in the fourth. However, before concluding that these individuals have undergone no change with age, it is necessary to perform longitudinal studies on the same individuals. Such studies as have been performed so far tend to validate the cross-sectional studies done previously. In this example it is probable that those individuals with a high cardiac output at age 75 had a proportionately high output at age 25.

When comparing subjects of different ages, the cross-sectional approach, there are two other potential sources of confusion. First, the various cohorts have had different environmental exposures and, second, the survivors represent a selected group. Without longitudinal studies it is not possible to determine if the change has been protective, or if the more severely affected individuals had a higher mortality, thus hiding an even greater average trend.

BODY SYSTEMS

Cardiovascular System

At least 40 percent of all individuals over the age of 65 years will die of cardiac disease, 15 percent of cerebrovascular disease, and possibly another 5 percent secondary to other types of vascular impairment. Since well over one half of all deaths are due to defects of the cardiovascular system, it is important to identify those changes that are age-related as opposed to those that are pathologic in origin. However, since, as will be seen later, the frequency of cardiovascular complications can be mathematically related to age, a number of gerontologists now question whether all cardiovascular "disease" that follows this pattern may not, in fact, be a manifestation of differential rates of aging. The cliche that we are as old as our blood vessels may be untrue in the implication that all aging changes stem from reduced blood supply but is certainly true in regard to the major causes of death.

Heart

SIZE. The concept that cardiac enlargement with age must indicate an underlying pathologic process has clouded the determination of actual aging change. It is now the concensus that there is myocardial hypertrophy with age per se. This amounts to an 8 to 15 percent increase in 24-month as compared to 12-month-old rats. In humans the left ventricular wall may be 25 percent thicker at age 80 than at age 30 years.

Areas of fibrosis are present and the overall collagen content is increased according to most, but not all, studies. In rates, there may be subendocardial and subepicardial concentrations of connective tissue, perhaps corresponding to subendocardial localization in humans. The heart valves become thicker and stiffer with age. Since myocardial cells are post-mitotic, replacement of lost fibers, as well as the increase in total muscle mass, is accomplished by hypertrophy of the residual bundles. In rats there is sclerosis of the coronary arteries, manifest by fibrosis of the media, thickening of the wall, and elastocalcinosis, but there is no narrowing of the lumina or atherosclerotic changes. In senile rats there is a reduction in the capillary to muscle fiber ratio and a decreased capillary density; however, this can be increased by exercise.

CELLS. The previously noted increase in volume of lipofuscin pigment may be appreciable, but its effect on cardiodynamics is unknown. On electron microscopic studies old hearts contained autophagic vacuoles, rarely seen in the mycardium of young animals, and some observers noted changes in the myofibers and the mitochondria.

RATE. *The resting heart rate* in man essentially is unchanged by age, and the question of resting stroke volume and cardiac output is clouded by whether or not cardiac catheterization is a "resting" state. However, there is no doubt that with a maximal load the cardiac rate and stroke volume are decreased and, therefore, the cardiac output is reduced. In both men and women this decrease amounts to about 40 percent between the third and eighth decades, or a little less than 1 percent per year. The time required for the heart rate to return to normal is prolonged.

A standardized measure of the limit of performance capacity is the maximal oxygen consumption (VO max). A number of studies now confirm that the maximal oxygen consumption declines with age at approximately the same rate as the cardiac output. The actual decline is to some extent influenced by obesity, reduced activity, and smoking. Oxygen uptake is identical in the young and old at equal work levels; thus the difference lies in *work capacity,* not efficiency of oxygen extraction.

OXYGEN UPTAKE. At maximal load the right and left ventricular end-diastolic pressures and the pulmonary wedge pressure are significantly higher in the aged. Since the central venous pressure is monitored routinely, it should be appreciated that these values may not necessarily reflect myocardial reserve in the recumbent position.

CARDIAC RESPONSE TO STRESS. Three factors are involved in the cardiac response to stress: an increase in the heart rate, an increase in myocardial contractibility, and the Frank-Starling mechanism (an increase in myofibrillar length with increased efficiency and increased ventricular volume). The *increase in the heart rate is impaired.* This may be due to increased connective tissue in the S-A and A-V nodes and in the bundle branches. Recent evidence indicates a decrease in the number of catecholamine receptors on the myofibers, which may have some relationship to the reduced rate response. Further, with age, the refractory interval between stimuli-causing mechanical response increases, although there is no increase in the electrical refractory interval.

A number of studies have suggested that with age both the isometric contraction and relaxation times are prolonged. Recent studies indicate that contraction depends upon the release of calcium from the sarcoplasmic reticulum to act upon the contractile proteins and relaxation requires that the calcium be removed from these proteins and taken up again by the sarcoplasmic reticulum. The release of calcium is slowed in age, not as a result of inadequate catecholamine concentration but to apparent lack of response, perhaps owing to the reduced number of receptors. The uptake of calcium during diastole is slowed by an age-related deficiency in the sarcoplasmic reticulum. Under these conditions a prolonged refractory period, and some limitation in cardiac rate, is understandable.

Studies of rat trabecula carnea, paced at 24 beats per minute in vitro in an isometric system, showed *no significant age-related difference in active tension or maximum rate of tension development.* Since there was no age difference in the active tension curves at all lengths up to that at which contraction tension was maximal, the Frank-Starling mechanism seems to be intact. There is evidence that there is less compliance, or relaxation of tension, with age. This stiffness may result from increased connective tissue or from changes in the myocardium itself; obviously it decreases myocardial efficiency.

CORONARY BLOOD FLOW. It is of considerable theoretic importance that studies of coronary flow in a group of rats showed that the maximal flow was decreased by an amount proportional to the degree of myocardial hypertrophy. Maximum oxygen extraction (86 percent) was identical in both young and old. Studies on oxidative phosphorylation are inconclusive. There is no evidence that the observed anatomic and physiologic changes can be attributed to a reduction in vascular perfusion.

ELECTROCARDIOGRAPHIC CHANGES. The normal electrocardiogram shows little change with age. There are small, inconspicuous but statistically significant, increases in the P-R, QRS, and Q-T intervals. There is also a decrease in the amplitude of the QRS complex, and, probably as a result of the noted left ventricular thickening, a left shift in the QRS axis. Since pathologic changes in the heart accumulate with age, comparable changes will be increasingly frequent in the electrocardiogram, but these should not be considered normal manifestations of aging.

Blood Vessels

Elastin gives the arteries their resiliency, a property that diminishes with aging, independent of atherosclerotic processes. The elastic fibers progressively straighten, fray, split, and fragment. These changes are associated with increasing deposition of calcium which has been termed elastocalcinosis. Both the media of the elastic arteries and the elastic lamina of the muscular arteries are involved in this process. At the same time, the increasing absolute amount of collagen in the vessels and the cross-linkage of collagen fibers into bundles of larger and larger size further compromises the vascular distensibility. In young arteries half the collagen is at maximum length with a 60 percent stretch, while in old arteries only a 30 percent stretch is possible. The increased volume of the aorta compensates in part for this lack of elasticity. However, the intra-aortic systolic pressure rises more abruptly as an increasing amount of blood is forced into the vessel.

PULSE-WAVE VELOCITY. The pulse-wave velocity reflects the decreasing elasticity of the blood vessels. The aortic pulse-wave velocity increases from 4.1 meters per second at age 5 years to 10.5 meters per second at age 65 years. The radial pulse-wave velocity is greater than the aortic pulse-wave velocity until age 65; thereafter the order is reversed. This change in velocity is independent of atherosclerosis, but Simonson and Nakagawa showed that pulse-wave velocity changes in patients with coronary artery disease were greater than were to be expected by age alone. This accelerated change could be due to the complicating effects of atherosclerosis or it could indicate that acceleration of the normal vascular changes predisposed to atherosclerosis. The aortic pulse pressure rises from the arch to the bifurcation in children but remains unchanged in old age. O'Rourke and his associates (1968) estimate that in youth 8 percent of the heart energy is lost in pulsatile work and that this increases to 17 percent in the aged because of the diminished elasticity.

The reduction in cardiac output with age results in reduced blood flow to the various organs, but this reduction is not symmetric. Flow to the brain and the coronary vessels is reduced proportionately less than is the total cardiac output, but flow to most other tissues (particularly the kidneys) is reduced more. The status of the splanchnic blood flow is uncertain, with values showing both a lesser and a greater than average reduction (Table 6-1).

The altered distribution of blood flow, as well as the increased peripheral resistance with age, could derive from either anatomic or physiologic causes. Anatomic changes which disproportionately reduce flow through a tissue would increase peripheral resistance. The usual mechanism, which regulates local blood flow and which controls peripheral resistance, is variation in arteriolar tone. Shock and his associates (1951) had shown that while the glomerular filtration rate and the renal plasma flow were linearly reduced with age, the latter decreased more rapidly than the former. Thus, the filtration fraction—the ratio of filtration rate to renal plasma flow—progressively increased with age. In their subsequent experiment they established baseline control values, then injected pyrogen to remove the effects of arteriolar spasm. The pyrogen produced no change in the glomerular filtration rate but caused a general increase in the renal plasma flow which was inversely proportional to age, and the filtration fraction became identical in all three groups (Figure 6-4). This reduction in the arteriolar resistance indicates that the prior resistance was functional, not anatomic, and that the vascular supply to the kidney remains proportional to renal mass.

More recent studies by Hollenberg and his associates (1974) support the opposite interpretation. In very extensive studies of normal kidney donors they were unable to reduce the difference in filtration fraction. Yet, surprisingly, their studies indicated

TABLE 6-1. Age changes in regional perfusion.

	Approximate Average Rate of Change (% per year)	
	Bender*	Landowne & Stanley†
Cardiac output	−0.75	−1.01
Cerebral flow	−0.35	−0.5
Coronary flow	−0.5	
Visceral flow (liver)	−1.1	−0.3 (−0.36)§
Renal flow	−1.1	−1.9
Remainder (by difference)		−1.3

* Bender, A. D.: J. Am. Geriat. Soc. 13:192, 1965.

† Landowne, M., and Stanley, J.: In Shock, N. W. (ed.): Aging—Some Social and Biological Aspects. Washington D.C., Am. Ass. Adv. Sci., 1960.

§ Flood, C., et al.: J. Clin. Invest. 46:960, 1967.

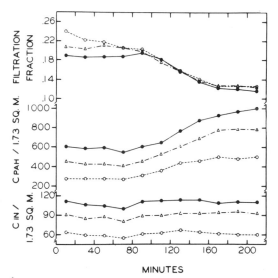

FIGURE 6-4. Changes in glomerular filtration rate (Cin), effective renal plasma flow (Cpah), and filtration fraction during the pyrogen reaction. Fifty-million killed-typhoid organisms were injected intravenously at 0 time. (From McDonald, R. K., Solomon, D. H., and Shock, N. W.: J. Clin. Invest. 30:457, 1951, with permission)

0—0, mean values for 14 subjects aged 70 to 85 years

<>—<>, mean values for 20 subjects aged 50 to 69 years

•—•, mean values for 20 subjects aged 20 to 49 years

that the aged were more sensitive to pressor substances, indicating that old arterioles are still capable of vascular control.

It is not unexpected that with increasing vascular rigidity the systolic blood pressure should increase with age. The diastolic pressure also increases with age, as it must if there is an increased peripheral resistance despite a reduced cardiac output. When a pressure pulse is applied to a rigid instead of an elastic tube in experimental systems the diastolic pressure falls proportionately and the mean pressure is unchanged.

Recent studies have revealed some very significant changes in the capillary walls. The capillary endothelial cells lie on a layer of collagen-like material, the basement membrane, which separates these cells from those of the tissues. The basement membrane gradually thickens from about 700 Angstroms in youth to 1100 Angstroms in old age. There are no direct physiologic data to correlate with this change, but it is not unreasonable to suspect that there is a resultant slowing in the exchange of nutrients and waste products across the capillary wall.

Excretory System

Kidney Structure

Each human kidney contains approximately one million nephrons at birth. These increase in size, but not in number, until maturity. A few nephrons normally are lost during maturation, but then the loss accelerates, so that between ages 25 and 85 years the number decreases by 30 to 40 percent. Recent micro-dissection studies show that the obsolescence starts as a sclerosis or scarring of the glomeruli, followed by atrophy of the afferent arterioles. These studies demonstrate that this process is not primary to the large vessels. In fact, the glomeruli in the deep cortex near the medulla (the juxtamedullary glomeruli) retain one capillary, which enlarges as the remainder of the glomerulus atrophies, and becomes a shunt between the afferent and efferent arterioles. These become the vasa rectal supplying the renal medullae. The atrophic nephrons are not replaced. Such compensation as occurs results from enlargement of the residual nephrons. Despite this, the net weight of the kidney decreases about 30 percent from maturity to old age.

Kidney Function

Since the number of functional units in the kidney is reduced with age, it is not unexpected that function also declines. Shock and his associates (1950) showed that the glomerular filtration rate de-

creased 46 percent from age 20 to age 90. At the same time the renal plasma flow (RPF) decreased 53 percent. The ratio between the filtration rate and the plasma flow, the filtration fraction (FF), increased as a result (see previous section). In Figures 6-5 and 6-6 Wesson has collected the results of a number of different studies, showing the decreases in the glomerular filtration rate and the renal plasma flow. Calculation of the filtration fraction from these data indicate that the increase may not occur until the sixth or seventh decades (Table 6-2). The data show that some quite old individuals may have better function than others considerably younger. In a recent longitudinal study of a large number of subjects, the individual trends paralleled those of the group; persons with extreme values had been at the extreme at earlier ages as well.

The fractional extraction of low concentrations of para-aminohippuric acid show no age-related decrease. The concentration of para-aminohippuric acid is determined simultaneously in the renal arterial and the renal venous blood and the fractional removal is calculated. The average ratios were 91.8

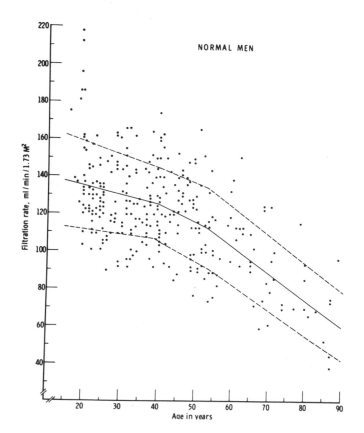

FIGURE 6-5. Age changes in glomerular filtration rate (Cin) of normal men (mean and one standard deviation). (From Wesson, L. G.: Physiology of the Human Kidney. New York: Grune & Stratton, 1969, pp. 98–99, by permission)

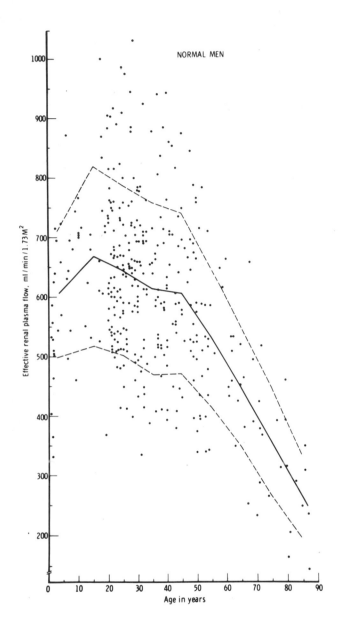

FIGURE 6-6. Age changes in effective renal plasma flow (PAH or diodrast) of normal men (mean and one standard deviation). (From Wesson, L. G.: Physiology of the Human Kidney. New York: Grune & Stratton, 1969, pp. 98–99, with permission)

percent and 91.1 percent in youth and old age, respectively. Thus, the ratio of the blood supply to the nephrons and to the parenchymal tissue remains constant despite the reduction in tissue supplied.

The reduced renal tubular cell mass is reflected by reduced maximal tubular functions. The reabsorption of glucose from the filtrate (Tm_G) is decreased 43.5 percent, and the maximum secretion of Diodrast (Tm_D) decreased 47.6 percent, and that of para-aminohippurate (Tm_{PAH}) by a similar amount, values which closely parallel the filtration rate. Thus, the

reduction reflects a reduced number, not a reduced function, of the individual cells. The ability to concentrate the urine declines moderately. The usual value for maximum specific gravity in youth is 1.032 which decreases to 1.024 at age 80. A similar decline in maximum osmolality is noted from 1040 mOs/L to 750 mOs/L between ages 20 and 80 years. Studies of urinary dilution reveal a decreasing C_{H_2O}, but when the C_{H_2O} is divided by the residual GFR, the value is constant, again reflecting a reduced cell mass. The administration of acid load produces a

Table 6-2. Average values for GFR, RPF, and filtration fraction (FF) by age and sex.*

Age	Women			Men		
	GFR	RPF	FF	GRF	RPF	FF
15	123	655	0.188	138	665	0.208
25	119	585	0.203	132	650	0.203
35	117	575	0.203	128	615	0.208
45	112	570	0.196	121	610	0.198
55	105	480	0.219	110	530	0.208
65	94	425	0.221	96	445	0.216
75	84	300	0.280	80	350	0.229
85				66	250	0.264

* The individual GFR and RPF values are derived from Figures 6-5 and 6-6 and are approximations. The filtration fractions are computed from these data.

comparable reduction in the serum bicarbonate and urinary pH at all ages. The rate at which the acid load is excreted is proportional to the residual GFR. There is a slight relative decrease in ammonia production with a proportionate increase in the titratable acidity. The response to base loads is also delayed and prolonged.

There is concern about the possible effects of the age-related reduction in renal function, especially in relation to drugs primarily dependent upon renal excretion. However, *50 percent residual function is quite adequate,* when it is realized that renal patients can be managed with functions as low as 5 and 10 percent of normal. It is important to realize that, because of the reduced muscle mass, less creatinine is produced and, as a result, the serum creatinine does not rise in proportion to the fall in renal function. Therefore when dosage is critical, *a creatinine clearance, not the serum creatinine alone, should be the criterion for renal function.*

Compensatory hypertrophy has become of considerable interest since the development of renal transplantation. Addis (1948) was the first to note that the capacity for such hypertrophy was inversely related to age. Many studies have been performed to determine the increase in function in humans and to determine the increase in renal mass in rats after nephrectomy. Some of the most elegant studies have been performed on kidney donors. There is a large increment kidney in size and function in three days which continues more slowly for three weeks, then there may be minor increases subsequently. In early maturity a residual kidney will demonstrate a 50 percent increase, in old age a maximum 30 percent increase. It is probable that early compensatory growth involves both cellular hyperplasia and hypertrophy, while the old kidney cells are capable only of hypertrophy. It is too soon to know if there is differential survival of young and old kidneys used in successful grafts, but the early data show a significantly greater success rate with the use of younger kidneys.

Respiratory System

IMMUNITY. There probably are several hundred viruses that can cause an upper respiratory infection; during childhood, immunities are built up against the common agents. The frequency of colds decreases from five or six per year to about two per year in early adulthood, and more slowly to one per year in old age. However, infections such as influenza, when they do occur, are associated with a rapidly increasing mortality with age.

STRUCTURE. The anteroposterior diameter of the chest increases with age. There is a progressive kyphosis, often complicated and exaggerated by osteoporosis and vertebral collapse, calcification of costal cartilages, reduced mobility of ribs, and partial contraction of inspiratory muscles. These factors combine to reduce the compliance of the chest wall and the force of the expiratory muscles. There is a gradual decrease in the number of alveoli because of progressive loss of interalveolar septi. The residual alveoli are larger, and there is dilatation of the bronchioles and alveolar ducts.

The aging lung becomes increasingly rigid and less likely to collapse when the chest cavity is opened. Yet a number of reports indicate that the elastin content increases with age and the total amount of collagen is unchanged. The loss of collagen in alveolar septa may be balanced by increased collagen in the residual vasculature, and this collagen would show increased cross-linkage and other age-related changes. However, despite the rigidity and failure to collapse, it may be for these reasons that the compliance of the aging lung probably decreases very little compared to the chest wall.

FUNCTION. The elevation of the ribs and flattening of the diaphragm results in a 50 percent increase in the functional residual capacity between the third and the ninth decades, and the residual volume increases 100 percent. As a result there is a partial inflation of the lungs at rest when compared to younger ages. Nevertheless, there is *no significant change in total lung capacity.* The dead space ventilation increases and approximately balances the decrease in oxygen requirement. As a result the resting tidal volume remains constant (Fig. 6-7). These changes are not sufficient to produce subjective or objective manifestations at rest, or to predict the ability to cope with stress.

There is a nearly linear decrease in the maximal breathing capacity (MBC) between the third and ninth decades. This test is difficult to perform and is affected by poor motivation. The forced expiratory volume correlates well and is a satisfactory substitute. Both tests depend on the ability to move air out of the lungs and on such factors as airway resistance, the compliance of the lung itself, and the characteristics of the thoracic cage, including rigidity, loss of muscular strength, and velocity of contraction. A simple but useful test is the ability to blow out a bookmatch at 6 inches with the mouth wide open. Failure indicates advanced functional impairment requiring further evaluation (Fig. 6-8).

Blood Gases

There is no change in the arterial pressure of carbon dioxide (PA_{CO_2}) between the ages of 20 and 80, but there is a 10 to 15 percent decrease in the pressure of oxygen. The oxygen saturation decreases about 5 percent. In the past, the decrease in arterial

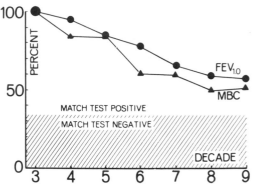

FIGURE 6-8. Percentage change in maximal breathing capacity (MBC) and forced expiratory volume (FEV) with age in normal subjects. (From Mithoefer, J. C., and Karetzky, M. S.: In Powers, J. D. (ed.): Surgery of the Aged and Debilitated Patient. Philadelphia: W. B. Saunders Co., 1968, with permission)

oxygen pressure has been attributed to a fall in pulmonary diffusing capacity. This would be compatible with the observed thickening of the basement membranes. Recently it has been proposed that if there were ventilation perfusion mismatching, unventilated capillaries would not be exposed to oxygen. The higher diffusibility of carbon dioxide would maintain its pressure constancy. In the low-pressure pulmonary system, gravity might cause dependent, basilar localization of blood flow. The basal portion of the lung is the best ventilated in the young and there is correspondence between ventilation and perfusion. Later, the increasing lung rigidity improves apical ventilation, there is relative basal alveolar collapse, and ventilation perfusion mismatching results. The constancy of the partial pressure of carbon dioxide suggests that alveolar ventilation is adequate. The extent to which the decreased arterial oxygen pressure is due to reduced diffusing capacity, to ventilation-perfusion mismatching, and to increased dead space will undoubtedly be resolved.

O_2 UTILIZATION. The maximal amount of oxygen utilized under stress is reduced 50 percent by age 80. Alveolar ventilation is adequate, since the partial pressure of carbon dioxide does not increase. However, the arteriovenous oxygen difference does not increase to the expected degree. Since this indicates underutilization of oxygen already in the circulation, it cannot be due to failure at the pulmonary level. Possible causes include failure of perfusion, delayed oxygen diffusion, or impaired oxygen utilization of the stressed tissues.

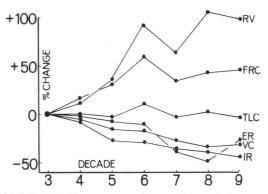

FIGURE 6-7. Percentage changes in static lung volumes in normal subjects at various ages compared to values found in the third decade of life. RV—Residual volume; FRC—Functional residual capacity; TLC—Total lung capacity; ER—expiratory reserve; VC—vital capacity; IR—inspiratory reserve. (From Mithoefer, J. C., and Karetzky, M. S. In: Powers, J. D. (ed.): Surgery of the Aged and Debilitated Patient. Philadelphia: W. B. Saunders Co., 1968, with permission)

Emphysema has much in common with the aging lung. The maximum breathing capacity and forced expiratory volume are decreased in both, the residual volume and the functional residual capacity are increased, the lungs are rigid and distended on autopsy, and the microscopic changes may be similar. However, the normal aged individual does not have the elevations in blood carbon dioxide and bicarbonate which are found in emphysema as a result of the functional obstructive characteristics.

Clinical Implications

The increased rigidity of the thoracic wall and the decreased strength of the expiratory muscles *decreases the propulsive effectiveness of the cough,* an extremely important clinical consideration. The *reduced cough efficiency, decreased ciliary activity in the bronchial lining, and the increased dead space all enhance the potential for mechanical and infectious respiratory complications of surgery and enforced bedrest in the aged individual.* Because of their potential severity, it is necessary to anticipate and prevent these complications whenever their potentiality exists.

Gastrointestinal System

STRUCTURE. Despite a wide variety of functional change described or implied, description of anatomic change in the gastrointestinal tract is limited. In view of altered motility, studies of myenteric nervous plexuses are lacking, and there is little reported on mucosal change. In the esophagus the embryonic columnar epithelium is replaced by squamous epithelium. In the aged, a return of columnar epithelium in the lower esophagus becomes increasingly common. Whether this represents an abnormal change or just aging has not been established. Similarly, *the increased frequency of hiatal hernia may be a manifestation of age change.*

Atrophic gastritis, intestinal metaplasia of the gastric mucosa, and gastric polyposis become more common. Although it is believed there is atrophy of the small intestine, there is no objective documentation. Small bowel x-ray studies are reported to show a coarser outline. The number of Peyer's patches, and the number of follicles within them, decreases. In the mouse the half time for the turnover of intestinal cells increases with age.

In the vermiform appendix there is fibrous atrophy of what was originally a large amount of lymphoid tissue, and the lumen becomes progressively obliterated from tip to base. *Diverticulosis of the sigmoid colon becomes common, and is present in at least one third of all individuals over age sixty.* Surprisingly, the aging colon shows thickening of the muscularis, rather than thinning. It is possible that segmental areas undergo periods of spasm, with resultant increases in the intraluminal pressure which then causes the mucosal blow-out. Autopsy studies of excised colons into which water is injected under pressure have shown that diverticuli can be produced by this mechanism in old, but not young, individuals.

MOTILITY. Studies of esophageal motility in nonagenarians showed that esophageal persistalsis followed only 50 percent of swallows, compared to 90 percent in young individuals. These investigations showed defects in deglutition and relaxation of the lower esophageal sphincter, delay of esophageal emptying, dilation of the esophagus, and an increase in nonpropulsive contractions. Such observations suggest that the older patient may have difficulty emptying the esophagus in the supine position and that this might not only affect nutrition but also contribute to the increase in aspiration as well.

Few reports of age-related changes in gastric and small intestinal motility were found, and studies in large bowel motility appear to be limited, despite the general assumption that constipation in the aged is due to decreased colonic peristalsis and possibly to decreased abdominal muscle tone.

Fecal incontinence increases in frequency with age and may occur in 20 percent of hospitalized geriatric patients. Brocklehurst (1951) found that a third of these patients had organic neurologic changes and another third were confused without neurologic signs. Rectal awareness of balloon distention was diminished in many of the incontinent patients, despite the increased frequency of evacuation. The sphincter appeared to have decreased tone by digital examination and the stool was frequently semiliquid.

Manometric examinations of the reflex responses of the internal and external sphincters have been performed. The internal sphincter is strongly contracted in the normal state and the external sphincter much less so. The older, incontinent persons had normal internal sphincter reflexes, but the external sphincter reflexes were absent and were thought to be the major factor in incontinence. Normally, the two sphincters function with a close complementarity which, for example, will allow for the passage of gas without the loss of stool. This competence obviously fails when incontinence appears.

SECRETION. *Saliva*. The volume of saliva, both stimulated and unstimulated, is greatly reduced and averages only a third of that produced in youth, contributing to the dry tongue of old age, and possibly to reduced taste sensation. Meyer and Necheles (1940) confirmed earlier work indicating that by age 50 there is a marked decrease in salivary ptyalin and with it failure of starch digestion, particularly to dextrin, the first step.

Gastric Acid. The secretion of both free and total gastric acid decreases with age. Since this is most marked in association with atrophic gastritis, and the incidence of atrophic gastritis rises with age, this type of gastritis could be either an aging or a pathologic process. Gastric atrophy also results in a decrease in the production of intrinsic factor; however, this is rarely sufficiently complete to cause pernicious anemia. The gastric secretion drops markedly between ages 40 and 60 years to about one fifth of earlier values; then it becomes stable.

Pancreatic Enzymes. Pancreatic amylase in fasting duodenal juice is decreased, but normal amounts are available after stimulation. Since older individuals often rely upon high carbohydrate diets, it is important to note that the pancreatic amylase, even in the absence of salivary amylase, seems adequate for carbohydrate digestion. The amount of pancreatic trypsin is also reduced but the lipase appears to be relatively stable. Thus, the older individual should, in most instances, be capable of digesting a normal dietary intake. However, the reported studies are by no means consistent, and further studies are necessary. Also, there is little clinical evidence that the stool contains significant amounts of undigested nutrients, although further studies are warranted.

ABSORPTION. Absorption is the most critical function of the gastrointestinal tract. A number of established and possible age-related factors could influence this function, such as the rate and degree of digestion, the integrity of the absorbing surface, the efficiency of the transport mechanisms, gastrointestinal motility, and alterations in vascular perfusion.

There is little information on *protein* absorption, although selective defects in amino acid absorption have been suggested. Glucose is absorbed by an active transport mechanism. *Glucose* absorption studies have been difficult to interpret because of changing glucose-insulin relationships. Determina-

tions of the rate of decrease of residual glucose in the rat intestine indicates a slower rate of absorption. This is supported by an apparent delay in the absorption of 3-methyl glucose and galactose. Xylose, which is absorbed by passive transport, also exhibits impaired absorption, although possibly not until very late in life. Two studies which showed that fat absorption was delayed, also showed that absorption could be accelerated by adding lipase to the fat meal, thus suggesting that the decreased rate is due to deficient lipase secretion. Persistently elevated chylomicron counts may be due to inactivity rather than age. Radioactive fat tolerance tests suggest that variations in blood lipid levels were most likely the result of impairment in metabolism or distribution of fat rather than of altered absorption. The question still seems moot.

Calcium absorption is in the proximal small intestine and may correlate with the secretion of gastric acid. There is agreement that *calcium absorption becomes impaired as a result of decreased active transport*. Iron is also absorbed in the proximal portion of the small intestine and also depends on gastric acid secretion. One animal study showed a decreased uptake of radioactive iron which was independent of iron need. Vitamin A tolerance curves are unchanged, although the peak blood level may be later, suggesting delayed absorption. It is probable that vitamins B_1 and B_{12} are less well-absorbed in old age, but there is no evidence that absorption is inadequate except in overt cases of pernicious anemia.

Liver

Calloway (1965) documented the known decrease in liver size by examining 400 livers obtained at autopsy. The peak average weight of 1929 gm in the fourth decade declined to 1000 gm in the tenth, with the most marked decline after the sixth decade. It remained constant at 2.5 percent of total body weight until the seventh decade and then dropped to 1.6 percent by the tenth. Cellular changes are so characteristic that in 46 of 50 attempts it was possible to identify young and old livers.

Studies on the effect of age upon rat liver regeneration showed maximal regeneration in the young animals. There was little difference in the response of mature and old rats at 15 days after partial liver extirpation.

The status of splanchnic, and thus of hepatic, blood flow is not clear. The data are about evenly divided so that, although the blood flow decreases with age, the fractional decrease may be greater than or less than the average decline in relation to the decrease in the total cardiac output. This important problem still requires critical evaluation. The clearance of bilirubin is not affected by age and there are *no significant differences* in the total serum bilirubin, SGOT, SGPT, and alkaline phosphatase values in young and old persons. Although there is an insignificant decrease in the total serum protein from 7.40 to 7.04 gm/100 ml, there was a significant difference in the A/G ratio, which was 4.04/3.06 gm/100 ml in the young subjects (average age 23) and 3.26/3.76 gm/100 ml in the old subjects (average age 79). The reduced serum albumin may represent failure of the liver to maintain youthful levels. The rise in globulin may represent accumulated immune experience.

The most critical studies of liver function have been those using the sulfobromophthalein (BSP) technique. Three components of the BSP clearance must be evaluated: storage by the liver cells and possibly by the RE cells, splanchnic blood flow, and a secretory transport maximum (Tm) comparable to the Tm observed in renal functions. Splanchnic blood flow determinations, like renal blood flow, must be made at load levels below the Tm, and require a constant infusion technique. There seems to be a concensus that there is a linearly decreased storage capacity with age, but that the secretory Tm is unchanged. The usual clinical BSP test utilizes a single injection, with determination of BSP blood levels at 30 minutes. Under these circumstances the reduction in the amount of BSP stored in cells with progressive age results in a higher blood level, which falsely suggests that the hepatic excretory function has diminished.

Gallbladder

Biliary stones are estimated to be present in 10 percent of men and 20 percent of women between the ages of 55 and 65 years, and to approach a frequency of 40 percent by the eighth decade. The mechanism of formation is probably the same as at all ages, but obviously the normal mechanisms of cholesterol stabilization and absorption become progressively less efficient.

Pancreas

The weight of the adult human pancreas averages 95 gm. Although several reports indicate that there is a significant loss with age, Calloway (1965) found no significant decrease whether expressed as absolute weight or as a percentage of total body weight. However, it has been reported that the fat content of the pancreas increases, which may mask loss of functional tissue. Microscopic and electron microscopic studies have shown metaplasia and proliferation of ductile cells, irregularities of size, arrangement and staining of parenchymal cells, and alterations in subcellular organelles. As noted in the sections on secretion, studies generally tend to indicate a decreased volume and concentration of enzymes, but sufficient for normal digestive functions. If the work of Rosenberg and associates (1966) reporting that there is no decrease in bicarbonate secretion is confirmed, there may be interesting implications. Since there is a decreased gastric acid secretion with age, the persistent pancreatic bicarbonate secretion may be the mechanism which reduces peptic ulceration with age.

Endocrine System

It is not possible to summarize the voluminous material on the relationship of aging and the hormones. The recent identification of the hypothalamic-releasing hormones adds a new dimension as yet barely touched. The following discussion focuses on those changes that are relatively well examined and which clearly have applicable clinical implications.

Pituitary Gland

The weight of the pituitary gland may decrease 20 percent in extreme old age, but the significance cannot be determined because the patients examined also had prolonged terminal illnesses. However, there is a marked decrease in the number of mitoses, decreased vascularity, increased connective tissue, a change in the proportion of cell types, and definite disorganization of the cellular organelles. The concentrations of adrenocorticotropic hormone (ACTH), thyroid stimulating hormone (TSH), growth hormone (GH), and luteinizing hormone (LH) seem unaltered. Follicle-stimulating hormone (FSH) increases in postmenopausal women but remains normal in men.

GH. Obesity is associated with reduced serum GH levels, and it is not entirely clear if the moderately decreased levels with age are real or the indirect effects of relative obesity. The GH surges during sleep tend to disappear. One study indicated that the GH response (increased blood levels) to insulin hypoglycemia was decreased, but two other studies showed normal response. The small decrease in the response to arginine appeared to be correlated with body fat content rather than to age. In general, the responses to GH were unchanged except for a failure to increase hydroxyprolinuria, to inhibit glucose consumption by red blood cells in vitro, and to increase urinary calcium.

TSH. Plasma TSH does not decrease with age, but several studies indicate that there is reduced TSH release on stimulation by thyrotropin-releasing hormone (TRH). This probably is due to impairment of the TSH release mechanism, since the pituitary content of TSH is normal.

ACTH. The plasma levels of ACTH and the diurnal cycle, with a morning peak, are the same in youth and old age. When the ACTH stress response is determined by the increase in plasma cortisol, several studies have noted that there is a clear but moderate decrease with age. However, there is disagreement not only on this point but also on whether the adrenocortisol response to ACTH is impaired with age. As yet no data are available using direct measurements of serum ACTH relating to stress and age. Metapyrone tests, which impair cortisol production and cause a positive feedback augmentation of ACTH production, and several tests that cause a negative feedback and a decreased ACTH production show this mechanism to be essentially intact with age.

FSH and LH. The amount of FSH in the postmenopausal pituitary is clearly elevated, but the status of LH is less clear. The blood level of FSH increases fifteenfold and that of LH threefold. In the postmenopausal state estrogens appear to have an impaired negative-feedback effect, and the elevated gonadotropins are not suppressed completely except with unphysiologically high doses. The gonadotropins increase much more slowly and less significantly in males. Apparently the feedback mechanism remains more intact in men than in women.

ADH. Although studies in rats show a decrease in antidiuretic hormone (ADH) with age, there is no such evidence for humans. There does seem to be an increased frequency of the syndrome of inappropriate secretion of ADH, particularly in diabetics treated with chlorpropamide.

Thyroid Gland

The thyroid gland probably does not change weight with age, although the frequency of clinical nodularity is increased. Microscopically there is fibrosis, cellular infiltration, and micro- as well as macronodularity.

The plasma T4, both protein-bound and free, is unaffected by age, but the plasma T3 decreases 25 to 40 percent after the sixth decade. Thyroxine-binding globulin rises slightly and thyroxine-binding prealbumin falls. As noted, TSH levels are unchanged.

The rate of radioiodine accumulation in the thyroid gland decreases with age at the 6-hour determination, but the differences at 24 hours are less clear. It is now believed that the reduced renal function of older persons results in longer retention of radioiodine, with a greater opportunity for late accumulation in the thyroid gland. Prolonged exposure thus compensates for a slower rate of uptake.

The normal plasma T4 concentration and the reduced radioiodine uptake by the gland suggests that the rates of destruction and replacement of thyroid hormone are slowed proportionately. Gregerman and his associates (1962) showed that the hormone degradation decreased 50 percent in the six decades between 20 and 80 years. The turnover rate averaged approximately 88 ng/day at age 20 and decreased to 42 ng/day at age 80. The reduced rate of T4 disposal probably is due to slowed hepatic metabolism, although reduced physical activity may also be a factor.

The thyroid response both to stress and to exogenous TSH is comparable at all ages. This ability of the aged thyroid to respond normally to stress implies that the age-related decrease in normal thyroxine turnover results from reduced peripheral need rather than from failure of thyroid response. The normal blood levels of both T4 and TSH indicate a physiologic balance and are evidence against either thyroid or pituitary insufficiency. However, the fall in the plasma T3 presents a theoretical problem. If T3 is the effective hormone, the failure of TSH to respond to the age-related decline is inconsistent. Yet the correlation of decreased oxygen consumption with decreased cell mass, and the absence of clinical manifestations makes the concept of senile hypothyroidism as a routine phenomenon difficult to accept.

Parathyroids

Past difficulties with parathyroid hormone (PTH) assay have resulted in conflicting interpretations of bone and renal stone disease. One recent report suggests that PTH decreases with age except in cases of osteoporosis, where it is increased. Estrogen is believed to protect against the demineralizing effects of PTH, and the postmenopausal decrease in estrogens may heighten the physiologic sensitivity to PTH.

Pancreas

Insulin. Studies by Andres and his associates (1967) indicate that there is constant decrease in the glucose tolerance with age. The average 2-hour serum glucose value is 30 mg percent higher at 75 years than the values derived from young adults. By such standards, more than half of these individuals must be considered diabetic. This phenomenon seems to be independent of age-related obesity, despite the fact that fat impairs the hypoglycemic effect of insulin. He suggests that arbitrarily, and until better information is available, an age-determined rating be established and that the top 7 percentile at each age be considered diabetic and the next 7 percentile potentially diabetic (Fig. 6-9).

The impairment in these tests may be the result of either a reduced insulin release from the pancreas or a reduced peripheral sensitivity to circulating insulin. Earlier studies suggested that the defect was a failure of peripheral utilization. Evidence has accumulated more recently indicating that there may

be a delay in insulin release by the beta cells and that, because higher blood glucose levels result, there eventually may be higher blood levels of insulin as well.

It is of interest that while the usual insulin assay at basal conditions shows similar total insulin levels, recent studies demonstrate that the less active proinsulin is a larger fraction of the whole in the older individual. The implications of this observation need further study.

Glucagon. Glucagon, which causes a rise in blood glucose, could have an effect on the glucose tolerance. One study on the effect of glucagon administration showed a delayed and reduced response with age. Another showed no difference in fasting levels or in response to intravenous arginine stimulation.

Adrenal Glands

The human adrenal gland shows no major gross changes with age, but microscopic alterations include cortical nodule formation, increased connective tissue and pigment, reduced lipid, and changes in intracellular organelles. There may be vascular dilatation and hemorrhages.

Glucocorticoids. The plasma level of cortisol and the normal diurnal cycle, high in the morning and low at night, persist at all ages. However, a variety of diseases will abolish the diurnal rhythm and, since multiple diseases are common with age, abnormal cycles may be more frequent. The secretion rate of cortisol is reduced 25 percent in old men and there is a comparable decrease in the urinary excretion rate.

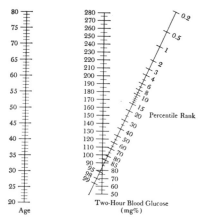

FIGURE 6-9. This nomogram enables the clinician to rank a response to the oral glucose tolerance test against the response of other individuals of the same age. (From Andres, R.: Hosp. Pract. 2:63, 1967, with permission)

The disposal rate of cortisol in elderly subjects was prolonged 40 percent, which is compatible with the constant blood level and reduced excretion. The combination of normal blood levels, reduced production rate, delayed degradation, and normal ACTH levels is comparable to the change in T4.

Several experiments have been performed to test the ability of the aging adrenal to respond to stress. The results have been variable, about equally divided between a normal and a reduced response. It has been suggested that given the normal level of plasma ACTH and the reduced output of cortisol, there must be some adaptation that might be a reduced adrenal responsivity.

Aldosterone. Both the blood levels and the urinary excretion of aldosterone decrease about 50 percent between youth and old age. The metabolic clearance rate drops 20 percent and the splanchnic extraction decreases from 96.3 percent to 89.7 percent. The increase in urinary excretion following sodium depletion is only 30 to 40 percent of the amount in young adults, and the secretion of renin shows a parallel age-related decrease. In a third of the women over the age of 70 the plasma urine levels are low and there is no response to sodium deprivation, postural change, or exercise.

Adrenal Androgens. The adrenal androgens make up the largest component of adrenal steroid hormone production, but their function is not known. The urinary excretion of 17-ketosteroids falls progressively to about one-half youthful values. The adrenal androgens, primarily dihydroepiandrosterone, decrease more rapidly than the total ketosteroids in both blood and urine. It is possible that this decrease is due to a reduced rate of production rather than to altered removal.

Epinephrine and Norepinephrine. Despite the differences in autonomic activity of young and old individuals, there is only one study of age-related changes in the urinary excretion of epinephrine and norepinephrine. In this study there was no age difference. There must be a large body of unpublished clinical data obtained in the routine survey of patients with potential pheochromocytoma.

In one study, the excretion of epinephrine and norepinephrine was determined in the urine following the injection of insulin which produced hypoglycemia as a stimulating mechanism. The norepinephrine excretion averaged 2.3 ng/minute in the old and 1.4 ng/minute in the young, but there was no significant change on stimulation. There was a marked increase in epinephrine excretion in the young group which peaked at 90 minutes. In the older group the response was much less marked but was still increasing at 180 minutes. These results should be qualified in view of the delayed responsiveness to insulin by older persons.

Gonads

Estrogens. Following ovarian atrophy after the menopause, there is no ovarian estrogen produced and the remaining estrogens are adrenal in origin. Despite a fall in the metabolic clearance rate, the plasma estradiol level drops to between 5 and 10 percent of prior levels, and the estrone to 25 percent, indicating an even lower rate of production. In males, estrogens are produced by the adrenal cortex and there is little age-related change.

Progestins. Progesterone is produced primarily by the ovary and placenta and to a lesser extent by the testis and adrenal cortex. The production and excretion decrease abruptly after the reproductive period. The production rate decreases about 60 percent between youth and old age. Pincus (1955) proposed that because progesterone is a precursor of cortisol, adrenal production is sustained.

Testosterone. Blood levels of testosterone probably decrease, but the reports are not unanimous. However, there is agreement that the metabolic clearance rate and the production rate have declined. The capacity of testosterone-binding globulin increases with age, further lowering the free testosterone. Figure 6-10 summarizes the changes in plasma hormones during aging in humans.

The Blood

Remarkably little change with age has been reported for blood and its components. Until at least age 80 there is no decrease in the blood volume, despite the decrease in active cell mass of the body. There are only very subtle changes in the red blood cells. Although anemia is frequent, it is always secondary. Red cell survival time is normal. A delay in replacement after bleeding is noted, but this may be due to iron depletion. Both the serum iron and iron-binding capacity are decreased moderately, and iron absorption is decreased. Unless iron deficiency can be ruled out, a primary failure of erythropoiesis cannot be established.

The number and distribution of the leukocytes are unchanged. The polymorphonuclear cells tend to be hypersegmented and there are fewer granules

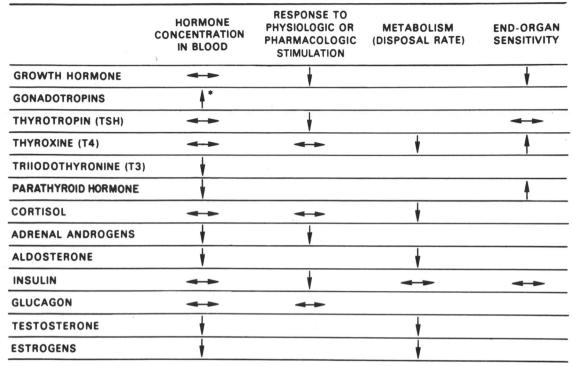

	HORMONE CONCENTRATION IN BLOOD	RESPONSE TO PHYSIOLOGIC OR PHARMACOLOGIC STIMULATION	METABOLISM (DISPOSAL RATE)	END-ORGAN SENSITIVITY
GROWTH HORMONE	↔	↓		↓
GONADOTROPINS	↑*			
THYROTROPIN (TSH)	↔	↓		↔
THYROXINE (T4)	↔	↔	↓	↑
TRIIODOTHYRONINE (T3)	↓			
PARATHYROID HORMONE	↓			↑
CORTISOL	↔	↔	↓	
ADRENAL ANDROGENS	↓	↓		
ALDOSTERONE	↓		↓	
INSULIN	↔	↓	↔	↔
GLUCAGON	↔	↔		
TESTOSTERONE	↓		↓	
ESTROGENS	↓		↓	

FIGURE 6-10. Changes of plasma hormones during aging in man. Symbols: ↑, increase; ↓, decrease; ↔, no change; *, postmenopausal. Blank spaces indicate that no data are presently available. (From Gregerman, R. I., and Bierman, E. L. In Williams, R. H., (ed.): Textbook of Endocrinology, ed. 5. Philadelphia: W. B. Saunders Co., 1974, p. 1069, with permission)

present. The leukocytosis of inflammation may be reduced. No reports of change in chemotactic response or of phagocytic capability were noted. There appears to be no significant change in the number of T or B lymphocytes, but there is a clear-cut reduction in immunosurveillance with age. The mechanism for this decrease is not known, and the experimental data are conflicting. Immunoglobulin production following antigenic challenge is reduced markedly. There is a progressive increase in total circulating gamma globulin owing to increases in IgG and IgA, since the IgM is decreased.

No change in platelet structure, number, or function has been observed except for a possible increase in adhesiveness. The few available studies of hemostasis and coagulation are conflicting and most aged individuals probably fall within the normal range for younger individuals. Fibrinogen does seem to be increased, but the evidence for hypercoagulability is not conclusive. There is, at the same time, no evidence of inadequate clotting factors.

The erythrocyte sedimentation rate can be markedly accelerated even in the absence of any evidence of disease. Values up to 40 mm per hour (Westergen) are not unusual (normal under 5 mm for men and 15 mm for women). This may be due to the age changes in plasma proteins, particularly the increase in fibrinogen.

Musculoskeletal System

Muscles

Muscles are composed of postmitotic cells and are dependent upon intact motor neuron innervation for survival. A progressive loss of muscle strength is a characteristic of aging. Careful studies reveal that there is a significant linear decrease in the number of muscle cells with age and that this decrease actually exceeds the loss of essential neural components. The loss exceeds the relative loss of total body mass as well. Some of this change is masked by an extracellular increase in interstitial fluid, fat, and collagen. Ultrastructural changes are extensive and complex. Lipofucin deposition is marked. The density of capillaries per motor unit is decreased.

Although oxygen utilization per unit of tissue is essentially unchanged, there is a significant reduction in the activity of half of the enzyme systems so far studied. There is a prolongation of contraction time, latency period, and relaxation period by about 13 percent and a decrease in the maximal rate of tension development. These correlate with the decrease in myosin ATPase activity. The decrease in motor function is compounded by poor motivation, deconditioning, malnutrition, endocrine change, and normal involution and, thus, may be difficult to interpret. Reconditioning will improve muscle function and efficiency at all ages, but the increment clearly decreases with age.

Joints

Joints are surfaced with cartilage, a poorly functional tissue that shows major deterioration as early as the third decade. These changes are probably the result of cumulated trauma and result in fraying and chipping. As the cartilage is eroded, the bone makes direct contact with bone and results in one form of degenerative arthritis with pain, crepitation, and limitation of movement. There is also loss of water from the cartilage which results in narrowing of the joint spaces, particularly of the intervertebral disks, and contributes to the loss of height.

In another form of degenerative joint disease, there is an irregular bony overgrowth at the edges of joints, presumably at sites of trauma. When this occurs on the fingers, usually of women, it may be only unsightly. When it occurs about the hip, the femoral head may become trapped, painful, and immobile. This is the most common cause for hip replacement. When it occurs on the vertebrae it may impinge on spinal nerves as they penetrate the intervertebral foraminae, causing severe pain (sciatica is a common example) and often a corresponding muscle weakness. Effective therapy for this common problem has not yet been developed.

Bone

Bone is a complex tissue that undergoes change throughout life. Starting before the age of 40 years in both sexes, there is a shift from an increase in bone mass to a progressive decrease. This is characterized by gradual reabsorption of the interior surface of long and flat bones and a slower accretion of new bone on the outside surface. Thus the long bones are externally enlarged but internally hollowed-out, the vertebral endplates are thinned, and the skull becomes slightly enlarged. At the same time there is a loss of the trabeculae. The end result is weaker bone that is subject to fracture.

Roentgen examination then shows the characteristic features of reduced bone mass, or osteoporosis, which is characterized microscopically by a loss of both bone salts and the supporting protein matrix. Modern experimental methods have established that aging bone loss is a universal phenomenon. Bone loss in the woman is approximately 25 percent and in men is 12 percent. Since in women this represents 750 gm loss from an original 3000 gm in the skeleton while in men it is only 450 gm from 4000 gm, it is obvious why osteoporosis is more apparent in women.

Osteoporosis may result from immobilization, failure to absorb calcium, excessive calcium loss from the bowel or the kidney, or a number of endocrine disorders that affect the protein matrix. None of these is demonstrably the cause of aging osteoporosis. Ovariectomy may accelerate and estrogen supplement may delay the process, but only for relatively short periods of time. There is little relationship to calcium intake. Changes in calcium balance are hard to detect, and balance is achieved on the normal intake of 8 to 12 mg/kg body weight per day.

Thinning of bone predisposes to fracture, particularly of the hip, vertebral body, shoulder, and wrist, and particularly in women. The most serious is fracture of the hip, which leads to immobilization and increased mortality. The cumulative risk of hip fracture at age 90 approaches 25 percent in women and 10 percent in men. Vertebral fractures with collapse cause back pain which usually resolves in several months. Shoulder and wrist fractures result from falls on the out-thrust arm; they are inconvenient but usually heal well.

All types of therapy have been attempted with little convincing effect. It seems probable to me that if there is progressive bone loss with age, the most marked osteoporosis would be seen in those with the least bone mass at the start. Thus, what is seen is the lower end of a distribution curve that is shifting to a reduced density. It would not be surprising, then, that therapy is ineffective.

There is considerable loss of height with age which is difficult to evaluate without longitudinal data. If the span of the outstreched arms, which does not change with age, is used to estimate mature height, it has been estimated that the average loss is 1.5 inches between ages 65 to 74, increasing to 3 inches by ages 85 to 94. This loss is due to multiple factors, decrease in intervertebral disk height, vertebral osteoporosis and collapse, kyphosis resulting from both these factors, and a characteristic knee flexion. Thus, the musculoskeletal system contributes greatly to the appearance of age.

Nervous System

The complexity of structure and function of the nervous system has made it difficult to develop a comprehensive view of the aging process in that organ. Only a few components are presented here. These include some that have significant implications or that may provide important or interesting leads.

Anatomic Changes

Nerve cells are postmitotic and, when lost from any cause, are not replaced. Studies of brain weight have shown a small but consistent loss of 6 to 7 percent from maximum at maturity to advanced old age. Most studies have been cross-sectional. Brain weight is affected by body size, and body size has increased for several generations. The significance of brain weight decrement has been challenged on these grounds, since the older brains must have come from smaller individuals.

However, painstaking studies by a number of workers has established that there is a significant loss of cells, which may be 45 percent in some cortical areas. In some senescent mice the loss is as much as two thirds. Cerebellar cell loss may be 25 percent. In much of the brainstem, cell loss seems to be relatively trivial. Cell loss is not always at the same rate, and certain areas may show acceleration at particular time. Thus, Brody (1970) found major losses from the superior frontal gyrus during the fifth decade. Even when cells are not lost, they may undergo changes that compromise function. The Scheibels (1977) studied the pyramidal cells in the third layer of the cerebral cortex. These cells showed a marked and progressive decrease in the number of interconnections between dendrites (Fig. 6-11). These observations have been confirmed and found in animals as well. The resultant reduction in the number and complexity of inputs implies major losses of function even for those residual cells.

At the cellular level many changes have been documented. The most extensively studied has been the intracellular accumulation of lipofuscin pigment. This major accumulation is in storage vacuoles and is quantitatively highly correlated with age. The amount per cell varies, but there can be sufficient to fill the cytoplasm and force the nucleus into an eccentric position. Despite the obvious and apparently significant nature of this material and the interest which it has engendered, it is not known if its presence has any actual effect upon cell function.

The previously enumerated changes would seem sufficient to account for senile dementia, yet intellectual function seems to be sustained out of proportion to the anatomic decrements. There are several anatomic lesions that have a high correlation with senile dementia, regardless of the age of onset. The most common are senile plaques and neurofibrillary tangles. The question of whether senile dementia is a manifestation of aging or a disease process has not been resolved. Age unquestionably is a major factor, since the age specific incidence increases geometrically. It is a major problem, with over one million persons requiring custodial care at the present time. Although it is not generally recognized, dementia is associated with a high mortality and might legitimately be considered a major cause of age-related death.

Brain Circulation and Oxygen Utilization

The circulation and oxygen utilization of the cerebrum are important physiologic components that have been well studied. The parameters generally examined include the cerebral blood flow (CBF) in ml/min/100 gm brain tissue, mean arterial pressure (MAP) in mm Hg, cerebral oxygen consumption rate ($CMRO_2$) as ml O_2/min/100 gm of brain tissue, and cerebrovascular resistance (CVR) expressed as mm HG/ml blood flow/min/100 gm of brain. The CVR is equal to the MAP divided by the CBF. A summary of data is presented in Table 6-3.

These studies by various authors are remarkably consistent, and there is a progression of values from age 17 years to age 80. During this period the MAP remained at 90 to 100 mm Hg. The CBF declined from 79 to 46 ml/min/100 gm of brain tissue. The $CMRO_2$ declined from 3.6 to 2.7 ml/min/100 gm of brain. The derived CVR showed a reciprocal increase from 1.3 to 2.1 mm Hg/ml blood/min/100 gm of brain. Hypertension increased the CVR but had little effect on oxygen utilization. There is a significant reduc-

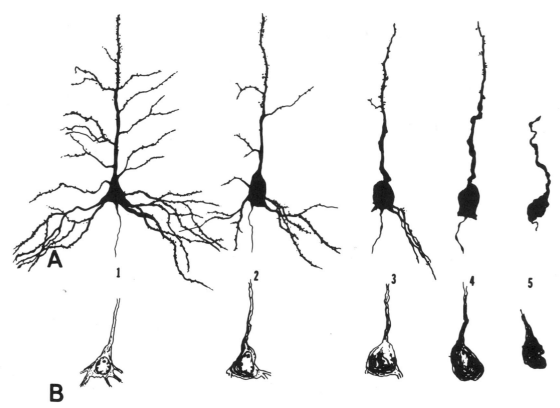

FIGURE 6-11 Progressive changes occurring in neurons of prefrontal neocortex with aging and senescence. *A*, Progressive changes as seen with golgi impregnation methods; *B*, Appearance of neurons stained by a reduced silver method to show neurofibrillary changes of Alzheimer. (From Scheibel, M. E., and Scheibel, A. B.: In Nandy, K., and Sherwin, I. (eds.): The Aging Brain and Senile Dementia. New York: Plenum Press, 1977, p. 41, with permission)

TABLE 6-3.   Effect of aging on cerebral hemodynamics and metabolism.*

	No. of Obser-vations	Age Range	Mean Age	MAP	CBF	CVR	CMRO$_2$
1*	4	17–18	17	97	79.3	1.3	3.6
2†	19	18–36	—	85	65.3	1.3	3.8
3§	25	20–44	29	91	52.0	1.8	3.1
4**	12	18–40	30	91	53.0	1.8	3.4
5*	12	18–47	32	94	57.5	1.7	3.2
6†	15	38–55	—	96	60.5	1.6	4.0
7§	23	45–75	56	101	46.0	2.2	2.9
8†	17	56–79	63	97	50.6	2.0	3.3
9**	23	45–86	68	95	46.0	2.1	2.7
10*	13	57–99	80	94	47.7	2.1	2.7

* Fazekas, Kleh, and Finnerty: Am. J. Med. 18:477, 1955.

† Scheinberg, et al.: Arch. Neurol. Psychiat. 70:77, 1953.

§ Heyman, et al.: New Engl. J. Med. 249:233, 1953.

** Shenkin, et al.: J. Clin. Invest. 32:459, 1953.

tion in cerebral blood flow and metabolism with aging. Patients with senile demential cluster at the lowest values of blood flow and oxygen utilization. Yet on an individual basis there is much overlap, and subjects without overt intellectual deterioration may be comparable with some who are totally incapacitated.

Nerve Conduction Velocity

The extensive use of electromyography as a diagnostic procedure has produced a mass of clinical data showing age-related changes in nerve conduction velocity. Nerve conduction velocity is most rapid in myelinated fibers and is roughly proportional to the diameter of the neuron. Most of the reported studies have been made of the motor conduction of the ulnar nerve. The velocity is quite slow in the newborn infant, and averages 30 meters/second. This increases rapidly so that at approximately three years of age almost all values are at the lower range of adult normal and maximum adult levels are achieved by age five. There is a variation between individual studies, but young adults have an average conduction velocity of slightly less than 60 meters/second.

From maturity the velocity decreases with age, especially after the fifth decade. By the eighth or ninth decade, values of approximately 50 meters/second are generally reported. This represents a decrease of approximately 15 percent. The conduction velocity is slightly greater in women than in men. No statistically significant difference has been noted between the dominant and nondominant extremities. One study of sensory conduction in the median nerve reported a 30 percent decrease in conduction velocity between the ages of 20 and 95 years. A significant decrease was also noted in both the motor and sensory latency between 20 and 80 years.

Sleep

Sleep is a phenomenon of great biologic and clinical importance. Four levels of increasing depth can be identified by electroencephalographic criteria and are numbered in increasing order. An additional level associated with rapid eye movements, known as REM sleep, is borderline in depth but is associated with the majority of dreams and has multiple unique physiologic characteristics. In infancy, deep levels 3 and 4 predominate and arousal is rare throughout the sleep cycle. With aging, level

3 and 4 become less prominent and brief arousals more frequent. By old age, there is little level 4 and there may be numerous brief arousals, although the total sleep time is only slightly reduced from young adulthood (Fig. 6-12). It is this frequent arousal that gives the impression of sleeplessness, even though in most instances actual sleep loss is minimal. Sedatives reduce latency to the onset of sleep and decrease the number of arousals. However, after a few days the pattern characteristic of the individual usually recurs and the sedative becomes ineffective. At this point, withdrawal may produce adverse effects even though the drug has lost its therapeutic value. With rare exceptions, sedatives should be used only briefly for specific situations. The elderly patient should be told that arousals are normal, but brief, and do not impair the effectiveness of the total sleep period.

Neurotransmitters

Perhaps the most active area of interest and study at present is that of the neurotransmitters. These include acetylcholine and epinephrine and their precursors and metabolites, as well as a variety of other compounds, both endogenous and exogenous, that interact with their metabolic pathways. The greatest interest has centered on the catecholamines (epinephrine-related compounds) and serotonin. These are all monamines, and their degradation is dependent, in part, on the activity of monamine oxidase (MAO). Recent investigations have shown that MAO and serotonin increase with age in the human brain, platelets, and plasma, while norepinephrine, the active precursor of epinephrine, decreases.

Current treatment of depression is based on the hypothesis, associated with considerable data, that depression is associated with decreased stores of catechols in the brain, and the use of MAO inhibitors, which block the MAO breakdown of catechols, is based on this rationale. The reciprocal increase of MAO and decrease of norepinephrine may explain the depression and apathy so often associated with aging. It also appears that steroid sex hormones also are necessary for adequate catechol function, and it is possible that the symptomatology of the menopause may be related to the abrupt reduction of estrogen production.

Parkinson's disease, or paralysis agitans, increases in frequency with age. Chemical studies show a decrease in dopamine, another epinephrine

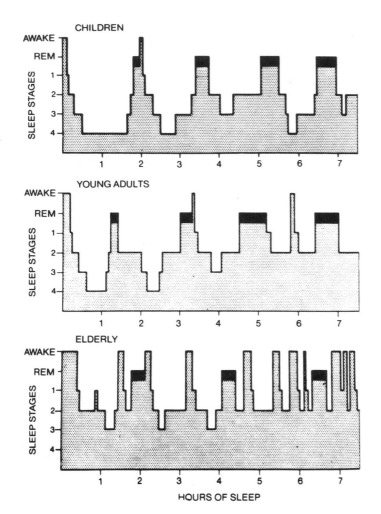

FIGURE 6-12. Changes in sleep cycle with aging. (Reprinted from Kales, A., and Kales, J. D.: Sleep disorders, by permission from the New Eng. J. Med. 290:487, 1974)

precursor, in the midbrains of these patients. This has been the rationale for the use of L-dopa which has had considerable success in controlling symptoms. It is obvious that expansion of this type of information will have considerable application to the explanation and amelioration of aging phenomena.

Sensory Organs and Sensation

The Eye

Visual acuity decreases with age. Friedenwald (1952) estimated, based on projections from available data, that blindness would be universal if survival were extended to 130 years. The actual amount of visual loss is variable. The major amount is due to cumulative damage to the transparent portions of the ocular system. However, there is also loss of the extent of the visual fields, decrease in the speed of dark adaptation, elevation in the minimal threshold of light perception, a greater proportionate loss of visual acuity in dim illumination, and reduction in the critical speed of flicker fusion.

The lens is formed by cells which, as they mature, lose their nuclei and cell membranes while their cytoplasm becomes crystalline and transparent. The lens continues to grow throughout life, although at a decreasing pace, as new cells develop surrounding the transparent nuclear region. Thus, the lens material in the core approaches the age of the individual, while the outer layers are progressively younger. With age the crystalline nucleus becomes progressively more rigid and discolored. Only the more recent portion near the surface is sufficiently soft and deformable to participate in accommodations, and as the ratio of the cortex to the nucleus becomes smaller, the ability to accommodate decreases. This process is remarkably uniform and predictable. Between ages 40 and 45 years, almost all individuals require corrective lenses in order to read and perform tasks requiring accommodation (Fig. 6-13). Whether the more or less complete opacification which occurs in cataract formation, and which markedly increases in frequency with age, is a pathologic process or a manifestation of differential aging, cannot be answered.

As the individual ages, a tilting of the lens above the vertical axis increases the power of the horizontal meridian, resulting in astigmatism with the major axis horizontal. The continued lens growth causes it to enlarge progressively toward the posterior surface of the cornea, reducing the depth of the anterior chamber. The resulting change in the optical nodal point, along with the continued growth and increased density of the lens nucleus, increases the refractive power of the lens and produces a relative

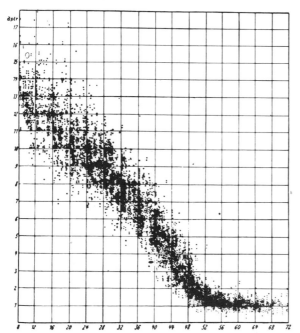

FIGURE 6-13. The accommodation capacity of the human eye in relationship to age. (From Friedenwald, J. S.: In Lansing, A. J. (ed.): Cowdry's Problems of Aging, ed. 3. Baltimore: Williams & Wilkins, 1952, p. 239, with permission)

myopia. The efficiency of the mechanism for reabsorption of the intraocular fluid decreases and, with the decreasing depth of the anterior chamber, may contribute to the increased frequency of chronic glaucoma in older individuals.

A well-known phenomenon, arcus senilis, is an age-related deposition of lipid which forms a white circle at the outer edge of the iris. Although it appears earlier in persons with hyperlipidemia, the impression that it is correlated with atherosclerosis has not been established.

The pupil becomes smaller and response to light and accommodation decreases. According to Howell, by age 85 only one third will respond to light and none will respond to accommodation. The ability to visualize the optic fundi becomes increasingly important with age, yet retinal examination becomes progressively more difficult.

The Ear

Audiometric studies indicate that the mean pure-tone threshold increases with age at all frequencies and for both sexes. There is little loss in sensitivity until the ninth decade at frequencies of 250 to 1000 cycles per second, and then only for men. There is a marked increase in the threshold at higher frequencies, again more significant for men, particularly after the age of 60. Most individuals over 60 have lost their serviceable hearing for frequencies above 4000 cycles.

The ability to hear and understand speech is more important than hearing pure tones. Although speech frequencies are relatively low, the ability to identify words is affected more than would be expected. Presbycusis, the aging changes in hearing, progresses from loss of discrimination to increase in speech-reception threshold to an increase in pure-tone threshold. Tinnitus does not seem to correlate with actual measured hearing loss. The auditory reaction time increases and becomes significant after 70 years. Age changes in vestibular function do not seem to have been examined.

Taste and Smell

The number of taste buds per papilla decreases from an average of 248 in children to 88 in individuals 74 to 85 years of age. Moreover, half of the buds in the older group are atrophic, and there probably is an 80 percent total reduction of functional units. Studies employing sugar, salt, quinine, and hydrochloric acid to test sensitivity for sweet, salty, bitter, and acid sensations have been equivocal. In order to obtain quantitative results, Hughes (1969) used a weak galvanic current which produces a definite metallic or acid taste when applied to the tongue. At a level of 10 microamperes 82 percent of a young group aged 20 to 30 had a positive response, compared to only 16 percent of an older group aged 62 to 96 years. Figure 6-14 shows the increase in the average taste threshold level with advancing age. Cigarette smoking had no effect, but pipe-smoking impaired the responses at all ages, and these individuals were excluded.

In one study, 89 percent of the young subjects had a normal smell sensitivity compared to only 22 percent of the old, a proportion comparable to that of taste (Table 6-4). Hughes (1969) comments that there is evidence that taste, smell, and hearing are appreciated in the parietal lobe at the inferior portion of the postcentral gyrus, and he suggests that losss of sensation with age may be due to cellular degeneration in this area.

Touch

No data could be found on changes in dermal sensation with age. However, histologic studies show a highly age-correlated decrease in the number of pacinian, Merkel's, and Meissner's corpuscles. Many of the remaining corpuscles showed marked disorganization and change. On the basis of these observations it would be reasonable to assume some reduction in the acuity of touch sensation. On the other hand, the free nerve endings underwent very little change, and the dermal sensation pain should be relatively much more intact.

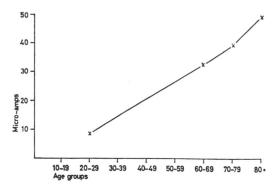

FIGURE 6-14. Increase in taste threshold level with advancing age. (From Hughes, G.: Geront. Clin. 11:224, 1968, with permission)

PERSPECTIVE

It was noted at the beginning of this chapter that survival to maturity is followed by a decreasing frequency of acute disease and an increase in chronic processes. Although myocardial and cerebral infarction are acute episodes and are frequent causes of disability and death, they follow upon the time-dependent development of atherosclerosis and other vascular changes. It was also noted that there is a growing conviction among gerontologists that the aging process is intrinsic and is independent of extrinsic (environmental) factors which may, however, accelerate the process. If this concept is true, it is necessary to reorient some aspects of social and research policy.

Figures 6-15 and 6-16 show the changes in survivorship that can be documented over a recent

Table 6-4. Age changes in ability to identify four common odorous substances.*

Age	No. of Subjects	Percentage of Subjects Who Smelled Nothing	Percentage of Subjects in Each Age Group Who Identified the Number of Substances Indicated				
			0	1	2	3	4
20–39	52	0	8	4	8	46	35
40–59	40	0	15	0	30	35	20
60–69	48	8	27	27	27	6	4
70–79	87	10	31	34	15	6	3
Over 80	63	29	29	24	19	0	0

From Anand, M. P.: Accidents in the home. In Anderson, W. F., and Isaacs, B. (eds.): Current Achievement in Geriatrics. London: Cassel, 1964, p. 239, with permission.
* Coffee, oil of almonds, peppermint, and coal tar.

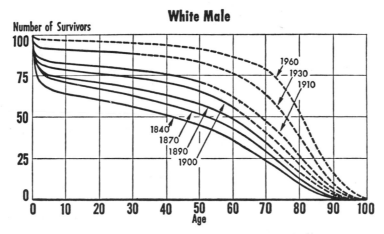

FIGURE 6-15. Survivorship of the white male in the United States, 1840 to 1960. (From Jacobson, P. H.: Cohort survival for generations since 1840. Milbank Memorial Fund Quart. 42:36, 1964, with permission)

period of human history. There is a consistent decrease in mortality at early ages and an increase into the postreproductive ages. However, while there is what is termed a squaring of the curve, the upper limits of survivorship have not been significantly altered. The magnitude of the change is shown in Table 6-5. Only 18 percent of women in 1600 survived to the reproductive age of 20, 11 percent completed the period, and approximately 3 percent reached age 65. In the developed countries today, over 97 percent reach age 20, 96 percent reach 40, 82 percent reach age 65, and 62 percent reach age 75. After this age, however, mortality increases rapidly.

An important concept was introduced by Ben-

Table 6-5. Survivorship of white women in percentage.

| | Age | | | | |
	1	20	40	65	75
Townswomen, York, 16th Century	45	18	11	3	
Aristocrats, England, 16th Century	82	70	58	11	
United States, 1900	89	79	68	44	7
United States, 1972	99	98	96	82	62

Data from Cowgill, U. M.: Sci. Am. 222:104, 1970, and the Statistical Abstract of the United States, United States Government Printing Office, Washington D.C., 1974.

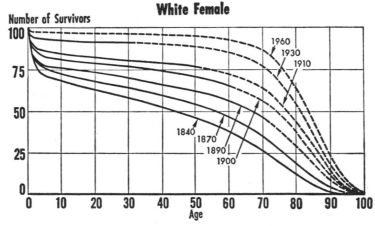

FIGURE 6-16. Survivorship of the white female in the United States, 1840 to 1960. (From Jacobson, P. H.: Cohort survival for generations since 1840. Milbank Memorial Fund Quart. 42:36, 1964, with permission)

jamin Gompertz, a British actuary, in 1825. Strangely, it was not until a relatively short time ago that his observation was recognized by biologists. His concept was that, after a high neonatal mortality, the death rate dropped to a nadir at the onset of puberty, and then increased. The important component was that at some point past maturity the risk of death increased geometrically; when age was plotted on a regular scale, but risk of death was plotted on a logarithmic scale, the result was a straight line. Thus, in advanced age the risk of death is related to age and is independent of specific cause. Figure 6-17 shows several Gompertz curves for women in Sweden since 1750. The excessive mortality caused by infection, malnutrition, accidents, and the hazards of childbirth are represented by the hump in the curve during childhood and early

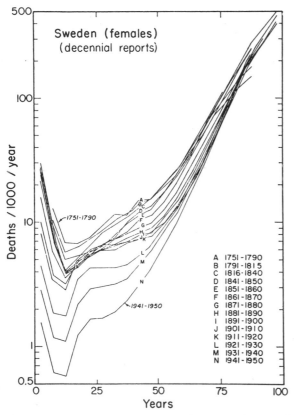

FIGURE 6-17. Age-specific mortality rates of Swedish women, 1751 to 1950, showing changing Gompertz curves. (From Jones, H. B.: In Birren, J. E. (ed.): Handbook of Aging and the Individual, p. 336. Copyright © 1959, Univ. of Chicago Press, Chicago. Used with permission)

maturity. As these causes have decreased, this anomaly has decreased, and the straight portion of the curve starts at earlier ages. However, while the straight portion is longer and starts at a lower level, it is steeper, so that at advanced age there is a limit to the potential for environmental improvement.

The fact of the Gompertz observation is well established and is true, with little modification, for almost all living organisms. The interpretation is subject to some variation. Many theories of aging have been proposed and are under investigation. Although interesting, it is not possible to examine these theories in this short chapter.

If aging is universal, why is there a variety in the causes of senescent death? I would like to present one formulation. It was postulated initially that after maturity the decremental changes exceeded the incremental changes in structure and function. We have seen a wide variety of such changes in the cells and in all organ systems. If we postulate that species survival depends upon reproduction and survival in a limited ecologic niche, then there would be an advantage if young individuals could compete successfully with older individuals once successful reproduction had taken place. Thus, aging need have no program, but rather, the exhaustion of a finely tuned program of repair. When we examine most chronic conditions and diseases of the aged, they can be plotted in individual curves identical with the Gompertz curve, that is, they show an age-related increase with a slope lower than, but parallel with, the overall curve. This observation is true for all of the vascular dependent conditions (heart disease, stroke, ischemic gangrene) as well as for cancer, senile dementia, arthritis, osteoporosis, and diabetes mellitus. It probably would be true of other age-related conditions if the data were available.

As a result of variations in constitution, plus the factor of specific environmental exposure, the deterioration of one system will be more rapid than another. For example, it is known that the level of blood pressure is associated with mortal risk and that, at any age, the lower the blood pressure, even within the so-called normal range, the longer the life expectancy. If the force of each systolic impact produces damage to the vascular wall, it is not unreasonable to anticipate an earlier manifestation of vascular decline with each increment in this force. The same would be true for each of the risk factors. Similarly, if neoplasia is due to a decrease in immune protection, which is known to decline with age, then the increased incidence of cancer with age is explicable.

If a carcinogenic factor were added from the environment, then the manifestation of neoplasia would be earlier.

Thus, the cause of death could vary, even though its specific manifestation was closely related to the aging process. It should be realized that, because of the geometric increase in frequency of each potential cause, the older the individual the more likely that if one cause is avoided (or successfully treated) another will shortly appear.

CONCLUSIONS

After maturity, there is an accelerating decrease in the rate of repair of the normal wear and tear of living. This is manifested by decremental changes in all tissues and their functions. This decrement progresses at different rates in the various organs, probably most related to genetic factors, but modified by environmental impacts. The reduction of violent environmental hazards has allowed these processes to become increasingly apparent.

As the result of the improving environment an increasing number of individuals is surviving to old age, although the life span, or maximal attainable age, has not been altered. These individuals and their medical care have become a primary problem for modern health services. Because there is a geometric increase in mortality with age, it is improbable that there will be a significant increase in the life expectancy of an aging population. This depends primarily on characterization of the aging process and maneuvers to make it slower. However, in the meantime, there is much that can be done to make this segment of life enjoyable, meaningful, and comfortable.

BIBLIOGRAPHY

Addis, T.: Glomerular nephritis, diagnosis and treatment. New York: Macmillan Co., 1948.

Andres, R.: Hosp. Pract. 2:63, 1967.

Bender, A. D.: The effect of increasing age on the distribution of peripheral blood flow in man. J. Am. Geriat. Soc. 13:192, 1965.

Brocklehurst, J. C. (ed.): Textbook of Geriatric Medicine and Gerontology. Edinburgh and London: Churchill Livingstone, 1973.

Brocklehurst, J. C.: A study of the bladder, rectum and anal sphincter in senile incontinent patients. In Incontinence in Old People. Edinburgh: E. S. Livingston, 1951.

Brody, H.: Structural changes in the aging nervous system. In Blumenthal, H. T. (ed.): Interdisciplinary Topics in Gerontology, Vol. 7. New York: Karger, 1970.

Calloway, N. O., Foley, C. F., and Lagebloom, P.: Uncertainties in geriatric data. II. Organ size. J. Am. Geriat. Soc. 13:20, 1965.

Cowgill, U. M.: The people of York: 1538–1812. Sci. Am. 222:104, 1970.

Davies, D. F., and Shock, N. W.: Age changes in glomerular filtration rate, effective renal plasma flow and tubular excretory capacity in adult males. J. Clin. Invest. 29:496, 1950.

Fazekas, J. F., Kleh, J., and Finnerty, F. A.: Influence of age and vascular disease on cerebral hemodynamics and metabolism. Am. J. Med. 18:477, 485, 1955.

Finch, C. E., and Hayflick, L. (eds.): Handbook of the Biology of Aging. New York: Van Nostrand Reinhold Co., 1977.

Flood, C., et al.: The metabolism and secretion of aldosterone in elderly subjects. J. Clin. Invest. 46: 960, 1967.

Friedenwald, J. S.: The eye. In Lansing, A. I. (ed.): Cowdry's Problems of Aging: Biological and Medical Aspects, ed. 3. Baltimore: Williams & Wilkins, 1952.

Gregerman, R. I., et al.: Thyroxine turnover in euthyroid man with special reference to changes with age. J. Clin. Invest. 41:2065, 1962.

Hayflick, L.: The limited *in vitro* lifetime of human diploid cell strains. Exp. Cell. Res. 37:614, 1965.

Heyman, A., et al.: The cerebral circulation and metabolism in arteriosclerotic and hypertensive cerebrovascular disease. New Eng. J. Med. 249:223, 1953.

Hollenberg, N. K., et al.: Senescence and the renal vasculature in normal man. Circ. Res. 34:309, 1974.

Hughes, G.: Changes in taste sensitivity with advancing age. Geront. Clin. 11:224, 1969.

Landowne, M., and Stanley, J.: Aging of the cardiovascular system. In Shock, N. W. (ed.): Aging . . . Some Social and Biological Aspects. Washington D.C.: Am. Ass. Adv. Sci., 1960.

McDonald, R. K., Solomon, D. H., and Shock, N. W.: Aging as a factor in the renal hemodynamic changes induced by standardized pyrogen. J. Clin. Invest. 30:457, 1951.

Meyer, J., and Necheles, H.: Studies in old age. IV. The clinical significance of salivary, gastric and pancreatic secretion in the aged. J.A.M.A. 115:2050, 1940.

O'Rourke, M. F., et al.: Pressure wave transmission along the human aorta. Changes with age and in arterial degenerative disease. Circ. Res. 23:567, 1968.

Pincus, G., et al.: Steroid metabolism in aging men and women. Recent Progr. Hormone Res. 11:307, 1955.

Reichel, W. (ed.): Clinical Aspects of Aging. Baltimore: Williams & Wilkins, 1978.

Rosenberg, I. R., et al.: The effect of age and sex upon human pancreatic secretion of fluid and bicarbonate. Gastroenterology 50:191, 1966.

Rossman, I. (ed.): Clinical Geriatrics. ed. 2. Philadelphia: J. B. Lippincott Co., 1979.

Scheibel, M. E., and Scheibel, A. B.: Differential changes with old and new cortices. In Nandy, K., and Sherwin, I. (eds.): The Aging Brain and Senile Dementia. New York: Plenum Press, 1977.

Scheinberg, P., et al.: Effects of aging on cerebral circulation and metabolism. Arch. Neurol. Psychiatry. 70:77, 1953.

Shenkin, H. A., et al.: The effects of aging, arteriosclerosis, and hypertension upon the cerebral circulation. J. Clin. Invest. 32:459, 1953.

Strehler, B. L.: Time, Cells and Aging, ed. 2. New York: Academic Press, 1977.

Wesson, L. G.: Physiology of the Human Kidney. New York: Grune & Stratton, 1969.

7

Laboratory Values

Lynne Talley

QUICK REVIEW

LABORATORY VALUES

		Sex	Over-70 Age Group*	Ranges† Standard‡
HEMATOLOGY	Hemoglobin	♂	10–17	13.5–18.0 gm/dl
		♀	10–16	12.0–16.0 gm/dl
	Red blood cell count	♂	3–5	4.6–6.2 10^6/mm^3
		♀	3–5	4.2–5.4 10^6/mm^3
	Hematocrit	♂	36–56	40–54%
		♀	30–54	38–47%
	White cell count	♂	4,250–14,000	4,500–11,000/mm^3
		♀	3,100–12,000	4,500–11,000/mm^3
	White cell differential	See discussion		
	Platelet count	See discussion		
	Erythrocyte sedimentation rate	See discussion		
		♂	< 50 yr	<15 mm/hr
			> 50 yr	<20 mm/hr
		♀	< 50 yr	<20 mm/hr
			> 50 yr	<30 mm/hr
SERUM CHEMISTRY	Albumin	♂	2.9–4.4	3.2–4.5 gm/dl (salt fractionation) or
		♀	3.0–4.3	3.2–5.6 gm/dl (electrophoresis) or 3.8–5.0 gm/dl (dye binding)
	Total Bilirubin	♂ & ♀	0.2–1.2	0.1–1.2 mg/dl
	BUN	♂	8–35	8–18 mg/dl
		♀	6–30	8–18 mg/dl
	Calcium	♂	9.1–10.6	9.0–10.6 mg/dl or 4.5–5.3 mEq/L
		♀	9.2–10.6	
	Cholesterol	♂	154–314	150–250 mg/dl
		♀	171–347	150–250 mg/dl

Continued on next page.

Quick Review (cont.)

SERUM CHEMISTRY
(Cont.)

	Creatinine	♂	0.8–1.6	0.6–1.2 mg/dl
		♀	0.6–1.4	0.6–1.2 mg/dl
	Creatinine clearance	♂	96.9	107–140 ml/min
		♀	96.9	87–107 ml/min
	Fasting glucose	♂	52–135	70–110 mg/dl serum or
		♀	58–135	60–100 mg/dl whole blood
	Glucose tolerance test	See discussion		
	Inorganic phosphorus	♂	2.1–5.0	{ 3.0–4.5 mg/dl or
		♀	2.7–5.0	1.8–2.6 mEq/L
	Potassium	♂	3.5–5.6	3.8–5.0 mEq/L
		♀	3.5–5.2	3.8–5.0 mEq/L
	Total protein	♂	6.0–7.9	6.0–7.8 gm/dl
		♀	5.9–7.7	6.0–7.8 gm/dl
	Sodium	♂	134–147	136–142 mEq/L
		♀	135–145	136–142 mEq/L
	Uric acid	♂	2.9–8.8	2.1–7.8 mg/dl
		♀	2.4–7.2	2.0–6.4 mg/dl
ENZYMES	Alkaline phosphatase	♂	2.0–15.3 KAU	1.5–4.5 U/dl (Bodansky) or
		♀	3.7–17.4 KAU	4–13 (King-Armstrong) or
				0.8–2.3 (Bessey-Lowry) or
				15–35 (Shinowara-Jones-Reinhart)
	LDH	♂	122.8–268.4	71–207 IU/L
		♀	133.6–250.2	71–207 IU/L
	SGPT	♂ & ♀	See discussion	1–36 U/ml
	SGOT	♂	0.2–38.1	8–33 U/ml
		♀	1.8–31.8	8–33 U/ml
	SCPK	♂	See discussion	55–170 U/L @ 37°C
		♀		30–135 U/L @ 37°C
URINALYSIS	Specific gravity	See discussion		1.016–1.022

* Each of these values is taken from one or more of the studies cited in the chapter.

† Ranges reported = ±2 Standard Deviations (95%) Values

‡ Standard ranges are from Davidshohn, I., and Henry, J. B. (eds.): Todd-Sanford Clinical Diagnosis by Laboratory Methods, ed. 15. Philadelphia: W. B. Saunders, 1974.

One of the problems faced by health care providers who work with the elderly is the lack of age-related standards with which to compare patient values. Those standards that are available have been largely standardized on relatively small samples of young healthy adults, frequently using only young men. When laboratory values for adults over 70 years of age are compared to the standards based on young adult samples, the question arises as to whether those values falling outside of the reported normal ranges are a reflection of illness or of normal age-related physiologic changes. Clearly, standards are required that are based on a population as similar to the person being tested as possible.

In this chapter age-related findings in commonly-used laboratory tests will be reported as literature documenting research on these tests could be located. Sex and age differences usually are fairly clear, with most studies in each test reflecting the same trends, if not the same precise values.

One difficulty in interpreting the data and evaluating the studies lies in the variety of methods used to select a "healthy" population. Some studies relied on questionnaires and others did physical examinations and laboratory work. Some ruled out any subject with current and/or past disease while others deleted those with abnormalities which are known to affect the laboratory value in question. Some studies allowed the ingestion of medications and others did not. In order to allow the reader who is interested to compare the research designs on these variables, the health characteristics of the group in each study are summarized in the annotated bibliography at the end of the chapter. Studies on institutionalized populations will not be reported in the tables, although the references will be cited for those who wish to do further exploration. One study (O'Kell and Elliott, 1970), which tested hospital admissions, is included for comparison.

Studies reporting on the largest populations, such as the Cutler study (1970) with a sample of 33,959 individuals (15,033 males and 18,926 females), are the ones presented in the tables. Findings from smaller studies have been added for further clarification or are used where large studies were not located.

Almost all studies on age-related effects on clinical laboratory values have used a cross-sectional methodology, that is, the individuals are not studied over time. Libow (1971) reported a longitudinal study on eight healthy survivors from an original study done at an 11-year interval; however, only a few tests were involved. With such a small group the trends only raised questions which need to be explored in further longitudinal research. Both cross-sectional and longitudinal designs involve difficulties such as the selective survival of a biologically superior group for the former and "learning" or "stress" during repeated testing for the latter.

Beyond these rather basic considerations on variables affecting findings, there are a myriad of other variables that are known to affect values on at least some tests. These include heredity, race, sex, age, socioeconomic environment, diurnal variation, circadian periodicity and season of the year (Winsten, 1975), geographic location (Reed, 1972), posture and time of the day (Roberts, 1967), and weight (Goldberg, 1973). Additionally, the laboratory method utilized for the same types of tests can greatly affect the values reported. Even the units reported may vary.

Still, given all these constraints, it seems valuable for nurses to have available data on what is known about age-related laboratory values. Such knowledge may lend perspective to interpretations they make of laboratory values in their case loads.

NOTE: All standard normal values referred to in this chapter are from Davidsohn, I., and Henry, J. B. (eds.): *Todd-Sanford Clinical Diagnosis by Laboratory Methods*, ed. 15. Philadelphia: W. B. Saunders Co., 1974.

ABBREVIATIONS AND SYMBOLS USED IN TABLES IN CHAPTER 7

>	greater than
<	less than
dl	100 milliliters
gm	gram
IU	International Unit
L	liter
m²	square meter body surface
mEq	milliequivalent
mg	milligram
gm%	gram percent or gm/dl
ml	milliliter
mM	millimole
mm³	cubic millimeter
μL	microliter
♂	male
♀	female
#	number
N	number of subjects
≤	less than or equal to
≥	greater than or equal to
C	centigrade

TABLE 7-1. Hemoglobin, red blood cell count, and hematocrit values.

Source	Age (years)	Sex	Number	Hemoglobin (gm/dl) Mean	Range	Red blood cell count ($10^6/mm^3$) Mean	Range	Hematocrit (%) Mean	Range
Shapleigh et al.		♂	50	14.1	—	4.75	—	42.1	—
(1952)	60–95	♀	50	13.7	—	4.71	—	40.8	—
Hobson and	60–	♂	22	14.4	—	—	—	—	—
Blackburn (1953)		♀	23	13.8	—	—	—	—	—
Hawkins et al. (1954)	61–70	♂	81	13.9	10.7 –17.1	—	—	—	—
		♀	55	12.9	10.2 –15.6	—	—	—	—
	71–80	♂	71	13.4	10.2 –16.6	—	—	—	—
		♀	71	13.0	10.1 –15.9	—	—	—	—
	81–90	♂	28	12.4	8.9 –15.9	—	—	—	—
		♀	33	13.0	10.5 –15.5	—	—	—	—
Orchard (1955)	65–95	♂	58	15.46	—	5.04	—	44.62	—
		♀	92	15.58	—	4.82	—	42.29	—
Borner et al. (1958)	74–92	♂	46	13.98	13.3 –14.7	4.41	4.2–4.7	47.4	40.5–54.3
Maekawa & Kinugasa	60–[a]	♂	110	14.2	11.4 –17.0	4.14	3.1–5.2	—	—
(1958)		♀	152	13.1	9.5 –16.7	3.93	2.9–4.0	—	—
	60–[b]	♂	50	15.3	12.3 –18.3	4.60	3.4–5.8	—	—
		♀	45	14.0	11.2 –16.8	4.33	3.4–5.3	—	—
Undritz & Bragatsch	65–91	♂	50	16.4	—	5.1	—	46.0	—
(1962)		♀	28	15.0	—	4.7	—	42.0	—
Parsons et al. (1965)	75–79	♂	16	14.61	10.9 –18.3	—	—	46.06	36.0–56.0
		♀	20	13.56	11.0 –16.1	—	—	43.55	36.2–50.9
	80–84	♂	5	13.64	10.5 –16.8	—	—	44.40	37.7–51.1
		♀	18	12.83	8.6 –17.0	—	—	41.71	29.5–51.0
Lederer (1966)	70–	♂	57	12.3	10.1 –14.5	4.12	3.2–5.1	—	—
		♀	63	12.0	10.2 –13.3	4.04	3.2–4.9	—	—
Burnett (1966)		♂	—	14.63	—	4.58	—	41.61	—
		♀	—	13.97	—	4.57	—	39.25	—
Myers et al. (1968)	65–	♂	81	13.6	10.6 –16.6	—	—	—	—
		♀	121	13.1	10.14–15.8	—	—	—	—
Libow (1963)	65–91	♂	47	15.0	14.0 –16.0	—	—	44.0	38.0–50.0
Miller (1939)	>60[c]	♂	160	14.3	12.0 –17.5	4.46	3.5–5.5	—	—
Fowler (1941)	65–80	♂	73	13.1	—	4.66	—	41.7	—
		♀	27	12.5	—	4.46	—	40.4	—
Shapleigh et al.	60–104	♂		14.1 (N475)	—	4.73 (N577)	—	43.7 (N266)	—
(1952)[d]		♀		13.5 (N265)	—	4.46 (N356)	—	40.5 (N212)	—
Standard Normal		♂		—	13.5 –18.0	—	4.6–6.2	—	40.0–54.0
Values		♀		—	12.0 –16.0	—	4.2–5.4	—	38.0–47.0

Adapted from Maekawa (1976, 153) with additional data from Libow (1963), Miller (1939), Fowler (1941), and Shapleigh, et al. (1952). References for this table are given in Maekawa (1976).
Notes: [a] living at home; [b] living in institution; [c] living in home for the aged; [d] combined data from 13 earlier studies

These values have implications for nursing practice. For example, decisions concerning hydration and salt intake are affected by knowledge of appropriate normal ranges for sodium at any given age. Enzymes such as SCPK, LDH, SGOT, and SGPT are used in assessment of status in cardiac, liver, and muscle diseases. Cholesterol levels change with age, yet still are used as indicators of risk of coronary disease. Elevations in blood sugar and changing responses to glucose tolerance testing confuse the assessment of the person for diabetes. Decline in kidney function in age and disease is reflected most sensitively by creatinine clearance, which declines with age. Age has implications for administration of drugs that are excreted by the kidney; there is a narrower range of safety and a need for a closer attention to possible signs and symptoms of toxicity with drug accumulation.

The laboratory tests have been placed in the sequence used on the Quick Review: hematology, blood chemistries (in alphabetical order), serum enzymes, and urinalysis.

HEMATOLOGY

Hemoglobin, Red Blood Cells, and Hematocrit

In general, the studies on hemoglobin, red blood cells, and hematocrit for older persons (Table 7-1) show wider ranges and lower values than the normal ranges for young adults. The values for older men continue to be higher than those for women, but the sex differences are smaller than in younger adults.

Many variables have been found to affect these values. Older persons with higher intelligence, periodic health examinations, and adequate health care tend to have higher levels. Elderly men living with their wives have higher levels than men living alone, presumably because their diets are more adequate. Elderly persons living at home and retaining social activity have higher levels than the aged living in institutions.

White Blood Cells (WBC)

The studies on age-related changes in the numbers and types of white blood cells are difficult to interpret because of the small numbers of persons studied and the varied findings. The mean WBC total count values in all studies fall well within the standard normal values; however, the range of counts extends both lower and higher than the standard range of 4500 and 11,000 in many of the studies (Table 7-3).

The differential counts showed no clear age-related change, except for an increased range of values.

Platelet Count and Blood Coagulation

In Maekawa's review he noted the difficulty in comparing various findings for platelet counts because the technique of measurement greatly affects the values found (Table 7-2). Many papers indicate no difference in the platelet count between the elderly and the young adult (Maekawa, 1976).

An increase in plasma fibrinogen level in the elderly is generally accepted (Maekawa, 1976), with two studies of persons 60 to 90 years old reporting averages of 485 mg/dl and 471 mg/dl (Maekawa, 1976, 155). Conflicting data have emerged concerning coagulation factors and activity, but no significant change in coagulation is seen in the healthy aged person that would give rise to serious disturbance (Maekawa, 1976).

TABLE 7-2. Platelet count (#/cm³).

| Standard Normal Values: | | | 150,000–400,000/mm³ | |
| Dameshek Method Normal Values: | | | 400,000–800,000/mm³ | |

Sex	Age	N	Mean	Range
♂*	60–95	50	732,000	255,000–1,392,000
♀*	60–95	50	781,000	330,000–1,430,000
♂ & ♀†	60–89	94		70,266– 175,000

* Shapleigh et al., 1952 (Dameshek Method)
† Puxeddu, 1927, cited in Shapleigh (Method not given)

Erythrocyte Sedimentation Rate (ESR)

The number of studies and subjects within the studies is small in the erythrocyte sedimentation rate (Table 7-4). Hayes (1976), in the most recent study located, combined males and females. His findings showed a progressive increase in ESR values with age and a decrease in the percentage of subjects who fell within the normal range. The conflicting results from researchers reporting only older subjects lend confu-

TABLE 7-3. White cell differential.

Author	Age range	Sex and no. of cases	Total WBC (mm³) Mean	Total WBC (mm³) Range	Basophils %	Eosinophils %	Bands or stabs %	Polys or segs %	Lymphocytes %	Monocytes %
Olbrich (1947)[a]	61–88	♂ 41	7020	4600–9000	0.0–3.0 / Mean 0.5	0.0–7.0 / Mean 2.3	0.0–1.0 / Mean 0.04	— / Mean 71.8	10.0–46.0 / Mean 22.9	0.0–8.0 / Mean 2.3
		♀ 48	7058	3200–12,809	0.0–4.0 / Mean 0.6	0.0–8.0 / Mean 1.9	0.0–1.0 / Mean 0.1	— / Mean 67.8	12.0–45.0 / Mean 27.0	0.0–8.6 / Mean 1.8
Etienne & Perrin (1908)[b]	80–96	♂ 20	8680	5600–12,800	1.0–2.5	1.0–2.5 / Mean 1.75	—	57.0–74.0 / Mean 67.1	18.0–36.0 / Mean 24.85	1.0–8.5 / Mean 5.1
		♀ 7	7371	5600–9200	—	—	—	—		
Newman & Gitlow (1943)	65–104	♂ 50	8330	5000–12,050	0.3–1.0[e] / 0.0–0.5	0.6–3.5[c] / 1.0–2.0	Mean 5.1 / Mean 4.2	Mean 60.2 / Mean 63.0	Mean 33.5 / Mean 33.8	0.7–2.0[e] / 1.0–2.1
		♀ 50	8170	5050–11,100						
Miller (1939)[d]	60–104	♂ 160	7700	4000–13,000	0.0–2.0 / Mean 0.7	0.0–8.0 / Mean 2.7	—	40.0–75.0 / Mean 57.5	15.0–50.0 / Mean 30.0	1.0–15.0 / Mean 7.8
		♀ none								
Gabbert et al. (1947)[e]	>70		—	2000–16,000	—	—	—	—	—	—
Fowler et al. (1941)[f]	65–80	♂ 73	7220	2900–12,450	0.0–3.0 / Mean <1	0.0–10.0 / Mean 2.8	1.0–13.0 / Mean 4.0	43.0–79.0 / Mean 60.2	11.0–48.0 / Mean 27.5	1.0–15.0 / Mean 5.4
		♀ 27	—	—						
Dobrovici (1904)[g]	67–81	♂ 11	—	—	—	1.0–1.5 / Mean 1.2	—	64.5–80.5 / Mean 73.0	13.5–30.0 / Mean 20.4	3.0–9.5 / Mean 5.4
		♀ none								
Dotti (1927)[h]	60–92	♂ 26	7039	4948–8602	0.0–3.5 / Mean 0.8	2.2–17.0 / Mean 4.6	—	30.5–67.4 / Mean 52.4	21.0–65.0 / Mean 37.9	1.0–9.5 / Mean 3.3
		♀ 35	5795	4000–7450	0.0–1.5 / Mean 0.3	0.5–5.0 / Mean 2.2	—	28.3–70.5 / Mean 55.6	22.0–54.4 / Mean 36.7	2.6–8.3 / Mean 5.2
Shapleigh et al. (1952)[i]	60–95	♂ 50	7730	4250–16,000	0.0–4.0 / Mean 1.1	0.0–9.0 / Mean 4.4	0.0–5.0 / Mean 1.4	28.0–86.0 / Mean 59.1	4.0–46.0 / Mean 23.5	4.0–26.0 / Mean 10.4
		♀ 50	6497	3150–10,350	0.0–3.0 / Mean 1.0	0.0–17.0 / Mean 4.7	0.0–8.0 / Mean 1.8	28.0–75.0 / Mean 55.6	11.0–62.0 / Mean 27.7	2.0–19.0 / Mean 9.1
Libow (1963)	65–91	♂ 47	6600	3800–9400	0.0–1.4 / Mean 0.44	0.0–7.2 / Mean 3.64	—	—	19.0–51.0 / Mean 35.09	0.0–8.5 / Mean 3.75
Normals				4500–11,000 Means	0–1 / 0.3	1–5 / 2.7	0–5 / 3.0	50–70 / 56.0	20–40 / 34.0	1–6 / 4

Adapted from Shapleigh et al. (1952).

Notes: [a] Tendency to increased lobulation and decreased granulation of WBC. No total segmented form values given; divided into number of lobes; [b] Morphology essentially normal. No sex differences in differential; [c] Range of averages of 5-year age increments from 65 to 94 years; [d] WBC essentially the same as in younger age groups; [e] Total WBC same in aged as in young adults; [f] Total WBC and differential normal; [g] Tendency to more mature cells in aged; [h] Total WBC normal, with increase in lymphocytes, decrease in monocytes and segmented forms; [i] Morphology normal

TABLE 7-4. Erythrocyte sedimentation rate (ESR) (mm/hr).

Age	Miller (1936) N	Miller (1936) % within normal range*	Eckerström (1949) N	Eckerström (1949) Mean	Olbrich (1948) N	Olbrich (1948) Mean	Olbrich (1948) Range	Shapleigh (1952) N	Shapleigh (1952) % within normal range*	Libow (1963) N	Libow (1963) Mean	Libow (1963) Range	Libow (1971) N†	Libow (1971) Mean	Libow (1971) Range
MEN‡															
20–29	—	—	—	—	—	—	—	—	—	—	—	—	—	—	—
30–39	2	100	—	—	—	—	—	—	—	Adult[a]	—	0–15	—	—	—
40–49	18	89	—	—	—	—	—	—	—	—	—	—	—	—	—
50–59	87	90	—	—	—	—	—	—	—	—	—	—	8[b]	16.9	0–41.1
60–69	243	85	—	—	34[c]	12.1	0–30.0	50[d]	17	47[e]	20.6	0–46	—	—	—
70–79	125	81	100[f]	6.3	—	—	—	—	—	—	—	—	—[g]	27.1	1.1–53.1
80+	20[h] 1[i]	85	—	—	—	—	—	—	—	—	—	—	—	—	—
WOMEN§															
20–29	—	—	—	—	—	—	—	—	—	—	—	—	—	—	—
30–39	—	—	—	—	—	—	—	—	—	—	—	—	—	—	—
40–49	—	—	—	—	—	—	—	—	—	—	—	—	—	—	—
50–59	—	—	—	—	—	—	—	—	—	—	—	—	—	—	—
60–69	—	—	—	—	33[j]	11.7	0–21.6	50[k]	8	—	—	—	—	—	—
70–79	—	—	100[l]	10.4	—	—	—	—	—	—	—	—	—	—	—
80+	—	—	—	—	—	—	—	—	—	—	—	—	—	—	—

Men and Women (Hayes, 1976)

N	Mean	Range	% within normal range*
23[m]	8.8	1–20	100
26	11.7	2–32	88
24	14.8	2–30	79
25	15.0	3–35	76
32	19.3	6–40	53
22	22.7	4–50	54
17	26.8	14–54	53

* Normal range utilized in these studies ≤20 mm/hr
† Values for eight healthy survivors from the 1963 Libow study
‡ Standard normal values: Men under 50 years <15 mm/hr; men over 50 years <20 mm/hr
§ Standard normal values: Women under 50 years <20 mm/hr; women over 50 years <30 mm/hr

Notes:
a Adult group represents the NIH Clinical Pathology Laboratory normal adult values
b 1956
c 60–88 yrs.
d 60–95 yrs.
e 65–91 yrs.
f ≥70 yrs.
g 1967
h 80–89 yrs.
i 90–99 yrs.
j 60–98 yrs.
k 60–95 yrs.
l ≥70 yrs.
m <30 yrs.

sion to the picture, although there seems to be a trend toward increasing values. Many normal older persons have been found to have high values even when compared to the age-adjusted values.

SERUM CHEMISTRY

Data are presented in chart form from four research studies involving large healthy populations of both men and women including those over 70 years of age. All data are reported in a similar manner for comparison. In addition, data from selected smaller studies dealing with each particular laboratory test are shown.

The reader is referred to a number of other studies which examined age-related changes in values for the entire screening battery but which did not include as old a population as those presented here or which reported values in a different format (Craig and Bartholemew, 1970; Cunnick, et al., 1970; Ludvigsen and Taylor, 1970; Reed, et al., 1972; Roberts, 1967). The data from these studies are incor-

porated into the discussions concerning each laboratory test.

Albumin

All of the studies located showed lowering values for albumin with increasing age (Table 7-5). In addition to the five reported on the table, several others agree with this trend (Altman, 1961; Craig and Bartholemew, 1970; Karel, et al., 1956; Keating, et al., 1969; Libow, 1963; Oeriu, 1964; Prusik, 1957; Rafsky, et al., 1952). Only Roof and her associates observed a different trend (1976).

Age-related differences found in younger years tend to disappear at about the sixth decade. In younger adults, men have higher albumin values than women; however, with the more gradual decline in women's values, are comparable later.

Most older persons studied still fell within the standard normal values with some reported values falling as low as 2.8 and 2.9 compared to the 3.2 to 3.8 lowest values in the standards (variation depends on method used).

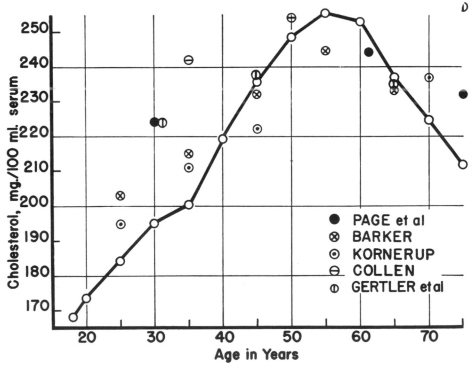

FIGURE 7-1. The mean total cholesterol concentration in the serum of healthy men at different ages. The open circles and connecting heavy line show the trend for 1492 men in the twin cities. (From Keys, A.: The age trend of serum concentrations of cholesterol and of S_f 10–20 (G) substances in adults. Journal of Gerontology 7:201–206, 1952, with permission)

TABLE 7-5. Albumin (gm/dl).

Men Age	Cutler et al. (1970)*			Cutler et al. (1970)†			Wilding et al. (1972)			Werner et al. (1972)		O'Kell & Elliott (1970)		
	N	Mean	Range	N	Mean	Range	N	Mean	Range	N	Mean	N	Mean	Range
20–29	586	4.03	3.3–4.8	1843	4.03	3.3–4.8	96	4.41	4.0–4.8	‡	4.52	507	4.4	3.2–5.6
30–39	943	3.95	3.2–4.7	2861	3.99	3.1–4.8	721	4.35	3.9–4.8		4.44			
40–49	1152	3.90	3.1–4.7	3958	3.91	3.0–4.8	1268	4.29	3.9–4.7		4.32	964	4.1	2.9–5.3
50–59	857	3.83	3.0–4.6	3656	3.84	3.0–4.7	1112	4.24	3.8–4.7		4.23			
60–69	314	3.70	3.0–4.4	2039	3.74	3.0–4.5	415	4.19	3.8–4.6		4.08	1077	3.8	2.6–5.0
70–79	68	3.64	2.9–4.4	676	3.66	2.8–4.5	105	4.13	3.5–4.7		4.03			
80+	—	—	—	—	—	—	—	—	—		—	205	3.5	2.3–4.7
Women														
20–29	1003	3.70	3.0–4.4	3016	3.70	3.0–4.4	72	4.30	3.9–4.7	‡	4.21	583	4.2	2.9–5.5
30–39	940	3.67	3.0–4.4	2998	3.69	3.0–4.4	193	4.24	3.8–4.7		4.11			
40–49	1292	3.62	2.9–4.3	4732	3.66	2.9–4.4	283	4.20	3.7–4.7		4.12	1546	4.0	2.8–5.2
50–59	1063	3.66	3.0–4.4	4638	3.69	3.0–4.4	278	4.18	3.8–4.6		4.10			
60–69	499	3.66	3.0–4.3	2763	3.70	3.0–4.4	229	4.15	3.7–4.6		4.07	1448	3.9	2.7–5.1
70–79	91	3.62	3.0–4.3	779	3.68	2.9–4.4	39	4.13	3.7–4.6		4.03			
80+	—	—	—	—	—	—	—	—	—		—	360	3.8	2.6–5.0

Standard normal values: 3.2–4.5 gm/dl (salt fractionation); 3.2–5.6 gm/dl (by electrophoresis); 3.8–5.0 gm/dl (by dye binding)
* No significant abnormality on physical examination
† Total group
‡ Total N > 3000 including men & women

TABLE 7-6. Total bilirubin (mg/dl).

Age	Wilding et al. (1972)			Werner et al. (1972)		Craig & Bartholemew (1970)			O'Kell & Elliott (1970)		
	N	Mean	Range	N	Mean	N	Mean	Range	N	Mean	Range
MEN											
20–29	96	0.64	0.0–1.3	*	0.72	955	0.52	0.29–0.75	507	0.7	0.2–1.2
30–39	721	0.65	0.0–1.3	—	0.65	1306	0.51	0.28–0.74			
40–49	1268	0.63	0.1–1.2	—	0.62	2349	0.47	0.24–0.70	964	0.6	0.2–1.0
50–59	1112	0.61	0.0–1.2	—	0.61	2130	0.49	0.27–0.71			
60–69	415	0.60	0.0–1.2	—	0.55	597	0.50	0.28–0.72	1077	0.6	0.2–1.0
70–79	105	0.68	0.0–1.7	—	0.67	—	—	—			
80+	—	—	—	—	—	—	—	—	205	0.7	0.2–1.2
WOMEN											
20–29	72	0.55	0.0–1.1	*	0.51				583	0.6	0.3–0.9
30–39	193	0.51	0.1–1.0	—	0.46						
40–49	283	0.54	0.2–1.1	—	0.47				1546	0.5	0.2–0.8
50–59	278	0.52	0.1–0.9	—	0.46						
60–69	229	0.49	0.0–1.0	—	0.48				1448	0.5	0.1–0.9
70–79	39	0.51	0.1–0.9	—	0.48						
80+	—	—	—	—	—				360	0.6	0.2–1.0

Standard normal values: 0.1–1.2 mg/dl
* Total N > 3000 including men & women

Total Bilirubin

In general, the studies of total bilirubin (Table 7-6) indicated no significant change in the total bilirubin values with age. Male values tended to be slightly higher than those of women. All values for the 70- to 79-year-old group fell within the standard normal range except for the males in Wilding's study who reached a high of 1.7 mg/dl as their upper range compared to a 1.2 normal.

Other research on total bilirubin includes work by Hodkinson (1977).

Blood Urea Nitrogen (BUN)

An increase in values in blood urea nitrogen was generally observed with advancing age for both men and women (Table 7-7). In addition, men consistently had higher values than women throughout the adult life span.

Calcium

Calcium values (Table 7-8) decline for men with increasing age; however, no change was found for women. In young adulthood, male values are higher than those for women but, after the fourth or fifth decade, the sex differences disappear. Even with the decline in men's values, almost all of the subjects in the 70 to 79 age group in these studies fell within the standard normal values.

For further references see Craig and Bartholemew (1970); *Documenta Geigy Scientific Tables* (1970); Goldberg, et al. (1973); Keating, et al. (1969); Roof, et al. (1976); Somerville, et al. (1977); and Williams, et al. (1978).

Cholesterol

The standard normal range for cholesterol is 150–250 mg/dl, although it varies with diet and age.

TABLE 7-7. Blood Urea Nitrogen (BUN) (mg/dl).

Age	Werner et al. (1972) N	Mean	Craig & Bartholemew (1970) N	Mean	Range	O'Kell & Elliott (1970) N	Mean	Range	Libow (1963) Age	N	Mean	Range	Libow (1971)* N	Mean	Range
MEN															
20–29	[a]	17.5	995	13.0	6.2–19.8	507	15	8.1–21.9	—	—	—	—	—	—	—
30–39	—	17.0	1306	13.6	6.9–20.3				Adult[b]	—	—	8–22	—	—	—
40–49	—	17.9	2349	14.2	7.7–20.7	964	16	7.3–24.7	—	—	—	—	—	—	—
50–59	—	18.9	2130	15.0	8.1–21.9				—	—	—	—	[c] 8	18.0	11.2–24.8
60–69	—	20.4	597	15.9	9.1–22.7	1077	18	7.6–28.4	65–91	47	17	11–23	—	—	—
70–79	—	18.1	—	—	—				—	—	—	—	[d] 8	19.0	4–34
80+	—	—	—	—		205	22	8.5–35.5	—	—	—	—	—	—	—
WOMEN															
20–29	[a]	13.8				583	12	5.2–18.8							
30–39	—	14.2													
40–49	—	16.3				1546	13	5.0–21.0							
50–59	—	16.9													
60–69	—	18.9				1448	16	5.9–26.1							
70–79	—	18.9													
80+	—	—				360	19	6.4–31.6							

Standard normal values: 8–18 mg/dl
* Values for eight healthy survivors from the 1963 Libow study

Notes:
[a] Total N > 3000 including men and women
[b] Adult group represents the NIH Clinical Pathology Laboratory normal adult values
[c] 1956
[d] 1967

TABLE 7-8. Calcium (mg/dl).

Age	Cutler et al. (1970)*			Cutler et al. (1970)†			Wilding et al. (1972)			Werner et al. (1972)		O'Kell & Elliott (1970)		
	N	Mean	Range	N	Mean	Range	N	Mean	Range	N	Mean	N	Mean	Range
MEN														
20–29	586	10.09	9.3–10.9	1843	10.08	9.2–10.9	96	10.03	9.3–10.8	a	10.20	507	9.5	8.6–10.4
30–39	943	9.99	9.2–10.8	2861	9.98	9.2–10.8	721	9.98	9.1–10.8		10.12			
40–49	1152	9.92	9.0–10.8	3958	9.92	9.1–10.8	1268	9.94	9.1–10.8		10.03	964	9.3	8.4–10.2
50–59	857	9.89	9.1–10.7	3656	9.90	9.1–10.7	1112	9.91	9.1–10.7		9.92			
60–69	314	9.80	8.9–10.7	2039	9.85	9.0–10.7	415	9.89	9.1–10.7		9.95	1077	9.1	8.0–10.2
70–79	68	9.84	9.1–10.6	676	9.88	9.0–10.8	105	9.90	8.9–10.9		9.83			
80+	—	—	—	—	—	—	—	—	—	—	—	205	8.9	7.8–10.0
WOMEN														
20–29	1003	9.83	9.0–10.7	3016	9.83	9.0–10.7	72	9.97	9.1–10.8	a	9.99	583	9.2	8.3–10.1
30–39	940	9.79	8.9–10.7	2998	9.79	8.9–10.7	193	9.85	9.1–10.6		9.87			
40–49	1292	9.75	8.8–10.7	4732	9.78	8.9–10.7	283	9.85	9.0–10.7		9.91	1546	9.2	8.3–10.1
50–59	1063	9.89	9.0–10.8	4638	9.88	9.0–10.8	278	9.98	9.2–10.8		10.01			
60–69	499	9.88	9.1–10.7	2763	9.91	9.0–10.8	229	10.05	9.2–10.9		9.96	1448	9.2	8.2–10.2
70–79	91	9.91	9.2–10.6	779	9.90	9.0–10.8	39	9.88	9.1–10.7		9.82			
80+	—	—	—	—	—	—	—	—	—	—	—	360	9.0	8.0–10.0

Standard normal values: 9.0–10.6 mg/dl; 4.5–5.3 mEq/L

* "No significant abnormality" on physical examination
† Total group

Notes: [a] Total N > 3000 including males and females

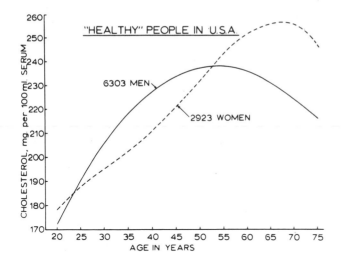

FIGURE 7-2. Averages for serum cholesterol of clinically healthy persons in the Twin cities area of Minnesota and at Tecumseh, Michigan. (From Keys, A.: Serum cholesterol and the question of "normal." In Benson, E. S., and Strandjord, P. E. (eds.): Multiple Laboratory Screening. New York: Academic Press, 1969, p. 170, with permission)

The studies show that cholesterol values rise with age. Many normal, clinically-healthy older men and women exceed these normal ranges. For example, Cutler, et al. (1970) reported values for 70- to 79-year-old males of 154–314 mg/dl and for women in this same age group, 171–347 mg/dl.

Summary graphs are presented here to demonstrate the age and sex effects on serum cholesterol. Effects of lifestyle and racial differences for those living in their country of origin have also been identified (Keys, 1969; Winsten, 1975).

Much of the research has been done using males. In Figure 7-1, Keys summarizes the data obtained in his study of 1492 men (indicated by the solid line)

and compares this with the values obtained by five other researchers. Longitudinal data confirm the shape of this curve (Keys, 1952; Libow, 1971; Thompson, et al., 1965).

Data from studies on clinically-healthy adults in the Minnesota and Michigan areas of the country illustrated sexual differences over the adult life span (Keys, 1969; Johnson, et al., 1965). Keys' data (Fig. 7-2) extended through the 75-year age group.

Johnson's data covered an extended age grouping beyond 75 years of age. His population included 33 men and 41 women between 75 and 79, and 25 men and 39 women 80-years old and over. Figure 7-3 shows cholesterol levels for all age groups.

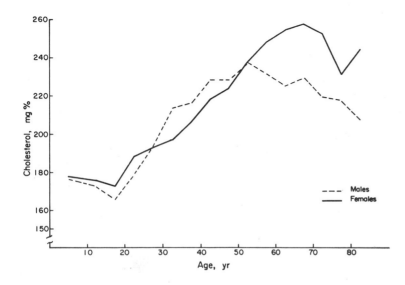

FIGURE 7-3. Mean cholesterol by age and sex, Tecumseh, Michigan, 1960. (From Johnson, B. C., et al.: Distributions and familial studies of blood pressure and serum cholesterol levels in a total community—Tecumseh, Michigan. Journal of Chronic Diseases 18:151, 1965. Used with permission of Pergamon Press, Elmsford, New York.)

TABLE 7-9. Creatinine (mg/dl).

Age	Cutler et al. (1970)* N	Mean	Range	Cutler et al. (1970)† N	Mean	Range	Wilding et al. (1972) N	Mean	Range	Rowe et al. (1976) Age	N	Mean
MEN												
20–29	586	1.08	0.7–1.4	1843	1.10	0.7–1.5	96	1.01	0.7–1.3	25–34	73	0.81
30–39	943	1.10	0.7–1.5	2861	1.12	0.7–1.5	721	1.02	0.7–1.4	35–44	122	0.81
40–49	1152	1.12	0.8–1.5	3958	1.13	0.7–1.5	1268	1.04	0.7–1.4	45–54	152	0.83
50–59	857	1.13	0.8–1.5	3656	1.15	0.7–1.6	1112	1.04	0.7–1.4	55–64	94	0.84
60–69	314	1.15	0.7–1.6	2039	1.18	0.7–1.7	415	1.05	0.7–1.4	65–74	68	0.82
70–79	68	1.19	0.8–1.6	676	1.23	0.7–1.7	105	1.10	0.7–1.5	75–84	29	0.84
80+	—	—	—	—	—	—	—	—	—	—	—	—
WOMEN												
20–29	1003	0.89	0.6–1.2	3016	0.89	0.6–1.2	72	0.79	0.4–1.1			
30–39	940	0.90	0.6–1.2	2998	0.91	0.6–1.2	193	0.83	0.6–1.1			
40–49	1292	0.93	0.6–1.2	4732	0.93	0.6–1.3	283	0.83	0.5–1.2			
50–59	1063	0.96	0.6–1.3	4638	0.96	0.6–1.3	278	0.84	0.5–1.1			
60–69	499	0.98	0.6–1.3	2763	0.99	0.6–1.4	229	0.89	0.6–1.2			
70–79	91	1.00	0.6–1.4	779	1.03	0.6–1.5	39	0.84	0.5–1.2			
80+	—	—	—	—	—	—	—	—	—			

Standard normal values: 0.6–1.2 mg/dl
* "No significant abnormality" on physical examination
† Total group

Creatinine

A small, but consistent, increase in creatinine with age was found in all studies for both men and women, with some values exceeding the standard normal range (Table 7-9). Values for men were slightly higher than those for women at all ages.

Additional references include Korenchevsky (1961); Libow (1963); and Libow (1971).

Creatinine Clearance

Creatinine clearance values decline with age. Rowe and his associates studied 548 normal men and found a decline of 44 ml/min in the mean values, though the values continued to remain within the normal range (Table 7-10 and Fig. 7-4).

From these data Rowe developed a nomogram for determination of age-adjusted percentile rank in creatinine clearance (Fig. 7-5). Further research is needed to confirm the accuracy of the nomogram using larger groups of men and including women as well, particularly since the standard normal values

TABLE 7-10. Creatinine clearance values.

Age	N*	Creatinine Clearance ml/min Mean Values
25–34	73	140.1
35–44	122	132.6
45–54	152	126.8
55–64	94	119.9
65–74	68	109.5
75–84	29	96.9

From Rowe, J. W., et al.: The effect of age on creatinine clearance in men: a cross sectional and longitudinal study. Journal of Gerontology 31:160, 1976, with permission.

* N = 543 males

Standard normal values ♂ 107–140 ml/min
♀ 87–107 ml/min

indicate sex differences. This variable is not taken into account in the present nomogram.

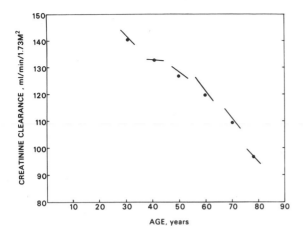

FIGURE 7-4. Comparison of cross-sectional age differences and longitudinal age changes in creatinine clearance. The dots represent the mean values for each age decade obtained from cross-sectional data. Longitudinal results are represented by line segments which indicate the mean slope of changes in creatinine clearance for each age decade. Lines are drawn with the midpoints at the mean clearance for each age decade, and with their lengths, along the abscissa, representing the mean time span over which the longitudinal data were collected for each age group. (From Rowe, J. W., et al.: The effect of age on creatinine clearance in men: a cross sectional and longitudinal study. Journal of Gerontoloty 31: 160, 1976, with permission)

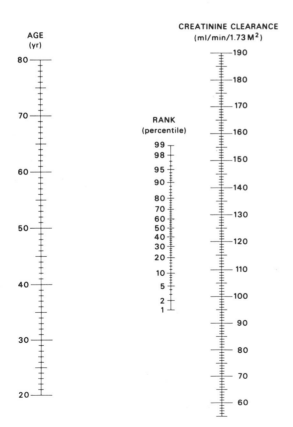

FIGURE 7-5. Nomogram for determination of age-adjusted percentile rank in true creatinine clearance. To use the nomogram: (1) Line up a straight edge with the person's age and creatinine clearance value. (2) Read the person's percentile rank at the point where the straight edge crosses the percentile rank line. (From Rowe, J. W., et al.: The effect of age on creatinine clearance in men: a cross sectional and longitudinal study. Journal of Gerontology 31:159, 1976, with permission)

TABLE 7-11. Fasting glucose (mg/dl).

Age	Wilding et al. (1972) N	Mean	Range	Craig & Bartholemew (1970) N	Mean	Range	O'Kell & Elliott (1970) N	Mean	Range	Libow (1963) Age	N	Mean	Range	Libow (1971) N	Mean	Range
MEN																
20–29	96	91.86	62.5–121.2	955	100	72–128	507	102	79.1–124.9	Adult[a]			65–110			
30–39	721	91.96	63.0–121.0	1306	104	76–132										
40–49	1268	94.14	61.1–127.1	2349	106	78–134	964	104	77.2–130.8							
50–59	1112	95.92	63.7–128.2	2130	107	78–136								8	75	63–87
60–69	415	96.68	60.2–133.2	597	109	80–138	1077	106	77.4–134.6	65–91	47	77	59–95			
70–79	105	93.63	51.8–135.4	—	—	—								8	85	69–101
80+	—	—	—	—	—	—	205	106	76.6–135.4							
WOMEN																
20–29	72	90.06	59.5–120.7				583	95	72.8–117.2							
30–39	193	92.73	65.3–120.2				1546	99	72.5–125.5							
40–49	283	94.26	64.6–123.9													
50–59	278	97.90	67.8–128.0				1448	104	72.8–135.2							
60–69	229	96.23	64.3–128.2													
70–79	39	96.46	57.8–135.2				360	106	73.3–138.7							
80+	—	—	—													

Standard normal values: 70–110 mg/dl (serum or plasma)
60–100 mg/dl (whole blood)

Notes: [a] Adult group represents the NIH Clinical Pathology Laboratory normal adult values

Fasting Glucose

While many normal subjects of all ages can be seen in Table 7-11 to exceed the standard normal ranges, older groups exceed them by the greatest amount. In his review of the effect of age on glucose tolerance, Reaven (1977) cited a small increase in fasting glucose levels beginning in young adulthood and involving approximately 2 mg/dl/decade. Other studies support this trend (Sandberg, et al., 1973; Williams, et al., 1978). Others reported either no change with age or an increase until the seventh decade and then a decline (Feldman and Plonk, 1976; Kimmerling, 1977; O'Kell and Elliott, 1970; and Wilding, et al., 1972). (For further studies, see also the references for the glucose tolerance test.)

Oral Glucose Tolerance Test (OGTT)

The postprandial glucose values increase with age, particularly those taken 1 to 2 hours after a 50 to 100 gm oral glucose challenge, as can be seen in Table 7-12. This table reports *mean* values, not the upper limits. All one-hour post-challenge mean

TABLE 7-12.   Oral glucose tolerance test (OGTT).

Study[a]	Glucose dose (g)	Source of blood[d]	AGE (YR) Young	AGE (YR) Old	Mean Blood Gluc.[e] (mg%) 1 HR Young	1 HR Old	2 HR Young	2 HR Old	Age Effect on Glucose Conc. (mg % per decade life) 1 hr	2 hr
1. U.S. Nat. Center Health Stat., 1964	50	V	18–24	75–79	100	166	—	—	12	—
2. Welborn et al., 1969	50	V	21–29	>70	86	135	—	—	10	—
3. Boyns et al., 1969	50	V	<24	>55	89	125	74	78	9	1
4. Nilsson et al., 1967	(50)[b]	C	20–39	60–79	111	154	—	—	11	—
5. Butterfield, 1966	50	C	20–29	70–79	125	194	86	121	14	7
6. Diabetes Survey Working Party, 1963	50	C	<29	>70	122	186	98	119	13	4
7. Hayner et al., 1965	100	V	16–19	70–79	100	177	—	—	13	—
8. Unger, 1957	100	V	18–29	50–59	—	—	99	131	—	11
9. Studer et al., 1969	100	C	25–34	65–74	—	—	98	127	—	7
10. Gerontology Research Center, 1972	(122)[c]	V	20–29	70–79	144	174	113	145	6	6

From Andres, R., and Tobin, J. D.: Endocrine systems. In Handbook of the Biology of Aging, edited by Caleb E. Finch and Leonard Hayflick. © 1977 by Litton Educational Publishing, Inc., p. 359. Reprinted by permission of Van Nostrand Reinhold Company, New York.
References for this table are given in Andres and Tobin (1972).

[a] In studies 3–6 and 8–10, glucose was ingested in the morning after an overnight fast. In studies 1, 2, and 7, subjects presented themselves for testing at various times of the day and at various time intervals after the last meal.
[b] 30 g glucose per m² surface area—50 g for man of average size.
[c] 1.75 g per kg body weight = 122 g per 70 kg man.
[d] V = antecubital venous blood; C = capillary blood.
[e] It should be stressed that these values should *not* be taken as the upper limits of normality. They represent mean values. Note that at 2 hours the *mean* value for the old subjects is equal to or exceeds 120 mg%, a level commonly taken to be the upper limit of normality.

Standard normal values   Fasting: 70–110 mg/dl
                          5 min: maximum of 250 mg/dl
                          60 min: significant decrease
                          120 min: below 120 mg/dl
                          180 min: fasting level

values for the old subjects exceed this upper normal range. Reaven (1977) reported studies that observed increases of from 3.5 to 14 mg/dl per decade. Glucose tolerance is one laboratory value that rises distinctly with aging on a consistent basis.

Some authors question the assumption that increasing GTT values with aging are purely ontogenetic. They suggest instead that the more direct cause is an age-related increase in weight (Kimmerling, et al., 1977; Reaven, 1977). This question has not been clearly resolved at this point.

One of the most useful tools available for interpreting GTT values at different ages is an oral GTT nomogram developed by Andres (Fig. 7-6).

Andres indicates that the percentile rank obtained on the nomogram compares the subject's values to those of age cohorts, with 50 percent being average. Percentages below 50 percent indicate increasingly poor performance in comparison to age mates. He proposes the category system shown in Table 7-13 for interpreting the GTT percentile as a standard for applying the diagnostic label of diabetes. He suggests that the table be used as a "rule of thumb" but believes future adjustments might be made in it.

For additional references on intravenous GTT

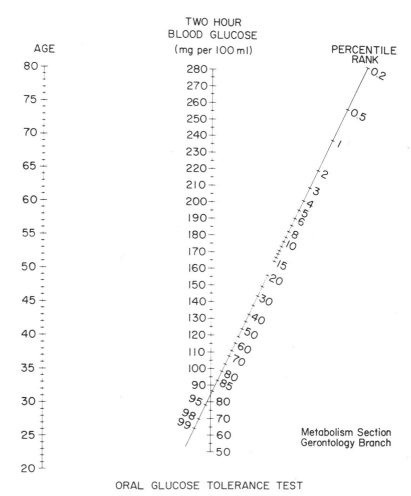

FIGURE 7-6.   Oral glucose tolerance test nomogram. To use the nomogram: (1) Line up a straight edge with the person's age and two-hour blood glucose value. (2) Read the person's percentile rank at the point where the straight edge crosses the percentile rank line. (From Andres, R.: Aging and diabetes. Medical Clinics of North America 55:841, 1971, with permission)

TABLE 7-13. Interpretation of glucose tolerance test percentile.

Age Group	Abnormal	Percentile Rank Borderline	Normal
20–29	0–2	3–4	5 and over
30–39	0–3	4–6	7 and over
40–49	0–4	5–8	9 and over
50–59	0–5	6–10	11 and over
60–69	0–6	7–12	13 and over
70 plus	0–7	8–14	15 and over

From Andres, R.: Aging and diabetes. Medical Clinics of North America 55:842, 1971, with permission.

and response of GTT to certain drugs see Andres (1971); Andres and Tobin (1972 and 1977); and Feldman and Plonk (1976).

Inorganic Phosphorus

The research located on inorganic phosphorus values in the elderly showed conflicting findings. In general, as with several other laboratory values reported in this chapter, inorganic phosphorus values range both higher and lower than standard normal ranges among the older age group. As can be seen on Table 7-14, some researchers reported no age-related changes, others indicated a decline for both men and women, while still others show for women an initial decline until the fifth decade and then an increase to above young adult levels. Older women tended to have higher values than did comparable male age groups.

For further references on inorganic phosphorus studies see Goldberg, et al. (1973); Hamilton, et al. (1956); Keating, et al. (1969); Somerville, et al. (1977); and Williams, et al. (1978).

TABLE 7-14. Inorganic phosphorus (mg/dl).

Age	Wilding et al. (1972) N	Mean	Range	Werner et al. (1972) N	Mean	Keating et al. (1969) N	Range	O'Kell & Elliott (1970) N	Mean	Range
MEN										
20–29	96	3.51	2.3–4.7	*	4.17	†	2.55–4.45	507	3.7	2.5–4.9
30–39	721	3.56	2.3–4.8		4.11		2.45–4.34			
40–49	1268	3.50	2.3–4.7		3.97		2.35–4.24	964	3.4	2.3–4.5
50–59	1112	3.51	2.3–4.7		3.87		2.24–4.14			
60–69	415	3.56	2.4–4.7		3.78		2.14–4.04	1077	3.4	2.3–4.5
70–79	105	3.62	2.2–5.0		3.78		2.04–3.94			
80+	—	—	—		—		—	205	3.4	2.1–4.7
WOMEN										
20–29	72	3.65	2.6–4.7	*	4.00	†	2.85–4.74	583	3.7	2.6–4.8
30–39	193	3.62	2.6–4.6		3.88		2.55–4.24			
40–49	283	3.60	2.4–4.8		3.87		2.55–4.25	1546	3.7	2.5–4.9
50–59	278	3.82	2.7–4.9		3.98		2.66–4.43			
60–69	229	3.85	2.8–5.0		4.02		2.79–4.65	1448	3.6	2.4–4.8
70–79	39	3.91	2.7–5.1		4.09		2.90–4.84			
80+	—	—	—		—		—	360	3.4	2.2–4.6

Standard normal values: 3.0–4.5 mg/dl; 1.8–2.6 mEq/L
* Total N > 3000 including men and women
† 298 men total; 278 women total

TABLE 7-15. Potassium.

Age	Wilding et al. (1972)			Josephson & Dahlberg (1952)			♂ & ♀ Age	Herbeuval et al. (1954)			Mean Range (mEq/dl)	
	N	Mean (mM/l)	Range	N	Mean (mg/dl)	Range		N	Mean (mg/dl)	Range		
MEN 20–29	96	4.34	3.7–5.0	23	18.67	14.6–22.8	Normal Adults	30	175.5	154.3–196.7	4.5	3.96–5.04
30–39	721	4.38	3.6–5.1	—	—	—	60–69	74	183.5	150.7–216.3	4.7	3.88–5.52
40–49	1268	4.39	3.6–5.1	—	—	—	70–79	88	185.8	145.4–226.2	4.76	3.74–5.78
50–59	1112	4.44	3.7–5.2	—	—	—	80–90	42	186.6	160 –213.2	4.78	4.10–5.46
60–69	415	4.49	3.7–5.3	60[a]	20.50	16.7–24.3						
70–79	105	4.55	3.5–5.6	54	19.90	16.4–23.4						
80+	—	—	—									
WOMEN 20–29	72	4.31	3.5–5.1	20	18.49	16.4–21.6						
30–39	193	4.29	3.5–5.1	—	—	—						
40–49	283	4.30	3.5–5.1	—	—	—						
50–59	278	4.37	3.6–5.2	—	—	—						
60–69	229	4.47	3.6–5.3	—	—	—						
70–79	39	4.33	3.5–5.2	54	20.03	16.4–23.6						
80+	—	—	—									

Standard normal values: 3.8–5.0 mEq/L   [a] 60–64 years

Potassium

The three largest studies used in Table 7-15 showed a slight increase in potassium with advancing age. Those subjects at the upper end of the range, particularly in the older ages, exceeded the upper end of the range for standard normal values.

Other research includes work by Korenchevsky (1961); Leask et al. (1973); Roberts (1967); Sweetin and Thomson (1973); and Videbaeck (1953).

TABLE 7-16. Total protein (gm/dl).

Age	Cutler et al. (1970)*			Cutler et al. (1970)†			Werner et al. (1972)	Keating et al. (1969)	O'Kell & Elliott (1970)		
	N	Mean	Range	N	Mean	Range	N Mean	Range	N	Mean	Range
MEN											
20–29	586	7.15	6.3–8.0	1843	7.17	6.3–8.0	‡ 7.67	6.2–7.7	507	7.1	6.1–8.1
30–39	943	7.08	6.2–7.9	2861	7.09	6.2–8.0	7.63	6.2–7.6			
40–49	1152	6.98	6.1–7.9	3958	7.02	6.1–7.9	7.51	6.1–7.5	964	6.9	5.8–8.0
50–59	857	6.95	6.0–7.9	3656	6.98	6.1–7.9	7.46	6.0–7.4			
60–69	314	6.90	6.0–7.8	2039	6.98	6.1–7.9	7.39	6.0–7.4	1077	6.8	5.7–7.9
70–79	68	6.94	6.0–7.9	676	7.01	6.0–8.0	7.51	5.9–7.3			
80+	—	—	—	—	—	—	—	—	205	6.6	5.4–7.8
WOMEN											
20–29	1003	6.97	6.1–7.8	3016	6.98	6.1–7.9	‡ 7.54	6.0–7.5	583	6.9	5.8–8.0
30–39	940	6.90	6.0–7.8	2998	6.94	6.0–7.8	7.49	6.0–7.4			
40–49	1292	6.85	6.0–7.7	4732	6.88	6.0–7.8	7.48	5.9–7.4	1546	6.8	5.7–7.9
50–59	1063	6.88	6.0–7.8	4638	6.92	6.0–7.9	7.49	5.9–7.3			
60–69	499	6.88	6.0–7.8	2763	6.95	6.0–7.8	7.35	5.9–7.3	1448	6.7	5.6–7.8
70–79	91	6.79	5.9–7.7	779	6.92	6.0–7.9	7.36	5.8–7.2			
80+	—	—	—	—	—	—	—	—	360	6.5	5.3–7.7

Standard normal values: 6.0–7.8 gm/dl
* "No significant abnormality" on physical examination
† Total group
‡ Total N > 3000 including men and women

Total Protein

Most studies reported a slight decline in the total protein with increasing age, corresponding to decreasing albumin levels (Table 7-16). All age groups in the studies, including the oldest subjects tended to fall within the standard normal values.

For additional references, see Goldberg, et al. (1973); Karel, et al. (1956); Libow (1963); Oeriu (1964); and Prusik (1957).

TABLE 7-17.   Sodium.

Age	Wilding et al. (1972) N	Mean (mM/L)	Range	Josephson & Dahlberg (1952) N	Mean	Range (mg/dl)	♂ & ♀ Age	Herbeuval et al. (1954) N	Mean (mgm/dl)	Range	Mean (mEq/dl)	Range
MEN							Normal					
20–29	96	140.52	134.6–146.4	22	356.3	298.9–413.7	Adults	30	3.34	—	145.0	—
30–39	721	140.49	135.2–145.8	—	—	—	60–69	47	3.29	311–347	143.0	135.4–150.6
40–49	1268	140.45	135.2–145.7	—	—	—	70–79	51	3.26	313–340	141.7	135.9–147.5
50–59	1112	140.56	135.1–146.0	—	—	—	80–90	26	3.26	301–351	141.7	130.7–152.7
60–69	415	140.51	135.0–146.0	60[a]	346.6	292.2–401.0						
70–79	105	140.28	134.0–146.6	54	338.6	306.2–371.0						
80+	—	—	—									
WOMEN												
20–29	72	139.80	134.5–145.1	20	359.6	293.0–420.2						
30–39	193	139.89	134.4–145.4	—	—	—						
40–49	283	140.02	134.6–145.4	—	—	—						
50–59	278	140.76	135.6–146.0	—	—	—						
60–69	229	141.19	135.6–146.8	—	—	—						
70–79	39	140.02	134.7–145.3	54	339.5	306.5–372.5						
80+	—	—	—									

Standard normal values: 136–142 mEq/L or mM/L
[a] 60–64 years

Sodium

The age-related changes in sodium are not clear, as evidenced by the three studies in Table 7-17. Two of these studies show a decline in mean values with age, while the third study shows there is no change. The 70 to 79 age group demonstrates a wider normal range than the standard normal values, and this extends both higher and lower than the standard.

For additional references see Korenchevsky (1961); Leask et al. (1973); Roberts (1967); and Sweetin and Thomson (1973).

TABLE 7-18. Uric acid (mg/dl).

Age	Cutler et al. (1970)*			Cutler et al. (1970)†			Wilding et al. (1972)			Werner et al. (1972)		O'Kell & Elliott (1970)		
	N	Mean	Range	N	Mean	Range	N	Mean	Range	N	Mean	N	Mean	Range
MEN														
20–29	586	5.50	3.1–7.9	1843	5.49	3.1–7.9	96	6.29	4.0–8.6	‡	6.23	507	5.9	3.2–8.6
30–39	943	5.47	3.0–7.9	2861	5.58	2.9–8.3	721	6.54	4.2–8.9		6.44			
40–49	1152	5.52	3.1–7.9	3958	5.61	3.0–8.2	1268	6.52	4.1–8.9		6.35	964	5.9	3.2–8.6
50–59	857	5.52	3.0–8.0	3656	5.65	2.9–8.4	1112	6.53	4.1–8.9		6.42			
60–69	314	5.39	2.9–7.9	2039	5.66	2.9–8.4	415	6.45	4.0–8.9		6.39	1077	5.7	2.8–8.6
70–79	68	5.84	2.9–8.8	676	5.82	2.9–8.8	105	6.41	3.1–8.8		6.19			
80+	—	—	—	—	—	—	—	—	—		—	205	5.9	2.6–9.2
WOMEN														
20–29	1003	3.87	2.0–5.7	3016	3.93	2.0–5.8	72	4.89	2.9–6.9	‡	4.66	583	4.6	2.2–7.0
30–39	940	3.82	2.1–5.5	2998	3.94	2.0–5.8	193	4.63	2.5–6.7		4.69			
40–49	1292	3.96	2.1–5.8	4732	4.09	2.0–6.2	283	4.66	2.6–6.7		4.97	1546	4.6	1.8–6.4
50–59	1063	4.18	2.3–6.1	4638	4.42	2.1–6.8	278	5.11	2.8–7.4		5.26			
60–69	499	4.42	2.2–6.7	2763	4.67	2.1–7.3	229	5.58	3.3–7.9		5.43	1448	5.0	2.7–8.2
70–79	91	4.83	2.4–7.2	779	4.91	2.1–7.7	39	5.22	2.7–7.7		5.20			
80+	—	—	—	—	—	—	—	—	—		—	360	5.2	1.9–8.5

Standard normal values: Men   2.1–7.8 mg/dl
Women 2.0–6.4 mg/dl
* "No significant abnormality" on physical examination
† Total group
‡ Total N > 3000 including men and women

Uric Acid

Age-related changes in uric acid, according to the studies found, are those of increasing values, particularly among women (Table 7-18). For the over-70 group, the upper ranges of values found (8.8 for men and 7.7 for women), exceeded the normal high range of the standards (7.8 and 6.4 for men and women respectively). Males at all ages have higher uric acid values than do females. It may explain their higher risk of gout.

For further studies refer to Gephardt, et al. (1964); Goldberg, et al. (1973); and Korenchevsky (1961).

ENZYMES

Alkaline Phosphatase

A gradual increase in serum alkaline phosphatase activity occurs in both men and women throughout life. The increase is more marked in women, tending to eliminate the sex differences of higher values among males in the earlier years (Table 7-19). Normal values in older healthy adults may be one to one-and-a-half times the standard normal values (Clark, et al. (1951); Winsten (1975).

Additional work is reported by Keating, et al. (1969); Somerville, et al. (1977); and Williams, et al (1978).

TABLE 7-19. Alkaline phosphatase.

Age	N	Wilding et al. (1972) Mean (KA units)	Range	N	Werner et al. (1972) Mean (U)	Keating et al. (1969) Range (IU)	Age	N	Clark et al. (1951) Mean (NPP units)	Range	N	O'Kell & Elliott (1970) Mean (mU/ml)	Range
MEN													
20–29	96	9.41	4.7–14.1	*	50.1	18.51–73.99	25–29	8	2.46	1.42–3.90	507	47	21.5–72.5
30–39	721	9.50	4.2–14.8		48.2	19.18–75.34	30–34	10	2.16	1.46–2.87			
							35–39	19	2.05	0.97–3.96			
40–49	1268	9.79	4.4–15.2		51.4	19.87–76.70	40–44	18	2.45	1.54–3.73	964	51	22.4–79.6
							45–49	12	2.21	1.23–3.44			
50–59	1112	9.98	4.1–15.8		55.5	20.58–78.08	50–59	55	2.39	1.13–5.29			
60–69	415	10.21	3.7–16.7		57.3	21.29–79.47	—	—	—	—	1077	54	22.9–85.1
70–79	105	8.64	2.0–15.3		56.8	22.02–80.87	—	—	—	—			
80+	—	—	—		—	—	80–84	29	2.91	0.84–6.02	205	56	23.7–88.3
							85–92	20	2.68	1.22–4.97			
WOMEN													
20–29	72	7.28	3.6–10.9	*	41.4	12.21–62.77	25–29	17	1.77	1.06–2.56	583	43	20.1–65.9
30–39	193	7.11	2.7–11.6		41.9	13.95–66.66	30–34	18	1.55	0.99–2.67			
							35–39	13	1.55	1.07–2.08			
40–49	283	7.75	2.6–12.9		43.2	15.82–70.67	40–44	10	1.66	1.25–2.39	1546	47	15.9–78.1
							45–49	—	—	—			
50–59	278	9.87	3.6–16.1		54.0	17.80–74.79	50–59	23	2.51	0.88–5.99			
60–69	229	10.66	3.7–17.6		61.7	19.90–79.04	—	—	—	—	1448	57	24.9–89.1
70–79	39	10.51	3.7–17.4		60.9	22.12–83.40	—	—	—	—			
80+	—	—	—		—	—	80–84	31	2.80	1.31–5.10	360	60	25.8–94.2
							85–92	18	2.91	1.73–6.35			

Standard normal values: 1.5–4.5 U/dl (Bodansky)
4.0–13.0 U/dl (King-Armstrong)
0.8–2.3 U/ml (Bessey-Lowry)
15.0–35.0 U/ml (Shinowara-Jones-Reinhart)
* Total N > 3000 including both men and women

Lactate Dehydrogenase (LDH)

In general, the data reflect an age-related increase in lactate dehydrogenase (Table 7-20). Differences in values between men and women are not clearly demonstrated.

For further reference, see Conconi, et al. (1963); Hesch, et al. (1976); Schiele, et al. (1974); and Williams, et al. (1978). Schiele's group found no significant age changes, while Conconi's and Williams' data support an age-related increase in lactate dehydrogenase.

Serum Creatine Phosphokinase (SCPK)

Standard normal values for serum creatine phosphokinase are:

♂ 55–170 U/L at 37°C
♀ 30–135 U/L at 37°C

Researchers studying serum creatine phosphokinase (SCPK) generally studied only small samples and did not report the specific values for different age groups; however, they reported that there were *no significant changes with age* (Hesch, et al. 1976; McCormick, 1976; Sweetin and Thomson, 1973; Thomson, 1968). In a larger study, Worthy and co-workers (1970) observed age-related changes in SCPK in 248 men and 268 women with highest values in the 40 to 49 year-old group in males and in the 60 to 69 year olds among the females. There are no data to indicate normal ranges for older persons. Sex differ-

TABLE 7-20. Lactate dehydrogenase (LDH).

Age	Werner et al. (1972) Mean N (U/l)	Davis et al. (1966) N	Mean U	Range	O'Kell & Elliott (1970) N	Mean (mU/ml)	Range	Munan et al. (1977) Age	N	Mean (IU/l)	Range
MEN											
20–29	* 145	—	—	—	507	115	61.1–168.9	25–34	182	177.8	115.3–240.3
30–39	153	—	—	—				35–44	131	186.0	116.4–255.6
40–49	148	19	252	130–374	964	123	65.4–180.6	45–54	137	187.8	115.2–260.4
50–59	159	32	262	134–390				55–64	101	187.3	121.3–253.3
60–69	159	102	254	140–368	1077	128	60.9–195.1	65–74	92	179.8	122.4–237.2
70–79	176	93	265	99–431				≥75	40	195.6	122.8–268.4
80+	—	18	254	172–336	205	135	69.9–200.1				
WOMEN											
20–29	* 138				583	109	62.9–155.1	25–34	216	164.5	89.9–239.1
30–39	143							35–44	162	174.0	97.6–250.4
40–49	148				1546	118	63.9–172.1	45–54	186	179.3	92.9–265.7
50–59	161							55–64	127	191.5	120.3–262.7
60–69	173				1448	131	70.9–191.1	65–74	104	192.9	117.3–268.5
70–79	163							≥75	43	191.9	133.6–250.2
80+	—				360	141	76.3–205.7				

Standard normal values: 71–207 IU/L
   80–120 Wacker units
   150–450 Wroblewski units
* Total N > 3000 including both men and women

ences were found by Worthy and coworkers (1970), McCormick (1976), and Thomson (1968), with males having consistently higher means and ranges.

Other researchers report elevated SCPK levels in some healthy persons (Emery and Spikesman, 1970) and elevations with exercise (Griffiths, 1966).

Serum Glutamic Pyruvic Transaminase (SGPT); Alanine Aminotransferase

The two studies reported on Table 7-21 included very small numbers of subjects, so it would be unwise

TABLE 7-21. Alanine/aminotransferase (glutamic pyruvic transaminase, SGPT) values for men and women.

	Conconi et al. (1963)				Hesch et al. (1976)		
Age	N	Mean	Range	Age	N	Mean	Range
20–45	20	17.2	6.6–27.6	—	—	—	—
51–64	21	8.6	0.0–18.4	—	—	—	—
65–74	28	7.3	0.0–15.3	Over 60	22	6.60	0.74–12.5
75–89	31	9.7	0.0–22.3	—	—	—	—

SGPT—Standard normal value 1–36 U/l

TABLE 7-22. Aspartate aminotransferase; serum glutamic oxalacetic transamenase (SGOT).

Age	Cutler et al. (1970)*			Cutler et al. (1970)†			Wilding et al. (1972) Mean			Werner et al. (1972)		O'Kell & Elliott (1970) Mean		
	N	Mean	Range	N	Mean	Range	N	(RF units)‡	Range	N	Mean (U)	N	(mU/ml)	Range
MEN														
20–29	586	18.59	0.0–48.4	1843	18.51	0.0–40.6	96	15.46	0.7–30.3	§	31.6	507	39	14.5–63.5
30–39	943	18.55	0.0–43.4	2861	19.85	0.0–48.9	721	16.34	0.4–32.3		32.9			
40–49	1152	18.79	0.0–35.8	3958	19.45	0.0–40.3	1268	16.52	1.1–32.0		33.9	964	38	17.0–59.0
50–59	857	19.26	0.0–43.1	3656	19.59	0.0–40.0	1112	17.07	0.4–33.8		34.8			
60–69	314	18.31	1.6–35.0	2039	18.96	0.5–37.4	415	15.97	1.4–30.5		34.7	1077	39	17.3–60.7
70–79	68	19.19	0.2–38.1	676	19.06	0.0–43.2	105	17.10	0.0–41.2		38.0			
80+	—	—	—	—	—	—	—	—	—		—	205	40	15.2–64.8
WOMEN														
20–29	1003	14.65	3.1–26.2	3016	15.21	0.0–31.8	72	11.01	0.0–22.5	§	29.2	583	33	15.0–51.0
30–39	940	14.99	3.5–26.5	2998	15.37	1.7–29.1	193	12.07	0.0–27.7		29.0			
40–49	1292	15.25	0.8–29.7	4732	15.80	0.6–31.0	283	11.95	0.0–26.8		30.4	1546	35	15.4–54.6
50–59	1063	17.23	0.0–44.8	4638	17.61	0.0–40.9	278	13.74	2.0–25.5		33.8			
60–69	499	16.95	4.1–29.8	2763	17.76	0.0–37.0	229	14.68	0.4–29.0		33.7	1448	38	16.2–59.8
70–79	91	16.83	1.8–31.8	779	18.20	0.0–46.7	39	15.31	0.0–32.6		30.4			
80+	—	—	—	—	—	—	—	—	—		—	360	41	19.7–62.3

Standard normal values: 8–33 U/ml
* "No significant abnormality" on physical examination
† Total group
‡ Reitman Frankel units
§ Total N > 3000 including both men and women

to draw conclusions from the data. In Conconi's study (1963), SGPT decreased with age, although all subjects fall within the standard normal range. For additional references see Sweetin and Thomson (1973) and Thomson (1968).

Serum Glutamic Oxalacetic Transaminase (SGOT); Aspartate Aminotransferase

There appears to be no age-related changes in SGOT values for males. However, values for females increase somewhat with age, achieving almost equal levels with males in some studies, but remaining a bit lower in others (Table 7-22). Subjects of all the studies showed a wider range of values than those cited in the standard normal values.

For additional references see Conconi, et al. (1963); Hesch, et al. (1976); Rose, et al. (1976); Sweetin and Thomson (1973); Thomson (1968); and Williams, et al. (1978).

URINALYSIS

Findings on urinalysis are not influenced by age in a clinically important way in healthy older persons (Lane, 1963; Rowe, 1977). Data are available on specific gravity of small groups of persons from 40 to 89 years of age, as illustrated in Table 7-23. Goldman (1971) cited a study indicating a maximum specific gravity of 1.032 in youth which decreased to 1.024 at age 80. The maximum urinary osmolality decreases from 1040 at 20 years to 750 at 80 years (see Chapter 6, p. 60).

SUMMARY

Changing laboratory values reflect the normal physiologic changes of aging as well as pathophysiologic problems. One of the challenges of working with older persons involves the valid interpretation of the changing states of the individual. All the tables in this chapter clearly point out that trends begin in the young adult (30 to 39 years group) and continue over the ensuing decades.

Many of the age-related changes in laboratory values discussed in this chapter are small, yet they indicate the importance of an awareness of *age standardized norms* when caring for the older person. Even where the mean value for a group of persons on any particular laboratory test changes only minimally with advancing years, the variance of the values also commonly increases, resulting in values for older persons at both ends of the range who could be labeled as having an abnormal or questionable laboratory result when actually they are still within the *normal limits for their age group.* Because normal individual differences in all parameters increase with age, it is important to evaluate carefully all the data available concerning the individual—behavior, self-experience, and signs and symptoms as well as laboratory values in the context of knowledge about normal changes with aging before making a judgment about what the laboratory values suggest.

A lower, or higher, normal range for a laboratory test in older individuals could mean that those people are closer to a level that indicates risks of serious problems. On the other hand, it could mean that the older person is able to tolerate lower or higher levels of that particular substance without getting into difficulty. Age-related changes occur gradually over many years, allowing many individuals' physiology to adjust to the altered levels without distress. Glucose tolerance and cholesterol values may be examples of changes to which the body adapts. There is no question that the interpretation is difficult. Research is continuing in an effort to clarify these issues.

TABLE 7-23.   Specific gravity of urine.

Age (yrs.)	Addis-Shervky concentration test	
	Number of persons in group	Specific gravity of urine
40–49	8	1.029 (1.0258–1.0362)
50–59	4	1.029 (1.0258–1.0316)
60–69	8	1.028 (1.0230–1.0308)
70–79	7	1.025 (1.0179–1.0327)
80–89	11	1.024 (1.0210–1.0281)

Adapted from Korenchevsky, V.: Physiological and Pathological Aging. New York: Hafner Publishing Co., 1961, p. 438, and Karger, Basel, 1961. The 1961 table was recalculated and abbreviated from Lewis and Alving: American Journal of Physiology, 1938, p. 123. Used with permission.

Standard normal values: 1.016–1.022 (normal fluid intake) 1.001–1.035 (range)

Nurses are in a critical position in interpreting laboratory values—to themselves and others. Their close contact with the patient and their skills in observation make it possible to synthesize many kinds of input about the patient. One crucial factor in making any judgments, however, must be that they do not rely upon their recall of normal values learned at an earlier time, normal values that apply to young people.

BIBLIOGRAPHY

Altman, P. L.: Blood and Other Body Fluids. Washington D.C.: Federation of American Societies of Experimental Biology, 1961.

Altman, P. L., and Dittmer, D. S. (eds.): Biology Data Book, Vol. III, ed. 2. Bethesda, Md.: Federation of American Societies for Experimental Biology, 1974.

Andres, R.: Aging and diabetes. Med. Clin. N. Am. 55:835–846, 1971.

Andres, R., and Tobin, J. D.: Endocrine systems. In Finch, C. E., and Hayflick, L. (eds.): Handbook of the Biology of Aging. New York: Van Nostrand Reinhold Co., 1977, p. 357–378.

Andres, R., and Tobin, J. D.: Aging, carbohydrate metabolism, and diabetes. Proceedings of the Ninth International Congress of Gerontology 1:276–280, 1972.

Bartuska, D. G.: Physiology of aging: metabolic changes during the climacteric and menopausal periods. Clin. Obstet. Gynecol. 20:105–112, 1977.

Brown, K. S., and Forbes, W. F.: A mathematical model of aging processes. III. Comments on the relative importance of serum cholesterol and blood pressure levels on mortality. J. Gerontol. 30:513–525, 1975.

Calloway, N. O., and Dollevoet, P. L.: Selected tabular material on aging. In Finch, C. E., and Hayflick, L. (eds.): Handbook of the Biology of Aging. New York: Van Nostrand Reinhold Co., 1977, p. 666–708.

Clark, L. C., Beck, E. I., and Shock, N.W.: Serum alkaline phosphatase in middle and old age. J. Gerontol. 6:7–12, 1951. (The 50 to 90-year-old group consisted of unselected residents of a hospital and home for the aged, and those below 50 years of age were parents in a research program. The latter group was screened by routine medical and laboratory examinations.)

Conconi, F., Manenti F., and Benatti, G.: Behavior of some enzyme activities in plasma in normal subjects in relation to age. Acta Vitaminologica 17:33–35, 1963.

Craig, J. L., and Bartholomew, M. D.: Blood profile ranges by age decades in 7,337 male employees. In Advances in Automated Analysis, Vol. III, Technicon International Congress, 1969. White Plains, N.Y.: Mediad, Inc., 1970, p. 105–114. (7,337 male employees of the Tennessee Valley Authority.)

Cunnick, W. R., et al.: Biochemical profiles in a healthy employee population: distribution of values classified by age and sex. In Advances in Automated Analysis, Vol. III, Technicon International Congress, 1969. White Plains, N.Y.: Mediad, Inc., 1970, p. 85–88.

Cutler, J. L., et al.: Normal values for multiphasic screening blood chemistry test. In Advances in Automated Analysis, Vol. III, Technicon International Congress, 1969. White Plains, N.Y.: Mediad, Inc., 1970, p. 67–73. (Total group: large population undergoing Automated Multiphasic Screening. Subgroup: "No significant abnormality" found on physical examination. This subgroup comprised from 32 percent of the total 30 to 39 age group, down to 11 percent for the 70 to 79 age group.)

Davidshohn, I., and Henry, J. B. (eds.): Todd-Sanford Clinical Diagnosis by Laboratory Methods, ed. 15. Philadelphia: W. B. Saunders Co., 1974, Appendix 3, p. 1376–1392.

Davis, R. L., et al.: Serum lactate and lactic dehydrogenase levels of aging males. J. Gerontol. 21:571–574, 1966. (Ambulatory residents of a V.A. Domiciliary free of overt acute disease and with no clinical or laboratory evidence of significant liver or renal disease.)

Diem, K., and Lentner, C. (eds.): Documenta Geigy Scientific Tables, ed. 7. Basel, Switzerland: Ciba-Geigy Limited, 1970.

Eckerström, S.: Sedimentation reaction in normal aged persons. Nordisk Medicen 11:471–472, 1949. (Screened by physical examination for diseases which might cause changes in sedimentation rate.)

Emery, A. E. H., and Spikesman, A. M.: Serum creatine kinase levels. Brit. Med. J. 2:790, 1970.

Feldman, J. M., and Plonk, J. W.: Effect of age on intravenous glucose tolerance and insulin secretion. J. Am. Geriatr. Soc. 24:1–3, 1976.

Fowler, W. M., Stephens, R. L., and Stump, R. B.: The changes in hematologic values in elderly patients, Am. J. Clin. Pathol. 9:700–705, 1941.

Gephardt, M. C., Hanlon, T. J., and Matson, C. F.: Blood uric acid values as related to sex and age. J.A.M.A. 189:1028–1029, 1964.

Gherondache, C. N., Romanoff, L. P., and Pincus, G.: Steroid hormones in aging men. In Gitman, L. (ed.): Endocrines and Aging. Springfield, Ill.: Charles C Thomas, 1967, p. 76–101.

Gofman, J. W., Young, W., and Tandy, R.: Ischemic heart disease, atherosclerosis, and longevity. Circulation, 34:679–697, 1966.

Goldberg, D. M.: Demographic and analytic factors affecting the normal range of serum enzyme activities. Clin. Biochem. 9:168–172, 1976.

Goldberg, D. M., Handyside, A. J., and Winfield, D. A.: Influence of demographic factors on serum concentrations of seven chemical constituents in healthy human subjects. Clin. Chem. 19:395–402, 1973.

Goldman, R.: Decline in organ function with aging. In Rossman, I. (ed.): Clinical Geriatrics. Philadelphia: J. B. Lippincott Co., 1971.

Gregerman, R. I.: The age-related alteration of thyroid function and thyroid hormone metabolism in man. In Gitman, L. (ed.): Endocrines and Aging. Springfield, Ill.: Charles C Thomas, 1967, p. 161–173.

Griffiths, P. D.: Serum levels of ATP: creatine phosphotransferase (creatine kinase)—the normal range and effect of muscular activity. Clinica Chimica Acta 13: 413–420, 1966.

Hamilton, J. B., Bunch, L., and Hirschman, A.: Serum inorganic phosphorus levels in males and females at progressive ages, with concomitant measurements of urinary ketosteroids and androgens in men. J. Clin Endocrin. Metabol. 16:463–472, 1956.

Hayes, G. S., and Stinson, I. N.: Erythrocyte sedimentation rate and age. Arch. Ophthalmol. 94:939–940, 1976.

Herbeuval, R., Cuny, G., and Manciaux, M.: Des électrolytes K et Na et de la pression osmotique du plasma par le delta cryoscopique. La Presse Médicale 62:1555–1556, 1954. (Subjects screened for diseases affecting the ionic equilibrium—they retained subjects with problems such as hypertension, arteritis, and hemiplegia.)

Hesch, R. D., et al.: Total and free triiodothyronine and thyroid-binding globulin concentration in elderly human persons. European J. Clin. Investigation 6:139–145, 1976. (Healthy subjects, none on drugs known to influence protein-binding of thyroid hormones.)

Hodkinson, H. M.: Biochemical Diagnosis of the Elderly. New York: John Wiley and Sons, 1977.

Hollingsworth, J. W., Hashizume, A., and Jablon, S.: Correlations between tests of aging in Hiroshima subjects—an attempt to define 'physiologic age.' Yale J. Biol. Med. 38:11–26, 1965.

Johnson, B. C., Epstein, F. H., and Kjelsberg, M. O.: Distributions and familial studies of blood pressure and serum cholesterol levels in a total community—Tecumseh, Michigan. J. Chronic Dis. 18:147–160, 1965.

Josephson, B., and Dahlberg, G.: Variations in the cell content and chemical composition of the human blood due to age, sex, and season. Scandinavian J. Clin. Lab. Invest. 4:216–236, 1952. (Healthy population, determined by questionnaire.)

Kagan, A., et al.: The Framingham Study: a prospective study of coronary heart disease. Federation Proceedings, 21:52–57, 1962.

Karel, J. L., Wilder, V. M., and Beber, M.: Electrophoretic serum protein patterns in the aged. J. Am Geriatr. Soc. 4:667–682, 1956.

Keating, F. R., et al.: The relation of age and sex to distribution of values in healthy adults of serum calcium, inorganic phosphorus, magnesium, alkaline phosphatase, total proteins, albumin, and blood urea. J. Lab. Clin. Med. 73:825–834, 1969. (Caucasian population, identified as healthy at routine physical examinations.)

Keys, A.: Serum cholesterol and the question of "normal." In Benson, E. S., and Strandjord, P. E. (eds.): Multiple Laboratory Screening. New York: Academic Press, 1969, p. 147–170.

Keys, A.: The age trend of serum concentrations of cholesterol and of S_f 10–20 ('G') substances in adults. J. Gerontol. 7:201–206, 1952. (Healthy men who remained healthy over four years when studied annually.)

Kimmerling, G., Javorski, W. C., and Reaven, G. M.: Aging and insulin resistance in a group of non-obese male volunteers. J. Am. Geriatr. Soc. 25:349–353, 1977.

Kohn, R. R.: Heart and cardiovascular system. In Finch, C. E., and Hayflick, L. (eds.): Handbook of the Biology of Aging. New York: Van Nostrand Reinhold Co., 1977, p. 281–317.

Korenchevsky, V.: Physiological and Pathological Aging. New York: Hafner Publishing Co., 1961.

Lane, M. H., and Vates, T. S., Jr.: Medical selection, evaluation, and classification of subjects. In Birren, J. E., et al. (eds.): Human Aging, A Biological and Behavioral Study. Washington D.C.: U.S. Department of Health, Education, and Welfare, 1963, p. 13–25.

Leask, R. G. S., Andrews, G. R., and Caird, F. I.: Normal values for sixteen blood constituents in the elderly. Age and Aging 2:14–21, 1973.

Libow, L. S.: Medical investigation of the processes of aging. In Birren, J. E., et al. (eds.): Human Aging, A Biological and Behavioral Study. Washington D.C.: U.S. Department of Health, Education, and Welfare, 1963, p. 37. (Physically healthy, socially independent aged group, including a subgroup in optimal health and a subgroup with mild asymptomatic disease—lab values were very similar between the two subgroups.)

Libow, L. S.: Medical factors in survival and mortality of the healthy elderly. In Granick, S., and Patterson, R. D. (eds.): Human Aging II, An Eleven-year Followup Biomedical and Behavioral Study. Washington D.C.: U.S. Department of Health, Education, and Welfare, 1971, p. 21–39. (For population description, see Libow, 1963.)

Ludvigsen, B., and Taylor, A.: Profile studies on the population of western South Carolina. Advances in Automated Analysis, Vol. III, Technicon International Congress, 1969. White Plains, N.Y.: Mediad, Inc., 1970, p. 15–24.

Maekawa, Tadashi: Hematologic diseases. In Steinberg, F. U. (ed.): Cowdry's The Care of the Geriatric Patient. St. Louis: C. V. Mosby Co., 1976, p. 152–166.

McCormick, C.: The normal range for serum creatinine phosphokinase. Irish J. Med. Sci. 145:86–91, 1976.

McGavack, T. H.: Endocrine ichnography of aging. In Gitman, L. (ed.): Endocrines and Aging. Springfield, Ill.: Charles C Thomas, 1967, p. 36–50.

Miller, I.: Normal hematologic standards in the aged. J. Lab. Clin. Med. 24:1172–1176, 1939.

Miller, I.: Blood sedimentation rates in middle aged and old people. J. Lab. Clin. Med. 21:1227–1230, 1936. (496 apparently normal old men tested during admission to hospital.)

Munan, L., Kelly, A., and Petitclerc, C.: Enzymatic activity patterns in probability population samples, serum lactate dehydrogenase. Am. J. Clin. Pathol. 68:587–591,

1977. (An area cluster probability sample of a national population—no health screening.)

Norris, A. H., Lundy, T., and Shock, N. W.: Trends in selected indices of body composition in men between the ages of 30 and 80 years. Ann. New York Academy Sciences 110:623–639, 1963.

Oeriu, S.: Proteins in development and senescence. In Strehler, B. L. (ed.): Advances in Gerontological Research, Vol. 1. New York: Academic Press, 1964, p. 23–85.

O'Kell, R. T., and Elliott, J. R.: Development of normal values for use in multitest biochemical screening of sera. Clin. Chem. 16:161–165, 1970. (All patients admitted to hospital in a certain time period. All values outside three standard deviations were excluded.)

Olbrich, O.: Blood changes in the aged. Edinburgh Med. J. 55:100–115, 1948. (67 Subjects, 34 men and 33 women. Characteristics of the population were not given.)

Prusik, B.: The importance of the composition of blood proteins in aged. Proceedings, 4th Congress of the International Association of Gerontology, Merane, Italy, 2:400–405, 1957.

Rafsky, H. A., et al.: Electrophoretic studies on the serum of 'normal' aged individuals. Am. J. Med. Sci. 224:522–528, 1952.

Reaven, G. M.: Does age affect glucose tolerance? Geriatrics August, 1977, p. 51–54.

Reed, A. H., et al.: Estimation of normal ranges from a controlled sample survey. I. Sex- and age-related influence on the SMA 12/60 screening group of tests. Clin Chem. 18:57–66, 1972. (Subjects clinically normal on physical examination.)

Roberts, L. B.: The normal ranges, with statistical analysis for seventeen blood constituents. Clinica Chimica Acta 16:69–78, 1967.

Roof, B. S., et al.: Serum parathyroid hormone levels and serum calcium levels from birth to senescence. Mechanisms of Aging and Development 5:289–304, 1976. (A mixed racial group (white, black, oriental) of "normal subjects.")

Rose, C. S., et al.: Age Differences in vitamin B_6 status of 617 men. Am. J. Clin. Nutrition 29:847–853, 1976.

Rowe, J. W.: Clinical research on aging: strategies and directions. New Engl. J. Med. 297:1332–1336, 1977.

Rowe, J. W., et al.: The effect of age on creatinine clearance in men: a cross sectional and longitudinal study. J. Gerontology 31:155–163, 1976. (Subjects screened by physical examination and a variety of clinical and laboratory tests.)

Sanadi, D. R.: Metabolic changes and their significance in aging. In Finch, C. E., and Hayflick, L. (eds.): Handbook of the Biology of Aging. New York: Van Nostrand Reinhold Co., 1977, p. 73–98.

Sandberg, H., et al.: Effects of oral glucose levels on serum immunoreactive insulins, free fatty acid, growth hormone, blood sugar levels in young and adult subjects. J. Am. Geriatr. Soc. 121:433, 1973.

Schiele, F., et al.: Determination of frequency values of total LDH as a function of individual variation factors. Zeitschrift für Klinische Chemie and Klinische Biochemie 12:228, 1974.

Shapleigh, J. B., Mayes, S., and Moore, C. V.: Hematologic values in the aged. J. Gerontol. 7:207–219, 1952. (60 to 95-year olds free from any known or recognized disease except for degenerative changes.)

Shock, N. W., and Yiengst, M. J.: Age changes in the acid-base equilibrium of the blood of males. J. Gerontol. 5:1–4, 1950.

Somerville, P. J., Lein, J. W. K., and Kaye, M.: The calcium and vitamin D status in an elderly female population and their response to administered supplemental vitamin D_3. J. Gerontol. 32:659–663, 1977.

Sunderman, F. W., and Boerner, F.: Normal Values in Clinical Medicine. Philadelphia: W. B. Saunders Co., 1950.

Sweetin, J. C., and Thomson, W. H. S.: Revised normal ranges for six serum enzymes: further statistical analysis and the effects of different treatments of blood specimens. Clinica Chimica Acta 48:49–63, 1973.

Thomson, W. H. S.: Determination and statistical analyses of the normal ranges for five serum enzymes. Clinica Chimica Acta, 21:469–478, 1968.

Thompson, L. W., Nichols, C. R., and Obrist, W. D.: Relation of serum cholesterol to age, sex, and race. J. Gerontol. 20:160–164, 1965.

Videbaeck, A., and Ackermann, P. G.: The potassium content of plasma and red cells in various age groups. J. Gerontology 8:63–64, 1953.

Werner, M., et al.: Influence of sex and age on the normal range of eleven serum constituents. Zeitschrift für Klinische Chemie und Klinische Biochemie 8:105–115, 1970. (Volunteers from the visitors to a health fair. Used only those having no previous disease and not taking medication. When this group was compared to the total population, the values were "almost identical.")

Wilding, P., Rollason, J. G., and Robinson, D.: Patterns of change for various biochemical constituents detected in well population screening. Clinica Chimica Acta 41:375–387, 1972. (A population of persons attending a well-population screening center. They were not screened for level of health but markedly abnormal results were excluded.)

Williams, G. Z., Widdowson, G. M., and Penton, J.: Individual character of variation in time-series studies of healthy people. II. Differences in values for clinical chemical analytes in serum among demographic groups, by age and sex. Clin. Chem. 24:313–320, 1978.

Winsten, S.: The Ecology of normal values in clinical chemistry. CRC Critical Rev. Clin. Lab. Sci. 6:319–330, 1975.

Worthy, E., Whitehead, P., and Goldberg, D. M.: Advantages and limitations of a simplified colorimetric assay for ATP: creatine phosphotransferase activity of human serum. Enzymologia Biologica et Clinica 11:193–210, 1970. ("Healthy" persons attending a well-patient screening clinic and "healthy" members of hospital staff.)

8

Oral Health Maintenance

James Bennett

The author's premise: Certified health care providers, especially those providing nursing or rehabilitative patient care, should be competent in the practice of oral health maintenance.

Perspectives

The mouth is a complex organ system which too often has been isolated from the rest of the body by nondental health care providers. To many patients the mouth is the virtual "soul" of existence in terms of the complex relationships involved, such as nutrition, communication, esthetics, sexuality, sociability, taste, and ubiquitous disease entities. It is an organ system that can suffer a wide gamut of diseases that afflict other body systems; likewise, it has problems unique to itself. Although dying from oral disease has become rare, virtually 100 percent of all adults suffer from some form of oral disease; individuals with natural teeth remaining may suffer from multiple oral problems. One of the most important perspectives for health care providers to appreciate is that most oral disease can be silent, chronic, and *painless* until a significant level has been attained.

New vistas in dentistry have been created in the areas of prevention and geriatrics. These two areas have a significant link inasmuch as the current surge in preventive dentistry will result in millions of persons' retaining significant numbers of natural teeth through their old age. Recent monographs and texts in prevention attest to the basic research that has provided strong rationale for disease control and preventive clinical practice (Bernier, 1975; Caldwell, 1977; Glickman, 1972; Kutscher, 1973; Muhlemann, 1976; and "Preventive Dentistry," monograph, 1972). It is only in recent years that Geriatric Dentistry, itself a young area of interest, has begun to adopt prevention along with the other important diverse areas relevant to geriatrics, such as medicine, nursing, and mental health. The dentist treating geriatric patients must often practice "rational serendipity," and often hesitates to share his innovations since they might be considered patchwork and less than ideal. Recent texts, however, attest to the progress being made in this area (Davidoff, 1972; Franks, 1973; and Lynch, 1977). There is no doubt that Nursing has long recognized the oral cavity as a problem area and, recently, Maurer (1977) provided an excellent review of the literature relative to oral hygiene and its clinical applications.

Myths, Attitudes, and Realities

There are many myths associated with the oral cavity, and the nurse should be aware of some that can be deleterious to an older person's oral health maintenance. It is difficult to overcome or combat attitudes and stereotypes that some adults adopt, especially when individuals in the professions help perpetuate such myths. The wholesale removal of teeth during the 1930s, for example, has resulted in an elderly population in whom prosthetic devices (dentures) predominate and in whom attitudes affect current national dental politics.

One of the prevalent myths is that, as we grow older, it is natural to lose the teeth just as one may lose hair, sight, hearing, and so forth. The vast majority of people lose their teeth as a result of *preventable* dental disease, while some teeth are lost because of trauma or because the dentist judges that salvaging some natural teeth will not be helpful to the person's dental, medical, or emotional health. In some families there is a cultural trend that the grandparents, the parents, and finally the children lose their teeth by the age of 30 years. It may become an ingrained expectation within such families that dentures are the "normal course of events."

It is never too late to teach an older person to maintain his oral health. Many elderly, for the first time in their lives, are beginning to maintain their mouths in an acceptable manner. The older person can and should, through consultation with the dentist, decide which teeth are to be maintained as long as possible. Once the older individual has decided to save as many teeth as possible, however, he is challenged to prevent disease in an oral environment that has already suffered from years of chronic dental problems.

Some professionals assume that "tooth loss is inevitable" for a different reason. There are some dentists who would advocate the removal of all natural teeth on persons entering long term care in a nursing home. They have observed and coped with the rampant disease processes that befall older persons when they become ill and debilitated in some homes. Such attitudes will disappear *only* when institutions are regulated by licensing agencies and when appropriate oral health measures are routine within a facility.

Attendant to the aging-tooth-loss myth is the "going to die" attitude which may be held by the patient, relatives, and professionals. The attitude in relatives is often expressed as "We are not going to sink one more penny in that mouth." This attitude runs counter to the elderly person's right to oral health maintenance. Much of the blame lies with our lawmakers and health care programs. Medicare is a prime culprit in this area since prevention of oral disease is not covered by the insurance plan. Consider the situation where a person with a minor skin rash will have coverage for

treatment, whereas an acute, debilitating disease of the mouth such as pyorrhea will not be covered.

A rather dangerous myth is that oral disease is painful; therefore, "if nothing is hurting, all is well." Low-grade, chronic disease may smolder for years with the individual's considering symptoms as insignificant because there is no pain. Oral cancer usually is silent in early stages (squamous cell carcinoma), while pain often denotes significant invasion of underlying tissues.

Another negative attitude is that fluorides are not beneficial to the older person. Some regard fluoride as a poison and, therefore, to be avoided at all cost. Children benefit most from fluorides in water and food; however, adults can benefit from the topical action of fluorides on the teeth. Topical fluorides are extremely important to patients who have received radiation to salivary glands and jawbones.

Proposed Standards

For persons under the health care of an institution or agency, the following basic standards are proposed for oral health maintenance:

1. The oral cavity is to be examined on any patient entering a licensed health care institution.
   a. Such assessments are to be entered into the patient's legal health record.
   b. Oral assessment should be performed at least one time per month in a chronic care setting, and more often if the patient's health situation is changing daily.
2. Oral health maintenance.
   a. All patients will have their mouths cleaned daily.
   b. Microbial and food debris will be removed from teeth, mucosa, and prostheses at least once per day.
   c. Dentures will be kept in clean water when not in the patient's mouth.
   d. Include oral care in the nursing plan.

In this chapter nurses are provided with information and materials to better fulfill the often avoided responsibility of oral health maintenance. Such responsibility is increasing for several reasons:

1. The maintenance of oral hygiene in an institutionalized situation is the responsibility of the nursing staff. The task is often delegated to a

person who has little understanding or skill to perform the task effectively.

2. Increasing numbers of elderly are maintaining more of their natural teeth for longer periods of time and expectations are rising on the part of relatives that when the older person enters into an institutional or home care situation, the teeth, mouth, and/or dentures are part and parcel to good, quality care.

3. Governing and advocacy groups are pushing and demanding higher levels of accountability and performance on the part of health care providers. As more written standards and peer review protocols are developed, oral health maintenance should be included in the audit parameters. Oral health neglect should carry the same weight of guilt or neglect as any other parameter.

4. With aging, the individual incurs risks of oral disease exacerbation as with other disease entities, particularly when the person is debilitated and cannot effectively care for the mouth. The sick, institutionalized person may find himself in the undesirable situation of suffering physical, emotional, and social problems related to the mouth. The stench from an unclean mouth will keep others away and may create shame and frustration in the patient.

The terms and explanations in this chapter's Glossary are intended to provide some basic background for understanding of subsequent material. See Figures 8-1 and 8-2 to supplement information. Bibliographic material should be used for more comprehensive and in-depth information.

GLOSSARY

Plaque—dental plaque: The microbial flora indigenous to the mouth. The microorganisms utilize food metabolites, particularly sucrose, and are considered to be the primary link in the production of dental caries and periodontal diseases. Daily removal of plaque is one of the key therapies in the prevention of dental disease.

Decay—dental decay—dental caries: The destruction of tooth structure (enamel and dentin) by interaction of dental plaque and metabolites, particularly sucrose.

Gums—gingiva: The soft tissues investing the teeth and forming an attachment to tooth structure.

Periodontium: The bone, collagen, and gingiva investing the teeth and maintaining them in the alveolar bone of the jaws. Disease of the periodontium is called periodontitis or pyorrhea.

Occlusion and articulation: The manner in which the teeth in the jawbones meet. The cusps of teeth in one jawbone ideally articulate with a fossa (depression) of teeth in the opposite jaw with which they occlude.

Tooth pulp—nerve: The inner tooth space is filled with soft tissues; namely nerves, connective tissues, and blood vessels. Disease of the pulp leads to inflammation and/or infection of the tissue. When this affects the end of the tooth root, inflammation, necrosis, and reparative efforts may result in abscesses, granulomas, and/or cysts.

Denturism: The fitting of prosthetic devices by a dental mechanic. Many state legislatures have had bills introduced to legalize such activity. Several very negative aspects of denturism are (1) the elderly are at high risk to suffer several significant oral diseases for which the dental mechanic is not competent to assess or treat; (2) the concept of denturism leads many people to believe that dentures are the ultimate answer to tooth loss and the inevitable result of aging; (3) all individuals should have routine oral health assessments, particularly older persons who run a higher risk of having oral cancer, abscesses and cysts of the jawbones, desquamative conditions such as pemphigoid or pemphigus, and other chronic conditions such as pernicious anemia or malnutrition.

Keratoses—hyperkeratoses—leukoplakia: Several disease conditions of the mouth produce excess keratin (tough protein substance). Low-grade chronic irritation may produce the callus, whereas higher levels may produce erosion and ulceration. Squamous cell carcinoma and lichen planus are two common keratin-producing diseases.

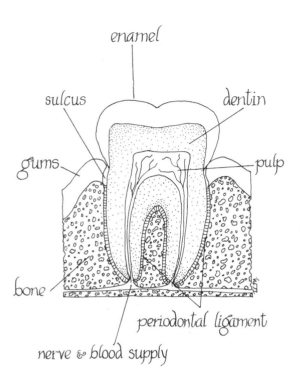

enamel

sulcus

dentin

gums

pulp

bone

periodontal ligament

nerve & blood supply

FIGURE 8-1. Major features of a tooth and investing tissues. The features of interest to the nurse are the enamel, sulcus, and gingiva. Features not shown are the epithelial attachment of the gingiva to the tooth and the cementum, which is a thin layer of calcified tissue covering the dentin of the tooth root. The periodontal ligament is made up of connective tissue (collagen) bands that secure the teeth to the bone (alveolar bone).

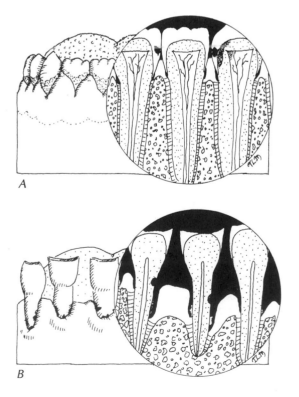

A

B

FIGURE 8-2. Contrast of the diseased dentition of a young person (*A*) with that of an older adult (*B*). *A,* The gingiva surrounds the crown (enamel) of the tooth and there are accumulations of dental plaque about the necks of the teeth. The teeth are close together and dental caries (decay) is shown occurring in the interspaces of the teeth. One carious lesion is shown involving the enamel and dentin and encroaching on the pulp. Early formation of calculus is occurring in several sulcular spaces. *B,* The gingiva, periodontal ligament, and bone have receded, leaving the tooth poorly supported. The enamel is markedly thinned owing to attrition and abrasion, and the pulp has filled in the inner chamber, leaving only a thin remnant of pulp in the root of the tooth. The teeth have separated as a result of periodontal disease (pyorrhea). Such conditions tend to exacerbate disease because of increased stresses during eating and accumulations of bacteria and food debris in the interdental spaces, caries, and periodontal pockets. Note the marked change in the size of pulp, the anatomic features of the crown (enamel), and the relationship of tooth to supporting tissues in diagrams *A* and *B*.

ORAL CHANGES WITH AGING

The mouth undergoes aging changes in its tissues just as do other body areas that are made up of bone, glands, nerves, muscle, connective tissues, and epithelia. In this parameter, therefore, similar forms of atrophy, decreasing function, and loss of regenerative cellular units are found. Teeth, being unique to the mouth, also undergo changes with the passage of time. The actual effect of aging per se is lost in the constellation of time/environment factors called "oral disease." In this section, some of the more generalized effects of time/environment are presented, while the more specific structural changes/problems are presented in the section under Oral Assessment (For more detailed information on so-called aging changes, refer to Franks, 1973; Kutscher, 1973; and Lynch, 1977.)

The general aging changes to be described are stereotypes of what we have come to expect to find in the aging mouth; however, stereotyping a patient for treatment planning purposes can result in inappropriate care.

Teeth

The natural teeth that survive into later periods of life tend to be darker with stress lines in the enamel that tend to accumulate stains. Usually the crown and root structure will have suffered varying degrees of abrasion and erosion, depending on the nature of the diet, toothbrushing habits, employment environment, and/or the degree of grinding (bruxing) the teeth. Sharp tooth edges that may lacerate the soft tissues are often produced by abrasion, tooth or filling fractures, and rampant decay. The loss of periodontium over many years usually leaves increasing amounts of root structure open to the environment and decreasing support for the teeth, resulting in a tendency for increasing mobility of the teeth. Such changes have often been used as reasonable excuse for removal of such teeth, even if the condition could possibly be maintained. The pulp of the tooth usually lays down calcified tissue on the walls of the pulp chamber until there is often only a small fragment of tissue left in the tooth root; this has significant implications on treatment. The condition of the tooth root reduces sensitivity of the tooth, and fillings may often be placed without anesthesia. If the crown of the tooth fractures as a result of trauma or caries, the nerve is often safe and may not require root canal therapy.

Chewing Efficiency

Chewing efficiency tends to decrease owing to loss of tooth units, reduced muscle strength, increased tooth mobility, and the obliteration of the anatomic marking (cusps) in the chewing surfaces. The latter factor is especially significant since, as the chewing surface flattens, it increases the stress to the tooth. Food is caught between broad, flat surfaces that do not incise in the normal manner.

The biting force gradually decreases from a high of about 300 pounds per square inch to 50 for those persons who retain their teeth. Those with dentures suffer additional losses of chewing power and so they end up with about one fifth the efficiency in food partitioning (Lynch, 1977).

Once tooth units are lost, there is a tendency for the alveolar bone to decrease in height. Osteoporosis also is significant in the decrease of alveolar bone. Along with the loss of tooth structure by chewing abrasion and/or the loss of alveolar bone beneath dentures, the mandible often collapses towards the maxilla. This results in the typical aged appearance of the chin's having moved toward the nose (loss of intermaxillary space). The alveolar bone of the maxilla tends to resorb in the anterior portion first, enhancing the chin-to-nose relation. The loss of intermaxillary space may lead to problems in the temporomandibular joint and accentuation of the commissures of the mouth. The latter condition is exacerbated when there is concomitant vitamin deficiency, microbial infection (called perleche), and/or chronic drooling.

Salivary Glands

Decreased salivary flow is common; it may be related to loss of acinar cell units in the glands, the use of some drugs, emotional reactions, or fever. The mucinous component may predominate over the serous, making the smaller amounts of saliva even less effective in removing debris from the mouth and probably contributing to increased retention by the tissues of food, cells, and bacteria. This retention effect is further aggravated in persons with significant neuromuscular defects in which the movement of the tongue is markedly decreased. Decreased salivation often is associated with the "burning mouth syndrome" which, in turn, has been related to such things as anemia, avitaminoses, moniliasis, emotional overlay, allergy, and drug toxicity. It is helpful if such drugs as phenothiazines, anticholinergics, and antihistamines can be reduced or eliminated. Stimulation of salivation by chewing sugar-free gum or sucking on sugar-free candies has been reported as helpful (particularly sour ones such as lemondrops). A recent suggestion to have the patient sip diet cola should be tried, however, the old standby of plain water sipped frequently may be better than nothing. Artificial saliva is now available; however, some patients prefer diet cola.

Mucosa

The mucosal tissues of the mouth in the elderly are particularly prone to changes relative to a significant cluster of factors: nutrition, drugs, and immunologic competency. The periodontium is probably the most vulnerable site relative to alterations in these factors.

The mucosa appears satiny, waxlike, or edematous with atrophy of the epithelial covering; it becomes more vulnerable to stress from coarse food textures, dentures, and oral hygiene measures. When medical and emotional problems are added to the cluster, the oral soft tissues are at high risk for disease. As the connective tissues become more fibrous and less vascular, healing is slowed and infection is more difficult to resolve. Candidiasis (moniliasis) is a common problem in the debilitated patient, especially where dentures are present.

Body Image

The emotional overlay to the oral cavity of elderly is not an easy parameter to evaluate. There are many instances where an elderly person won't eat or socialize when his dentures are being repaired. Males are not as overtly sensitive about esthetics as females and are more likely to request that diseased teeth be removed. Males also are more likely to be edentulous without prosthetic replacement and to have developed the ability to masticate food on toughened, healthy gingiva and alveolar bone. Females are more likely to require some form of esthetic restoration, and several patients have requested that they be allowed to die with at least one natural tooth in their mouth.

Mental health problems in older adults are well documented, and the dentist must interact often with the patient whose mouth has become the emotional target or whose oral problems are intermixed with the emotional problems. One of the more difficult types of patients to deal with is the person who is anxious, fearful, or under heavy stress and is clenching or bruxing (grinding) his teeth.

Nutrition

Nutrition may be a major key in the so-called aging of oral tissues, since there is such a complex effect in the process of chewing, tasting, sensing, and finally swallowing. The systemic effects of foods are well known, however, the local effect of various foods is also important. Nizel (1976) relates important oral conditions to the quality and quantity of food intake.

The implications for daily living found in changes in the oral cavity and in nutrition are of interest to nurses who deal with patients in either institutional or home care settings. The change in chewing power may explain the decreased interest in meat as well as the "tea and toast" syndrome. It certainly suggests the need to carefully select and prepare foods so that compensation is made for the lost ability to chew food effectively. Lynch (1977, 590) suggests that denture wearers should chew each bite of food longer but reports they do not. Therefore, nurses may be helpful in alerting older persons, particularly denture wearers to the need to alter chewing/eating patterns, i.e., consciously chewing food longer and eating more slowly. The nurse can inquire about the person's usual diet and style of food preparation. If appropriate, she can recommend cooking styles that incorporate longer cooking, adding water, or other forms of tenderizing food so as to make the loss of chewing power less of a health hazard.

The friability of tissues may suggest checking on the patient's comfort in eating foods with coarser textures such as raw vegetables, fruits, and coarse ground grains.

Thus, in checking the nutritional patterns and status of the older person the nurse will be interested in (1) chewing capability; (2) symptoms associated with decreased salivary flow that would suggest more frequent eating, drinking, or mouth rinsing; and (3) ability of the soft tissues to withstand the abrasion of coarse hard foods.

Drugs

Drugs can affect oral tissues directly or indirectly. The mouth also can be used as a barometer of certain drug reactions, particularly when toxic or allergic responses occur. For example, when the immunologic system is suppressed, as in chemotherapy for oncologic diseases, the mouth may be the initial site of infection. The person's comfort and his ability to ingest food and communicate can be severely compromised.

DENTURES AND ASSOCIATED NURSING MANAGEMENT

Types of Dentures

TRANSITIONAL DENTURES. Transitional dentures, like immediate dentures, are designed to be worn immediately after final tooth extraction. The idea is to provide temporary dentures during the transitional period when bone and soft tissue heal and shrink. Because of the rapid change in that part of the mouth that supports the dentures, there is some loosening and settling of the dentures. When this period of healing has slowed down (a few months after final extractions), the dentist may construct conventional dentures to replace the transitional dentures.

The advantages of transitional dentures are similar to those of immediate dentures, i.e.:

1. There is no need for a toothless period of healing.
2. The denture acts as a splint during healing.
3. Artificial teeth can be placed so as to appear similar to natural teeth (as with immediate dentures, the patient must be prepared for some additional time and expense).

Transitional dentures often do not have any posterior teeth; simple bite blocks are substituted. The patient has an opportunity to practice with a simple chewing system during healing and tissue change. The patient's experiences with transitional dentures often are useful in deciding the design of the replacement conventional dentures.

As with any dentures, transitional dentures function best in the mouth of someone willing and able to adjust to a suddenly-introduced artificial part of the body. The care and upkeep are similar to that discussed under conventional dentures.

IMMEDIATE DENTURES. Many times, when the diagnosis has been made for complete dentures and the patient has one or more front teeth remaining, the dentist may decide to construct an immediate denture. There are advantages to be gained if only one cuspid, or any front tooth, is remaining in the upper arch. If there are several front teeth remaining, it is possible to set the artificial teeth exactly like the originals.

With immediate dentures, the patient need not go through the toothless period of healing. This is especially advantageous for business men and women who must meet the public. With immediate dentures there is, less pain from extractions because the denture acts as a splint over the extraction wounds and aids healing.

There are some disadvantages to immediate dentures. The patient should be prepared to meet the additional time and expense involved. The bony structure of the mouth changes rapidly when the teeth are removed, thus necessitating a rebase within a few months. During the time the bone is resorbing, the denture will become loose and adjustments will be necessary as it continues to settle. Therefore, the patient must "limp along" during this healing period before the final impression for the rebase can be made. The advantages of immediate dentures seem to outweigh the disadvantages.

Care of immediate dentures is the same as that for conventional dentures. The patient who gives his denture the care and upkeep that any mechanical device should have will receive maximum comfort and usefulness from them.

PARTIAL DENTURES. The advantages of a partial denture are many. The remaining natural teeth help stablize and "hold in" the partial denture. Likewise, the partial denture helps to stablize and support the remaining natural teeth. The cast metal framework is designed to hold the denture on the teeth at strategic places. If, however, the natural teeth do not provide the retentive areas required, alterations of the teeth will be necessary. This consists of selective reshaping of the teeth, restoring the teeth with either silver amalgam or gold or finally crowning the tooth or teeth involved. All these natural teeth should be sound and free of decay. If the teeth are lost, the partial denture will also become useless.

Because a partial denture is made to fit closely against the natural teeth, it must be kept immaculate. Therefore, it must be brushed after each meal. A spiral clasp brush is ideal for cleaning the metal framework. The bristles will get into areas where food particles are most damaging. A regular denture brush should be used for the areas of the partial denture with teeth.

Some people have misconception that a partial denture will cause dental decay. This is not true. The lack of cleanliness of the partial denture causes the decay problem.

Learning to Live with Dentures

Modern materials and techniques enable dentists to make natural-looking dentures that function quite well. However, it takes time to become accustomed to them.

Learning to live with dentures can present a variety of challenges to older persons. Even replacing old dentures with new ones creates difficulties. Most people make a smooth transition from natural teeth to dentures; however, some find it difficult and others impossible. What can be done for one cannot always be done for another. The condition of the person's mouth determines how a denture is made.

MOUTH AND DENTURE CARE. It is very important to keep both the mouth and the dentures clean. The dentures should be removed at night, cleaned, and placed in a container of water. They should also be cleaned after every meal. A good brush, soap, and water should be used. It is wise to scrub them over a basin of water so they will not break if they are dropped.

First time dentures, or new dentures, will not always fit the mouth immediately and there may be sore spots. The dentist will adjust the dentures for better fit. If the mouth becomes very sore the dentures should be removed to give the mouth a rest.

LEARNING TO TALK WITH DENTURES. Learning to talk with dentures is a gradual process. The fullness felt in the lips and cheeks is caused by additional plastic denture material that replaces the bone. The patient will eventually adapt to the fullness and it will be ignored.

DIET AND NUTRITION. The soft tissues under dentures must be kept in good health. Prime factors are diet and nutrition. The occurrence of nutritional deficiencies in older persons is not uncommon (see Chapter 9). All denture wearers should be warned that mouth tissues will suffer if good dietary habits are not followed. The soft tissues under dentures are subject to constant and severe pressures. Maintaining normal levels of protein and Vitamins B and C becomes more than usually important. Meat, a common source of protein, will need to be prepared in such a way as to make it tender and easy to chew (see Chapter 9 for other ways of meeting these nutritional needs).

EATING HABITS AND PATTERNS. New eating habits and patterns have to be established since new neuro-muscular patterns are required to chew and swallow with dentures. Persons with new dentures should begin with foods that are easy to chew. Taking small bites is also important and food should be cut into smaller-than-normal pieces. The food should be worked onto the chewing surfaces on each side. An up-and-down chewing motion may be easier than a side-to-side rolling motion. Biting into solid foods such as bread, corn on the cob, and apples can often better be done using the side teeth rather than front teeth, although some persons have good success with a variety of chewing patterns and many kinds of foods.

DENTURE MAINTENANCE. Dentures tend to become loose and illfitting over a period of time as the bone and soft tissue atrophy. When this occurs dentures not only fail to function effectively but also damage the oral tissue. They should be rebased, relined, or remade to fit properly periodically.

NURSING IMPLICATIONS

The status of oral health and its impact on life-style and activities of daily living is an important aspect of nursing assessment and management with older people, particularly where deficits in coping behavior and support systems have been identified. This is true whether the individual is healthy or ill and whatever the health care setting is in which nursing care is being delivered.

Aging takes its toll on the mouth as well as the rest of the body. Because the mouth is involved in so many activities of daily living—eating, fluid intake, breathing, appearance and self-concept, communication and interpersonal relations—nursing attention to oral health is important.

Except in acute problems, oral health is an area that has been neglected or delegated to others by many nurses. Given the risks of oral problems with increased age and the many activities of daily living impinged upon by oral problems, it is an area of health nurses cannot afford to ignore or minimize as they participate in the older person's health care.

Assessment and Management

The nurse who cares for an older person over a period of time wants to know the following:

1. The actual status of the teeth and mouth.
2. The patient's perception of that status and concerns about it.

3. The skills and resources employed to maintain oral health and those being avoided or used ineffectively.
4. Patterns in lifestyle that are barriers to oral health (mouth care, diet, fluids, smoking, lack of professional care).
5. The importance of the mouth/teeth to the patient in terms of body image, communication, food preferences, finances, and so forth.
6. Adjustments being made in lifestyle because of changes in oral structures (including dentures) and satisfactions with these adjustments.
7. Strategies being used to manage oral problems such as pain, abrasions, halitosis, dry mouth, and denture fit.

The nurse may approach this assessment initially by pursuing the subjective and objective data systematically, focusing on the mouth. She may gather the data when associated problems are reported or when there is evidence that the person has not had dental care at appropriate intervals. Assessment should include a visual screening of the oral cavity as well as gathering of subjective data. Ultimately the nurse's data on a patient's oral status and management patterns should be an identifiable portion of the nurse's knowledge about the patient to whom care will be delivered on a maintenance basis (as opposed to one or two contacts for specific delegated tasks).

Nursing management areas may include (1) assistance with dietary planning, equipment, or techniques for more effective daily oral care; (2) assistance in planning and skills associated with patient self-care of specific problems such as protecting damaged or friable oral tissues, dry mouth, bad breath, cracked lips, etc.; and (3) locating resources for professional dental care needs.

In the Institutional Setting

Mouth care and skin care are areas of nursing responsibility, particularly in institutional settings. However, frequently these are areas where nurses delegate functions, including assessment, to untrained personnel and then fail to either teach or supervise that personnel.

Leadership nursing management in oral health programs for the elderly within institutional settings include the following:

- establish mouth care as a priority activity
- anticipate potential mouth problems and work

to prevent them if possible (drugs, fever, mouth breathing, dentures, restriction of oral fluids, etc.)
- give good mouth care or see that it is given
- teach patient self-care where appropriate
- supervise food and fluid intake
- know how to use equipment and techniques of oral care
- teach personnel the kind of oral care that is to be given
- refer and/or secure care from dentist/dental hygienist as needed
- evaluate outcomes of the total oral health nursing management, improve the program, and reevaluate at regular intervals.

Evaluation of the Patient's Response

Evaluation of the individual patient's response to nursing management of oral health will be associated with the degree to which the older person does the following:

1. Acquires the necessary knowledge and skills to care for teeth, dentures, and other oral tissues effectively.
2. Acquires and uses needed services and support systems for maintaining oral health or adjusts as effectively as possible to the lack of them. (funding for dental care is limited under many insurance plans and free dental clinics or care frequently is inaccessible.)
3. Adjusts the diet and lifestyle to accommodate to oral changes in a way that is still personally satisfying.
4. Maintains as comfortable and healthy a mouth as circumstances permit.
5. Retains or regains the desired body image, lifestyle, and interpersonal relationships that may have been endangered by oral problems.
6. Asks for information and understands impact of medications on salivary flow, teeth, and other oral tissues.
7. Communicates his oral problems to health providers so that they may influence the proposed treatment plans.

Processes Associated with Oral Health Maintenance

Oral health maintenance has the following implications for any nondental health care provider:

1. Insure daily oral hygiene as part of the total patient nursing care.
2. Provide assessment of the mouth at intervals of time appropriate to the patient's health status and his ability to care for himself.
3. Provide advocacy linkage to dental care when problems are detected.
4. Provide oral hygiene measures to patients who are unable to care for themselves adequately; assess the effectiveness of such measures. The dentist or physician may provide specific written orders customized to an individual patient. (This is uncommon at present.)
5. Realize that oral health measures and prevention are only relative; chronic oral disease may be contained for years but never entirely prevented or eradicated.

Oral disease and problems are usually multifactorial; however, it is estimated that 95 percent of the problems are related to those factors that are within the scope of the nursing profession to monitor and/or manage. These are:

1. Microorganisms⟶dental decay; periodontal disease; other inflammatory and infectious conditions of soft tissues and bone. The agents can spread to other areas of the body, particularly the heart, from the mouth.
2. Nutrition⟶dental decay; tissue resistance to infection and trauma; inadequate intake in quality and quantity.
3. Trauma⟶ill-fitting dentures; sharp edges to teeth; sharp metal and acrylic edges associated with prostheses; improper use of cleaning devices.

Oral Assessment

Assessment of the mouth should be carried out using the following guidelines:

1. *Ask* the patient (or someone close to him) about:
   a. pain, sore areas, or different sensations in the mouth
   b. bleeding, oozing, or altered taste perceptions
   c. loose teeth, sharp edges or ill-fitting (ill functioning) appliances
   d. swellings, bumps, or lumps of recent origin
   e. ability to chew, swallow satisfactorily? (It is common for neuromuscular and taste perceptions to diminish with aging.)

2. *Look* at the person's mouth and perioral areas for the following:
   a. changes in the skin, lips, and tissue tone and appearance
   b. palpate neck areas for enlarged glands or nodes
3. *Look into* the mouth using tongue blade and flashlight; systematically check all oral structures for the following:
   a. changes in the normal form, appearance, or texture
   b. inflammations, ulcers, bumps, bleeding, swellings, or draining fistulae
   c. mobile teeth, ill-fitting dentures, or broken teeth or appliances
4. *Enter* findings in the patient record.
5. *Notify* dental personnel when appropriate.

The following section presents the major oral sites and the more common problems that may arise. (See Franks, 1973; Kutscher, 1973; Lynch, 1977, and Orofacial Anatomy, 1977, for more detail about anatomy, physiology, pathology, and/or treatment. This section is not exhaustive.)

Lips and Adjacent Perioral Areas

The lips are covered by a keratinizing mucosa that is smooth and free of the adnexal structures found in the adjacent skin. Normally there is a definite demarcation between the perioral skin and the deep red vermillion border of the lip. In some persons there may be deep indentations at the corner of the mouth (lip pits) which may appear as enlarged pores. Several problems may arise in the perioral area (Table 8-1).

Cheeks, Vestibules, and Floor of Mouth

The cheeks, vestibules, and floor of the mouth are covered by a nonkeratinizing mucosa that is normally smooth and reddish. The continuity is interrupted by such normal structures as parotid ducts opening opposite the maxillary second molars and the mandibular ducts opening into the floor of the mouth just beind the mandibular anterior teeth. Problems concerning this area are listed in Table 8-2.

Teeth and Investing Tissues

Normally there are 32 teeth in the adult mouth, but most adults usually are missing significant num-

TABLE 8-1. Problems in the perioral and lip area.

Problem	Etiology	Signs and Symptoms	Management
Chapping of lips	Dehydration, fever, severe illness	Cracking and drying of surface epithelium	Apply emollients, e.g., Vaseline
Angular cheilosis	Loss of intermaxillary space, avitaminosis, moniliasis, drooling	Deep fissuring at corners of mouth, cracking and pain on opening mouth	Apply emollients, improve nutritional status, apply antifungal ointment
Keratosis of lips	Chronic irritants, e.g., sunlight and smoking	Buildup and thickening of keratin. May cycle if benign. Cannot be differentiated from malignancy	Apply emollients for several weeks. Biopsy if resolution does not occur
Squamous cell carcinoma	As above	Lower lip most common site. Several lesions may be present; induration	Medical management
Recurrent herpes labialis	Reactivation of virus by stress of various types	Small vesicles which may occur in clusters and form scabs or crusts on lips	Emollients; lactobacillus therapy such as buttermilk may help
Purse string mouth	Loss of intermaxillary space, loss of all natural teeth with no routine prosthetic replacement	Fibrous constriction of the oral opening making it increasingly difficult to place dentures. Loss of normal lip movement	Physical therapy may be of value if the person can cooperate

TABLE 8-2. Problems in the cheeks, vestibule, and floor of the mouth.

Problem	Etiology	Signs and Symptoms	Management
Chewing and biting cheeks and inner lip	Unconscious habit, stress	Whitish, fragmented bits of keratin lying attached to mucosa along the line of biting	Create awareness of biting pattern to change behavior
Snuff keratosis	Holding snuff in one vestibular area regularly for many years	Thickened, folded, leathery change in mucosa; may be keratotic, fissured, and indurated in undergoing malignant change	Stop holding snuff in this area; biopsy if lesion persists
Erosions, ulcers, vesicles	Microorganisms, trauma, allergy, and dystrophies such as pemphigus and pemphigoid	Loss of normal surface characteristics of the epithelium; inflammatory reaction; often painful	Milk of magnesia mouth rinses, drug therapy per physician or dentist. Fluids and diet that do not further irritate or traumatize the area
Xerostomia (dry mouth)	Age-related loss of salivary gland units, drugs, psychosomatic	Dry mouth, burning sensation, small amount of viscous saliva; tissue may be leathery, red, or poor tone, friable	Frequent rinsing of mouth with water, adequate fluid intake. Reflex salivary stimulation with food, sugar free gum, sugar free (sour) candy
Squamous cell carcinoma	Chronic irritants, viral, decreased immunologic competence	Often a combination of red, thickened mucosa with irregular patches of keratin.	Requires biopsy if supportive therapy and removal of irritants is not helpful

bers. Often these are replaced by fixed bridges, removable partial dentures, or complete dentures. The key assessment parameters are the following:

1. Can the person masticate?
2. Is the person satisfied with the existing esthetics and ability to talk?
3. Is there significant disease present?

The investing tissues of the teeth often undergo dramatic changes with aging (Table 8-3). The gingiva may become reddened and lose normal stippling. The epithelium becomes thinned and friable.

Tongue

The tongue is basically a mucosomuscular organ intimately related to taste, swallowing, food control in chewing, talking, and nonverbal communication. The dorsum of the tongue is covered by an irregular mucosa made up of papillary projections of various sizes and shapes ranging from the hairlike filiform papillae, the fungiform papillae on the anterodorsal aspects that are rounded formations, and the circumvalate papillae, the large mushroom formations forming a v-pattern on the posterior dorsum of the tongue. Taste buds are numerous within the sulcular formations at their bases.

The papillae tend to become sparser with aging (Table 8-4). They are extremely sensitive, however, to undernutrition and certain disease states such as sprue and pernicious anemia. The tongue often becomes more fissured with age, analogous to loss of substance and muscle tone.

Hard and Soft Palate

The hard palate divides the oral and nasal cavities and is covered by a firm, smooth, keratinizing mucosa, while the soft palate is a mucosomuscular extension that is vital to swallowing. The uvula is the final midline extension of the soft palate. Minor salivary glands are common in both areas while a rounded bony protuberance in the midline of the hard palate (torus palatinus), occurs in a high percentage of adults. Rugae in the anterior hard palate form an individualistic pattern and may assist in manipulation of food.

The mucosa of the palate is firmly attached to the bone and highly susceptible to trauma (Table 8-5). With aging the decrease in vascularity and increased fibrous tissue leads to slow healing.

Maxilla, Mandible, and Temporomandibular Joint

The temporomandibular joint and the jawbones make up a complex and unique system that is at high risk to suffer damage from trauma and the arthritic, osteoporotic changes of aging (Table 8-6). The alveolar bone supporting the teeth is especially susceptible to metabolic oral disease and hormonal changes associated with aging.

TABLE 8-3. Problems of the teeth and investing tissues.

Problem	Etiology	Signs and Symptoms	Management
Dental caries	Inappropriate diet, microorganisms, poor plaque control	Decay of crown (enamel, dentin) and exposed root with deep and rapid destruction; the total crown often lost	Utilize plaque control measures; modify diet; apply topical flouride frequently; professional care
Periodontal disease: periodontitis, gingivitis	Microorganisms, inappropriate diet, change in immunologic competency	Redness, swelling, and easy bleeding of gingiva. Mobility of affected teeth. Pain on chewing and cleaning mouth	Daily hygienic procedures; improved diet. Professional care on recurring, routine basis
Abrasion and erosion; erosive loss of tooth structure	Bruxism (toothgrinding); improper use of toothbrush. Abrasive particles in work environment, chronic acidic oral environment	Flattened enamel surfaces. Ditched areas at neck of tooth. Rapid loss of tooth height with reduced intermaxillary space. Smooth cup-shaped depressions where teeth do not contact	Professional care required
Dystrophies of gingiva	Stress, allergy, drug toxicity, hormones, nutrition	Swelling, redness, tenderness, loss of stippling	Bland mouth rinses/diluted non-astringent mouth washes. Professional treatment

TABLE 8-4. Problems of the tongue.

Problem	Etiology	Signs and Symptoms	Management
Varicosities (underside of tongue)	Unknown cause. Possibly result of congestive heart failure	Enlargement of veins tortuous and clustered	No treatment indicated
Hairy tongue	Drug therapy such as antibiotics or long term use of hydrogen peroxide	Long extensions of filiform papillae—brown, yellow, or black. Entrapment of food debris, bacteria	Reduce drugs if possible. Brush tongue daily. Can trim "hairs" with scissors
Glossodynia (painful tongue)	Undernutrition, allergies, infection, stress	Spontaneous, burning pain	Improve nutrition if needed. Bland mouth rinses. Frequent sips of cool water
Geographic tongue (migratory glossitis)	Unknown etiology—may be related to stress, allergy, and undernutrition	Irregular red areas surrounded by hyperkeratotic borders. Lesions tend to change size and shape	Bland/diluted mouth rinses for itching
Squamous cell carcinoma	High levels of irritants, particularly alcohol and tobacco	Usually occurs on lateral border, especially where it joins the retromolar area and tonsillar fossa. Irregular indurated lesions that may be keratotic	Refer to physician or dentist for biopsy and management.

TABLE 8-5. Problems of the hard and soft palate.

Problem	Etiology	Signs and Symptoms	Management
Ulcerations, erosions	Trauma, heat, chemical reactions (hard palate)	Raw, painful defects in mucosa, usually less than 1 cm. in diameter.	Intraoral emollients (e.g., Orabase and Benzodent as over the counter drugs and Kenlogin Orabase with prescription)
	Allergy, toxicity, infection (soft palate)		May require professional intervention
Nicotine stomatitis, other keratoses (may lead to squamous cell carcinoma)	Heavy smoking, particularly cigars and pipes; spicy foods	Heavy buildup of keratin with red pinpoint pattern of inflamed salivary ducts	

TABLE 8-6. Problems in the maxilla, mandible, and temporomandibular joint.

Problem	Etiology	Signs and Symptoms	Management
Arthritis and degenerative joint disease (osteoarthritis)	Osseous remodeling, spur formation, degeneration and possible ankylosis	Pain in joint and muscles, limited motion with associated crepitus and clicking (use stethoscope over area). Long standing complaint. May be unilateral.	Analgesics, moist heat, professional care to restore appropriate dental arch relations
Myofacial pain syndrome	Occlusal dysharmony. Emotional overlay with tension and nervousness	Pain and tenderness in masticatory muscles, limited movement of mandible, clicking and crepitus with difficulty in chewing, possible subluxation. Bruxism.	Muscle relaxants, emotional support, professional help for occlusal adjustment with acrylic bite splints. Physiotherapy

Oral Hygiene Measures

Oral hygiene can be defined as the removal of bacterial, food, and cellular debris from the mouth by any means that do not damage the tissues and by means that enhance the health of the soft tissues and teeth. For those providing nursing and supportive care to edentulous patients, the procedures may be simple and completed in a few seconds; for the patient with natural teeth and/or prosthetic appliances the procedures may take up to 5 minutes (once a day) to perform an acceptable cleaning. The following procedures should take only a few minutes when practiced with sincerity:

1. Removal of gross food/debris. Have the patient swish and spit water or mouth rinse thoroughly. The care provider will desire to wear a disposable glove if the hand is to be placed in the mouth during cleaning procedures. When food tends to lodge in the vestibules, on the tongue, or on the teeth, a moistened 4 × 4 cotton pad should be carried around the mouth and the debris removed gently. Several swabbings may be necessary if the mouth has been neglected. (We have even added a mild soap to the sponge when you can't bear to look until the third swabbing.)

2. Brush any natural teeth (or root tips), tongue (dorsum), palate, and gingiva with a soft, polished bristle toothbrush (Fig. 8-3). Do not use a cheap hard-bristle toothbrush in any mouth. Be sure that any and every tooth surface accessible to the brush is thoroughly cleaned of dental plaque (remember that plaque is almost invisible). Toothpaste helps freshen the mouth and if it is flouridated helps prevent decay. Patients with atrophic conditions of the mucosa will often not tolerate the more popular toothpastes. Soda or milk of magnesia may provide adequate cleaning.

3. For tooth and sulcular areas not covered by the brush, particularly between teeth, use unwaxed floss, or in the case of wide interdental spaces, use a 3-strand nylon yarn (Fig. 8-4).

4. Dentures should be brushed clean once a day. When left out of the mouth the appliance should be kept in water. Change the water daily since in about four days it is called "soup." Dentures should be marked by some identification means; permanent

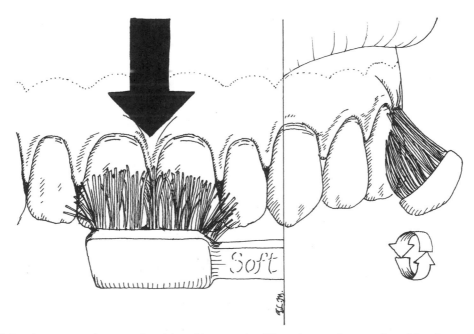

FIGURE 8-3. An appropriate mode of brushing teeth. All surfaces of enamel and tooth root that can be reached by the bristles of a soft toothbrush should be cleansed by eight to ten strokes that generally move in a gum-to-crown direction. Also, short vibratory strokes should be employed to introduce the bristles into the gingival sulcus. In older persons, the sulcus is a particularly vulnerable area for root decay and continuing periodontal disease.

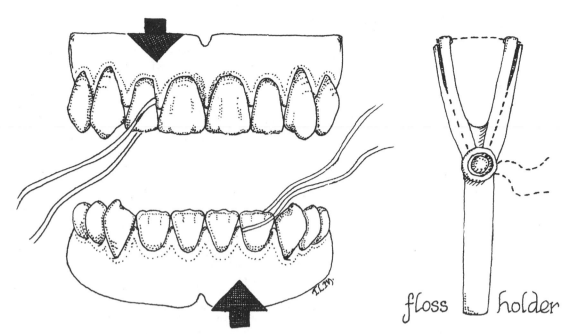

FIGURE 8-4. An appropriate method of using dental floss. The interproximal spaces can be cleaned with floss, yarn, string, toothpicks, and other devices. It is important not to damage the tissues investing the teeth any more than necessary. Floss (yarn) is placed to the depth of the sulcus, wrapped around that portion of proximal tooth structure, and pulled tangentially and upward. The movement is then repeated in the opposite sulcus of the same interspace. All interspaces should be treated thusly in a thorough, sequential manner. The floss should never be sawed back and forth at the neck of the tooth. Floss holders are available so that the nurse does not have to place her hands in the patient's mouth.

name tags imbedded in a clear acrylic are most satisfactory. When a patient's mouth becomes extremely sore beneath a denture, the denture should be kept out of the mouth until professional help arrives. Soft, temporary plastics can be placed by the dentist while evaluating the situation. All denture wearers should leave the prostheses out of the mouth several hours a day; many elderly have great difficulty in this since they have developed an ingrained habit of continual wear (especially if their spouse has been sensitive about dentures). Ultrasonic cleaning may be carried out on prostheses that are acrylic and/or metal; however, when teeth are cemented to the metal, do not use ultrasonics.

5. Other oral hygiene measures may be prescribed by the dentist, who should also teach the correct use of the device or preparation. Some of the devices are:

a. Water jet: A jet spray of water (or mouth rinse) that removes gross debris from the mouth; it does *not* adequately remove plaque. The water jet also tends to stimulate the soft tissues. If used incorrectly, it can produce further problems.

b. Mechanical aide: A large toothpick mounted on a plastic handle can be used to remove dental plaque from the gingival sulcus and from between the teeth.

c. Rubber tip: This is a pointed rubber tip, usually mounted on one end of the toothbrush. It stimulates the gingiva and aids in the removal of interdental plaque.

d. Interdental brush: A small, round brush that fits between wide interdental spaces.

e. Mouth rinses: Warm water with salt may still be the best rinse; however, some (cardiac, kidney) patients may not tolerate it well. Several commercial preparations may act as oral emollients, but they do not prevent plaque formation.

f. Electric toothbrushes (see Appendix 8-1).

EVALUATION OF THE ORAL HEALTH PROGRAM

From the Dentist's Perspective

Nurses should routinely evaluate the effectiveness of the oral health practices being performed by persons in their charge. Consultation and training should be sought from dental personnel so that evaluation is meaningful and will meet the standards of adjudicating agencies. However, it is to be realized that in the face of an acute stomatitis or an uncooperative patient, the level of oral hygiene will be compromised.

When a mouth has been cleansed daily over a period of time, it should appear as follows:

1. Dental plaque should not be apparent about the teeth. (Dyes should not be used to determine the presence of plaque.)
2. The tissues should be relatively firm about the teeth, and there should be no bleeding when brushing and flossing. (This may be compromised by certain medical problems or drug therapies.)
3. The patient should appreciate the feeling of a clean mouth; likewise the patient will be aware of roughness and improper techniques. This may be minimized if the patient is urged and guided in caring for his own mouth with assistance given as needed. Proper types of toothbrushes are specially important.

When evaluating an oral health program, there are several important parameters to consider:

1. Is there an inservice program and is it effective? (I have found that one-on-one training is the best; group training is often ineffective.)
2. Will relatives or volunteers help with oral health maintenance? Some spouses have been very effective in cleaning the teeth.
3. Are you utilizing dental personnel? At present it is very probable that most institutions do not have an effective oral health program, a key reason being the unavailability of dentists and hygienists.

The Nursing-Dental Interface

When dental personnel enter an institutional situation, they should carry out the following activities:

1. Check in with the main desk to inform per-

sonnel of their presence (with a preceding phone call).
2. Go over the patient's chart; talk with nursing personnel familiar with the patient.
3. Write all findings, plans, etc., in chart; oral hygiene measures should be specifically written.
4. Obtain approval of responsible parties before providing definitive care.
5. Assist in the training and assessment of oral health maintenance.

ANNOTATED BIBLIOGRAPHY

Accepted Dental Therapeutics, ed. 37. Chicago: American Dental Association, 1977.

Bernier, J. L., and Muhler, J. C.: Improving Dental Practice Through Preventive Measures, ed. 3. St Louis: C. V. Mosby Co., 1975. (This recent edition presents both basic diseases process and the rationale for the recommended preventive measures. In addition it covers the use of preventive procedures in the major categories [specialties] of dental practice.)

Butler, R. N., and Lewis, M. I.: Aging and Mental Health, Positive Psychosocial Approaches, ed. 2. St Louis: C. V. Mosby Co., 1977. This recent monograph should be required reading for anyone practicing in Geriatrics. A small paragraph on the need for dental care, however, does not reflect the psychological importance of the oral cavity.)

Caldwell, R. C., and Stallard, R. E.: A Textbook of Preventive Dentistry. Philadelphia: W. B. Saunders Co., 1977. (A recent and thorough text on preventive dentistry. Both the basic and applied perspectives are thorough in their treatment. This book is recommended as an excellent resource for nurses.)

Davidoff, A., Winker, S., and Lee, W. H. M.: Dentistry for the Special Patient; The Aged, Chronically Ill and Handicapped. Philadelphia: W. B. Saunders Co., 1972.

Franks, A. S. T., and Hedgegard, B.: Geriatric Dentistry. Oxford, England: Blackwell Scientific Publications, 1973. (This text reviews the major physical and emotional changes associated with aging. Dental practices for aged are described; however, the section on preventive dentistry is too brief.)

Glickman, I. (ed.): Symposium on preventive dentistry. Dental Clin. N. Am. 16:4, 1972. (This monograph gives a good perspective of applied preventive dentistry in the private office. Emphasis is placed on the control of dental plaque with some interesting perspectives in radiation, chemoprophylaxis, oral cancer, and prosthodontics.)

Kutscher, A. H., and Goldberg, I. K.: Oral Care of the Aging and Dying Patient. Springfield, Ill.: Charles C Thomas, 1973. (This text was derived from a Conference of the same name; it is a smorgasbord of topics and issues with subject redundancy. It is very humanistic in all perspectives and of particular interest to the nurse is the pharmacologic perspectives.)

Lynch, M. A. (ed.): Burket's Oral Medicine, ed. 7. Philadelphia: J. B. Lippincott Co., 1977. (This is an excellent resource text covering anatomy, pathophysiology, diagnosis, and treatment of oral diseases and oral problems. It also has extensive reviews of the major categorical areas in pathology as well as systemic pathology, particularly the organ systems with important relations to oral diseases.)

Maurer, J.: Providing optimal oral health. Nurs. Clin. N. Am. 12:4, Dec. 1977. (This article is a special feature that reviews oral structure, physiology, oral assessment, and methods and agents for oral hygiene. It gives a nursing perspective of using oral cleansing agents and reflects the serendipity required in coping with low oral hygiene.)

Muhlemann, H. R.: Introduction to Oral Preventive Medicine. Bunch und Zeitschriften-Verlag "Die Quintessenz," 1976. (An excellent monograph presenting the basic dental sciences and epidemiologic information associated with preventive dentistry. The conceptual models of common dental disease and their control is very nicely presented.)

Nizel, A. E.: Role of nutrition in the oral health of the aging patient, in Symposium on Nutrition. Alfano, M. C., and De Paola, D. P. (eds.): Dental Clin. N. Am. 20:3, 1976. (This chapter has an excellent review of common problems of the elderly that may be related to nutrition. Nutritional needs and the management thereof are detailed. The entire monograph is recommended to the nursing profession.)

O'Malley, K., Judge, T. G., and Crooks, J.: In Avery, G. S. (ed.): Geriatric Clinical Pharmacology and Therapeutics in Drug Treatment. Adis Press (Sydney, Australia) and Publishing Sciences Group Inc. Littleton, Mass., 1976.

Orofacial Anatomy, Block Drug Company, Inc., Jersey City, N.J., 1977. (A Trans-Vision Dissection of the Oral Cavity.)

Preventive Dentistry, Crest Professional Services Division, Proctor and Gamble Co., Cincinnati, Ohio. 1972. (A concise monograph on the basis and application of preventive dental measures by a group of leaders in modern dentistry.)

Appendix 8-1 follows on page 128
Appendix 8-2 is on page 134

APPENDIX 8-1

Excerpts from
"A Manual of Oral Hygiene for Handicapped
and Chronically Ill Patients"

Introduction

The handicapped or chronically ill patient frequently has complex dental problems such as sore gums, loose teeth, illfitting dentures, and an unclean mouth. Most of them have not had dental care for many years and have had little instruction of the importance of caring for their mouths.

Patience and skill are needed in persuading such patients to take an active interest in their oral health. The crippling and immobilizing effects of diseases often make normal procedures for oral hygiene difficult or impossible. Health service personnel can help these patients with a variety of services that will ensure clean, healthy, and more comfortable mouths.

Tissues of the mouth in the handicapped or chronically ill person, especially the aged patient, are oftentimes tender and painful to the touch. Tender loving care is needed. A too aggressive approach to mouth care can lead to severe oral problems.

The handicapped patient is proud of his ability to adapt to his condition. Give assistance at first if necessary, but the patient should be motivated to develop a good oral hygiene program within his own capabilities.

Dental care includes not only periodic professional dental care by the dentist or dental hygienist, but also *daily oral hygiene procedures.* Both the patient and attendant must work together in establishing and maintaining the cleanliness of the mouth. Healthy mouths are important to the patient's general health, comfort, and happiness.

Each patient needs his own toothbrush, either hand or electric. The brush should be labeled with the patient's name in indelible ink, nail polish, or an inscribing tool can be used for this purpose. A recommended toothbrush has:
—straight handle with flat brushing surface
—soft nylon bristles
—head (bristle part) small enough to reach all areas of mouth easily

Care of Toothbrush

1. Rinse the toothbrush with clean, cold water after use to remove any retained food and toothpaste.
2. Store the toothbrush in a light, airy place to dry thoroughly.

Circulated by the Oregon Dental Association and Dental Health Section of the Oregon State Health Division.

3. Any empty water glass or toothbrush holder can be used to store the toothbrush.
4. Replace the toothbrush when the bristles become loose, bent, broken, or worn.

Electric toothbrushes may be as effective as hand toothbrushes in maintaining cleanliness of the mouth. Electric toothbrushes may be especially helpful for the handicapped or seriously ill patient who cannot effectively clean his own mouth with a hand toothbrush or who must have his teeth cleaned by an attendant. The same electric toothbrush handle can be used for several patients; however, each patient must have his own toothbrush head labeled with his name. Toothbrush heads for electric toothbrushes usually need replacement more frequently than hand toothbrushes.

Brushing with an electric brush follows the same technique as brushing with a hand brush. The electric toothbrush is *not* turned on until it is placed in the mouth. A recommended method of toothbrushing with an electric toothbrush is:

1. Wet the bristles of the toothbrush with water and place a *small* amount of dentifrice on them.
2. Place the brush in the mouth with the bristles directed toward the side of the teeth.
3. Turn on the electric toothbrush *after* placing it in the patient's mouth.
4. Hold the bristles of the brush lightly against *side* of teeth so that both the teeth and gums are cleaned. Start on back teeth on one side and continue around entire mouth to back teeth on other side on both upper and lower teeth. (See manufacturer's instructions.)
5. Brush the tongue side as well as cheek side of the teeth.
6. Brush approximately two teeth at a time, holding the brush in the same place for three seconds, before moving on to the next area. Be sure to clean each area of the mouth thoroughly.
7. Brush chewing surfaces of teeth by holding brush for three seconds on each two teeth.
8. Extend the tongue and lightly brush top surface.
9. Rinse the mouth thoroughly with water.

Adaptation of Toothbrush

Many patients with physical handicaps or chronic diseases have special problems in maintaining their oral hygiene. Special adaptations of toothbrushes may be necessary to meet their needs. Inexpensive materials to make the special toothbrush adaptations can be obtained from variety, hardware, grocery, and hobby stores. The following examples illustrate several toothbrush modifications.

Patients with Arthritis, Chronic Diseases of the Joints, or Limited Hand Movement

A wide elastic band can be taped to toothbrush handle for persons who are unable to close their hands (Fig. 8-5). The band should be tight enough to hold brush snugly and avoid slipping.

Patients with Cerebral Palsy, Central Nervous System Disorders, or Partial Hand Mobility

Toothbrushes may be easier to control for these patients if they have an oversized handle made by building up with self curving plastic from a hobby shop. A dentist can be helpful in recommending the proper plastic. Another method for enlarging a toothbrush handle is:

1. Purchase bicycle handbar grip (rubber or plastic) and small sack of quick setting paster of paris. Mix small amount of very thick plaster. Fill bicycle grip with wet plaster. Cover hole in end of grip with adhesive tape to present plaster from running out hole. Push toothbrush handle into grip and hold until plaster hardens (few minutes). Clean excess plaster off handle with damp cloth before plaster hardens. (Fig. 8-6)
2. A sponge hair roller slides easily over a toothbrush handle.
3. A band of Velcro, wrapped around the hand, grips the toothbrush handle. Velcro adheres to itself. Band around hand, slip in toothbrush.

These adaptations are also useful in enlarging the handles of spoons and forks. A temporary method for enlarging a toothbrush handle is to push handle through middle of a soft rubber ball after piercing ball with sharp object.

Another temporary method is to glue a short piece of plastic tubing to the toothbrush handle (Fig. 8-7).

Proper size handle can be determined by wrapping suitable material (wrinkling aluminum foil, ace bandage, styrofoam) around handle until comfortable size is reached (Fig. 8-8).

Patients with Limited Arm Movement

To make the handle longer, cut the bristle portion off an old brush and attach this handle to handle of a new toothbrush. Secure with strong cord or plastic cement (Fig. 8-9).

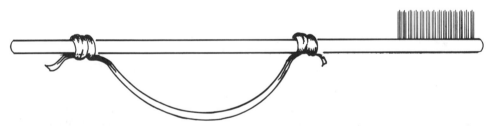

FIGURE 8-5. Toothbrush handle with elastic band.

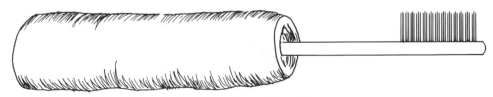

FIGURE 8-6. A sponge hair roller enlarges a toothbrush handle.

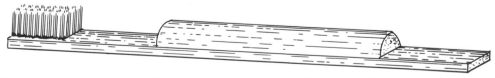

FIGURE 8-7. A short piece of plastic tubing glued to the toothbrush handle.

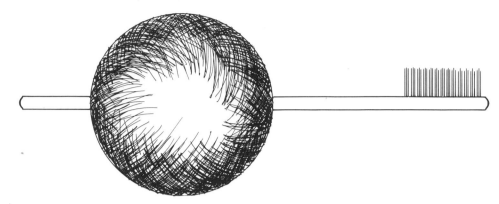

FIGURE 8-8. Wrinkled aluminum foil around the handle gives a better grip on the toothbrush.

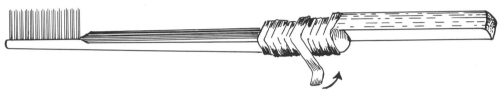

FIGURE 8-9. The handle of an old toothbrush attached to the present toothbrush provides a longer handle.

For an extra long handle, attach brush to plastic rod or comparable material of desired length. Plastic toothbrush handle can be curved if desired by heating gently (Fig. 8-10).

Patents With No Movement of Limbs

A long-handled T-shaped device with bristles facing two directions can be used (Fig. 8-11). The patient must retain some head movement.

Oral Hygiene for Denture Patients

Oral hygiene practices do not stop with the loss of natural teeth. Cleanliness of dentures is important for the patient's health and comfort. Dirty dentures can cause sore mouths and "denture breath." Food, stain, and calculus (tartar) collect on dentures (false teeth) the same as they do on natural teeth.

Dentures and removable partials should be brushed after each meal and rinsed in (cold) running water before replaced in the mouth. The mouth should be brushed with a soft nylon toothbrush and rinse with warm water before replacing cleaned dentures.

Patients should be encouraged to wear their dentures during the day. However, it is recommended and especially desirable to remove the dentures each night for the *chronically ill* patient, to give a rest to the denture-supporting tissue (gums). When the dentures are left out of the mouth for any length of time they should be *placed or stored in water*. This practice will prevent drying and warping of the dentures.

Cleaning of the Soft Tissues

Gauze strips and pads may be most helpful for cleansing the soft tissues of the mouth, the ridges of the jaw of the edentulous patient (patient without any teeth), also those patients with lost tooth spaces and those with chronic gum tissues when use of toothbrush may be contraindicated. The gauze should be wrapped around the under finger and pressed gently over the soft tissues of the mouth.

Cleaning Dentures

Remember—dentures are very fragile and costly to replace.

1. Fill the washbowl ⅓ to ½ full of water and hold denture near surface of water. A washcloth at the bottom of the bowl will prevent denture from breaking if it is accidentally dropped.
2. With a denture brush, brush both inside and outside of denture.
3. Rinse with cold running water before replacing denture in *clean* mouth.
4. Metal clasps that fasten PARTIAL dentures to natural teeth need to be brushed well on inside of clasps to remove stains and food particles.

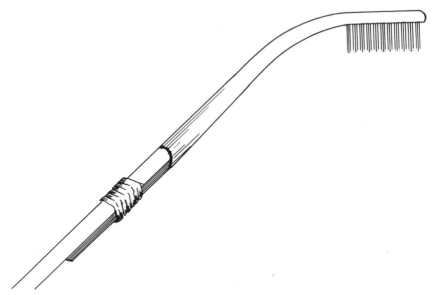

FIGURE 8-10. A plastic rod extension and a curved handle on the toothbrush.

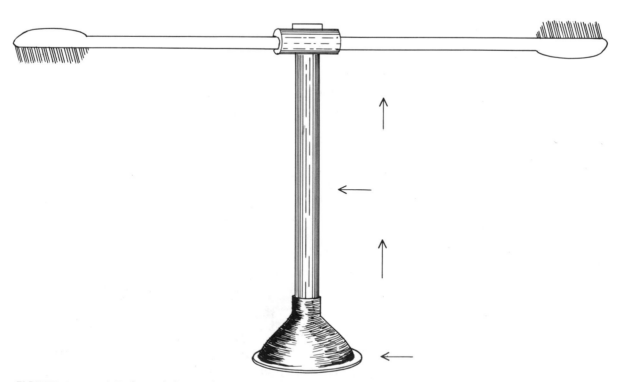

FIGURE 8-11. A T-shaped device for patients with no movement of limbs.

Stains and Odors

To remove stains and odors from dentures, soak denture overnight in glass of water with one teaspoon of laundry chlorine bleach (Clorox). *Do not* use pure bleach as pink base of denture may loose its color. *Do not* use Clorox solution on any appliance with metal as the metal may tarnish.

Caution: If a bleaching agent is used—dilute—and use with care as noted above.

Hard Deposits

To remove hard deposits on denture, soak denture overnight in white vinegar. (Brown vinegar may stain the pink base of the denture.)

Denture cleaning aids are commonly available from drug, grocery, and variety store. (However, the American Dental Association *does not* recommend the use of liquid denture cleaners that claim to be effective without the use of a brush.)

Labeling Dentures

Identification of each patient's dentures may be a major problem in a hospital or nursing home. One simple method of labeling dentures is to type the patient's name on a small piece of thin paper (onion skin) and attach paper to cheek side of denture with clear fingernail polish. One or two coats of polish should be applied over the paper to protect the label against moisture in the mouth.

A commercial denture labeling product is available at drug stores. When new dentures are made, the patient should request that his name be placed on the new dentures.

Procedure for Denture Patients Incapable of Caring for Themselves

The denture is removed from the patient's mouth by exerting pressure on the side of the denture. After cleaning, wet the denture with cool water before replacing it in the patient's mouth. Holding the sides of the upper denture, replace the denture gently in the patient's mouth. Holding the sides of the lower denture, slide into proper place and position with fingers in corner of mouth. Remove dentures from mouth of a patient who is having a convulsion, is unconscious, or is disturbed.

Denture Brushes

A stiff or hard bristle toothbrush, hand brush, or denture brush are satisfactory for cleaning dentures. Each patient should have his own brush. Special clasp brushes for partial dentures are available to clean inside the metal clasps.

Denture Brush—Adaptation

Suction cups may be attached to bottom of a hand brush for patient with use of only one arm to brush his own dentures (Fig. 8-12). The hand brush is attached to the bottom of a sink with the suction cups to keep it from slipping. The patient cleans both sides of the denture by rubbing these surfaces against the brush.

Cleansing Agents for Dentures

Dentures may be cleaned with the aid of a denture brush and (1) hand soap, (2) baking soda, or (3) commercial denture cleaning preparation.

Dentifrices and Mouthwashes

Dentifrices

Dentifrices (toothpastes or powders) make toothbrushing more pleasant, but are not necessary for plaque removal. Fluoridated tooth pastes are recommended for their action in preventing tooth decay.

Baking soda (two parts) and salt (one part) in a 4 ounce glass of water may be used with a *physician's approval* as a substitute for commercial dentifrice. It is *contraindicated* for patients on a "low salt" or "salt-free" diet.

Mouthwashes

Except for medicated mouthwashes prescribed by a physician or dentist for a specific disease, mouthwashes are merely solutions having pleasant tastes and odors. Mouthwashes may be useful in removing food particles loosened during toothbrushing and flossing. However, water is satisfactory for this purpose.

Oral Hygiene for Special Patients

Patients Confined to Bed

The patient's own toothbrush, a glass of water, and a small basin should be located within the patient's reach.

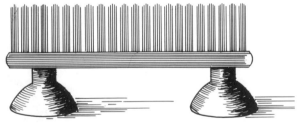

FIGURE 8-12. Denture brush made from a small hand brush.

The water is used to moisten the toothbrush and rinse the mouth. The basin is used for water discharge after rinsing. Cold water should *not* be used as it may cause pain while rinsing.

Patients Who Are Semicomatose

A coating may form on teeth even though the patient is not taking food by mouth. The teeth and gums should be lightly wiped four to six times a day with a swab of mineral oil and oil of lemon. A swab moistened with hydrogen peroxide may also be used. *It is very important* to clean and lubricate the semicomatosed patient's mouth to prevent the mouth tissues from drying. The patient's lips may be lightly lubricated with vaseline to prevent drying and cracking.

APPENDIX 8-2

SAMPLE CONTRACT BETWEEN DENTAL GROUP AND INSTITUTION

This agreement is entered into this _____ day of _____, _____, by and between the

Geriatric Dental Group, hereinafter called the G.D.G. and _____,
hereinafter called the Contractor.

    Whereas the Contractor has need of particular services relating to the dental care of its patients and whereas the G.D.G. is willing to undertake such care they agree to the assumption of the following responsibilities.

Responsibilities of the G.D.G.

A. To provide a dental team, which will visit the Contractor on mutually determined periods of time. The team will be composed of those personnel necessary to carry out a primary dental care program which will include:

1. Performing a complete oral examination upon each new patient.
2. Emergency dental care.
3. Indicated dental treatment (i.e., to alleviate pain, infection, disease progression).
4. To restore esthetics and function based on the clinical judgment of the dentist.
5. Annual oral examinations of participating residents.
6. Patient education in areas of oral hygiene.
7. Inservice training for nurses and nurse's aides regarding oral health maintenance.
8. Consultations as requested by administrative staff.
9. Written orders in patient charts as necessary for daily oral care.

B. To keep a daily diary of the team's activities with copies provided monthly to the Contractor. This record will show which patients have been seen, treatment rendered, and fees for Contractor's billing purposes. All welfare patients and their fiscal management will be the responsibility of the G.D.G.

C. To participate in regular evaluation of the program and to negotiate desirable changes with the Contractor.

Responsibilities of the Contractor.

A. To provide space, utilities, and consumable supplies as needed by the dental team (i.e., 2 × 2 gauze, tongue blades, cotton rolls, cotton swabs, toothbrushes, floss, etc.).

B. To provide staff support for coordination of training at all levels and making arrangements for staff inservice training. Daily oral hygiene is a nursing care responsibility and all staff members will participate in and support training programs to maintain an optimum level of oral care within the facility.

C. To act as a liaison between patients, dental team, and responsible parties of the patients.

D. To participate in regular evaluations of the program and to negotiate desirable changes.

Payment.

    The G.D.G. will bill the contractor per following schedule for services performed:

Dentist, Dental Hygienist, and Assistant(s)	$ /hour
Dentist and Assistants	$ /hour
Dental Hygienist and Assistants	$ /hour
Dentist and Dental Hygienist	$ /hour
Dental Hygienist	$ /hour

Daily diaries will reflect the variable team composition and the time spent as such.

In the event of nonperformance of any of the provisions or conditions of this contract, the G.D.G. will pursue all legal remedies available to it under the law. This contract can be terminated at any time by either party upon 30 days notice in writing.

Geriatric Dental Group

_____

_____

_____

Contractor

_____
Business Name

_____
Address

_____
Authorized Signatory

_____
Federal Identification No.

_____
Date

9

Nutrition

Bonnie Worthington

"Nutrition" has been defined in a variety of ways. The broad definition by the American Medical Association may be selected as most useful for this presentation in that consideration is appropriately given to the multitude of factors which necessarily are involved. According to AMA, "Nutrition is the science of food, the nutrients and other substances therein, their action, interaction and balance in relation to health and disease, and the process by which the organism ingests, digests, absorbs, transports, utilizes and excretes food substances. In addition, nutrition must be concerned with social, economic, cultural and psychological implications of food and eating." (Simko and Dolitz, 1973)

It is clear from this elaborate definition that consideration of nutrition as it relates to healthful living involves recognition of the variety of roles that food plays in the lives of individuals. Attention will be given in this discussion to the diverse meanings of foods in our society. Basic to discussion of this topic, however, is the critical need for food and its constituent nutrients for support of life itself as well as for growth, tissue repair, and resistance to infection. The nutrients in food are clearly vital to support of basic biochemical and physiologic mechanisms in the human body; each individual must provide his body with its basic needs or suffer the consequences of suboptimal performance.

BASIC NUTRIENT REQUIREMENTS OF OLDER ADULTS

Before examining in depth the specific nutritional needs of elderly persons, emphasis must be placed on the reality that individuals cannot be pooled or lumped into what is called the "old age group." Clearly, this tendency makes for convenience in discussing the needs of older people but common sense strongly supports the concept of increasing individuality with increasing age. As rough guidelines, however, for assessing nutritional needs of groups and for planning dietary programs for the elderly, the Recommended Dietary Allowances of the National Academy of Sciences serve a useful purpose (Table 9-1). It must be remembered, however, that the actual nutritional status of groups of healthy people or individuals must be judged on the basis of physical, biochemical, and clinical observation combined with observations of food or nutrient intake. If the RDAs are used as reference standards for interpreting records of food consumption, it should not be assumed that malnutrition will occur whenever the recommendations are not completely met. Conversely, it is important not to assume that nutritional adequacy is insured by fulfilling the recommended dietary allowances.

The concept of individuality has particular relevance for the aged. The overwhelming majority of elderly people have one or more chronic illnesses, such as atherosclerosis, digestive upsets, malabsorptive phenomena, rheumatologic disorders, osteoporosis, obesity, alcohol addiction, lack of teeth or poorly fitting dentures, and a whole host of other medical and psychologic problems. Certainly the aged person hardly represents the healthy reference man indicated in the Recommended Dietary Allowances. It is, therefore, a real challenge to health professionals not only to identify and manage the great variety of medical problems of the "aged" but

TABLE 9-1. Recommended Daily Dietary Allowances for persons over 51 years of age, revised 1974 (Designed for the maintenance of good nutrition of practically all healthy people in the USA)

	Males	Females
Calories (kilocalories)	2400	1800
Protein (grams)	56	46
Vitamin A (International Units)	5000	4000
Vitamin D (International Units)	No recommendation	
Vitamin E (International Units)	15	12
Ascorbic Acid (Vitamin C) (milligrams)	45	45
Folic Acid (milligrams)	0.4	0.4
Niacin (milligrams)	16	12
Riboflavin (milligrams)	1.5	1.1
Thiamine (milligrams)	1.2	1.0
Vitamin B_6 (milligrams)	2.0	2.0
Vitamin B_{12} (micrograms)	3.0	3.0
Calcium (grams)	0.8	0.8
Phosphorus (grams)	0.8	0.8
Magnesium (grams)	0.35	0.3
Iron (milligrams)	10	10
Zinc (milligrams)	15	15
Iodine (micrograms)	110	80

Adapted from information from the Food and Nutrition Board, National Academy of Sciences, National Research Council, Washington, 1974.

also to determine and establish an appropriate nutritional program that will insure individual nutrient adequacy, particularly in the face of these multifaceted problems. By no means does this imply that the Recommended Dietary Allowances should be disregarded but instead that they should serve as a guideline upon which individual nutritional status is estimated and dietary recommendations are prescribed. In the final analysis, nutritional requirements (like most other needs) represent individual characteristics.

Caloric Requirements

A calorie is a measure of the energy-producing content of food in units of heat. The energy needs of an individual are influenced by a variety of factors including basal metabolism, amount of sleep, and degree of physical activity. Additionally, the body requires energy for the synthesis of body tissues, the operation of basic biochemical processes, and the regulation of appropriate body temperature.

With increasing age, a gradual reduction in energy requirement takes place. Part of this reduction reflects a reduction in basal metabolism result-

ing from the loss of functioning body cells. The cells that remain continue to demand the same nutritional support as cells from younger persons. In addition, a reduction in daily physical activity is commonly observed in the aging individual. This has been clearly documented in studies involving both men and women. Because of the decrease in physical activity with age, basal metabolism represents a higher proportion of the total energy needs of elderly persons than of young adults who are physically more active.

Because of the decrease in physical activity and basal metabolism with age, calorie intake should be reduced gradually as persons become older. The Food and Nutrition Board of the National Academy of Sciences has recommended that calorie allowances be reduced by 5 percent between ages 22 and 35, by 3 percent per decade between ages 35 and 55, and by 5 percent per decade from ages 55 to 75. A further decrement of 7 percent is recommended from age 75 and beyond.

In practice, calorie needs of individuals may vary according to age, sex, basal metabolism, size, occupation, environment, hormonal balance, and physical activity patterns. Total calorie intake should be adjusted to a level that will prevent both overweight and underweight. Both problems are common among the aged with overweight and obesity afflicting the greatest percentage. In one study of 100 individuals aged 65 and over in Boston, 48 percent of the men and 59 percent of the women were 10 percent or more above their desirable weight (Howell and Loeb, 1969). Of 200 persons over 65 years of age who were referred to the Outpatient Nutrition Clinic at Ohio State University, 68 percent were 10 percent overweight and only 8 percent were more than 10 percent underweight (Howell and Loeb, 1969). The incidence of overweight and obesity peaks in the fourth decade for women and in the sixth decade for men. This trend toward successive lower body weights in decades from 50 years to 70

years and older not only may reflect decreases in food intake but also may represent the change in makeup of the population groups with the survival of the physically fit. Since studies of body composition of adults suggest that the proportion of body fat to body weight may increase with age, a desirable goal might be to avoid this nonbeneficial compositional change by attempting to maintain a desirable body weight for height throughout life (Table 9-2).

Generally the problem of obesity in older adults is a result of the persistence of unrestricted liberal eating habits in conjunction with reduction in energy expenditure. Gluttony usually is not the cause and people who claim that they eat no more than they used to are largely correct. Often the gain in weight

TABLE 9-2. Average height–weight table for persons 65 years of age and over.

Height in Inches	MEN					
	Ages 65–69	Ages 70–74	Ages 75–79	Ages 80–84	Ages 85–89	Ages 90–94
61	128–156	125–153	123–151			
62	130–158	127–155	125–153	122–148		
63	131–161	129–157	127–155	122–150	120–146	
64	134–164	131–161	129–157	124–152	122–148	
65	136–166	134–164	130–160	127–155	125–153	117–143
66	139–169	137–167	133–163	130–158	128–156	120–146
67	140–172	140–170	136–166	132–162	130–160	122–150
68	143–175	142–174	139–169	135–165	133–163	126–154
69	147–179	146–178	142–174	139–169	137–167	130–158
70	150–184	148–182	146–178	143–175	140–172	134–164
71	155–189	152–186	149–183	148–180	144–176	139–169
72	159–195	156–190	154–188	153–187	148–182	
73	164–200	160–196	158–192			

Height in Inches	WOMEN					
	Ages 65–69	Ages 70–74	Ages 75–79	Ages 80–84	Ages 85–89	Ages 90–94
58	120–146	112–138	111–135			
59	121–147	114–140	112–136	100–122	99–121	
60	122–148	116–142	113–139	106–130	102–124	
61	123–151	118–144	115–141	109–133	104–128	
62	125–153	121–147	118–144	112–136	108–132	107–131
63	127–155	123–151	121–147	115–141	112–136	107–131
64	130–158	126–154	123–151	119–145	115–141	108–132
65	132–162	130–158	126–154	122–150	120–146	112–136
66	136–166	132–162	128–157	126–154	124–152	116–142
67	140–170	136–166	131–161	130–158	128–156	
68	143–175	140–170				
69	148–180	144–176				

Adapted from a table by Master, A. M., et al.: J.A.M.A. 172:658, 1960.

is gradual with the addition of about two to three pounds per year. If this pattern persists from age 20 to age 50, a person may weigh 40 to 60 pounds more than he did as a youth.

Excess body weight by no means indicates that a person is in satisfactory nutritional status. The liberal ingestion of "empty calories" is the basis for weight gain in large numbers of individuals. Foods rich in empty calories include processed fats, refined sugars, and the many products produced from these materials. Consumption of these foods, which are almost devoid of protein, essential minerals, and vitamins, decreases the appetite for the intake of foods high in nutritive value and conducive to maintenance of health.

Needless to say, dietary counseling is essential for the older person who has laid down undesirable adipose tissue. Because activity generally is limited, the restriction of calories to bring about weight loss must be carefully planned so that the diet supplies adequate amounts of the essential nutrients. To achieve a loss of one pound of body fat per week, a reduction in daily intake of 500 calories is required. Moderate exercise may also assist in increasing expenditure of calories to a limited degree. Whatever program is devised, its success will relate directly to the ease with which it can be adapted to the lifestyle and established food habits of the patient in question.

Protein

Protein (and its constituent amino acids) is required by the body for synthesis of body proteins and other nitrogen-containing substances. Since humans are unable to synthesize about ten of the amino acids, these must be present in the diet for maintenance of life and health. Since proteins are vital structural and regulatory components of the body, it is not hard to understand that older people feel better and have fewer complications from acute and chronic illnesses when they ingest a diet adequate in protein content. Unfortunately, the self-selected diets of elderly individuals are sometimes deficient in this nutrient.

While difference in opinion is known to exist about protein and amino acid requirements of the elderly, considerable evidence supports the idea that elderly persons utilize dietary proteins quite effectively for protein synthesis and deposition of protein reserves. A recent study by Young and Scrimshaw at MIT (1975) showed that healthy elderly people achieve nitrogen equilibrium over the same range of protein intakes as reported for young men and women. From their limited data, the minimum protein needs of older persons do not appear to increase with advancing years if health is maintained.

Dietary protein derives from a number of food sources which basically can be classified as animal or vegetable materials. Animal protein foods, such as meat, fish, poultry, milk, eggs, and cheese, contain protein with a nice balance of essential amino acids and thus these protein sources are called "complete proteins." Vegetable proteins also are significant in the daily diet and largely derive from a variety of plant products like wheat, corn, soybeans, and rice. Because the essential amino acid composition of these proteins is not as appropriate for the needs of humans as that of animal proteins, vegetables are said to contain protein which is partially complete or incomplete. It should be remembered however, that combinations of vegetables that contain an amazingly well-balanced pattern of essential amino acids can be developed. Several good collections of recipes for such vegetarian dishes are available in most bookstores (Lappe 1971 and 1975). Those elderly persons who maintain an enthusiasm for cooking might profit immensely from including some of these food combinations in their diets.

Not only is it necessary for the essential amino acids to be present in the diet but also they must be available to the body tissues simultaneously and in proper proportions for utilization. This necessitates that some degree of regularity be established in presenting a balanced amino acid pattern to body tissues. The protein needs of most older people generally will be met if approximately 10 to 15 percent of the daily calorie intake is derived from protein. This need is easily met by the daily inclusion of two glasses of skim milk and an average portion of meat or meat alternate in the diet. These along with the small amounts of protein found in other common foods will serve to meet daily needs. However, culture, personal preference, oral problems, and a variety of other factors may serve to make the above recommendation useless; in such cases, other acceptable sources of dietary protein need to be identified and included in the diet on a regular basis.

Carbohydrates

Under most conditions carbohydrates provide at least 50 percent of the total calorie content of the diet. Anywhere from 50 to 75 percent of total calories should come from this source with 10 to 15 percent of the calories from protein and 10 to 40 percent of the calories from fat. Carbohydrates thus represent a very important source of energy for the body, and attempts to reduce carbohydrate intake drastically in an effort to lose weight are potentially harmful.

When dietary carbohydrates are drastically reduced, several things can happen. First, loss of tissue proteins (amino acids) will occur to make up the calorie deficit if one exists and to maintain blood sugar concentration at appropriate levels. Second, mobilization of fat may occur with a concomitant increase in blood cholesterol and triglyceride. Third, a significant loss of sodium and water via the kidneys may take place with the consequence of potential development of dehydration and renal damage. Even 10 percent of dietary calories from carbohydrate can overcome most of these problems. The human is known to exhibit a wide range of adaptability and thus no specific requirements for dietary carbohydrate have been defined.

Of significance, however, is the observation that some aged persons consume excessive amounts of *refined* carbohydrates because they usually are less expensive than other foods. Diets rich in refined carbohydrates not only may limit intake of other important nutrients but also they frequently will contain excessive calories. Complex carbohydrates are qualitatively much better in that the concentration of calories per unit of food is less, the content of other nutrients usually is higher, and the presence of fiber is probably vital to maintenance of health of the gastrointestinal system.

With relation to fiber it is interesting to note that constipation may easily develop in individuals with a poor intake of dietary fiber. Constipation is known to occur in at least 25 percent of older patients and many reasons have been cited as potentially influential. Among the factors believed to be contributory are the following:

1. Lack of fiber in the diet to stimulate peristalsis
2. Abuse of laxatives
3. Decrease in fluid intake
4. Decrease in motor tone and motor function of the bowel
5. Blunting or loss of the defecation reflex as a consequence of neglect of the urge to defecate
6. Organic lesions such as poor dentition, anorectal lesions inducing spasm of the anal sphincter, tumors and prolonged immobilization associated with fractures or paralysis

7. Medications such as sedatives or tranquilizers, antihypertensive and ganglionic blocking agents, narcotics, and calcium carbonate antacid

Poor dietary fiber intake accompanied by excessive laxative use is by far the circumstance of greatest significance; efforts to improve dietary composition and reduce laxative abuse should be aggressively made by all health professionals who care for older individuals in institutions or other community settings. Foods and beverages that aid in preventing constipation are summarized in Table 9-3.

TABLE 9-3. Foods and fluids which aid in the prevention and management of constipation.

Foods with bulk (fiber)
    Vegetables (especially raw)
    Fruits (especially raw)
    Whole grain cereal products
    Bran (in moderation)
    Legumes
    Nuts
Prunes and prune juice
Water (at least 6 glasses per day)
Benefit is also achieved by regular meal patterns, regular time for elimination, sufficient rest and relaxation, and adequate exercise

Fats

The diet of the typical American is high in fat. Recent statistics indicate that more than 41 percent of the daily calorie intake is obtained from this source. This fat is derived largely from animal sources but increasing use of vegetable oils in recent years is contributing to a slow change toward intake of less animal fat (saturated fat) and more vegetable fat (largely unsaturated fat). Fat is needed by the body for various reasons. Fats serve as a vehicle for the fat-soluble vitamins A, D, E, and K; they also reduce the amount of acid secretion and muscular activity of the stomach. They make the body feel full and appease hunger; they also increase the palatability of food and facilitate cooking. For these reasons, fats may be nutritionally, physiologically, and psychologically important to people. There is no conclusive proof, however, that they are an essential part of the adult diet other than their contribution of essential fatty acids which are needed in small amounts (2 to 4 percent of calories) each day.

A basic problem in our society is not one of fat deficiency but rather one of excessive fat consumption. Multitudes of research studies have indicated that high intake of dietary fat and/or cholesterol is directly correlated with incidence of atherosclerosis. In advanced industrialized societies the complications of atherosclerosis are the immediate cause of death of 50 percent of individuals. The lesion of atherosclerosis involves the formation of a fatty material in the inner lining of the arterial walls. This fatty material is rich in cholesterol and thus the lesions have long been associated with blood and dietary cholesterol. It is now well documented that deposition of cholesterol appears earlier and is more severe in those individuals whose blood cholesterol values are elevated. The level of blood cholesterol has been shown to depend on a variety of factors including genetic endowment, hormone interrelationships, psychic status, and diet. In the past two decades, a number of techniques have been discovered which will manipulate the blood cholesterol levels. One of the most promising of these has been the unexpected observation that, although the cholesterol level is difficult to regulate by manipulation of the total or fat-derived calories, it can be lowered by ingestion of an increased amount of unsaturated fatty acids. It is not necessary to reduce the total amount of fat to produce this effect, although this move seems advisable (Gotto, et al., 1974).

Despite the ability to reduce serum cholesterol level by dietary change and other methods, there is as yet no clear evidence that by doing so there is significant reduction in atherosclerosis and its complications. Although this is discouraging on the surface, it should be remembered that atherosclerosis takes time to develop and it may take a comparably long time before the prophylactic manifestations of a blood-lipid-lowering regimen become evident. Regardless of the outcome, this information has caused critical evaluation of the amount of eggs, dairy products, and fatty meats that should be in an optimal diet at all ages. The consensus is that fewer than 35 percent of dietary calories should be derived from fat and that the fat which *is* consumed should contain significant proportion of polyunsaturated fatty acids (Gotto, et al., 1974).

Practically speaking, calories as well as fats can be reduced in a variety of ways. Substituting fish, poultry, and lean meat for other meats, rich dairy products, and eggs will contribute significantly to reduction in fat intake. (Maintenance in the diet of *low-fat* dairy products is sensible in the long run,

however, since much nutritional value is obtained from the protein, riboflavin, calcium, and other nutrients which these foods contain.) The substitution of polyunsaturated margarines for butter and the use of vegetable oil instead of hydrogenated shortenings and standard salad dressings is also advisable. Avoidance of fatty desserts is particularly effective in reducing not only fat intake but sugar and calorie intake as well. There is no need for an individual to make these dietary changes overnight. This is very difficult for most people to accomplish; a much better approach to take is a gradual introduction of several new items into the diet each week as the fat-rich foods are gradually withdrawn or restricted in amounts.

It seems appropriate to insert a word of caution about working with people toward major dietary change. *Reasonable dietary changes for a man of 40 may not necessarily be right for the man of 90.* If a person has done well for 90 years on a particular diet (high-fat or otherwise), there seems little reason for him to institute change at this point. Diet therapy must be individualized. Recognition of the multitude of factors that influence eating patterns is basic to the planning and implementation of *any* special recommendations for dietary modification. Common dietary alterations are outlined at Table 9-4; the skilled clinician finds a workable means of squeezing these restrictive adjustments into the existant dietary patterns of elderly patients.

Vitamins

Vitamins are required by all humans throughout life, basically to allow for efficient operation of a variety of metabolic processes. Deficiency in one or more vitamins, consequently, impairs functionality of the biochemical processes which support physiologic activities. As a person grows older, need for each of the vitamins remains, and the level of need is largely comparable to that of younger individuals.

Unfortunately, the diets of many aged individuals are inadequate in terms of regular vitamin intake from natural sources. Data from the Ten State Nutrition Survey, conducted in the late 1960s and early 1970s, indicate that many older persons are poorly nourished. Sixteen percent of the population over 60 years of age showed serum vitamin C levels that were seriously low. Almost 40 percent of older individuals who were sampled consumed less than half the amount of vitamin A considered to be adequate (Hodkinson, 1975).

TABLE 9-4. Modification of daily menus for special diets.

BLAND
  Avoid highly seasoned foods
  Avoid fried foods
  Avoid raw vegetables and fruits, except ripe banana;
    avoid those with seeds, skins, and hulls such as
    raspberries, apples, corn, and any other that may
    cause distress
  Avoid whole grain cereals and breads
  Avoid pastries and rich desserts

LOW SALT
  Avoid adding salt (sodium chloride)
  Avoid all smoked, cured, or canned meats
  Avoid frozen fish fillets, lobster, shrimp, crab, clams,
    and oysters
  Avoid cold cuts and cheeses
  Avoid obviously salted foods such as potato chips,
    crackers, pickles, bouillon
  Avoid condiments and seasonings that contain salt
    such as catsup, celery salt

LOW SATURATED FAT
  Limit animal fats such as fatty meats, bacon, butter,
    cream
  Use predominantly veal, fish, and poultry
  Drink skim milk
  Limit cheese to dry or lowfat cottage cheese
  Use polyunsaturated fats such as safflower oil, corn
    oil, soybean oil, or margarines made predomi-
    nantly from these oils
  Avoid mixed dishes containing butter, whole milk,
    cream, and most cheeses

HIGH ROUGHAGE
  Use whole grain breads and cereals
  Use more raw and cooked fruits and vegetables
  Drink more water
  When more roughage is needed, eat a raw vegetable
    at both dinner and supper and a bran cereal daily

DIABETIC
  Eat only foods allowed and in amounts allowed
  Don't skip meals
  Avoid all desserts and sweets unless they are specifi-
    cally allowed by your doctor
  Avoid beer, wine, and other alcoholic beverages
  Avoid "special dietetic foods" other than canned fruits
    unless instructed otherwise

LOW CHOLESTEROL
  Limit animal fats such as fatty meats, bacon, butter,
    cream, whole milk, egg yolk, and cheeses, except
    dry cottage cheese
  Use predominantly veal, fish, and poultry
  Limit organ meats such as kidney, liver, heart, tripe,
    sweetbreads
  Limit clams, lobster, shrimp, oysters, and crab
  Use polyunsaturated fats such as safflower oil, corn
    oil, soybean oil, or margarines made predomi-
    nantly from these oils
  Avoid mixed dishes containing butter, whole milk, egg
    yolk and most cheeses

Adapted from Meal Planning for the Golden Years, General Mills, 1966.

Nonspecific symptoms such as fatigue, weakness, and mild paralysis may result from prolonged inadequate vitamin intake. Both the poor and the elderly who have severely restricted their diets without physician's advice may be especially prone to the development of vitamin deficiencies. Additionally, individuals with chronic diseases are especially susceptible. Since a number of vague complaints of ill health, suboptimal performance, impaired resistance to infection, poor wound healing, and other qualities may improve by the elimination of vitamin deficit, effort should be made to provide appropriate counseling about means of improving dietary input of specific vitamins. If dietary improvement seems unlikely or long in coming, supplementation with appropriate, low-level multivitamin preparations is often desirable.

Unfortunately, there are surprisingly few well-controlled studies of the effects of vitamin supple-mentation on health of the elderly. By far the best effort is a controlled, two-year study of chronically ill, hospitalized elderly patients (Taylor, 1968). In this population, 95 percent showed some sign of nutritional deficiency and 90 percent had low serum levels of vitamin C and thiamin. It was found that those patients receiving supplementary vitamin B complex and vitamin C showed highly significant improvement in physical and mental condition, although this improvement took up to one year to develop. When the vitamins were discontinued, signs of deficiency reappeared in about six months in many of the subjects, even while they were provided the general hospital diet which was designed to be complete in all nutrients.

Many older persons take vitamin supplements on their own initiative with the hope that improved health and vitality will develop. Often physicians recommend vitamin supplements for patients of advanced age without any real knowledge about their nutritional status. Classic vitamin deficiency diseases (i.e., beriberi, pellagra, scurvy) are infrequently seen in developed countries today but subclinical deficiency is hard to prove or disprove. To suggest that vitamin deficiencies cause most debilitation states in the elderly is unscientific but to disregard the fact that they do cause some is naive.

Unfortunately, elderly individuals who choose to use vitamin supplements may not be the ones with deficient diets. Several surveys have been conducted to judge dietary adequacy of older persons who regularly took vitamin supplements. Not surprisingly, it was found in one study that half of the vitamin users were consuming a completely adequate diet. Of the respondents whose diets were poor, (less than ⅔ of the RDA) only one in four such people were using vitamin supplements that covered all of their vitamin shortages. Only two out of four persons were using preparations which provided some, but not all, of the nutrients in which their normal diets were deficient. One fourth of the people whose diets were rated as poor were using the wrong supplements, that is, replacing none of the vitamins or minerals that their normal diet lacked (Howell and Loeb, 1969).

Some older people need to be warned not to depend exclusively on vitamin preparations to provide for all of their nutritional needs. Elderly people sometimes think that vitamin supplements take care of all nutritional problems or even all health problems. This certainly is not the case and such neglect of total individual requirements for maintenance of health most surely will lead to deterioration in nutritional status in some circumstances. Among elderly people who eat an ample diet, there is little evidence that supplementary protective vitamin therapy is required. Adequate medical and dietary histories and an awareness of the importance of nutritional status are required to insure that the individual is ingesting a balanced regimen.

A rational approach, then, to the use of vitamin preparations by the elderly must take into account their special problems and needs. Realistically, a diet with less than 1500 calories, in particular if it is poorly planned, is likely to be deficient in some vitamins. Under such circumstances, supplementation with a low-level, *appropriate* vitamin preparation may be justified. Common sense must be used in the selection of a vitamin supplement. For example, if a regular source of vitamin C can be identified in the diet, there is likely no need to include this vitamin in the supplement. Similarly, if milk or milk products are consumed on a regular basis, additional amounts of vitamin D are unnecessary.

Consideration should always be given to the possible danger associated with the indiscriminate use of vitamin supplements. Available information suggests that water-soluble vitamins are generally nontoxic, even in large doses, since the body is believed to excrete excesses in the urine. Several cases have been reported, however, of adverse responses to large doses of vitamin C, niacin, vitamin B_6, and folic acid. The fat-soluble vitamins, A and D, have long been recognized as toxic in large amounts. Vitamins E and K may produce similar problems but only recently have case reports appeared in the scientific literature; complaints associated with vitamin E excess include nondescript diarrhea, nausea, discomfort, fatigue, and other nonspecific symptoms. Some trace elements in vitamin preparations may be toxic if dosage is excessive and an additional problem might be the creation of significant vitamin imbalances by the use of single vitamin preparations. Without doubt the greatest danger in the use of vitamin supplements is failure to recognize and treat the underlying disease or other problems that caused the deficiency state to begin with.

Minerals

A number of minerals are required by the body to allow for normal operation of most chemical processes and adequate development of skeletal tissues. Most mineral elements are well distributed in food with the exception of iron and calcium. These minerals frequently are consumed in inadequate amounts by the elderly, and the incidence of iron deficiency anemia and skeletal problems is consequently high in this age group. Therefore, special attention must be paid to calcium and iron intake and ideally appropriate and acceptable food sources of these nutrients can be included in recommendations for dietary improvement.

Calcium

The long term effect of inadequate dietary intake of calcium relative to losses is demineralization of bone. A slight imbalance, when sustained over a long period of time can cause sufficient mineral loss to produce radiographically demonstrable osteoporosis. This concept might be best illustrated according to Lutwak (1974) by considering a hypothetic woman 50 years of age and weighing 65 kg. Weighing about the same at age 20, her skeleton would have contained about 1500 gm of calcium. Her average daily dietary intake of calcium is 0.4 gm, about 45 percent of which (0.18 gm) actually is absorbed. Daily losses are urinary calcium (0.1 gm), endogenous fecal calcium (0.15 gm), and dermal calcium (0.02 gm), for a total loss of 0.27 gm per day. This leaves a negative calcium balance of 0.09 gm per day. Over 30 years, 985.5 gm of calcium is lost, depleting the total body calcium to 515 gm or about a third of the original total.

In simple terms, osteoporosis may be defined as a condition of too little bone. Radiographically, it cannot be diagnosed until about 30 percent of the bone mineral has been lost. By this stage, mechanical instability of bone and subsequent fracture may have occurred. Recent surveys have indicated that approximately 30 percent of women over the age of 55 and men over the age of 60 have had sufficient bone loss to have resulted in at least one fracture (Lutwak, 1974). Other studies have also indicated that under various circumstances of demand, calcium is preferentially mobilized from bones with high trabecular content such as vertebrae and jaw. Consequently the clinical manifestations of osteoporosis would be expected to appear earliest in these bones. According to recent epidemiologic studies, at least 12 million women in the United States have sufficient osteoporosis to have produced vertebral fracture (Lutwak, 1974).

Research into the problem of osteoporosis has been extensive and much controversy still exists about etiology. Diets low in calcium have been associated with poor calcification of bones in a variety of animals and frequently the jaw has been found to demonstrate early resorption. In a prospective study involving dogs, institution of a low calcium diet led to loss of alveolar supporting bone in the jaw followed by loosening of the teeth, traumatization of the gingivae, exudation and hemorrhage—a typical picture of paradentosis (Henrikson, 1968). Demineralization occurred simultaneously but at a slower rate in other bones of these animals. Subsequent repletion studies indicated that remineralization occurred effectively in all bones with earliest effects apparent again in the jaw. Remineralization of jaw resulted in complete reversal of paradentosis (Krook, et al., 1971).

Subsequent work involving humans strongly suggested that the same phenomenon very likely occurred in this species as well (Krook, et al., 1972). Examination of autopsy material of patients with periodontal disease revealed the simultaneous presence of generalized osteoporosis in other parts of the skeleton and focal areas of parathyroid hyperplasia. This information suggested that in man, as in experimental animals, paradentosis was an early manifestation of osteoporosis and resulted from chronic low-degree secondary nutritional hyperparathyroidism.

In a later study involving patients with periodontal disease of various types but with no systemic osteoporosis, calcium supplement or placebo was provided for 12 months (Lutwak, et al., 1971). Bone density of the radius, ulna, and os mentis was measured at monthly intervals in all patients by the photon densitometric procedure. No significant increases in bone density occurred in the ulna or radius in either group of patients. Measurements of the os mentis, however, demonstrated a significant increase in bone density in the patients receiving calcium supplements, with no changes seen in those on placebo. These data suggest that the demineralization of the jaw seen in paradentosis can be reversed by dietary calcium supplements.

These human studies along with the previous animal work allow one to hypothesize that periodontal disease can be a manifestation of early osteoporosis, occurring five to ten years before significant bone mineral has been lost from other portions of the skeleton. Furthermore, this demineralization may be reversible by dietary calcium supplements and thus may provide a means for early detection of osteoporosis when treatment success may be expected.

While the insufficient intake of calcium (and/or vitamin D) in the diet probably is associated with deterioration in bone structure, the ratio of calcium to phosphorus may be more important than the actual amount of calcium that is provided. While blood calcium levels do not vary much with alteration in calcium intake, an increase in dietary intake of phosphate results in a rise in the serum inorganic phosphorus concentration. This may be demonstrated to be a postprandial response but it can also result in a rise in the fasting morning values. This rise in inorganic phosphorus concentration has been shown in normocalcemic persons and in animals.

To continue a bit further with this discussion, after this initial rise in inorganic phosphorus, there is a secondary fall to normal or below-normal levels, which can be ascribed to stimulation of parathyroid hormone secretion as a result of postprandial fall in the serum calcium level. This secondary fall occurs because any increase in serum phosphorus tends to raise the calcium-phosphorus product significantly; comparable increases in the serum calcium level do not elicit this response to the same degree, simply because the concentration of serum calcium is greater than that of serum phosphorus. If the mathematic product exceeds the formation product of calcium and phosphate, calcium level decreases.

In adult humans, living on diets typical of developed societies, the dietary intake of phosphorus is usually at least two to three times that of calcium, regardless of milk consumption. For instance, with an average American diet, a person who does not drink milk ingests about 300 mg of calcium and 700 mg of phosphorus daily, and a milk drinker ingests about 900 mg of calcium and 2000 mg of phosphorus. Consequently, in the majority of adults there will generally be a mild increase in the serum phosphorus concentration after each meal with a resultant stimulation of parathyroid hormone. This response may be slight or even invisible because of other rhythms of parathyroid hormone secretion; nonetheless, it will contribute to bone loss. Phosphate-induced bone loss has been shown experimentally in a number of animals (Jowsey, et al., 1974.)

Therefore, to prevent bone loss, the ratio of calcium to phosphorus intake should probably approximate 1 in the adult and more than 1 in the growing person. The most commonly used foods contain a great deal of phosphorus and almost no calcium (bread, cereal, meat, potatoes), while very few foods contain considerable calcium and no phosphorus (sesame seeds, pancake syrup, seaweed). Many vegetables, milk, and processed cheese contain slightly more calcium than phosphorus, but the ratio is almost 1.

Since bone loss appears to begin at about age 25, calcium supplementation might be started at this time and continued for the rest of life. That calcium supplements have been effective in reducing bone resorption by suppressing parathyroid hormone secretion has been demonstrated in persons with osteoporosis; there is every reason to believe that calcium supplementation would be effective preventive therapy in normal persons. Enrichment of selected processed foods with calcium salts might be a better approach than supplementation in the form of pills.

Comparative nutritional studies in various animal species indicate that the average calcium requirement is related to body weight of the species (Lutwak, 1974). The 800 mg of calcium required per day by humans is approximately 11 mg per kg body weight and this is probably lower than that for other animals. Since the efficiency of calcium absorption, however, is inversely related to dietary intake, a plateau of maximum calcium absorbed is most likely achieved at dietary intakes greater than 1000 mg per day (Table 9-5). A preliminary recommendation might be made therefore, of 1000 mg of calcium per day as optimum intake for the prevention of osteoporosis.

Thus it may be said that the high incidence of osteoporosis found in the population over age 50

TABLE 9-5. Relationship between calcium intake and absorption in humans.

Dietary Intake (mg/day)	Percent Absorption ($\pm$ S.D.)	Absorbed Calcium (mg/day)
Below 150	59.3 $\pm$ 49.6	89
150– 300	38.1 $\pm$ 22.5	114
300– 400	35.2 $\pm$ 21.8	141
400– 600	27.1 $\pm$ 24.7	163
600– 800	26.5 $\pm$ 21.8	212
800–1000	23.9 $\pm$ 22.5	239
1000–1200	27.5 $\pm$ 16.6	330
1200–1400	20.9 $\pm$ 46.6	293
1400–1600	24.9 $\pm$ 23.0	398
Above 1600	25.2 $\pm$ 23.8	504

Modified from Lutwak, L.: Continuing need for dietary calcium throughout life. Geriatrics 29:171, 1974.

may be related to long term low calcium intake. Although some people can adapt to relatively low calcium intake, there are others who continue to excrete large quantities of calcium in the urine in spite of low intake, indicating poor utilization in the body. Calcium balance tends to become negative with aging and there are many patients with osteoporosis who are in negative calcium balance. This may relate in part to reduction in the ability of the intestine to absorb calcium, impairment in the ability of the renal tubules to reabsorb calcium, and decreased physical activity which may promote increased urinary excretion of calcium. Increasing the calcium intake, if the total protein and other nutritional intake is adequate, usually will restore calcium balance. *Increasing the calcium content of the diet will not necessarily prevent or retard development of osteoporosis.* Much more research in this area is required at the biochemical and developmental level in order that the specific relationship between diet and bone integrity can be clarified.

Iron

A number of nutrients are required for blood cell formation and deficiency of any of them can compromise synthetic activities and, thereby, lead to the development of anemia. Iron deficiency is the most common problem, especially among individuals with low incomes and/or chronic diseases. The usual case of iron deficiency is related to a combination of poor dietary iron intake plus chronic blood loss, poor absorption and/or inadequate utilization of iron by the body. Low consumption of iron-rich foods may relate to poor appetite, unusual dietary habits, poor knowledge about iron-containing foods, and/or inappropriate food selection owing to insufficient funds (Jukes and Borsook, 1974).

Iron deficiency is characterized by hypochromic microcytic anemia with serum iron less than 50 mcg per 100 ml and iron binding capacity increased to levels of 450 to 650 mcg per 100 ml. Iron deficiency is most commonly diagnosed by the finding of low hemoglobin value in the blood and by reduction in size of erythrocytes. When poor iron intake is found to be involved, dietary correction should be instituted whenever possible. Sufficient iron-containing foods like leafy green vegetables, meats, legumes, and egg yolks should be incorporated into the diet on a regular basis. Sometimes iron supplementation may be needed on at least a temporary basis. Ferrous salts are the most readily absorbed source of iron and ferrous sulfate, ferrous fumarate, or ferrous gluconate are usually regarded as appropriate in this respect. But they are not without problems.

While iron deficiency may be the most common diet-related cause of anemia in the elderly, deficiency of folic acid and vitamin B_{12} should also be recognized as important. Deficiency of these vitamins, singly or simultaneously, may lead to the development of macrocytic or megaloblastic anemia. The incidence of this type of anemia in the elderly is especially high as compared to its presence in younger segments of the population (Meindok and Dvorsky, 1970).

Folic acid is present in many foods but the extent to which it is utilized varies with different foods. The availability of food folate in man has been shown to be relatively high in bananas, lima beans, liver, and brewer's yeast; the availability of folic acid is lower in orange juice, romaine lettuce, egg yolk, cabbage, defatted soybean, and wheat germ. The difference in availability probably relates to the fact that most food folic acid is present in conjugated form and, in some foods, release of free folic acid from its conjugated condition is difficult.

For many years, a strong prejudice existed against the use of dietary supplements of folic acid. This was due to the fact that large doses of folic acid produce a hematologic response in pernicious anemia without correcting the vitamin B_{12} deficiency that leads to neurologic degeneration. As a result, the addition of folic acid to food supplements, like over-the-counter vitamin preparations, was forbidden by the FDA at levels higher than 0.1 mg. In 1973, the FDA revised its regulations so that folic acid may be added to food supplements on the basis of 0.4 mg of the Recommended Dietary Allowance for adults. The usual therapeutic dose, oral or parenteral, is 1.0 mg daily. The upper limit of folic acid in dietary supplement preparations that can be sold without prescription is 0.8 mg daily. Use of folic acid supplements may be desirable in the elderly if dietary patterns are poor and cannot be changed, if malabsorption exists, or if drugs that interfere with the use of folic acid are being taken.

Vitamin B_{12} is unique among nutritional factors in that it requires a carrier protein, intrinsic factor, to take it from the intestinal tract into the body where it functions in a variety of biochemical processes or deposits in the liver. Intrinsic factor normally is present in gastric secretions. Individuals with pernicious anemia, however, do not produce intrinsic factor and these individuals show symptoms of vitamin B_{12} deficiency even when the diet contains a good supply of the vitamin. A deficiency of intrinsic factor is always accompanied by achlorhydria, but achlorhydric individuals are not necessarily deficient in intrinsic factor. Nevertheless, the presence of achlorhydria or a history of gastric resection is a good basis for advising an increased intake of vitamin B_{12}. The Recommended Dietary Allowance of vitamin B_{12} is 3 to 5 mcg. It is not present in vegetable foods: liver, meat, and fish are good sources. Vitamin B_{12} is commercially available in pharmaceutical preparations and in nutritional supplements in which it is supplied as a pure vitamin produced by fermentation. Intrinsic factor may also be supplied in pharmaceutical preparations alone or in combination with vitamin B_{12}, or the vitamin B deficiency may be corrected by injecting the vitamin at regular intervals or by supplying larger doses by oral administration. This latter method is rarely used but it is probably the cheapest. Patients who are secreting acid gastric juice can utilize the usual complement of dietary vitamin B_{12}, about 3 mcg daily, that occurs in a typical mixed diet of natural foods including animal products.

Sodium

Sodium is another mineral vital to maintenance of life in the human organism. It serves many functions as an ion in the fluid milieu of the body; one of its most significant roles is to assist in the regulation of fluid balance. The daily sodium requirement is unknown but a sufficient amount is easily obtained from almost any selected diet. More frequently, excessive amounts of sodium are consumed on a regular basis. The kidneys are helpful in dealing with this circumstance such that urinary excretion of sodium increases when diet excess occurs. It appears, however, that in some individuals who are genetically predisposed to hypertension, excessive sodium consumption may serve to contribute to the severity of their hypertensive disorder (Gordon, 1974).

Excessive intake of sodium in relation to intake of potassium may, therefore, lead to the elevation of blood pressure in some individuals. Up until about a decade ago, the major therapeutic measure that was instituted consistently in all cases of hypertension was the reduction of sodium intake by more or less rigorous restriction of salt in the diet. In certain areas, even the amount of sodium chloride in the drinking water was taken into consideration. This method of treatment probably reached its most ex-

treme form in the Kempner Diet which consisted largely of rice supplemented with fruits and vegetables. The response of the patients to this diet was promising but many were unable to tolerate it for long periods of time. As a continuous mode of therapy for a lifetime, it was out of the question.

Fortunately, the pharmaceutical industry investigated a series of diuretics and found that some were extremely efficient in producing marked diuresis and also effective natiuresis. Chlorothiazide, furosemide, and ethacrynic acid are three such drugs which produce a sharp increase in excretion of both sodium and potassium. The availability of these drugs has been a major contribution to the management of essential hypertension and largely has eliminated the need for severe dietary restriction of sodium. Avoidance of excessive sodium intake, however, is a reasonable measure to assist in prevention and management of hypertensive disease. Foods with high to moderately high sodium composition are in the following list:

1. Processed, smoked, or cured meats and fish (ham, bacon, corned beef, cold cuts, frankfurters, sausage, tongue, salt pork, chipped beef)
2. Salted foods (potato chips, nuts, popcorn)
3. Meat extracts, bouillon cubes, and meat sauces
4. Vegetable salts and flakes (onion, garlic, or celery salt; celery and parsley flakes)
5. Prepared condiments, relishes, Worchestershire sauce, catsup, mustard, pickles, and olives
6. Sodium in various additive compounds (sodium benzoate, monosodium glutamate)
7. Breads and bakery products (unless prepared specially for low-sodium composition)
8. Frozen fish fillets and shellfish (except oysters)
9. Prepared flours, flour mixes, baking powder, and baking soda
10. Frozen vegetables, especially peas and lima beans; sauerkraut in any form
11. Most canned meat and vegetable products unless specially prepared without salt
12. Some canned fruit (pears, figs, applesauce)
13. Butter, cheese, and peanut butter (unless unsalted)

Potassium

Potassium is the major cation in the intracellular fluid and a significant component of the extracellular fluid compartment as well. Potassium (along with sodium) is involved in the maintenance of normal water balance, osmotic equilibrium, and acid-base balance. It also acts with calcium in the regulation of neuromuscular activity. Any circumstance which significantly increases or decreases the level of potassium in the extracellular fluid may be regarded as indicative of serious disturbances in muscle biochemistry since change in the extracellular concentration of potassium occurs late in the process of potassium depletion.

Potassium deficiency is not likely to develop in healthy individuals under normal circumstances. Potassium is widely distributed in foods and the average intake is estimated to be 0.8 to 1.5 gm per 1000 calories. An adequate intake of milk, meats, cereals, vegetables, and fruits will provide adequate potassium. Significant food sources of potassium are the following:

- Legumes
- Potatoes
- Whole grains
- Winter squash
- Leafy vegetables
- Milk
- Meats

Certain fruits, such as the following, are potassium-rich foods:

- Bananas
- Dried prunes, apricots, dates, peaches
- Raisins
- Cantaloupe
- Citrus fruits

Excessive loss of extracellular fluid may result in potassium deficiency, especially in the elderly. The loss may be due to vomiting, diarrhea, excessive diuresis, or prolonged malnutrition. In these conditions, potassium from the intracellular fluid is transferred to the extracellular fluid. The serum potassium level is low and ionized potassium excretion is increased. In hypokalemia (low serum potassium), cardiac failure can result from depletion of ionized potassium in heart muscle. Prevention of potassium deficiency is of considerable importance in overall management of any patient with persistent gastrointestinal disorders, diuretic use (e.g., chlorothiazide, acetazolamide), or adrenocortical hormone therapy. Consumption of foods rich in potassium should be recommended (unless contraindicated by accompanying problems) and, in some cases, potassium supplementation of the diet may be required.

Fluid

Water or fluid is not often thought of as food but it probably is the most important single compound required by the body. Water is essential for maintaining an environment for all chemical reactions within the body and also is vital for the functioning of urinary excretory mechanisms and for prevention of constipation. So significant is water that it constitutes about two thirds of the weight of an adult; it also is present in all body secretions and is involved in regulation of body temperature. While the body usually can survive for many weeks without food, death will occur in less than a week when an individual is totally deprived of water.

Consequently, enough fluids should be consumed on a daily basis to allow for normal 24-hour urine volume of about 1 to 1½ quarts. The sensation of thirst will generally provoke intake of sufficient fluid, but elderly individuals, especially those with chronic illness, may lose this regulatory capacity. Both familial and cultural patterns may serve to de-emphasize the drinking of water.

In institutions where mealtime is regulated, fluid needs of some individuals may not be met if much time elapses between dinner and breakfast. Dehydration may easily develop overnight, especially if dinner has been served early and breakfast served late. Therefore it may be desirable to routinely provide an evening fluid snack, or at least water, to prevent the potential serious problem of water deficit.

FACTORS THAT DETERMINE NUTRITIONAL NEEDS

To a large extent, the nutritional needs of the older adult are related to the problems of nutritional balance. Nutritional balance is not solely a matter of appropriate nutrient intake but many other factors participate in altering the circumstance of nutritional equilibrium. Factors that serve to prevent achievement of balanced nutritional status include interference with food intake, modification of intestinal absorption, interference with storage and utilization, increase in urinary and fecal excretion, and change in nutrient requirements.

Interference with Food Intake

Many factors in isolation or in combination with each other lead to reduction in food intake among the elderly. Since *low income* prevents the purchase of an adequate diet for many elderly persons, this factor may be of prime significance in limiting the available food supply in the home. Additionally, however, *loss of teeth* and use of poor-fitting dentures along with age-related *loss of the senses of smell and taste* may have important effects on dietary intake. The sensory losses may render food monotonous, unattractive, and uninspiring. Oral problems may lead to the adaptation of a soft diet high in refined carbohydrate and low in protein. *Physical handicaps* may contribute to either primary or secondary loss of motivation by older persons in preparing meals, thus leading to the dependance on high-priced convenience foods or fad diets and ultimately the acceptance of a variety of dietary restrictions. In addition, certain *disorders of the esophagus* prevalent in the aged (such as spasm, cancer, or hiatus hernia) may retard the passage of food into the stomach. Such conditions may remain hidden to caretakers or attending health professionals until the individual progresses to the point of obvious deterioration in health.

As far as disorders of the oral cavity are concerned, these have frequently been considered a major factor in poor eating habits of aged people. By age 60, about 45 percent of people in the United States have lost all their teeth. Some studies, however, have indicated that satisfactory dentition was not necessarily required for maintaining good nutritional status as determined by height, weight, skinfold thickness, hemoglobin level, and other factors. Totally edentulous individuals are capable of gumming food surprisingly well and lack of teeth may not be a significant factor in compromising nutritional status (Anderson, 1971). Probably more important than whether or not teeth or good dentures are present and utilized is the overall adequacy of the diet available to the individual. It has been observed that regardless of dentition, many older persons, particularly those in institutions, will consume nutritionally important foods if given satisfactory opportunity to do so.

Alcoholism may also contribute to reduction in food intake in the aged (Howell and Loeb, 1969). Recent psychiatric studies indicate that alcoholism may be common, particularly in metropolitan areas, but often denied by both older persons and their families. The high caloric value of alcohol tends to satiate the appetite, reduce food intake, and lead to deficiency of essential dietary components, particularly protein. In the past, a variety of vitamin deficiencies were quite common, especially involving the B-complex, however, the frequency of obvious clinical manifestation of vitamin deficiency has decreased in recent years, probably owing to widespread availability of vitamin-enriched bakery products and improved preventive care by health professionals.

Depression also is common in the elderly and may lead to anorexia or complete refusal of food. The severe depressive states often respond to appropriate treatment although this may involve tremendous effort and may even necessitate shock therapy and tube feeding. Treatment of anorexia in the senile, deteriorated patient is even more difficult and often is unsuccessful under the best of circumstances.

Modification of Intestinal Absorption

A variety of phenomena associated with the aging process may interfere with the absorption of nutrients from the intestine. Significant changes include atrophy of the salivary glands with an accompanying loss of enzymes, gastric achlorhydria, a decrease in the production and delivery of digestive enzymes of the stomach, pancreas, and small intestine, and diminished production and release of bile from the liver and gallblader. Some of these changes may be the result of normal aging, while others may relate to the presence of pathologic conditions.

Drugs may also affect food absorption and interact with nutrients in a variety of ways. Mineral oil, for example, is an effective laxative because it is not absorbed. Since it is not absorbed but is able to bind fat-soluble vitamins, these vitamins may be lost in the stool and fat-soluble vitamin deficiencies may eventually develop. Additionally, numerous drugs are known to promote malabsorption as a result of their irritating or destructive effect on the intestinal mucosa or their interference with normal epithelial cell renewal.

Interference with Storage and Utilization

Diminished storage and utilization of nutrients from food may occur with aging for several reasons. There may be a diminished or altered endocrine pattern leading to impaired metabolism. With aging there may be a loss of cells involved in the utilization and storage of nutrients; there may also be loss of structural units which produce the enzymes required for these processes. Additionally, diminished efficiency of delivery by the vascular system may develop because of intrinsic changes within that system and because of the increase in fibrous tissue which accumulates in many organs; this latter condition may create a barrier between capillaries and the parenchymal cells of affected body tissues.

Increase in Urinary and Fecal Excretion

The aging process, in general, is not associated with significant increases in excretory losses from the body other than the possible passage through the large bowel of undigested food because of impaired digestion and absorption. There may develop in some old patients, however, a considerable loss of protein in the urine as a consequence of kidney disease. At the same time, there is also a loss of potassium and intracullular water with aging but there is no evidence that this is related to increased excretion.

Change in Nutrient Requirements

Most of the diet is utilized to provide energy for body functions. Energy-producing food constitutents include carbohydrates, fats, and those proteins not needed for maintenance of structural and regulatory proteins of the body. The components of the diet required for maintenance and repair of structure and regulation of biochemical processes include nine or ten essential amino acids (constituents of proteins), several unsaturated fatty acids, vitamins, and minerals. During the aging process, the body's need for some of these nutrients changes in accord with changing physiologic activities, exercise patterns, and overall lifestyle. Conditions of nutritional deficiency or excess may develop if eating patterns are not adjusted to accommodate the change in body needs.

In addition to the normal changes in nutrient requirements related to advancing age, many diseases produce a hypermetabolic state which may create a dietary need in excess of intake. Fevers of any type, especially if prolonged, consume excess calories and produce tissue wasting and weight loss if dietary intake is not increased to cover the calorie requirement. Persistent fevers, even of a low-grade type, may produce the same result. The most common cause of emaciation or cachexia, however, is malignancy. Cancer causes tissue wasting which seems excessive in many circumstances for the increased metabolic activity that exists. This phenomenon may be due to preferential requirement by the tumor for particular amino acids which if found in short supply in the diet will be leached from available lean body stores.

THE SIGNIFICANCE OF FOOD BEYOND ITS NUTRIENTS

Fulfillment of the need for food is a significant concern in the management of patients at all stages of the life cycle. Beyond the basic role of food in providing for physical sustenance and growth, however, food and foods take on special meanings in the lives of most people. Eating is an important activity that serves to meet not only physiologic requirements but also to fulfill basic psychologic, sociologic, and emotional needs of individuals. Recognition of the significance of food and eating in the cultural patterns of aging persons is critical to development of workable recommendations for improvement of health through modification of dietary practices.

Discussion of cultural patterns in relation to diet encompasses a variety of dimensions. For the practitioner who needs to understand fully what determines behavioral patterns of people, it is particularly important to be consciously aware of ethnicity, regional or urban-rural cultures, socioeconomic status, and age-appropriate behavior.

Ethnic Factors

Ethnicity includes those characteristics of behavior and habit that are part of national or ethnic custom. Ethnic patterns in food preference and use serve to consolidate group identity. Adherence to traditional patterns is particularly strong in connection with social and/or religious ritual. Culture defines those foods that are "good" and those which are not. Culture determines a group's perception of individual foods such that some highly nutritious food items may be considered good only as dogfood and totally unacceptable for human consumption.

Ethnic foods may be unsuitable for the aged only if they are medically contraindicated or if they consistently exclude necessary nutrients. The high fat diets of some Middle-European cultures and the high starch diets of Southern Europeans are cases of dominance in the diet but not necessarily inappropriate except as they may contribute to obesity. Soul foods of black Americans also may contain excessive fats and a very low lean-protein content. Research on obesity, especially among women 55 to 70, indicates that ethnic diets contribute greatly to the persistence of weight problems.

It has been established by anthropologic studies, however, that indigenous foods and their manner of preparation and combination typically represent "good" nutritional balance for a particular native group. It is the imposition of alien food forms or preparation methods that most often subverts the inherent balance existent in a traditional diet of a group of people.

Regional or Urban-Rural Cultures

There are traditional types of foods within the United States which are identified with certain areas of the country and which long-time residents of such areas associate with "home." For elderly persons, it is likely that the reintroduction of such foods in a social situation would have a positive reinforcement value. Presentation of foods from "down home" may encourage reminiscences, now considered a psychologic benefit in the aged's adjustment to the final stage of their life cycle. The exchange of memories may, in turn, facilitate the development of new interpersonal ventures, so necessary where old friends and many relatives have been lost.

Socioeconomic Status

Socioeconomic status is not strictly considered as "culture"; however, class often interacts in culture-like ways with, for example, rural origins of a migrant group of ethnic group identity. The concept of a *culture* of *poverty* appears to have considerable practical reality as one observes and programs for those elderly who have lived their entire lives far below a minimum standard of living accepted as tolerable in this society. The class identification of certain foods may serve a detrimental function in the diet of poor people. Status may be sought by selective purchase of high carbohydrate, processed foods thought to be preferred by the upper class.

Age-Appropriate Behavior

Of interest is the finding by social scientists that another culture-like input in the behavior of older persons is the expectation held by the aged as to how they should act, that is, what behaviors are appropriate or inappropriate to their chronologic level. These *shoulds* are reinforced by attitudes of younger adults such that a picture develops in the mind of young and old of appropriate *normal* behavior for old people in a particular culture. Age-appropriate behaviors relate especially to food choice and dietary habits since these are very often associated with the changed body image of the elderly. Older people, especially women, tend to be quite conscious about the internal and external states of their bodies and thus tend to develop protective attitudes in response to visible aging and body dysfunction. The dysfunctions or malfunctions may be real, imagined, or exaggerated. In any case, food selection and rejection is often justified by an appeal to the needs of the body. Areas of likely concern are related to digestion, constipation, tissue rejuvenation, blood, and muscle tone (fatigue).

The popularity of iron supplements among the elderly, for example, has been said to relate to the age-appropriate belief that high iron concentrations in the blood can reduce fatigue associated with aging. The reality that the fatigue of old age may mask (or be generated by) depression, cumulative social loss, or disease (none of which is affected by iron supplements) should create concern among health care professionals. Likewise, concern should also exist about the high use of health foods among older persons. This recognized practice also suggests the widespread interest among the elderly for maintenance of body image through acceptable age-appropriate dietary behavior. Efforts should be made to counter myths about "bottled health" and "magic foods." The elderly person should be advised on how to spot a "quack."

FIVE WAYS TO SPOT A "QUACK"

1. He claims to have a special or secret formula, product, or pill which prevents or cures disease.
2. He assures you a quick cure.
3. He bases his case on case histories and testimonials to promote his remedy.
4. He constantly challenges the medical profession to investigate his claims.
5. He claims authentic medical doctors persecute him or fear his competition.

IMPLICATIONS FOR EATING HABITS
OF THE AGED

Because of the multitude of roles that food plays in the lives of most people, feeding patterns and food preferences should be recognized as basic to happiness and survival. In particular, as far as the elderly are concerned, eating is remembering, eating is life-giving, and eating is relating.

Eating is Remembering

The aged person who uses "food for thought" as a means of gaining comfort in the present from reminiscence of the past is less concerned with the life-giving qualities of food and more concerned with the symbolic meanings of food. Eating habits that appear "unhealthful" to the nurse or nutritionist may be serving an important adaptive function for the aged person. Thus there may be conflict between the primary goal of the nutritionist and the aged person who is being served. The imposition of the nutritionist's needs may, if not handled cautiously, undermine the intrapsychic needs of the person to be served. While there is no easy solution to this conflict, it can be handled by a sensitive awareness of how particular eating habits play an adaptive function for the person. The older person can "have his cake and eat it too" if enough of the meaning of foods or particular detrimental routines to the individual are meshed into a more sensible nutritional regimen.

It may be more difficult, on the other hand, to introduce a beneficial food into a nutritional regimen when confronted with a lifetime of food aversions. Efforts to convince an aging person through a rational discussion that a new food might actually be rather tasty to him or indeed agree with him physically cannot help but conflict with persistent lifetime taboos and stereotypic attitudes. For example, the woman in her 70s with the common problem of constipation who says, "I don't eat cheese because it is constipating," is not about to be convinced that cheese is the obvious source of improved health. In her advanced age, such stereotypes form a convenient way of dealing with the world, a world which seems manageable and comfortable by just such reassuring perceptions. The heroic task of introducing new foods into the diet of a younger person is made even more difficult in working with the aged.

Eating is Life-Giving

When we are confronted with body deterioration, the primary function of food as bodily maintenance becomes of increasing importance. Here, also, magical solutions that take the form of food as recuperative agents or as restoring youth are sometimes sought by the aged. In the extreme, this magic is seen in food faddism and in hoarding behaviors where having an immediate access to a particular food offers reassurance. Part of the institutionalization process has been seen to *depersonalize* the individual by restricting his free access to food. Some nursing homes and hospitals in the United States have instituted a 24-hour food availability system by providing refrigerators and cupboards for free snacking. Although psychologically of benefit, this type of program, if inadequately supervised, could lead to poor diet in the aged.

For the community-dwelling aged an important aspect of the mechanism of food as reassurance may be shopping for and purchasing food in which the process of "gathering and storing" enhances feelings of life-maintenance. The more supportive an aged individual can be of his established food-related activities, the more likely that person is to maintain an optimistic outlook of his remaining life and a motivation to maintain his health.

Eating is Relating

Securing, preparing, and consuming food are activities basic to family relationships. Most of the elderly in today's society have actively participated in home-based food activities and have enjoyed the mealtime as a period for family discussion. In most cases the wife has performed her maternal function of preparing and serving the food to her family; the husband typically has enjoyed the role of provider and consumer. Sex-role identification generally is well solidified such that when age-related losses reduce the opportunity for these activities, the corresponding identifications are weakened. Consequently, to facilitate the maintenance of these identifications, it may be necessary to find substitutes in the form of activities and persons which replace significant others. Where the elderly come together in senior centers, the opportunity for reestablishing and reaffirming their sex roles in food preparation and serving should be supported when possible by the practitioner. Similarly, in a home care program it may be easier to prepare all meals for the elderly widow who needs a special diet; this service, however, may be depriving her of the personal meanings inherent in food activities. Likewise, for persons who are unable to work for their food, effort should be made to locate an activity which might partially satisfy their needs.

While maintenance of these food-related or meal-related activities is satisfying for most elderly people, several cross-cultural studies have shown that the need to maintain these activities is of less importance than the need to feel one is comfortable and secure. Fulfilling of the need for security may relate more to relationships with children than to spouse, especially if the spouse has died. Eating may thus become part of an intergenerational conflict where inadequate eating may function to arouse concern of a daughter, who may feel guilty about her caretaking relationship with a parent. The comment that "she doesn't eat enough to keep a bird alive" may reflect a generational conflict that must be handled if the elderly parent is to receive nutritional requirements. In a situation where the daughter is of an advanced age herself, especially if the mother is in her 70s or 80s, then inventive techniques geared toward the more elderly person may, by necessity, include therapeutic help for both.

Inadequate food intake as a plea for attention must be understood in the context of feelings of loneliness and of isolation and desolation. When faced with loneliness, food can become a solace, because it facilitates memories; on the other hand, the rejection of food may relate to a plea for immediate attention and caring. Often this plea is part of the paranoid behavior of the aged where the covert or unconscious message is, "If you really loved me you would care for me and make me well again." Whereas all efforts made to reduce these irrational feelings seem to be unsuccessful and all efforts to ameliorate the nutritional inadequacies appear to fail, the very contact between the provider and the elderly person may be relieving of feelings of loneliness and isolation.

Because of the multitudes of meanings that food has for aged individuals, part of the goal of any nutrition program for older people should be to keep them not only physically alive but also socially and psychologically active. This means that a good nutrition program for the aged includes more than the proper balance of nourishing food, even nourishing food adapted to the individual's past tastes and prejudices and taboos. It includes at least some opportunity for the meaningful social involvement and

some opportunity for individual planning and choice of both food and social involvement to suit varying personality types. Recent government-sponsored demonstration projects on the nutrition of the aged have paid careful attention to the multiple facets of the eating experience. Some of these programs and ideas are further discussed in the remainder of this chapter.

ASSESSING DIETARY PATTERNS AND NUTRITIONAL STATUS

The nutritional evaluation of the individual is as important as any other aspect of a thorough evaluation and consequently involves the acquisition of as much relevant information as possible. Effort should be made to identify significant factors known to adversely influence nutritional well-being. The evaluation must include a thorough physical examination, with special emphasis on those clinical signs that have been associated with malnutrition in humans. Of particular importance are neurologic findings and examination of the skin, eyes, and oral cavity including the tongue, lips, gums, and teeth. In addition, selected and relevent biochemical data must be accumulated to confirm or extend the clinical judgment derived from the physical and nutritional evaluation. Particular attention must be given to the latent aspect of nutritional deficiency which frequently is present but extremely difficult to define in concrete observations.

Most circumstances of nutritional deficiency are rather complex in the manner by which they develop (Fig. 9-1). Primary nutritional deficiency disease may occur solely because of inadequate dietary intake but this is rare unless the poor diet persists for a long period of time. More commonly, especially in the elderly, such factors as malabsorption, decreased utilization of nutrients, increased excretion and destruction of nutrients, and increased nutritional requirements related to genetic or metabolic factors must be considered. The typical sequence of events in the development of clinical malnutrition is the initial desaturation of tissue content of various nutrients. Usually this is evidenced by biochemical alterations in the blood, urine, and biopsy specimens. As tissue depletion proceeds, biochemical deficits may become increasingly manifest. It should be recognized, however, that these biochemical changes in the blood, like clearcut observable clinical changes attributable to malnutrition, seldom develop in well-

Dietary Deficiency of Nutrient(s)
(evaluated by diet record
and diet history)

*Conditions Which Compromise
Nutritional Status:*

–digestive disturbances
–malabsorption
–excessive urinary
   excretion
–increased metabolic
   requirements

(evaluated by medical
history and physical
examination)

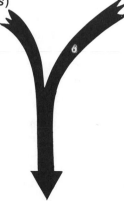

*Gradual Loss of
Nutrients from
Body Tissues*
(sometimes observed
by assay of blood,
urine, tissue specimens,
X rays)

*Biochemic Changes
in Body Tissues*
(evaluated by tissue assay
for enzyme activity,
assessment of
basal metabolic rate,
and metabolite levels)

*Anatomic Changes from
Prolonged Nutritional
Deficit*
(apparent in physical
examination)

Death

FIGURE 9-1. Sequential steps in the development of "malnutrition."

defined stages but rather present in a series of gradations in which the duration of the deficit is most important. *Clinical manifestation of nutritional deficiencies never appear as black or white problems but more often present as a spectrum of irregularities appropriately assigned to the "gray zone"* (Table 9-6).

If the circumstance of malnutrition continues long enough, the classic anatomic and pathologic lesions or signs of deficiency disease become obvious (Table 9-6). At this point of severe deprevation, complete responses to nutritional rehabilitation usually are slow. Clearly, then, it is important to diagnose malnutrition before the full-blown deficiency condition develops.

To summarize the above ideas, the basic principles underlying the evaluation of nutritional status are not much different from those used in general medical evaluation of a patient. The nutritional evaluation is based on (1) observing the general appearance of the individual, (2) obtaining a complete medical, personal, and social history, (3) recording an accurate diet history, either elaborate or concise, (4) completing a thorough physical examination, including measures of body weight and height, and (5) compiling pertinent laboratory data as they relate to suspected nutritional deficits.

As far as biochemic or laboratory data are concerned, several basic principles deserve attention in establishing guidelines for sensible lab workups. First, laboratory assays should be carefully selected to answer specific questions that exist about the patient's nutritional status. Second, the lab work should provide substantiation of the clinical judgment or remove lingering doubt. Third, a number of do-it-yourself procedures may save time and costs for both patient and health care staff. A simple urinalysis, evaluation of a blood smear, and microscopic

TABLE 9-6. Clinical syndromes associated with deficiencies of specific nutrients.

Calories: Underweight, underheight, weight loss, lethargy, anemia, edema, marasmus

Protein: As above, fatty liver, kwashiorkor

Fat: Dermatoses in infants (essential fatty acid deficiency), deficiencies of the fat-soluble vitamins A, D, E, and K

Vitamin A: Growth failure, follicular hyperkeratosis, night blindness, xerophthalmia, keratomalacia

Vitamin D: Rickets, tetany, osteomalacia

Vitamin E: Unknown, macrocytic anemia

Vitamin K: Decreased plasma prothrombin activity with prolonged coagulation time and hemorrhages

Thiamine: Anorexia, beriberi, polyneuropathy, toxic amblyopia, heart disease, the ophthalmoplegia of Wernicke's syndrome

Riboflavin: Photophobia, corneal vascularization, angular stomatitis, glossitis, dermatitis

Niacin: Pellagra, dermatitis, glossitis, diarrhea, mental confusion and deterioration, encephalopathy

Pyridoxine: Anemia, convulsions (infants), polyneuropathy, seborrheic exzema

Pantothenic acid: Nutritional melalgia (burning feet syndrome)

Folic acid: Glossitis, macrocytic anemia, megaloblastic anemia of infancy, megaloblastic anemia of pregnancy

Vitamin B_{12}: Glossitis, macrocytic anemia, peripheral neuropathy, combined system diseases (posterolateral column degeneration), mental changes and deterioration

Biotin: Seborrheic dermatitis

Choline: Unknown

Inositol: Unknown

Carnitine: Unknown

Ascorbic acid: Scurvy, scorbutic gums, subperiosteal hemorrhages, petechial hemorrhages, anemia, impaired wound healing

Iron: Anemia, achlorhydria, glossitis

Iodine: Simple goiter

Fluorine: Dental caries

Calcium: Osteomalacia, a role in the production of senile osteoporosis has been suggested but not proved

Magnesium: Neuromuscular irritability, tetany

Potassium: Alkalosis, muscle weakness and paralysis, cardiac disturbances

Salt (NaCl): Anorexia, nausea, vomiting, lassitude, asthenia, muscle cramps, circulatory collapse

Water: Thirst, dehydration, oliguria, mental changes progressing to coma

Adapted from Goodhart, R. S., and Wohl, M. G.: Manual of Clinical Nutrition. Philadelphia, Lea & Febiger, 1964.

study of the stool for the presence of fat can be completed rather easily in an office or clinic. Fourth, the importance of appropriate timing of lab tests should be fully recognized. A fasting blood sample should be just that and assessment of vitamin level in the bloodstream or urine has no value if the therapeutic provision of vitamins has already begun. Lastly, at least two points should be established sequentially in a series of laboratory evaluations to determine the progress of the illness or the effects of therapy.

The Diet History

The diet history may turn out to be the most important piece of information available in completing a routine evaluation of nutritional condition. Unfortunately, recording an accurate diet history is not always easy and usually requires considerable time and patience. One aspect of this procedure which may prove to be especially valuable as a screening mechanism is the listing of foods in major categories and determining the number of times per week that the patient consumes them. This process may easily identify the individual who tends to follow some fad diet, who restricts his diet to only several foods, who ingests significant amounts of "empty calories" like alcohol and sugar, or who follows highly unusual dietary practices that exclude important foods or food groups. Generally speaking a balanced dietary regimen best fulfills daily needs and such a dietary pattern should provide no more than 20 to 25 percent of daily calories from a single food. It is also important to inquire about eating habits and the distribution of meals, particularly the omission of certain meals, such as breakfast, and the type and frequency of snacks. Some people do not regard between-meal snacks as "food" and frequently do not report these as part of their daily diet. Obtaining this important information by careful questioning is important if accurate overall assessment of nutrient intake is to be secured.

NUTRITIONAL STATUS OF THE ELDERLY IN DEVELOPED SOCIETIES

Nutritionists generally agree that the diets of elderly individuals often are nutritionally inadequate and that this adversely affects their nutritional status and health. This concensus is supported by results of a number of nutrition studies including the recently published findings of the Ten State Nutrition

Survey (Howell and Loeb, 1969). Dietary studies indicate that the aged often have a low intake of vitamins and minerals, particularly iron, calcium, ascorbic acid, and B vitamins (especially folic acid). The recent Ten State Nutrition Survey indicated iron deficiency anemia is more prevalent in persons over 60 years of age than in younger people whose daily iron requirement is believed to be higher (American Dietetic Association, 1970; Stewart, 1972).

One interesting study of elderly persons in rural Pennsylvania clearly demonstrates the kinds of findings that have arisen from a series of studies on this age group (Guthrie, 1975). Two coexisting populations were studied. Members of Group I were eligible for food assistance while members of Group II were not. Information obtained related to social, economic, and educational background, frequency of intake of selected foods in the basic four food groups, nature and extent of home production of food, self-ratings of health status, nature and extent of use of nutritional supplements, and participation in food assistance programs. The adequacy of dietary intake was compared with income, age, number in household, sex, education, self-rating of health, ability to chew food, special medical restrictions, and sources of dietary advice. Less than two-thirds of the Recommended Dietary Allowances is considered inadequate intake.

In comparing the two income groups, the lower income group had significantly less protein, iron, and riboflavin in the diet. Women tended to have less adequate intake of iron. Subjects in two-person households consumed less vitamin A. Of the families eligible for food assistance, those who made use of it tended toward a more adequate diet. Nutrient intake was not found to be related to dental health, self-ratings of health, or to dietary restrictions.

Looking at the whole group, the following dietary inadequacies were found: 63 percent were deficient in calcium and vitamin A, 27 percent in protein, 18 percent in iron, 45 percent in calories, riboflavin, and vitamin C, and 42 percent in thiamine. One can draw one of two conclusions from this data: either the standard of adequacy is unrealistically high or the older poor in this area have marginal to serious nutritional deficiencies.

One further item of interest in the above study was the comparison of Group I subjects (those eligible for food assistance) to families at a similar poverty level living in the same area which had members of all ages. The older group showed a significantly less adequate intake of calories, protein, thiamine, and riboflavin than the other representatives of the families as a whole. One might conclude from this as well as substantial amounts of other data that the elderly in our society are at particular high risk for exposure to diets of inferior value and the development over time of clinically obvious malnutrition.

Other investigations of the nutritional status of the institutionalized elderly have been conducted in recent years. One study directly compared the food choices of institutionalized with a group of independently-living elderly (Clarke, 1975). The nutritional score was determined by measuring the intake of eight nutrients and comparing it to two thirds of the RDA. On this basis, the nutritional score did not correlate to place of residence, age, or sex. The average intake was above two thirds of the 1968 RDA for all nutrients except for calcium. Again, individual scores varied widely. Only one half of those studied consumed two thirds of the RDA for all nutrients.

A study of private nursing home patients showed many of the same tendencies (Miller, 1971). The food offered by the staff was above the 1974 RDA for all nutrients studied, but individual food choices showed many deficiencies. The most noteworthy were inadequacies in calcium and iron intake. Many patients were reported to be anemic upon examination.

The hearings of the Select Committee on Nutrition and Human Needs of the U.S. Senate identified the elderly as one of the groups particularly vulnerable to malnutrition, especially the substantial segment of this group with low income (Stewart, 1972). This important committee recommended that special consideration be given to the plight of the elderly and that workable ideas be formulated to help solve current problems as they exist. The White House Conference on Food, Nutrition and Health in 1969 evidenced additional concern for the nutrition of the aged, and the 1971 White House Conference on Aging made Recommendations to improve the quality of nutrition and the food supply particularly for those in the low income or poverty category (Watkin, 1970).

EFFORTS TO SOLVE NUTRITIONAL PROBLEMS OF THE ELDERLY

Recognition of the serious problem of malnutrition among the elderly increased during the 1960s to the point where significant government involvement developed. The Department of Health, Education and Welfare became increasingly involved in 1965 and, by 1973, under Title VII of the Older Americans Act, The Administration on Aging instituted the National Nutrition Program for the Elderly (National Clearing House on Aging, 1974).

The overriding goal of this massive undertaking was to provide inexpensive, nutritionally-sound meals to older Americans. Additionally, however, the program was designed to reduce the isolation of older people by offering them an opportunity to participate in community activities which combine food and friendship. As the amended form of the Older Americans Act stated:

Many older persons do not eat adequately because (1) they cannot afford to do so, (2) they lack the skills to select and prepare nourishing and well-balanced meals, (3) they have limited mobility which may impair their capacity to shop and cook for themselves, and (4) they have feelings of rejection and loneliness which obliterate the incentive necessary to prepare and eat a meal alone. These and other physiological, psychological, social and economic changes that occur with aging result in a pattern of living which causes malnutrition and further physical and mental deterioration.

To cope with this national problem of widespread concern, nutrition projects have been established throughout the country which provide at least one hot meal per day, five days a week, to older citizens (60 and over) and their spouses (any age). The meal must provide one third of the Recommended Dietary Allowance for each nutrient and, if this regulation is met, the USDA provides ten cents worth of commodities toward each meal served. Meals are prepared and served in group settings if at all possible. Meal sites include schools, churches, community centers, senior citizen centers, public housing, and other public and private facilities where other social services may also be available. Outreach programs to identify persons most in need of services (as well as transportation to meal sites) are also part of the program's responsibilities.

The nature and format of the individual programs now in existence depends on the composition and orientation of community personnel and resources. The aim of such assistance is to provide supplemental or enabling services to the older person who has the capabilities to function alone if this is desired. A typical group of elderly persons includes a wide range of individuals with a variety of needs; their physical and mental capabilities may not be the prime considerations. In such a group one might find the following: the older man who is widowed and has never prepared meals for himself; the person with a disabling illness that is not completely incapacitating but does cause pain in undertaking meal preparation activities; the person who always has had meals of his own "cultural derivation" and who is now faced with trying to maintain a special diet as a result of disease condition or weight problem; and the individual in dilapidated housing whose cooking equipment is less than optimum and whose mental or physical state involves a safety hazard. A number of other examples could be cited. Some of thse individuals may require other community services in the home such as public health nursing and nutrition services and the home economics and related services of voluntary health, social, and civic agencies.

Mechanisms by which the older person learns of a community service often are rather haphazard. The federal and state governments are now actively supporting community coordination efforts by adding their own supplemental and enabling programs to activities such as information and referral centers. Frequently, however, the local governments and suprapublic agencies are trapped in the apathy and rigidity of their local agencies and personalities. Program planners need to carefully screen the potential personnel and facilities in their own area so that matching of services with needs of the people can be accomplished. At the present, very little federal and state money is available for planning in advance of programming.

Special facets of the federally-supported nutrition demonstration-research-projects are basic to the success which many of these projects have appreciated. Among the supplemental provisions are the following:

1. Auxiliary services such as transportation, dental care, and counseling on individual dietary requirements to make it possible for older people to use the services.
2. Research projects to gain new knowledge on such matters as dietary needs and habits of older persons.
3. Social settings designed for personal adjustment and adequacy of diet.
4. Tools and appliances for food preparation, handling, and storage which older persons can use with greater safety and ease.
5. Unit cost analyses of different systems for improving diets.
6. Settings conducive to eating meals with others.
7. Surplus or donated foods or food stamps from the USDA.

The nutrition projects funded under Title VII began serving hot meals to the elderly in July 1973. Since then they have grown from 32 holdover projects from research and demonstration days to 680 projects in operation at the end of August 1975. These new projects comprise over 4700 meal service sites. Projects and sites are managed by a total staff of over 65,000 of whom about 10,500 are paid and 54,500 volunteers. At the end of its second year of operation, the Nutrition Program was serving about 270,000 meals daily and had enrolled as participants almost 1.5 million Americans 60 years of age or over (National Clearing House on Aging, 1974).

Organization of the individual nutrition projects and administration of the federal funds is handled by the separate state agencies on aging unless another agency is designated by the Governor and approved by the Secretary of Health, Education and Welfare. This administering body makes grants to or contracts with public and nonprofit organizations for actual provision and delivery of the meals. Advisory assistance is available through the state agency to assist with consumer problems and overall planning for provision of high-quality nutrition services at the local level.

Most nutrition projects funded under this program primarily serve low income elderly persons and spouses who are determined to be in greatest need of nutrition services. Effort is made by the governing state body to see that awards are made to initiate projects to serve minority groups and individuals with limited English-speaking abilities within the state. Meal sites are required to be located in urban areas that have heavy concentrations of target-group elderly and in rural regions where high proportions of elderly eligibles reside.

Payment for meals obtained in the nutrition projects is not required and no one is turned away because of lack of funds. Participants *do* have the opportunity, however, to pay part of the cost of the meal if they wish. The project directors must establish either a range of contributions or a single flat sum as a suggested contribution by participants. Each participant determines for himself what he is able to contribute and collection of money is handled confidentially.

While the National Nutrition Program does not specifically provide support for home-delivered meals, meals can be delivered to homebound elderly persons as part of a larger group meals project where appropriate or necessary. Currently about 10 to 15 percent of meals are home delivered and frequently this aspect of the program is called Meals on Wheels. White this type of feeding arrangement does not provide an effective mechanism for socialization and contact with the outside world, it does help meet the ongoing nutritional needs of persons who otherwise would be inadequately nourished or forced to reside in an institution where assistance was close at hand.

In the United States the first Meals on Wheels program originated in January 1954. This was sparked by the request of the Health and Welfare Council in Philadelphia. The Lighthouse, a Red Feather settlement house, began the program for an area of approximately five square miles. On five days a week, one hot and one cold meal per day were delivered to identified persons who were homebound.

The aims of this portable meals program were quite specific and were beautifully defined by Martin Keller and Charlotte Smith (Howell and Loeb, 1969). These authors state:

> The prevention of institutionalization is a basic aim in preventive medical and public health programs. In every community, there are people who can be helped to live successfully in their own homes by a number of simple services. Aside from the salutary benefits of relative independence, there is a distinct economic advantage (to the community) in the extension of such services.

The further point is made that the provision of such meals would prevent malnutrition and allow these persons to continue living at home. They are needed, then, and:

> . . . aside from their virtue, such programs serve to elevate the level of the community action in the general area of the health of the aged and in chronic disease control. They can serve as a direct way into larger, more comprehensive programs.

The authors take great care in pointing out:

> . . . that in the enthusiasm generated by (portable meals) programs, the fundamental aim may be overlooked. *The object is to increase the independence of the recipient. Unless the activities are constantly reviewed with reference to this objective, the program may, instead, foster dependency.*

Portable meals are not designed for persons who can leave their homes and dine in restaurants, for those who can shop for food and prepare adequate meals for themselves, or for those who can obtain family or neighbor help in doing so. Their particular value may exist during periods of convalescence, especially where earlier hospital discharge would be feasible.

Specific portable meals programs have some common features, although there are variations in the administrative aspects based on local need and available resources. One survey indicated that 22 such services studied had the following characteristics:

1. A typical portable meals program is a community service, most often located in a metropolitan area.
2. The average number of persons served is approximately 20 to 40 per day, with the midday and evening meals being delivered five days a week, Monday through Friday.
3. The program has the professional assistance of a dietitian, a nutritionist, or a home economist.
4. The meals are prepared in an agency kitchen and modified diets are provided.
5. Various vehicles transport the meals to the recipient's home and a fee for service is charged according to the person's ability to pay.

A home-delivered meals program is only one part of a comprehensive approach to providing food to older persons in the community and must be viewed in this context. To be sure, it is a very important service and can be critical to survival for the person who needs it. It may be that the prevention of dependency requires that some recipients evolve from portable, home-delivery meals to counseling of family and neighbors in food preparation assistance, to neighborhood group meals, and to self-responsibility as the person's autonomy improves.

EDUCATIONAL AND CONSULTATIVE SERVICES FOR THE ELDERLY

All nutrition programs administered under the Older Americans Act are required to include an educational component. There is concern, however, for the effectiveness of this aspect of the program and the limited skills in communities for designing sound educational evaluation. The problem of appropriate teaching materials is a prime concern. There are many prepared written materials on nutrition and age, special diets, and other topics. They are often randomly distributed to older persons, even though they may not be tailored to this population or even readapted for special aged subgroups. These materials may be of better use in the training of aides than in reshaping the eating habits of the elderly directly.

Appropriate nutrition guidance for a given geriatric patient needs to be highly individualized—physical, psychologic, socioeconomic, and cultural factors must all be recognized as highly relevant. To provide the most effective counseling, the answers to a number of questions must be obtained. The following questions may prove helpful in development of a more complete picture of the individual patient who needs advice:

1. What are the patient's physical limitations?
2. Is he able to plan for his food needs?
3. Does he know what his food needs are?
4. Is he physically able to shop for his food?
5. Does he have a convenient means of transportation?
6. Can he handle the food himself and get it back to his residence?
7. If he has special nutritional needs or limitations, is. he able to read and understand labels on food packages?
8. Does he understand his condition and needs well enough to follow dietary directions?
9. If he cannot shop for food himself, what other options are open to him?
10. What are his housing arrangements?
11. Does he live alone or with others?
12. If he can't take care of himself, will those with whom he lives take over this responsibility?
13. Are they capable of this responsibility? Are they willing to accept it?
14. What facilities are available for food storage, refrigeration, preparation, cleanup, and garbage disposal?
15. Is the patient able to use the facilities to prepare an adequate diet?
16. What kinds of utensils are available?
17. Have the utensils been rearranged to be within easy reach.
18. Is there a pleasant place to eat comfortably?
19. Are there enough dishes and tableware for attractiveness and sanitation?
20. Does the person have someone with whom he can eat?
21. What is the person's usual eating pattern?
22. Is there an eating pattern?
23. Are there foods which are disliked or don't agree with the patient?
24. Have any dietary limitations been prescribed?
25. What food items are eaten in a representative day (24-hour recall)?

This series of questions provides much information to the health care worker who needs to counsel the patient about nutrition. Using this data and knowledge of nutritional needs of the elderly, the counselor can make reasonable suggestions in tune with the patient's physical condition, lifestyle, and unique circumstances. A daily food guide, such as that seen in Table 9-7, may be useful in discussing diet with some individuals. Budgeting tips may also be very informative (Table 9-8 and accompanying box). In some circumstances, however, the use of these materials may be awkward and other educational tools may serve the purpose more effectively. The skilled nutrition counselor is always on the lookout for well-designed nutrition education materials. The development of a repertoire of approaches and methods will serve the educator well in the real world where folks are amazingly different in their response to specific educational experiences.

Teaching nutrition and consumerism to an elderly group is an exciting and rewarding experience if it is done properly with a thorough understanding of the audience before starting. The nutrition education experience must be based on the awareness that older persons come to the learning experience as voluntary participants, mature adults with a wealth of past experiences, special interests, training, and expertise, and not as young impression-

TABLE 9-7. Daily food guide.

MILK, CHEESE, ICE CREAM—2 or more cups daily
  Leading source of calcium and riboflavin; excellent source of high-quality protein and vitamin A; lesser quantities of other nutrients.

  May be taken in many forms: fresh whole or skim, reconstituted dried whole or skim, evaporated, buttermilk, whole or skim cheese, ice cream.

  If calories or fat, or both, are restricted, skim milk fortified with vitamin A may be used.

  The calcium equivalent of 1 cup of milk is 1⅓ oz. cheddar cheese, 1 lb. cream cheese, ¾ lb. creamed cottage cheese, 1 scant pint ice cream; with restricted calories or fat, either skim or lowfat milk is the best source of calcium.

MEAT, FISH, POULTRY, EGGS, DRY BEANS AND PEAS, NUTS—2 or more servings daily
  Meat, poultry, and fish are of particular value for high-quality protein and also provide iron, thiamine, riboflavin, and niacin; at least 1 serving daily.

  Eggs are a source of high-quality protein, iron, vitamin A, thiamine, riboflavin, and vitamin D; 4 or more weekly unless cholesterol is restricted.

  Nuts and dry beans and peas contain good protein, iron, and some B vitamins; protein value is enhanced if some animal protein is served with them.

GRAIN PRODUCTS—4 or more servings daily
  Provide significant quantities of iron, thiamine, riboflavin, and niacin if made with whole grain or restored or enriched with minerals and vitamins; included breads, cereals, noodles, macaroni.

VEGETABLES AND FRUITS—at least 4 servings daily
  Should include at least 1 serving daily of fruit rich in vitamin C and at least 3 or 4 servings per week of vegetables rich in vitamin A value.

Fruits particularly rich in vitamin C are oranges, grapefruit, and tomatoes; the vitamin C equivalent of 1 orange is ½ grapefruit, 4 oz. orange or grapefruit juice, 10 oz. tomato juice, ½ medium-sized cantaloupe, ½ to ¾ cup fresh strawberries, 1 cup shredded raw cabbage, ½ cup broccoli, ¾ to 1 cup dark green leaves from kale, spinach, or brussel sprouts, or a small green pepper.

Vegetables rich in vitamin A value (dark green and deep yellow vegetables) also provide some riboflavin, iron, and calcium; chard, collards, kale, spinach; carrots, yellow winter squash, pumpkin, sweet potatoes; broccoli; green peppers.

Potatoes provide some of several minerals and vitamins, including iron, thiamine, riboflavin, and vitamin C and can be eaten every day.

Other vegetables and fruits; 1 to 3 or more servings should be used daily to total at least 4 servings of fruits and vegetables per day.

FATS AND OILS—some butter or margarine daily
  Butter and margarine are rich in vitamin A.

  All fats and oils are high in calories and should be used sparingly if calories are restricted

  Some authorities recommend reduction of the total quantity of fat in the American diet, with an increase in the proportion of polyunsaturated fats and oils and a decrease in the proportion of saturated fats; in general, the use of fat as salad oil (especially corn, cottonseed, safflower, sesame, and soybean oils) and soft corn-oil margarines in preference to animal fats such as meat fat, cream, butter, and cheese, is encouraged.

SUGARS AND SWEETS—can be used sparingly to add flavor
  Sugars, jellies, jams, syrups, molasses, honey, and candy essentially provide calories for energy.

Adapted from Young, C. M.: Nutritional counselling for better health. Geriatr. 29:83, 1974.

able students. For this reason, they are ready to learn different things. In short, the adult learner will probably be most interested in knowledge that is of immediate usefulness.

  If effective learning is to take place, the instructor must stimulate an interest in the subject of nutrition. Since learning depends on attention, retention, and recall, the instructor's greatest ally is the individual's desire to learn. Interest in the subject aids in the mental organization necessary for attention and retention. The first session is extremely important in getting off on the right foot. It should be carefully

planned and given advance publicity. Large attractive posters may be placed in strategic places in the community or dining room of a program site so that everyone is aware of the upcoming event. The title of the nutrition class should not be too general or too dull. Many interesting presentations can be labeled with provocative titles that will help to attract the appropriate audience to the gathering.

  The best ideas for discussion topics come from the elderly themselves. Clearly they are most responsive to information which meets their specific needs rather than abstract or generalized information

TABLE 9-8. Suggestions for cutting down food costs within each food group.

MEAT OR MEAT SUBSTITUTES

Dry beans, peas, and nuts are the cheapest sources of protein and iron.

Cheaper meat cuts are nourishing: beef brisket, beef or pork liver, stew meat, ground meat, chuck roast, frankfurters, and heart.

Poultry, dry peas or beans, peanut butter, cheese, and some fish cost less than many meats.

Canned fish and native fresh fish are often good buys.

B and C grade eggs are good for cooking, baking, and scrambling; these grades and brown eggs are more economical.

BREADS AND CEREALS

Bread and cereal products are one of the cheapest sources of B vitamins.

Commercial bread usually costs less than bakery bread or rolls. Compare prices by weight.

Day-old baked goods are good buys.

Compare cereal prices. Sugared cereals often cost more than unsugared varieties.

FATS

Margarine costs less than butter.

Some brands of margarine and oil are cheaper than others.

VEGETABLES AND FRUITS

Green and yellow vegetables and citrus fruits are the most economical sources of vitamins A and C.

Fresh fruits and vegetables are cheapest in their peak harvest seasons.

Canned or frozen fruits, juices, and vegetables are often cheaper than fresh. Watch for specials and price differences between brands.

Lower grades of canned fruits and vegetables (B and C) are nutritious and usually cost less, best if used in mixed dishes.

There is less waste when you buy amounts small enough to use completely.

MILK

Milk and Cheddar-type cheese are the cheapest sources of calcium and certain B vitamins.

Dry skim milk costs less than fresh milk.

Large boxes of dry skim milk cost less per quart than small boxes.

Adapted from Meal Planning for the Golden Years. General Mills, 1966.

HELPFUL HINTS TO STRETCH FOOD DOLLARS

1. Plan your meals and snacks before you shop.
2. If possible, shop for a week at a time for your food needs.
3. Plan to buy staples such as flour, sugar, and corn meal only once or twice a month in larger and less expensive sizes.
4. Eat before you shop! If you are hungry when you go shopping, you will probably "buy on impulse" items you don't need.
5. You can save time by arranging your food list in the same way as the food is found in your store.
6. As you plan your menus, check newspaper ads for weekly specials. However, buy only if you can save money by buying an item you need and if the store is near you. *Note:* Don't drive 3 miles to save 3¢.
7. Remember that nonfood items are necessary perhaps, but they are not a part of your food bill.
8. Use discount coupons only if they are for things you really need.
9. Keep a list of commonly purchased food items and compare regular and sales prices. Remember: sometimes so-called specials are not really specials.
10. Learn new ways to use inexpensive high nutritional foods. However, if you will not eat the food and you throw it away, it is not a savings.
11. Beware of some so-called budget recipes in women's magazines or in the newspapers that start with low-cost main dish and then "fancy them up" with costly rare spices, nuts, etc.
12. You usually pay more for convenience. Plan to save money whenever possible by doing your own cutting, grating, mixing, seasoning, and cooking.
13. Skillet "helper" dinners are costly. Usually you can put the ingredients together yourself and get twice as much food for the same money.
14. Plan to use moderate-sized portions of high cost items, such as meat.
15. Plan to drink water when you are thirsty. It's the cheapest thirst quencher there is. (Leave the over-priced "sugar-loaded" or artificially sweetened sodas and fruit drinks on the grocery shelf.)
16. Shop on days when you get the best buys and freshest foods at your store. Often this is toward the end of the week. However, some stores offer savings at the beginning of the week to encourage early shopping.
17. Plan to shop when you are not rushed or distracted.

not concretely related to their immediate concerns. Thomas Elwood of the American Association for Retarded Persons polled the participants in a Senior Citizens Health Education Program to determine the nutrient-related issues they were most concerned about (Elwood, 1975). As can be seen in Table 9-9, topics related to nutrition and health, cholesterol, and weight control were often indicated with some degree of interest apparent for food labeling, food storage, and food preparation. In another effort to determine the nutrition-related interests of the elderly, Elizabeth Marks of the University of Maine at Farmingham conducted a survey to determine those topics that would be of the most value and interest to an elderly population. The 31 topics listed in Table 9-10 were identified by a selected group of elderly meal site participants as topics in which they may be interested. The ten topics designated with an asterisk received the greatest number of responses. It is clear from the listing of discussion topics that creativity was built into the titles and likely provided much stimulus to the potential audience.

Just how effective the final educational product happens to be relates directly to the enthusiasm,

TABLE 9-9. Questions asked by participants of a Senior Citizen health education program.

Subject of Question	Number of Questions
Cholesterol	105
Dietary supplements	43
Food composition	30
General aspects of nutrition	22
Weight control	20
"Health" foods	18
Sugar and artificial sweeteners	16
Fruit juices	15
Food handling and storage	14
Meal preparation	14
Preservatives and additives	11
Nutrition and health problems	8
Calorie intake	7
Nutrition and the heart	6
Fraudulence	5
Community services	5
Other (miscellaneous)	31
TOTAL	370

From Elwood, T. W.: Nutritional concerns of the elderly. J. Nutr. Educ. 7:50, 1974. Reprinted with permission.

TABLE 9-10. Nutrition topics of interest to an elderly population

Topic	Concept
The First Impression	Labelling and packaging practices
Cook for One*	Single serving recipes and economy measures for a single person
Making Tea and Toast a Complete Meal	Simple additions to the tea and toast meal to make it nutritionally balanced
Meal in a Glass or Cup	Preparation of a simple, nutritious meal in a cup
Fruit with a Flair	Use of fruit as a colorful, tasty addition to any meal
Eating with or Without Dentures	Planning menus to accommodate individuals with or without dentures
Shopping for One*	Guidelines for the individual who shops for him/herself only
Digestibility of Food	Overeating—focus on food groups and characteristics of each group
What Happened to the "Good Old Days"?	Availability of food and food sources
Fads and Fashions in Nutrition	Research related to current diets and food practices
Budget Wisdom	Sharing of guidelines for food spending
Meals Steals*	The thrifty use of leftovers
Tipping the Scales	Underweight/overweight
Enjoyable Eating	Controlled and modified diets
Bottled Health	Vitamins, prescribed diets
Listen to Your Body	Distresses suffered from eating particular foods
One-ly in Place of Lone-ly	Alone at mealtime
The Spice of Life*	Adding zest, color, flavor garnishes to meals
A Token Suggestion	Small quantity recipes
Snappy Snack*	Nutritious between-meal snacks
I Never Promised You an Herb Garden	Growing and using herbs in the kitchen
Stop Those Cereal Blues	Adding variety to cereal

Topic	Concept
Foster, the Food Detective	Indicators for freshness—date code, etc.
Anything You Want to Be	Humorous look at conflicts and absurdities about diet that beset senior adults
The Name of the Game*	Differences between food brands
Sensible Cooking for Senior Adults*	Preparing a simple, colorful cookbook with recipes for senior citizens
Streaking Through the Supermarket*	A quick look at the supermarket from the senior adult's point of view
Chowder Power*	Quick tricks with soups, chowders, stews
Meat Measures*	Ways to economize on use of meat, poultry, fish
The Salad Bar	Use of salads as taste teasers
Potatoes on the Half Shell	Misconceptions about the potato

Adapted from Nutrition Education for the Older American. New England Gerontology Center, Durham, New Hampshire, 1975.

* Topics indicated with asterisk are those which attracted the most attention.

skill, sincerity, and creativity of the teacher. It takes more than just a list of relevant topics and an understanding of the subject matter to develop a program that is truly outstanding. There are absolutely no limits to what an active thought process can come up with in designing an interesting mechanism of presenting nutrition information. Practice inevitably improves one's abilities in this area and generally it also reduces the difficulty involved in development of subsequent presentations. In a nutshell, a good nutrition educator knows the audience and the subject matter well and exercises to the fullest creative talents in the development of interesting, provocative, and relevant programs for the elderly.

CONCLUDING COMMENTS

The purpose of this chapter has been to describe the importance of food and its constituent nutrients in maintaining health and happiness of the elderly. Recognition of the multiple roles of food in the lives of individuals is vital to the effective planning for optimum nutritional support of groups or of group members. Specific nutritional needs of the aged are similar in most respects to those of younger persons. These needs must be met, however, in a dietary pattern that consists overall of fewer total calories than was required in previous years. Care must be taken to avoid excesses of calories, fat, sodium, and other nutrients. Likewise, close attention must be paid to nutrient composition of selected foods and aggressive action needs to be taken to provide for nutritional support under adverse conditions. Whatever the case, the secret to successful work with or management of senior citizens relates directly to the "quality of life" they can be led to enjoy. Food is basic to the fulfillment of health, socialization, cultural ties, and other pleasures. Thus, quality of life is dependent upon the availability of appropriate foods to satisfy diverse lifestyles and unique physiologic demands.

REFERENCES

American Dietetic Association. The American Dietetic Association position paper on nutrition and aging. J. Am. Diet. Assoc. 57:448, 1970.

Anderson, E. L.: Eating patterns before and after dentures. J. Am. Diet. Assoc. 58:421, 1971.

Balacki, J. A., and Dobbins, W. O.: Maldigestion and malabsorption: making up for lost nutrients. Geriatrics 29:157, 1974.

Berman, P. M., and Kirsner, J. B.: The aging gut. II: Diseases of the colon, pancreas and gallbladder, functional bowel disease and iatrogenic disease. Geriatrics 27:117, 1972.

Caster, W. O.: The nutritional problems of the aged. University of Georgia, Athens, Ga., 1971.

Clarke, M. J.: Food choices of institutional and independent-living elderly. J. Amer. Diet. Assoc. 66:600, 1975.

Council on Foods and Nutrition, American Medical Association: Nutrition teaching in medical schools. J.A.M.A. 183:955, 1963.

Davidson, C.: The nutrition of a group of apparently healthy aging persons. Am. J. Clin. Nutr. 10:181, 1962.

Dreizen, S.: Clinical manifestations of malnutrition. Geriatrics 29: 97, 1974.

Drummond, J. F.: Clinical and laboratory diagnosis of nutritional problems. Dental Clin. N. Am. 20:585, 1976.

Elwood, T. W.: Nutritional concerns of the elderly. J. Nutr. Educ. 7:50, 1975.

Esposito, S. J., Vinton, P. W., and Rapuano, J. A.: Nutrition of the aged: review of the literature. J. Am. Geriatr. Soc. 17:790, 1969.

Exton-Smith, A. N.: Physiological aspects of aging: relationship to nutrition. Am. J. Clin. Nutr. 25:853, 1972.

Gordon, E. S.: Dietary problems in hypertension. Geriatrics 29:139, 1974.

Gotto, A. M., Scott, L., and Manis, E.: Prudent eating after 40. Relationship of diet to blood lipids and coronary heart disease. Geriatrics 29:109, 1974.

Gutherie, H. A.: Nutritional practices of elderly poor in rural Pennsylvania. Gerontologist 12:330, 1975.

Hendrikson, P. A.: Periodontal disease and calcium deficiency. Acta Odontol. Scand. Suppl. 50, 26:1, 1968.

Hodkinson, H. M.: Nutrition of the elderly. In An Outline of Geriatrics. New York: Academic Press, 1975.

Howell, S. C., and Loeb, M. B.: Nutrition and aging: a monograph for practitioners. Gerontologist, Part II, 9:1–122, 1969.

Jowsey, J: Osteoporosis: its nature and the role of diet. Postgrad. Med. 60:75, 1976.

Jowsey, J., Resiss, E., and Canterbury, J. M.: Long-term effects of high phosphorus intake on parathyroid hormone levels and bone metabolism. Acta Orthop. Scand. 45:801, 1974.

Jukes, T. H., and Borsook, H.: Nutritional management of the anemic geriatric patient. Geriatrics 29:147, 1974.

Justice, C.: Dietary and nutritional status of elderly patients. J. Am. Diet. Assoc. 65:699, 1975.

Krehl, W. A.: The influence of nutritional environment on aging. Geriatrics 29:64, 1974.

Krook, L., Lutwak, L., and Henrikson, P. A.: Reversibility of nutritional osteoporosis: physiochemical data on bones from an experimental study on dogs. J. Nutr. 101:233, 1971.

Krook, L., Whalen, J. P., and Lesser, G. V.: Human periodontal disease and osteoporosis. Cornell Vet. 62:371, 1972.

Kutscher, A., and Goldberg, I.: Oral Care of the Aging and Dying Patient. Springfield, Ill., Charles C Thomas, 1973.

Langan, M. J., and Yearick, E. S.: The effects of improved hygiene on taste perception and nutrition of the elderly. J. Gerontology 31:413, 1976.

Lappe, F. M.: Recipes For a Small Planet. New York: Ballantine Books, 1975.

Lappe, F. M.: Diet For a Small Planet. New York: Ballantine Books, 1971.

Lutwak, L.: Continuing need for dietary calcium throughout life. Geriatrics 29:171, 1974.

Lutwak, L., Krook, L., and Henrikson, P. A.: Calcium deficiency and human periodontal disease. Isr. J. Med. Sci. 7:504, 1971.

Lyons, J., and Trulson, M. J.: Food practices of older persons living at home. J. Gerontology 11:66, 1956.

Mayer, J.: Aging and nutrition. Geriatrics 29:57, 1974.

Meindok, H., and Dvorsky, R.: Serum folate and vitamin B$_{12}$ levels in the elderly. J. Am. Geriatr. Soc. 18:317, 1970.

Miller, M. B.: Unresolved feeding and nutrition problems of the chronically aged. Gerontologist 2:329, 1971.

National Clearing House on Aging. National nutrition program for the elderly. U.S. Dept. of Health, Education and Welfare, Office of Human Development, Admin. on Aging, Washington D.C. 1974.

National Research Council, Food and Nutrition Board. Recommended Dietary Allowances, ed. 8. National Academy of Sciences, Washington D.C., 1973.

Nutrition Education for the Older American. New England Gerontology Center, 15 Garrison Avenue, Durham, N.H. 03824, 1975.

Pelcovits, J. J.: Nutrition to meet the human needs of older Americans. J. Amer. Diet. Assoc. 60:297, 1972.

Piper, G. M., and Smith, E. M.: Geriatric nutrition. In Working With Older People. A Guide to Practice. The Aging Person: Needs and Services. U.S. Dept. of Health, Education and Welfare, Washington D.C., 13:15, 1970.

Sherwood, S.: Sociology of food and eating: implications for action for the elderly. Am. J. Clin. Nutr. 26:1108, 1973.

Simko, M. D., and Colitz, K.: Nutrition and aging: a selected annotated bibliography, 1964–1972. Admin. on Aging, U.S. Dept. of Health, Education and Welfare, Washington D.C., 1973.

Skillman, T. G., Hamwi, G. J., and May, C.: Nutrition in the aged. Geriatrics 15:464, 1960.

Steinkamp, R. C., Cohen, N. L., and Walsh, H. E.: Resurvey of an aging population—fourteen year follow-up. J. Am. Diet. Assoc. 46:103, 1965.

Stewart, M.: White House Conference on Aging—Report of the nutrition section. Nutrition Program News, Mar–April, 1972.

Swanson, P., et al.: Food intakes of 2,189 women in five north central states. Iowa Agricultural and Home Economics Experimental Station Research Bulletin, 468, 1959.

Taylor, G. F.: A clinical survey of elderly people from a nutritional standpoint. In Exton-Smith, A. N., and Scott, D. L. (eds.): Vitamins in the Elderly. Bristol, England: John Wright and Sons, 1968, p. 51.

Troll, L. E.: Eating and aging. J. Amer. Diet. Assoc. 59:456, 1971.

U.S.D.A. Consumer and Food Economics Research Division. Agricultural Research Service. Food Consumption and Dietary Levels of Older Households in Rochester, New York. Home Economics Research Report No. 25, Washington D.C., 1965.

Watkin, D. M.: A year of developments in nutrition and aging. Med. Clin. N. Am. 54:1589, 1970.

Watkin D. M.: Nutrition and aging. Am. J. Clin. Nutr. 25:807, 1972.

Weir, D. R., Houser, H. B., and Davy, L.: Recognition and management of the nutrition problems of the elderly. A guide to practical clinical aspects of aging.

U.S. Dept. of Health, Education and Welfare, Washington D.C., 4:267, 1967.

Whanger, A. D.: Vitamins and vigor at 65 plus. Postgrad. Med. 53:167, 1973.

Young, C. M.: Nutritional counselling for better health. Geriatrics 29:83, 1974.

Young, V. R., and Scrimshaw, N. S.: Nutrition needs of the elderly. Nutrition Notes, December 1975.

10

Drug Use

Marianne Ivey

Geriatric pharmacology has become increasingly important to health professionals from several disciplines. It is commonly accepted that as the number of medications taken by an individual increase so do drug interactions and adverse reactions.

The over-60 age group buys and uses *more than two times* the amount of drugs used by the middle-aged population. The average range of medications is six to ten different drugs per patient. It is no wonder that special attention should be paid to the drug use of the elderly. This concern needs to be felt not only by physicians who prescribe and monitor intermittently and pharmacists who dispense and offer consultation but also by nurses who concern themselves with day-to-day living of the person consuming these medications and living with the effects.

There are reasons other than absolute numbers and amounts why medications tend to become a problem for the elderly person. The older person's body is undergoing physiologic changes that have an impact on both the medication-taking pattern and drug effects. Failures in the cardiovascular system are a classic example of normal aging and chronic disease that cause increased drug taking. Normal decreases in renal function and renal disease exemplify the changes that can produce changes in medication effect as accumulation of drugs excreted by the kidney increases with growing risks of drug toxicity.

The activity of taking drugs is in itself a problem that may be exacerbated with age. Some difficulties arise when elderly persons take their own medications. Some common problems include:

- Failing eyesight and difficulty in reading labels.
- Failure to recall side effects and to report them with either too rigid compliance or attribution of symptoms to other conditions.
- Carelessness in following a drug regimen.
- Differing beliefs about medications resulting in noncompliance.

PROBLEMS OF THE ELDERLY HAVING IMPACT ON DRUG USE

Increased use of drugs because of more chronic diseases.

Adverse drug effects potentiated by physiologic changes of aging.

Increased risk of drug interactions owing to increased numbers of drugs being ingested.

Erratic or dangerous drug-taking behavior because of vision and memory changes.

Lack of money to purchase needed drugs.

Similarity of drug side effects to manifestations or normal aging.

Failure to adequately monitor the responses to drug and drug-taking practices.

Use of over-the-counter drugs in addition to prescriptions without informing doctor or nurse.

Failure to reevaluate ongoing need for the drug, or drug dosage.

Seeing more than one physician and purchasing drugs at more than one pharmacy so no one has an accurate drug profile.

Discontinuance of drug by the patient without consultation.

Using medications shared by other persons who had similar conditions.

Trusted home remedies and ethnic health practices can also interact with prescribed medication to generate other-than-desired results.

Even when drugs are not self-administered, there may be problems related to failure of health providers to determine actual need for the drug prior to prescription. Once the drug regimen has been started, failure to monitor drug effects and side effects may result in ineffective treatment or iatrogenic disease. For example, antianxiety drugs and sedatives produce high risk in terms of over-utilization and failure to monitor side effects.

The monitoring of side effects in the elderly is more complex than with other age groups. Some older persons may be unable to notice and report their symptoms and concerns. Additionally the signs and symptoms associated with drug side effects may be closely related to manifestations of aging, posing problems for the person who takes the drugs as well as the professionals who are supposed to be monitoring response.

AGE-RELATED PHYSIOLOGIC CHANGES AND DRUG ACTIONS

Several things happen to drugs after they are ingested. Drugs taken by mouth must be:

- *absorbed* from the gastrointestinal tract into the bloodstream
- *distributed* around the body
- *metabolized* into a different and/or less toxic product
- *excreted* by kidney, lungs, or colon

These four activities often are altered in the elderly because of age-related physiologic changes.

Absorption

The absorption of drugs can be said to be erratic in the elderly. This may make it difficult to determine the correct dose since absorption may not be consistent. Warfarin is a drug that presents this ongoing problem. Another situation where absorption is modified is in the case of drugs that are weakly acidic. Here absorption takes place in the stomach and proximal bowel. The normally decreased production of hydrochloric acid in the stomach, or more serious decreases (achlorhydria), causes drugs such as aspirin and barbiturates to be less well absorbed.

Distribution

Drugs are often stored following absorption in parts of the body (including some that are modified by aging). Two important storage areas that are changed are fat and protein. Normally, stored drugs are released into the bloodstream at a rate that retains a concentration level. However if, as in the case of the elderly, the proportion of fat increases while body fluid and lean body mass decrease, there is a lowering of metabolically-active tissue. Drugs that are fat soluble will tend to remain stored in fat. The end result is that the *intensity of the drug action is decreased but the duration is increased.* Thus, in long term administration of fat-soluble drugs, there is a higher risk of accumulation and eventual toxic effects. Examples of commonly-used fat-soluble drugs include phenobarbital, diazepam, and chlorpromazine.

Distribution of other drugs within the body is determined by the amount of protein, particularly serum albumin. In any person, part of an absorbed drug will be bound to protein and part of it will be unbound in the bloodstream. It is the unbound drug that is active in producing the drug effects. It is also the unbound drug that can be excreted through the kidneys. With serum albumin levels lower in many elderly one might expect some alterations in drug availability. However, the effect of this lowered protein has not been fully investigated.

One can expect both greater or less than the expected response to the drug on the basis of distribution. It is difficult if not impossible to predict what will happen with different drugs in patients with various conditions of health and illness. Close surveillance by the patient and health providers is advisable.

Metabolism

Generally, drugs are metabolized into less toxic products. All absorbed drugs pass through the liver. Some remain unchanged but many are transformed into water-soluble compounds that can then be excreted by the kidneys.

This metabolism of drugs in the liver is accomplished by microsomal enzymes, with the duration of action and intensity of drug effect dependent largely on the number of these enzymes and their rate of functioning. These enzymes are proteins and, since the elderly often have a decreased production of protein, it is postulated that this is a cause for modified metabolism of drugs seen in older patients. The end result is that unmetabolized drugs continue to exert their effect.

Abnormal prolongation of effect is a particular risk in drugs that are quickly deactivated by the liver in the younger age group—meperidine, barbiturates, propranolol, and tricyclic antidepressants. With a drug like phenylbutazone there is an increase in the half life of the drug (t ½), which leads to accumulation of this very toxic medication with resultant gastrointestinal bleeding and/or depletion of platelets and white blood cells. This in turn sets the patient up for generalized hemorrhaging and infection.

On the other side of the coin, with a drug such as allopurinol that requires full metabolism to achieve the therapeutic effect, reduced effectiveness may occur.

In effectively monitoring drug effects in the elderly it becomes important for nurses to familiarize themselves with the relationship of metabolism of drugs in relationship to their effects (there is no other way to develop an awareness of the increased risk their patients are encountering) and set themselves to observe for early toxic effects of accumulation or lack of drug effectiveness.

Excretion

Although there are several routes for excretion of drugs, kidneys are the primary route of elimination. For some drugs, such as cardiac glycosides and some antibiotics, they are the only route.

Excretion via the kidneys takes place by glomerular filtration, tubular secretion, and tubular reabsorption. The cardiac glycosides (e.g., digoxin) and aminoglycoside antibiotics (gentamicin and kanamycin) are excreted unchanged by glomerular filtration. Because the number of functional tubules in the parenchyma of the kidney and glomerular filtration decreases about 30 percent in the elderly, these drugs and others including tetracycline, phenobarbital, and sulfonamides have decreased excretion and accumulate to potential toxicity.

Acid-base balance is also involved in the excretion of drugs, particularly in tubular reabsorption. If a weakly acidic drug is given when the urine is very acidic, reabsorption from the tubule back into the bloodstream is increased. This causes greater drug effect than expected with a given dosage. A similar enhancement of drug effect can occur when a weakly basic drug is given to a person whose urine is alkaline because of taking antacids. An example of this

would be the combination of quinidine and sodium bicarbonate.

Thus, even in normal elderly persons, the risks of accumulation are present through slowed or incomplete metabolism in combination with inefficient, slowed excretion. When the additional factors of dehydration, congestive failure, urinary retention, and other conditions are added, singly or in combination, the risks of toxicity rise significantly.

ADVERSE REACTIONS

Adverse drug reactions appear to occur in the elderly more frequently than they do in the younger adult. In a study done by pharmacists and pharmacologists on 6000 consecutive hospital admissions, 3 percent were found to be admitted as a result of adverse drug effects. Of the 180 patients 40 percent were over 60 years of age (Caranasos, et al., 1974).

Prescription Drugs

Certain drugs were at higher risk for causing iatrogenic disease. If aware of these, the nurse or others who monitor patient response can help in prioritizing monitoring efforts or alerting patients to be observant and conscientious in reporting. In the previously-mentioned study the following eight drugs caused 33 percent of the adverse effects: digoxin, aspirin, warfarin sodium, hydrochlorothiazide, prednisone, vincristine, norethindrone, and furosemide. All of these drugs produce high risk of iatrogenic disease.

Clinicians should suspect that several of these drugs would be culprits for the elderly on the basis of the characteristics shown in Table 10-1. A person taking any of these drugs should be monitored on a continuing basis by professionals. In addition, where appropriate, the older person should be helped to become a more accurate self-monitor and reporter, as should his family members.

Over-the-Counter Drugs

Prescription drugs are not the only ones that cause serious side effects in the elderly. Over-the-counter (OTC) drugs, seen by lay persons and some professionals alike as being innocuous, carry some iatrogenic risks.

The previously-mentioned study found three OTC drugs to have been associated with adverse

TABLE 10-1. Characteristics of some prescription drugs.

Characteristics	Drugs
Significant toxicity (narrow margin of safety) for any age group	digoxin, prednisone, vincristine
Excretion in unchanged state by kidney	digoxin
Erratic absorption patterns	warfarin
Common and long term utilization	digoxin, diuretics, aspirin, tranquilizers, antihypertensives
Side effects that mimic age-related signs and symptoms	diuretics, aspirin (tinnitus with hearing loss)
Common interaction with other drugs or diet	digoxin, warfarin, aspirin, diuretics, antacids, tranquilizers

reactions: antacids, antidiarrheals, and bromide-containing drugs. (The bromide-containing drugs have since been taken off the market, and so the concern now is with any remaining supplies in the older person's medicine chest.)

ANTACIDS. Antacids have the capacity to cause difficulties in multiple areas of body functioning. They can produce diarrhea, constipation, edema, kidney stones, respiratory distress, and complications to already existing renal disease. Side effects of various OTC drugs are listed in Table 10-2. (See also Table 15-1.)

Perhaps the side effects given in Table 10-2 are common because of their easy availability and because lay persons and health professionals often are unaware of the differences in ingredients in various products and, therefore, unaware of the associated risks. Professionals and consumers need to know about products and their relationship to the individual's health status as a basis for choosing and using wisely. A book published by the American Pharmaceutical Association, *APHA Handbook on Non-Prescription Drugs* (1976), probably is the most informative book on over-the-counter medications.

Antacids also inhibit the effects of other drugs including Butazolidin, tetracycline, penicillin G, sulfonamides, nalidixic acid, nitrofurantoin, Dicoumarol, coumarin, Panwarfin, and iron. This indicates, for nurses, the importance of spacing of drugs to minimize interaction when two or more are needed or the teaching of patients to space their drugs (Goldenberg, 1969).

ANTIDIARRHEALS. Drugs that are used to decrease diarrhea have two side effects. They interfere with absorption and may cause constipation. These drugs effect therapy for diarrhea by adsorbing toxins; however, they are not that discriminating and, in the process, may adsorb desired prescribed medication elements as well. Digoxin, for example, is at high risk. A nursing implication would be to give the medications at separated times, allowing a four to six hour interval between ingestion of the two drugs.

TABLE 10-2. Over-the-counter antacids and their possible side effects.

Side Effects	Products that May Contribute To It
Diarrhea	Maalox®
Constipation	Amphogel®
Edema related to sodium content	Krem®
Kidney stones related to absorbable calcium	calcium carbonate
Respiratory problems associated with aluminum-binding phosphate	Basaljel®

DRUG RISKS IN TREATMENT OF PARTICULAR DISEASE STATES

The elderly fall victim to some diseases in which drug therapy is used for treatment or maintenance. The treatment itself, in many instances, poses risks. Nurses need to be aware of these risks as a basis for monitoring older persons and helping them and their families to manage with the most effective results and minimal dangers. The diseases themselves will be treated fully in other chapters. Here the focus will be upon common drugs used, the risks of side effects, and possible alternatives of management.

Cardiovascular Disease

The diseases in this category which require chronic and/or multiple drugs are congestive heart failure, arteriosclerotic heart disease, arrhythmias, and hypertension.

Congestive Heart Failure

The mainstays of congestive heart failure management are digitalis glycosides and diuretics. Both are taken over long periods of time; both create side effects that must in turn be managed.

The digitalis glycosides have very narrow margins of safety—the *therapeutic dose is not very different from the toxic dose.*

Blood Levels
Therapeutic 0.5–1.5 ng/ml
Toxic   2.5–3.0 ng/ml

The potential for digitalis toxicity is greatly increased by allowing the potassium blood level to fall below 3.5 mEq/ml. This toxicity often shows up as ventricular arrhythmias. Low potassium could commonly occur in the elderly person because of concurrent use of potassium depleting diuretics and/or potassium-poor diets. (See Chapter 9 for high potassium foods).

Side effects of digitalis glycosides have been found to present themselves somewhat differently among the elderly. They do not follow the classic pattern of signs and symptoms. *Acute fatigue and loss of strength* are prominent symptoms. Anorexia may be the presenting symptom rather than nausea and vomiting (Hay, 1973). This anorexia may be hard for the nurse or patient to separate from a normally small appetite, so it is important to gather data on any decrease from usual eating habits.

Mental signs and symptoms are also early indicators—sometimes the first (Hay, 1973; Lely, et al., 1972; Wedgwood, 1973). It has been suggested that digitalis glycosides affect the neuronal cells in a way similar to their effect on cardiac cells (Miller and Forker, 1974). Signs and symptoms of toxicity manifested by the central nervous system include visual disturbances, difficulty reading, headaches, dizziness, drowsiness, nervousness, and agitation (Lely, et al., 1972; Ness, 1977).

Changes in cardiac rate and rhythm are also important. A pulse below 60 or above 100 has long been considered the classic sign of digitalis toxicity; however, bursts of tachycardia are also significant.

Changes in rhythm from regular to irregular (bigeminal, trigeminal beats, p.v.cs) or the reverse (a shift from irregular to regular) should raise the suspicion of drug toxicity for the person on digitalis glycosides (Hay, 1973; Herrman, 1966).

It was mentioned earlier that digitalis excretion is impaired because of age-related decreased renal function. As a general rule, persons who are 65 years of age or older might be expected to require 0.125 mgm/day of digoxin rather than 0.25 mgm/day for younger people. After a week's therapy a blood level, drawn just before the next dose, should be done to determine if the digoxin level is in the therapeutic range. If digoxin levels are not available the symptoms and signs should be monitored, including apical/radial pulse.

Digitoxin is another cardiac glycoside commonly given for congestive heart failure. Its dosage is different, as is its metabolism and excretion. In persons with poor renal function it becomes very long acting (with a half-life greater than nine days).

Because digitalis glycosides and diuretics are frequently used together, the drug interaction of the diuretic-induced hypokalemia that potentiates digitalis toxicity should be monitored. (See pp. 156 and 378 for signs and symptoms). Monthly potassium blood levels are helpful. If hypokalemia occurs, a potassium supplement must be given. A high potassium diet may help in preventing hypokalemia, but it is not very effective in treating it once it occurs. The bad taste of the potassium discourages long term compliance. Effervescent forms or combining them with fruit juices or soda helps. They also are very irritating to the stomach so should be taken with food.

Angina Pectoris

Angina pectoris and other associated symptoms of arteriosclerosis are commonly treated with drugs. Nitrates are frequently used for these cardiovascular diseases. The elderly are much more sensitive to the hypotensive effects of nitrates than are those who are younger. Several cases are known where nitroglycerin-induced vasodilation and subsequent hypotension was sufficient to cause the patient to black out and fall. On the other hand, nitroglycerin may be quite ineffective with patients who are already experiencing maximum stimulation for vasodilation from lowered O_2 tensions and arteriosclerotic constraints that limit vasodilation possible. For such persons the nitroglycerin may have a positive placebo effect or none at all. Lower doses should be tried (1/200 gr to 1/150 gr or 0.3–0.4 mg) before 1/100 gr or 0.6 mg.

The storage of nitroglycerin is very important in protecting its potency. It should be kept in its original small glass container, tightly capped with no cotton, paper, or any other material in the container. Nitroglycerin should not be put in pill boxes with other drugs. Improper storage allows for the vaporization of the drug and loss of potency.

Nitroglycerin has been physically and chemically manipulated into long-acting dosage forms. However, the standard sublingual nitroglycerin is still the most dependable and effective way to give nitrates. It is also the least expensive.

Arrhythmias

Arrhythmias often are treated with very potent drugs. An example is propranolol (Inderol®). Propranolol is a beta-adrenergic receptor-blocking drug —it blocks the effects of epinepherine and norepinepherine on the heart, reducing tachyarrhythmias caused by the catecholamines.

One of the problems with this drug occurs when it is given to the patient who has heart failure concurrent with the arrhythmias. Since the failing heart is caused to function by the action of epinephrine and norepinephrine, the blocking action of propranolol may cause further deterioration. Another problem occurs when propranolol is given to persons with obstructive pulmonary disease (see Chapter 13). Beta-adrenergic stimulation causes bronchioles to dilate, allowing for better movement of air. Propranolol-caused beta blockage may easily cause aggravation of obstructive respiratory disease.

Care must also be taken in administering propranolol to patients with insulin-dependent diabetes. Since propranolol masks the symptomatic response to low blood sugar (e.g., tachycardia), hypoglycemia may be missed until it becomes very serious. Propanolol also induces mental depression in some individuals.

Propranolol is currently being used for more and more conditions ranging from angina to tremor. The actions and side effects of the drug must be kept in mind and considered together with the person's other health problems and forms of treatment; the key is to start with low doses (10 mg b.i.d.).

Procainamide is commonly used for arrhythmias. It may cause hypotension, particularly if it is given parenterally. Procainamide in high dose has also caused a lupus-like syndrome of rash, joint aches, fever, and, in some cases, pulmonary effusion. Both procainamide and quinidine, another drug frequently used in arrhythmias, accumulate in renal failure and may require a dosage reduction.

Hypertension

Treatment of the elderly hypertensive patient differs in some important ways from that of the younger person: (1) reduction in blood pressure should be gradual to prevent infarction of the brain; (2) much lower doses of antihypertensive drugs may be adequate; and (3) higher risks of side effects are present.

The following are some drugs nurses may encounter in the medical management of hypertension. (For additional information see Chapter 19.) Because many of these drugs may be used concurrently, additional vigilance is needed in monitoring the therapy of hypertensive patients.

Reserpine. Effective in reducing hypertension and requires only one dose per day (where compliance is a problem). Its disadvantages make it less a drug of choice. It causes *depression* (even at low therapeutic doses) severe enough to cause suicidal ideations and attempts. This side effect is due to its action in reducing catecholamines in the brain. It also may cause *diarrhea* and *reactivate ulcers* in persons with histories of peptic ulcer disease.

Hydralazine. Reduces blood pressure by direct vasodilation. However, the decreased pressure in turn causes reflex tachycardia which may precipitate chest pain in patients with a history of angina. If hydralazine is the only drug that will control the blood pressure, propranolol may be added to prevent the tachycardia and, thus, the angina.

Clonidine (Catapres). Brings the danger of rebound hypertension when doses are missed. The rebound pressure levels may be sufficient to cause CNS complications.

Prazosin (Minipres). Acts very much like hydralazine; however, it does not seem to precipitate angina and may, therefore, be more useful in the person with arteriosclerotic heart disease.

Methyldopa (Aldomet). In combination with a thiazide diuretic this is a common form of treatment. Side effects include nasal stuffiness, sedation, and some depression.

Diuretics. A diuretic should be combined with nearly every antihypertensive agent. Often diuretics are the first class of drugs tried with other anti-hypertensives added to it. The combination allows one to use less of the more potent drugs and combats the sodium retention caused by many of the hypertensive agents when they are used alone (see Chapter 19, page 18). Thiazide diuretics (Diuril, Hydrodiuril) are the least expensive for therapeutic results. Furosemide (Lasix) and ethacrynic acid (Edecrin) (more potent loop diuretics) deplete electrolytes such as potassium, are more expensive, have potential for serious side effects (deafness with ethacrynic acid), and generally are reserved for persons with refractory edema.

1. *Schedule diuretics* in the morning and afternoon, avoiding the evening to minimize nocturia. The exception is the person with renal disease. The prone position facilitates urine production and the action of the diuretic. Urinary incontinence for the person on diuretics suggests need to review medication profile for the presence of long acting diuretics such as chlorthalidone since these contribute to incontinence.

2. *Renal disease* would be a reason to avoid or use cautiously the potassium-sparing diuretics (e.g., triamterine and spironolactone). They create high risk of hyperkalemia. Medication profiles should be reviewed also to be certain that potassium supplements are not being used with potassium-sparing diuretics. This type of diuretic is only mildly antihypertensive and should not be used alone in treatment of high blood pressure.

While nurses usually are not responsible for prescribing medications, they do have a role in helping patients to monitor their drug-taking behavior. Given an older person's trust they can learn about medications that have been saved from other times, those that have been given to them by a friend, and so forth. Then nurses can develop a realistic drug profile and help the patient to understand how to manage his medications with the least amount of risk. Pharmacists may be involved in this role also in providing counsel and drug information to the patient and/or his family. Nurses and pharmacists can contribute to each other's communication to facilitate the patient's well-being and coordinated care.

PSYCHIATRIC DISEASE AND EMOTIONAL DISTURBANCES

Insomnia, anxiety, depression, and schizophrenia are commonly experienced by the elderly. In addition, health care professionals and family members of the elderly person assume these problems exist, even when they may not. Drugs are commonly used to treat these problems and, since the elderly handle these drugs poorly, psychotropic drugs have become a major problem.

Insomnia

Insomnia is often a label placed on a complaint of the older person, whereas the real problem is often a change in sleep patterns. Lifestyles may have changed to permit such things as late rising and daytime naps, actions that spread the sleep cycles differently within the 24-hour period. The expectation of retaining an earlier pattern of six to eight hours of uninterrupted sleep at night becomes unrealistic. They may then demand, or others may suggest, sedatives. Lack of achieving a desired sleep pattern may also result from other physical problems such as drinking stimulants before retiring, a full bladder or rectum, joint discomforts, or breathing difficulties. Pressing sedatives on a person at this time rather than dealing with the underlying problem is poor nursing management.

Sometimes the choice of a sedative-hypnotic for the older person is difficult. Flurazepam (Dalmane®) is commonly used in any age group. In the elderly this drug must be used with care since it has a half life of 50 to 100 hours. Because of this, a small dosage (15 mg) may be quite adequate. It has been noted that use of this drug has been associated with the symptoms of organic brain syndrome in many elderly persons. When the drug is stopped their memories clear and they become less confused and more reality-oriented.

Among sedatives the drug of choice may be chloral hydrate. One advantage is that it does not appear to modify the rapid eye movement (REM) stage of sleep as many of the barbiturates do.

Anxiety

Anxiety is another problem commonly reported by individuals in older age groups. The drugs commonly prescribed for this are the barbiturates, benzodiazepines (Valium® and Librium®), and sometimes the phenothiazines (Mellaril®, Thorazine®, and Stelazine®). Drugs in this latter category are potent and would seem best reserved for treatment of psychoses.

Some clinicians consider barbiturates contraindicated in the older person because they cause nocturnal restlessness and morning hangover, which leads to slurred speech, inattentiveness, and unsteady gait. They also are particularly dangerous in patients with pneumonia and cerebrovascular accidents because they depress the respiratory center and change physical systems which are used to monitor patient progress.

Used in small doses, barbiturates can be effective and inexpensive sedatives. It should be remembered that barbiturates have different half lives and routes of excretion. For example, phenobarbital has a half life of about 30 hours and, therefore, can be taken once daily or with small multiple doses. Phenobarbital is excreted by the kidney and is not a wise choice for the person with poor renal function.

Valium® and Librium® are relatively safe drugs in many patients; however, they are overused. The following are guidelines for their rational use:

1. Use only intermittently to avoid need for increased doses to achieve desired result.
2. Use the smallest dose that is still effective (e.g., Diazepam 2 mg rather than 5 mg).
3. Give with the half life in mind (Librium half life is 36 hours; therefore it is inappropriate to give t.i.d. or q.i.d. after the third day when the blood levels are in a steady state). Frequency should be reduced to q.d. at that time. Valium half life ranges from 12 hours

with single doses to 60 to 70 hours when the person has been on multiple daily doses for a period of time.
4. Decrease dosage gradually rather than stop abruptly when person has been on these drugs for a prolonged period.

Many persons will themselves reduce their antianxiety drugs when they no longer need them. The nurse needs to be alert to the medication-taking preferences and previous medication-taking lifestyle of the individual.

Alcohol in the form of wine is an excellent antianxiety agent. In addition it may be an appetite stimulant, a vasodilator, and facilitator of social interchange. It becomes important for the nurse to check on the previous role alcohol has played in the person's life before recommending this however. (See Chapter 11, Alcoholism.)

Depression

Depression frequently is reported in the elderly and is sometimes treated with drugs. Tricyclic antidepressants (Elavil®, Tofranil®, Aventyl®, Petrofran®, Sinequan®), although effective for some forms of depression, have side effects related to their anticholinergic activity, as indicated in Table 10-3.

Dosages of tricyclic antidepressants for the older person should be started at very low levels. They may need to be increased to gain the desired effect; how-

TABLE 10-3. Side effects of tricyclic antidepressants.*

Anticholinergic Activity	Side Effects
Decreased salivary flow	Increased risk of tooth cavities and loosening denture fit
Slowed gastrointestinal activity	Constipation; possible paralytic ileus if much peristaltic action has been lost in aging
Urinary retention	A problem, particularly to the elderly male with prostatic hypertrophy
Mydriasis	Blurry vision (may clear up with continued use)
Congestive heart failure**; palpitations	Some cardiac deaths have occurred with use of these drugs
Postural hypotension	Dizziness; fainting when getting up
Sedation	Reduces insomnia
Wide mood swings	

* Most of these side effects also occur with antipsychotic agents and anticholinergic drugs used to treat Parkinson's disease or to prevent extrapyramidal reactions.

** Sinequan, in recent research, seems to cause the least amount of cardiac toxicity.

ever, they take about three weeks to become effective and do have a 24-hour half life so the patient may need support while waiting for the drug to alleviate the depression (See Chapter 25, p. 512). Up to 300 mg per day of doxepin (Sinequan) have been used without ill effects; however this is a very high dose. At dosages in this range extrapyramidal effects may also be seen (e.g., tremor, pill rolling of thumb and fingers) and it may be necessary to add an anticholinergic agent. Given the 24-hour half life, they may be given on a once-a-day basis. If doses of 30 to 100 mg are given, all of the drug may be taken at bedtime. This tends to increase the compliance in self-care and is convenient for institutionalized persons. The bedtime timing also causes most of the inconvenient side effects, such as dry mouth and blurry vision, to occur while the person is sleeping. On the other hand, if the dosage is in excess of 100 mg daily, the medication should be divided into b.i.d. or t.i.d. patterns, since the postural hypotension could have dangerous consequences for persons who must get up during the night.

Tricyclic antidepressants can serve as a sedative as well, particularly Elavil and Sinequan, so they can be useful where insomnia is a problem. Where wide mood swings are a problem a different type of antidepressant may be tried, either another one in the tricyclic class or one of an entirely different structure such as amphetamines.

Schizophrenia

Schizophrenia is seen throughout all age groups and the elderly are no exception. Since the antipsychotic drugs of the phenothiazine class as well as butryophenones (Haldol) and thioxanthines (Navane) have anticholinergic activity, they have the same side effects as listed in Table 10-3. But, in addition, these agents have an alpha-adrenergic receptor-blocking activity which causes postural hypotension. Safety dictates that persons taking these drugs, and those who care for them, be conscious of the need to change positions gradually to allow for adjustment to the changed pattern of blood flow.

These drugs have a sedative effect; therefore caution should be observed when other central nervous system depressant drugs are given concurrently. Patients with chronic obstructive pulmonary disease are at particular risk.

The phenothiazines may decrease the seizure threshold, thereby increasing the need for higher doses of anticonvulsants to maintain seizure control.

This class of drugs also affects the temperature-regulating mechanism of the hypothalamus, so that the person takes on the temperature of the environment—in cold environments they become chilled and in warm environments they can become overheated and experience heat strokes.

The other significant side effects of the phenothiazines are the extrapyramidal reactions that they produce:

1. *dyskinesias:* stiffening of muscles such as in the neck and tongue; oculogyric crisis; cogwheel rigidity of arms
2. *akathesia:* Inability to sit still
3. *parkinsonism:* Pill rolling of thumb and finger; drooling; shuffling gait; and masked facies

The elderly suffer most from the parkinsonian symptoms. Treatment consists in lowering the dose, changing drugs, or adding an anticholinergic drug such as Cogentin®. Addition of more anticholinergic activity will contribute to the side effects already present in the phenothiazines; therefore, the lowest effective dose of anticholinergic drug should be used and it should be discontinued after three months since the extrapyramidal symptoms in 90 percent of patients will have abated by this time.

Risks of side effects can be predicted on the basis of categorizing the drugs in terms of high and low dose types (Table 10-4). Thorazine® and Mellaril® whose doses are 50 mg or above fall into the high dose type. Stelazine® or Haldol® where dosages are more commonly in the 1 to 10 mg range are considered a low dose group. The usefulness of this classification may be shown by the following example. If you have an elderly patient who has an irritable heart you would tend not to choose Mellaril®

TABLE 10-4. Categorization of side effects in antipsychotic drugs.

	Drug	
Side Effects	High Dose Type	Low Dose Type
Sedative effects	Moderate to high	Low
Extrapyramidal effects	Low	High
Effects on blood pressure and heart	Moderate to high	Low
Anticholinergic effects	Moderate to high	Low

which has a record of causing arrhythmias particularly at doses around 200 mg and you might choose to use Haldol® which is shown to have little effect on the heart. On the other hand, if extrapyramidal effects are a particular problem for the elderly patient, then Mellaril® may be the drug of choice and Haldol®, which has a high incidence of associated extrapyramidal effects, should be avoided.

One last caution is warranted regarding the use of antipsychotic medications in the elderly. Tardive dyskinesia resulting in repetitive actions, particularly of the tongue or other facial movements, is a long term use effect in younger patients, but it seems to occur as a function of age rather than length of use in the elderly. Even worse—the problem becomes more severe if the drug is stopped. Therefore, prevention is important. These guidelines should be used:

1. Use antipsychotic drugs only with the psychotic (not the anxious).
2. Use the lowest effective dose, even though it may seem homeopathic.
3. Allow for drug-free periods of two to three days.
4. Discontinue the drug for a test period after two to three months to see if the person can maintain control without the drug.

BONE AND JOINT DISEASE

Salicylates are the agents of first choice in most patients with inflammatory joint disease. Again the key to their safe use in the elderly is the dosage. The activity and excretion of aspirin are influenced by renal function. If a large dose of salicylates is being used, as is often the case, toxicity may occur. Unfortunately, the characteristics of aspirin toxicity are often misinterpreted as the aging process itself. The symptoms of aspirin toxicity are ringing in the ears, deafness, confusion, and irritability.

Aspirin also is irritating to the gastric mucosa, inhibits vitamin K, and inhibits facilitation of blood-clotting and of platelet aggregation. These three activities set the person up for greater risk of gastrointestinal bleeding. Therefore, aspirin should be taken with food, e.g., meals or milk, and/or an antacid.

Other drugs used to treat joint problems should be used in the elderly with great caution. These include Phenylbutazone (Butazolidin®) and oxy-phenbutazone (Tanderil®). The side effects of these drugs are dependent on the dosage and duration of therapy. In any age side effects are common and reportedly occur more frequently in women than in men. The half-life (46 to 72 hours) may increase as much as 29 percent in persons over 65 years, so the dosage should be decreased by about one third. These drugs should not be taken in dosages greater than 300 mg per day for longer than a month. The most life threatening of its side effects are the blood dyscrasias (aplastic anemia, agranulocytosis). It can also cause gastrointestinal bleeding and sodium retention with attendant added stresses for the individual at risk for congestive failure or hypertension. These drugs should be administered with carefully selected patients under *close medical management and supervision.*

Steroids, sometimes used in younger persons for control of inflammatory joint disease, are rarely indicated for management of joint and bone problems of the elderly where degeneration is the predominate phenomenon. Side effects of steroids are the same at all ages.

INTESTINAL PROBLEMS

For drugs used with constipation and diarrhea, see Chapter 16.

CONCLUDING COMMENTS

From the pharmacists' perspective there are several things health care providers should keep in mind when participating in the health care of the older person who requires or is taking medications:

1. Dosage is a key. Therapy must often be started at what might seem to be homeopathic doses.
2. As the number of different drugs used in the same patient increases, the likelihood of drug interaction increases. The medication profile must be reviewed specifically to avoid serious interactions.
3. Side effects occur more commonly in the elderly because of their aging physiologic system. Keeping the dosage low may prevent many side effects.
4. Side effects of many drugs mimic the conditions that often occur in the aging process—

confusion, irritability, forgetfulness, anxiety, depression, anorexia, constipation, and urinary retention. Before attributing these symptoms to "old age," review the medication profile to determine if a drug may be the causative agent.

5. Actively encourage a team approach among nurse, physician, pharmacist, and older person to facilitate more rational drug therapy.

BIBLIOGRAPHY

Aagard, G. N.: Drug therapy in the aged. Post Grad. Med. 52:115–119, 1972.

APHA Handbook on Non-Prescription Drugs, Washington D.C.: American Pharmaceutical Association, 1976.

Avery, G.: Drug Treatment, Sydney, Australia: ADIS Press, 1976.

Block, L. H.: Drug interactions and the elderly. U.S. Pharmacist 2:46–55, 1977.

Chapron, D., and Lawson, I.: Drug prescribing and care of the elderly. In Reichel, W. (ed.): Clinical Aspects of Aging. Baltimore: Williams & Wilkins, pp. 13–32, 1978.

Crooks, J., et. al.; Pharmacokinetics in the elderly. Clin. Pharmacokinetics 1:280, 1976.

Davis, R. H.: Drugs and the Elderly. Los Angeles: Andrus Gerontology Center, University of Southern California, 1973.

Grunebaum, H. L.: The Practice of Community Mental Health. Boston: Little, Brown, & Co., 1976.

Hanan, Z. I.: Geriatric medications: how the aged are hurt by drugs meant to help. RN, 57–59, January 1978.

Hansten, P.: Drug Interactions. Philadelphia: Lea and Febiger, 1976.

Lawson, I., and Chapron, D.: A basic pharmacopeia for geriatric practice: a review of the FSASHP formulary. Reichel, W. (ed.): Clinical Aspects of Aging. Baltimore: Williams & Wilkins, pp. 33–34, 1978.

Use of Digitalis in the Elderly

Arbeit, S., et al.: Recognizing digitalis toxicity. A.J.N. 77:1935–1947, 1977. (General Reference and Continuing Education Unit.)

Hay, D. R.: Treatment of heart failure. Drugs 5:318–331, 1973.

Herrman, G. R.: Digitoxicity in the aged: recognition, frequency, and management. Geriatrics 21:109–122, 1966.

Huffman, D.: Clinical use of digitalis glycosides Am. J. Hosp. Pharm. 33:179–185, 1976. (Abnormal cardiac rhythm among most common signs and symptoms.)

Lely, A. H., et al.: Non cardiac symptoms of digitalis intoxication. Am. Heart J. 83:149–151, 1972.

Miller, S., and Forker, A.: Digitalis toxicity—neurological manifestations. J. Kans. Med. Soc. 8:263–264, Passim, 1974.

Ness, P.: Incidence and Clinical Manifestations of Unrecognized Digitalis Toxicity in a NH setting. Unpublished Master's Thesis, University of Washington, Seattle, 1977.

Wedgwood, J.: Cardiovascular disease in the old. Brit. Med. J. 3:622–626, 1973.

Part 3

High Risk Pathophysiology in the Elderly

Introduction to Part 3

Part 3 addresses selected health problems that are of high risk in people over 70 years of age. The conditions included are those that are commonly seen by nurses and significantly involve nursing management in an ongoing way. The list is not exhaustive. For instance, the behavioral problems of older people, although they are common and do require nursing management, are not included in this selection.

Long term care is the perspective that is taken, even though many of the conditions have acute stages. Much of the inhospital management included in other texts will not be found here. The majority of the elderly who have health problems do not spend much time in acute care facilities. Instead, much of their living with health, aging, and illness is done in noninstitutional settings. This reality suggests that nursing management, whether offered in a hospital, long term care facility, clinic, or home care setting, must consider long term self-care as well as living in some degree of independence with the presenting health issues and problems. The focus of Part 3, then, is on nursing management in both acute and chronic stages of disease with ongoing daily living in mind.

The chapters on pathophysiology and associated nursing management have been organized in two ways. Some chapters address conditions by organ or system—gastrointestinal, musculoskeletal, genitourinary, hearing, skin, and vision. In other chapters focus is placed on a particular condition often affecting multiple organs and systems—alcoholism, cancer, diabetes, hypertension, and stroke. In either case, the chapters are presented alphabetically within the section for ease of location.

The outline followed in each chapter or each condition within a chapter is comparable and in the same sequence. This was done to make information about particular aspects of any condition easy for the clinician to locate. So, while the writing styles of the contributors and content vary, a conscious effort has been made to avoid an anthology approach. This is not a collection of articles about conditions, but a series of chapters written by experts in which the sequence and format within which they address their specialty area has been held fairly constant.

Another assist to the nurses who are using this book as an ongoing aid in caring for elderly patients in their case load is the *Quick Review*. Here readers can find an overview of critical knowledge, crucial observations of risk factors or signs and symptoms, and guides to management and evaluation. It offers no depth but simply a check list for basic and important aspects of nursing management.

In all instances an effort has been made not to neglect the basic dynamics of the condition; however, the focus in applying this knowledge has been predominantly nursing, not medical, management. It is assumed that medical management is better addressed in medical texts. The reader is also referred to basic texts on each subject to deal with information that is not age-related. What is presented here is based upon the assumption that the reader has some information about the topic.

The bibliographies for each chapter include not only references cited but also articles and books that will address the topic in greater depth or sophistication for the reader who wishes more advanced or extensive treatment. In addition, where literature has been developed for patients and their families, these have been included in a separate listing. References that address development of community resources are also included in some chapters.

It is our intent in Part 3 to place in the reader's hands enough information and ideas to enable her to become increasingly effective and creative in participating in the nursing management of these common health problems among older people.

11

Alcoholism

M. Edith Heinemann and Kathleen Smith-Di Julio

QUICK REVIEW

ALCOHOLISM

DESCRIPTION	Dependence on alcohol to the point that it interferes with mental and physical health and social and economic well-being.
ETIOLOGIC FACTORS	Socioeconomic factors such as loss of loved ones, low income, poor health status, and feelings of alienation. Biologic and cultural influences under investigation.
HIGH RISK	Some increase in over-65 age group, elderly widowers, those facing major change in lifestyle.
DYNAMICS	Central nervous system depression. When rate of consumption chronically exceeds rate of metabolism (¾ oz whiskey/hr) tolerance raises threshold of CNS sensitivity to alcohol leading to physical dependence.
SIGNS AND SYMPTOMS	Response to alcohol: From initial decreased inhibitions→ clumsiness→ staggering- anger-weeping→ confusion stupor→ coma→ death. *Early:* Increasing urgency to drink to relieve tension; onset of memory blackouts; surreptitious drinking *Late:* Cannot stop drinking; becomes isolated and lonely; neglects eating; problems with family/friends
COMPLICATIONS	CNS-tolerance/dependence with withdrawal symptoms, gastritis, nutritional deficiencies, cirrhosis, congestive heart failure. Fluid-electrolyte imbalance: diureses with rising blood levels, fluid retention with decreasing levels. Magnesium deficiency. Respiratory alkalosis. Hematopoietic: increased risk of infection and bleeding. Osteoporosis.
DIFFERENTIAL DIAGNOSIS	Some signs of alcoholism confused with symptoms of aging, e.g., falls, malnutrition, tremors; strokes confused with withdrawal. Organic brain syndrome. Early/late alcoholism
PROGNOSIS	*Early onset:* Poor as a result of social maladjustments and physiologic complications. *Late onset:* Good, if no psychiatric complications.
MANAGEMENT	Confrontation. Deal with denial using facts re discrepancy between patients words and actions. Avoid arguments. Abstinence for early onset alcoholic, reduced drinking and management of stresses that triggered the drinking for late onset. Foster adequate nutrition. Treat loneliness and alienation.
EVALUATION	Abstinence from alcohol. Improvement in physical status. Effective participation of lifestyle without alcohol.

Alcoholism is a destructive and devastating phenomenon at any age, but it has unusually tragic consequences when it occurs during old age. At that time of life it adds to the often existing burdens of ill health, bereavement, and loneliness, sapping the person of already-diminishing physical and emotional energies. It has been said that old age is a time during which man can be at his best. It is the time when he is freed from the task of making a living, from the anxieties of holding a job, and from the need to please others. The older person has the chance to make living his main business and to use time in the most pleasurable and creative way possible. Instead, the person who has become addicted to alcohol is trapped in the pursuit of drinking. He uses most of his energies to satisfy the need for alcohol. Thoughts and actions are centered on this substance, the person becomes enmeshed in a cycle of drinking to feel good and drinking to ward off withdrawal. As a consequence of this addiction process, he becomes increasingly isolated from family and friends, economically destitute, and physically ill. Alcoholism in the elderly hastens the process of aging and shortens the span of life.

As is the case with many other disease processes, alcoholism can be prevented; when it does occur it can be arrested and treated. In fact, treatment of alcoholism in some elderly has been found to be more effective than in younger persons. However, in order for treatment to become instituted, alcoholism must be identified and the person must be helped to become convinced of his need for therapy.

Nurses are in a singularly advantageous position to make an impact on the problem of alcoholism. In all of their areas of service they encounter the alcoholic person and their professional preparation causes them to be particularly well-prepared for the issues involved in the treatment of this illness phenomenon. A basic problem in the genesis of alcoholism for many persons is an inability to cope with stresses of daily living. It is the essence of nursing to assist people in coping with such stress.

Prerequisite to effective nursing function is an understanding of the identified health problems and of the people who are affected. It is our intent in this chapter to provide information leading to such understandings related to alcoholism in the elderly.

Definition

Alcoholism has been difficult to define, largely because it most likely is not a single disease entity.

Etiologic factors, the course of the disease process, and responses to treatment vary from person to person and the constellation of symptoms are experienced differently. It is a progressive illness, usually developing over a period of from 5 to 20 years. Among the elderly it can be a disease of long standing or of recent onset. Since the duration of the disease presents different management problems and prognoses, it becomes important to determine the time of its onset.

Regardless of these variations, some common definitions and criteria for diagnosis have been developed. The World Health Organization, for instance, defines *alcoholics* as "those excessive drinkers whose dependence upon alcohol has attained such a degree that it shows a noticeable mental disturbance or an interference with their bodily and mental health, their interpersonal relations, and their smooth social and economic functioning; or who show the prodromal signs of such developments." (World Health Organization, 1952).

Perhaps the most significant step in defining alcoholism has been the establishment of "Criteria for the Diagnosis of Alcoholism," formulated by a committee of the National Council on Alcoholism (Criteria Committee, 1972). The committee viewed these criteria as a means for promoting early detection, providing a uniform nomenclature and preventing overdiagnosis. These criteria, articulated on three diagnostic levels, have been widely used and have provided a more uniform basis for diagnosing alcohol problems. (See Fig. 11-1 later in chapter.)

Some experts differentiate between problem drinkers and alcoholics. For those readers who wish to make this distinction, *problem drinking* was defined in the first special report to Congress, *Alcohol and Health,* as "Repeated episodes of intoxication or heavy drinking which impair health, and consistent use of alcohol as a coping mechanism in dealing with the problems of life to a degree of serious interference with an individual's effectiveness on the job, at home, in the community. . . ." (U.S. Department of Health, Education, and Welfare, 1971).

In line with the definitions above, and for the purposes of this chapter, the terms *alcohol abuse, problem drinking,* and *alcoholism* will be used to indicate varying levels of impairment of functioning as a result of alcohol consumption.

Etiologic Factors

No one cause for the development of alcoholism has as yet been identified. Studies have implicated psychologic states and sociocultural and biologic factors.

PSYCHOLOGIC STATES. The use of alcohol to decrease tensions, to provide fulfillment of unmet psychologic needs, and the preexistence of certain personality types have all been implicated as predisposing factors in development of alcoholism. Investigations have not, however, resulted in many definitive findings because of difficulties in assigning causal relationships between alcoholism and psychologic states, difficulties in defining those events that have existed prior to the development of alcoholism and those that are its consequences, and problems in measuring psychologic attributes. While it is generally accepted that psychologic stresses contribute to the development of alcoholism, they have not been identified as causal factors. This relationship is especially evident in elderly persons who have losses of loved ones, income, and health and who feel alienated, useless, and isolated.

SOCIOCULTURAL FACTORS. Observations of similarities and differences in drinking rates and rates of alcoholism between cultural groups have led to the investigations of sociocultural effects on drinking behavior. The way alcohol is introduced to members of a social group and the prescriptions for its consumption and for its misuse are viewed as factors influencing the development of alcohol problems.

It has been noted that Italians, for instance, who commonly use wine with meals and who reject intoxication, have a relatively low rate of alcoholism, while the French, who likewise use large quantities of wine but have less well-defined directions for its use, have high rates. Societal practices that encourage drinking as an acceptable mode of behavior may result in strong pressure to drink, thus favoring the development of alcoholism in those persons who have a predisposition for this disease. Such speculations raise important questions but have so far provided no definitive answers.

BIOLOGIC FACTORS. Investigations in this area include such things as abnormalities of body functioning such as glucose metabolism, food allergies, differences in metabolism, and the possible existence of genetic factors. While investigations of biologic functioning suffer from the issue of not being able to establish whether associations existed prior to or as a consequence of alcoholism, studies of genetic links have produced some interesting findings. For instance, studies of adopted children indicate that children of alcoholics are more likely to have alcohol problems than children of nonalcoholics despite being separated from their parents in early life

(Goodwin, 1976). Also, identical twins were found to be more concordant for heavy drinking than fraternal twins.

While biologic variations in responses to alcohol appear to be genetic in origin, there is no direct evidence as yet that innate factors contribute to the development of alcoholism.

Prevalence

Age is a factor in the prevalence of alcoholism. Some recent studies point to the existence of a relatively serious problem in the older age group.

GENERAL POPULATION. A household survey conducted in the Washington Heights section of Manhattan showed peaks of alcoholism in two age groups. Prevalence in the 45- to 54-year age group was found to be 23 per 1000 persons. However, a second peak of 22 per 1000 persons occurred in the 65- to 74-year age group (Bailey, et al., 1965). This study further showed that elderly widowers were most vulnerable with a rate of 105 per 1000 persons, five times the rate of the other peak ages (Zimberg, 1974).

In addition, the elderly alcoholic constitutes a significant proportion of those who are arrested for minor offenses. In San Francisco 82.3 percent of persons charged with drunkenness were 60 years of age and older (Zimberg, 1974).

HEALTH CARE SEEKING POPULATION. Relatively high rates of alcoholism among elderly persons have been observed in patient populations of psychiatric hospitals, outpatient mental health clinics, medical-surgical wards of general hospitals, and nursing homes. In a survey of 543 patients admitted to a psychiatric ward at San Francisco General Hospital, 28 percent were found to have serious drinking problems (Zimberg, 1974). Similarly, Kramer reported alcoholism to be present at the 30 percent level for ages 55 to 64 in a study of 279 state and county mental health hospitals (Kramer, 1969). In this same study a decrease in alcohol problems to 9 percent of this population was reported for those 65 to 74 years of age and a further decrease to 1 percent for patients over 75. Gaitz's study of 100 patients admitted to a county psychiatric ward at Baylor Hospital in Houston, Texas, resulted in a surprisingly high prevalence of alcoholism of 44 percent (Gaitz, 1971). A 17 percent rate of alcoholism was reported in patients seen in a mental health center in suburban Rockland County, New York (Zimberg, 1974).

Studies of patients admitted to general hospital medical wards indicate rates of alcoholism from 15 to 38 percent for men and up to 40 percent for women (Zimberg, 1974). A prevalence study of patients newly admitted to medical wards of Harlem Hospital Center in New York, for instance, showed that 63 percent of males and 35 percent of females in the 50- to 69-year age group were alcoholic. In the age group 70 and over, five of nine male patients and none of the female patients were alcoholics (Zimberg, 1974). However, a survey in England suggested that there was a higher chance of encountering drinking problems among elderly women than men (Rosin, et al., 1971). Review of nursing home populations indicated that alcoholism exists in about 20 percent of the residents (Graux, 1969).

While estimates vary widely for prevalence rates of alcohol problems among the elderly from a low of 2.2 percent found in a random population sample in New York City (Bailey, 1965) to a high of 82 percent of patients arrested for drunkenness in San Francisco, they suggest that alcohol problems among the elderly do indeed exist and that they appear to be more prominent than was formerly suspected. It has been estimated that alcoholism is present in about a million people over the age of 55 (Cohen, 1975).

HIGH RISK POPULATION. Among the elderly, certain groups are at higher risk for developing alcoholism than others. This includes those who have faced or must contemplate major relocations in their life-style such as change of housing, change of interpersonal environment, or retirement from valued, meaningful work with the accompanying loss of status and power. The nurse must be alert to the possibility of increased alcohol consumption accompanying such stresses. Efforts to deal with the problems that may generate drinking behavior become important for prevention of, as well as recovery from, alcohol problems.

Dynamics

The varied and complex effects of alcohol on the body are due primarily to changes in the function of the central nervous system. While the exact pharmacologic mechanisms are unknown, the overall effect is a depressant one depending on dosage, and increasing in severity as the blood alcohol level rises.

ABSORPTION. The rapidity with which the blood alcohol level increases and the resultant changes in functioning depend upon the speed of alcohol's absorption from stomach and small intestine and the drinking history of the individual. No age related differences in the metabolism of alcohol are known presently. The presence of food retards the rate of absorption, while carbonated water in the form of mixers, will speed it up.

METABOLISM. Alcohol is metabolized in the body at the fairly constant rate of 10 to 15 ml per hour. The typical drink contains a "shot" of spirits (1 oz of 40 to 50 percent alcohol), a glass of wine (4 oz of 12 percent alcohol), or a pint of beer (12 oz of 5 percent alcohol) (U.S. Department of Health, Education and Welfare, 1971).

As persons drink at a rate faster than the alcohol can be metabolized, it accumulates in the blood and results in ever higher concentrations. This results in evidence of intoxication. Chronic consumption of large amounts of alcohol over long periods of time results in an increased rate of metabolism. It also causes an altered state of sensitivity of the central nervous system to the effects of alcohol known as *tolerance.* Tolerance permits high blood alcohol concentrations to occur which result in the development of physical dependence. Physical dependence is characterized by the appearance of withdrawal symptoms upon cessation of alcohol intake.

ALCOHOL BLOOD LEVELS AND BEHAVIOR. In the naive drinker perceptible changes in mood and behavior occur at blood alcohol levels of 0.40 gm percent (U.S. Department of Health, Education, and Welfare, 1971, p. 38). Combining knowledge about expected symptoms at certain blood alcohol levels in the naive drinker (Table 11-1) the nurse can make estimates as to the patient's level of tolerance. For ex-

TABLE 11-1. Expected symptoms at specific blood levels.

Blood Level %	Behavior
0.05	Judgment and restraint loosened; individual feels carefree
0.10	Voluntary motor action becomes clumsy
0.20	Entire motor area of brain is measurably depressed. Staggering; may lie down; easily angered; may shout or weep
0.30	More primitive areas of brain dulled; confusion and possible stuporousness
0.40 0.50	Coma; possible death due to respiratory blocking effects on medulla

ample, a patient exhibiting symptoms of clumsy motor movement with a blood alcohol level of 0.40 percent shows high tolerance to alcohol.

TOLERANCE. Effects of alcohol on the alcohol-dependent person differ. In contrast to the initial euphoric aspects of intoxication experienced by the normal drinker, the alcoholic becomes more tense and anxious. Moreover, the alcohol-dependent person, with the presence of tolerance, can drink very large quantities without obvious behavioral impairment. He can perform accurately complex behavioral tasks at blood alcohol levels several times as great as those that would lead to behavioral impairment in light and moderate drinkers. It is this phenomenon, namely the ability to raise blood alcohol concentrations to high levels and to maintain these high concentrations for a prolonged period of time, which causes the development of physical dependence and pathologic changes in the tissues of organs.

PHYSICAL DEPENDENCE. Physical dependence is an adaptive process in the central nervous system. In contrast to the phenomenon of tolerance, which is evidenced as more alcohol is consumed, physical dependence becomes manifest when the drug (alcohol) is withdrawn, resulting in the appearance of withdrawal symptoms. The most prominent features of the syndrome are tremulousness, hallucinosis, seizure activity, and the most severe and sometimes fatal phenomenon of delirium tremens. It is of special interest to nurses, who care for patients during withdrawal crises, that both the intensity and advancement of the symptoms as well as time of onset can be predicted.

Characteristically, drinking in the early stages is intermittent, becoming more frequent and gradually more prolonged. Early significant landmarks of ensuing alcoholism are (1) constant drinking for relief of tension and anxiety, (2) increase in alcohol tolerance, (3) onset of memory blackouts, (4) surreptitious drinking, (5) urgency to drink, and (6) increasing dependence on alcohol. With the persistence of continued heavy drinking, physical dependence becomes manifest as early morning tremors and agitation, requiring a morning drink for relief of these symptoms. The person has now become addicted to alcohol.

Progress toward the chronic stage is characterized by (1) inability to stop drinking, (2) loss of outside interests, (3) work and money troubles, (4) difficulties with family and friends, (5) neglect of food, (6) feelings of guilt, remorse, and depression,

and (7) intense loneliness. The individual enters either the stage of continuous drinking, in which he remains in a more or less constant state of inebriation, or a vicious cycle of drinking bouts, each ending in acute withdrawal and leading to the next bout.

Tolerance during the chronic stage decreases and a host of pathologic conditions are demonstrable. Although the mechanism for the decrease in tolerance is not understood, it is thought to be related to diffuse brain damage (Kissin and Begleiter, 1974, p. 25).

Progression to chronicity characteristically takes from 12 to 20 years. Elderly persons, who began drinking late in life, may experience a telescoping of this period.

Signs and Symptoms

The subjective and objective data that suggest a diagnosis of alcoholism are comparable across age groups. While alcoholism and problem drinking have been used interchangably in this chapter, some experts do differentiate; therefore, the criteria for data gathering and diagnosing of either is offered.

Manifestations of Problem Drinking

The following history, behavior, and physical status should lead to diagnosing an individual as a problem drinker:

> A lifestyle in which major accidents, job and family difficulties and/or other traumas have been related to the abuse of alcohol.
> The presence of acting-out behaviors at the time of drinking such as aggressive outbursts, sexual affairs, job absenteeism, wife-beating.
> Absence of demonstrable physiological tissue damage specific to the diagnosis of alcoholism.
> Patterns of alcohol consumption less compulsive in nature than those of chronic alcoholism (Forrest, 1975, p. 59).

In the absence of therapeutic interventions, it is estimated that 70 percent of problem drinkers will eventually qualify for the diagnosis of alcoholism (Forrest, 1975, p. 63).

Manifestations of Alcoholism

According to the "Criteria for the Diagnosis of Alcoholism," the diagnosis of alcoholism is definite when one or more of the major criteria of Diagnostic Level I are satisfied (Fig. 11-1).

Problems in Diagnosing Alcoholism

Alcoholism is not effectively diagnosed, particularly among the elderly. There are several reasons for failure to recognize the problem.

LOW PROFESSIONAL AWARENESS. Health professionals have been found to have notoriously low levels of awareness of the presence of alcoholism and are prone to miss the diagnosis in persons who do present themselves to health agencies. Schuckit (1975), for instance, reported that over half of the diagnoses that were missed in a study of 50 male patients aged 65 and over admitted to medical and surgical wards at the La Jolla VA Hospital were either alcoholism or depression.

SHIELDING OF ALCOHOLIC PERSONS BY THEIR FAMILIES. The elderly alcoholic is often shielded by his family. In an effort to protect the older person, the family tends to deny that drinking constitutes a problem and hides the elderly person's difficulty. This kind of misplaced affection in a sense encourages the older person's excessive drinking, causing him to become increasingly more dependent on alcohol and to become physically ill. It also keeps the person from contact with potential sources of help.

In addition, the person who senses difficulties with alcohol is reluctant to admit to the presence of a drinking problem, and even more reluctant to present himself for treatment. Fears that such acknowledgment will rob him of the substance he views necessary to life as well as threat of increased rejection and isolation from friends and relatives are among reasons to avoid seeking help. There are others who, because of physical disability, are unable to leave their home unaided and cannot present themselves for help.

DECREASING ALCOHOL CONSUMPTION. An unrecognized fact that causes a failure to diagnose the elderly alcoholic is related to using the quantity of alcohol consumed as a criterion. Older people, especially those who have been heavy drinkers for many years, tend to have a lower tolerance for alcohol than younger people. This means that some may have a serious drinking problem even though their consumption of alcohol is less than that of younger alcoholics.

Differential Diagnosis

The prevalence of alcohol problems in the elderly, estimated to be 20 to 30 percent of those in treatment for either medical or psychiatric conditions, warrants routine screening for the existence of such problems in all elderly persons admitted to health agencies.

MANIFESTATIONS OF ALCOHOLISM

Physiologic Dependence
  gross tremors
  hallucinosis
  withdrawal seizures
  delirium tremens

Tolerance to Effects of Alcohol
  blood alcohol level more than 150 mg/100 ml without gross evidence of intoxication
  consumption of a fifth of whiskey or equal amount of wine or beer daily for two or more days by a 180-lb individual

Alcohol-Associated Illnesses
  alcoholic hepatitis
  alcoholic cerebral degeneration

Behavioral, Psychologic, and Attitudinal Indices
  drinking despite strong medical contraindications known to patient
  drinking despite strong, identified social contraindications (marriage disruption because of drinking, arrest for intoxication, driving accidents while intoxicated, and so forth)

FIGURE 11-1.   Criteria for diagnosis of alcoholism, Diagnostic Level I.

Problems

The diagnosis of alcoholism or alcohol problems frequently is missed by confusing the effects of alcohol with symptoms of old age. Rosin and Glatt (1971), for instance, described common symptoms of a group of elderly people referred to a psychiatrist because of drinking problems as those of social isolation, falls, malnutrition, general physical deterioration, and dementia. All of these could have been mistaken as symptoms of aging.

In assessing an elderly person who presents with any complaint, specific attention must be focused on physiologic signs that may indicate aging or an illness but might be a consequence of excessive alcohol intake. Hypertension, for example, is a frequent accompaniment of aging but is also a very clear manifestation of withdrawal form alcohol. Confused behavior may be a function of arteriosclerotic brain disease or it may be an indicator of Wernicke's encephalopathy. An uneven gait may be either a limp caused by some type of physical impairment or it may be an indicator of intoxication.

Differential Diagnosis of Early and Late Onset Alcoholism

Upon closer examination of the elderly population with alcohol problems, two quite distinct groups can be identified. Those who have had a lifelong history of excessive drinking and those who have started drinking heavily late in life. These two groups of people differ in several ways, but particularly in their state of physical wellness and, therefore, in potential responses to therapeutic interventions.

EARLY ONSET OF ALCOHOLISM. When one considers that alcoholism has been described by some authors to be a self-limiting disease, then the existence of a sizeable group who survived and continue their alcoholic drinking may come as a surprise. As described previously, social and moderately-heavy drinking tends to decline in old age because of such factors as lack of money, different social patterns following retirement, and a decline in desire for alcohol. The elderly person who has been drinking all his life appears to be one with remarkable resistance to have survived the long term effects of alcohol. Almost all persons who fall into this category, however, have one or more of the consequences of chronic heavy drinking, such as neurologic and vascular disturbances, organic brain syndrome, or liver diseases (Graux, 1969; Pascarelli, 1974; Rosin and Glatt, 1971).

There are conflicting reports about the extent to which disabilities exist among the elderly who show heavy alcohol consumption throughout most of their lives. Very few studies are available concerning such comparisons. Still it appears that elderly alcoholics do have serious disturbances in most of their areas of life functioning.

LATE ONSET OF ALCOHOLISM. Representing a second population of elderly alcoholic persons is that group that begins drinking heavily in old age. Drinking and the use of other depressants become ways of dealing with the stresses of aging such as loss of spouse, retirement, and other serious dislocations. It is important to recognize and treat these conditions. If no complicating factors are involved, such as chronic brain syndrome, depression, or paranoia, the prognosis is extremely good. When the stressful circumstances are alleviated, the person readily responds to treatment (Pascarelli, 1974; Zimberg, 1971). Thus it becomes important for the nurse to identify the conditions contributing to the drug intake and, if possible, alleviate them.

Complications and Consequences of Chronic Excessive Alcohol Use on the Body

The multiple and serious pathophysiologic disturbances resulting from chronic alcohol abuse are consequences of direct and indirect effects on cells and physiologic mechanisms of the body. Serious disturbances occur in the nervous system, the gastrointestinal system, the heart, the muscles, the blood, and the bloodforming organs. The mechanism that is in part responsible for these effects is the development of tolerance. As was discussed previously, tolerance is characterized by a reduced sensitivity of cells to the effects of a drug, in this case alcohol, allowing large quantities of the drug to be consumed and to circulate in the bloodstream. Damage to cells is a consequence of prolonged exposure to high alcohol concentration.

CENTRAL NERVOUS SYSTEM. Prolonged use of large amounts of alcohol affect the central nervous system in 100 percent of the alcoholic population (Gitlow, 1970). Disturbances resulting from the effects on the nervous system include the development of tolerance and physical dependence. Some of the normal diseases of the aged are made more severe in the older alcoholic person.

Tolerance. As discussed previously, tolerance is a state of altered sensitivity of the central nervous system to alcohol and is common to the chronic use of all addictive drugs. The nurse should be alert to the following two major symptoms of this phenomenon:

1. The need to ingest larger quantities to produce changes in feelings and behaviors formerly attained with smaller amounts.
2. The capacity to drink very large quantities without showing impairment in functioning.

Physical Dependence. The appearance of withdrawal symptoms, as previously discussed, is time-dose related. The occurrence of the more severe ones can be suppressed with proper management. Therefore, the nurse must take a careful history of the person's recent alcohol use and ascertain the time the last alcohol was consumed. (Questions on the Nursing History at the end of the chapter.) The nurse should be alert to the following signs and symptoms described as major and minor by Wolfe and Victor (1971):

Minor Withdrawal Syndrome
  Tremors and diaphoresis: 6 to 8 hours after cessation of drinking.
  Hallucination, convulsion, and mild disorientation: 10 to 30 hours after cessation of drinking.
Major Withdrawal Syndrome
  Delirium tremens: onset 60 to 80 hours following drinking.
  Profound disorientation, including misinterpretations and misidentifications.
  Fever.
  Tachycardia.
  Severe diaphoresis.
  Restlessness, tremors, jactitation.
  Vivid hallucinations.

While the majority of patients experience only the manifestations of the minor syndrome, those that develop delerium tremens are indeed very sick. This phenomenon, in the untreated state, carries with it a mortality rate of 12 to 15 percent (McNichol, 1970).

Other Associated Conditions. Other central nervous system disorders are the Wernicke-Korsakoff syndrome related to thiamine deficiency in the presence of alcoholism, Marchiofava Bignami disease, cerebellar cortical degeneration, amblyopia, myelinolysis, central pontine myelinolysis, pellagra, and so forth.

The more prevalent Wernicke syndrome is characterized by clouding of consciousness and paralysis of eye muscles, the latter giving rise to diplobia. Korsakoff's psychosis, usually succeeding the Wernicke syndrome, produces disturbances in short-term memory, coupled with a tendency to make up for the deficit by substituting imagined occurrences.

Alcoholic polyneuropathy is a nutritional disorder in alcoholics, occurring primarily in undernourished persons. It occurs in greatly varying severity from no complaints of symptoms to those of weakness, paresthesias, and pain. Symptoms are always symmetric, tending to develop from distal to proximal distribution, with legs being affected prior to arms. The administration of thiamine in addition to nutritious diets results in amelioration of symptoms and usually in recovery from the condition.

GASTROINTESTINAL SYSTEM. Prolonged alcohol consumption affects many components of the gastrointestinal system. Secondary complications are a result of direct work on the organs and/or nutritional deficiencies.

Inflammatory responses. Irritating effects of alcohol cause direct local injury to the digestive system in the form of esophagitis, gastritis, and enteritis. The malabsorption syndrome, a consequence of chronic alcohol use, gives rise to various nutritional deficiencies.

Liver and pancreas are seriously affected by chronic alcohol abuse. While fatty liver occurs in anyone ingesting moderate amounts of alcohol for several days, the more serious conditions of alcoholic hepatitis and cirrhosis may occur with increased frequency in persons drinking heavily over long periods of time. Fatty liver is a reversible process, but hepatitis and cirrhosis result in permanent changes. Alcoholic cirrhosis occurs in about 10 percent of alcoholic persons and is a most serious, generally irreversible process.

Pancreatitis may also occur in either acute or chronic form. It is characterized by severe abdominal pain. The reversibility of this abnormality depends on the degree of damage.

Malnutrition. By drinking, the elderly alcoholic person may have begun to satisfy a large proportion of calorie requirements, which normally decrease with age. This trend must be reversed if health is to be restored. The association between malnutrition and alcoholism gives rise to a host of disease conditions: hematopoietic disorders such as macrocytic anemia and thrombocytopenia and neurologic disorders such as Wernicke-Korsakoff syndrome, polyneuropathy, pellagra, and beriberi heart disease.

The clinical appraisal of the nutritional status is best achieved in a comprehensive nutritional assessment.

CARDIAC SYSTEM. Alcoholic cardiomyopathy, a direct effect of alcohol on the heart muscle, and nutritional heart disease in the form of beriberi heart disease, occur with a history of alcohol abuse. Clinical characteristics of alcoholic cardiomyopathy include symptoms characteristic of left- and right-sided congestive heart failure (Chapter 13). Abstinence from alcohol and the treatment of congestive heart failure usually results in improvement of the condition.

FLUID AND ELECTROLYTE BALANCE. Fluid and electrolyte imbalances are common situations among alcoholics. Given the renal changes of aging, the elderly alcoholic can be expected to have even greater problems than the younger one (see Chapter 6, p. 59). Situations in which the nurse needs to be suspicious of fluid and electrolyte problems include when the individual is (1) withdrawing from alcohol; (2) drinking cheap wine and beer as a substitute for the more expensive, concentrated hard liquors; or (3) vomiting, having diarrhea, or not eating much.

When blood alcohol concentrations are *rising* the individual will have *increased* urine output (diuresis). Stable or *decreasing* blood alcohol levels are associated with fluid *retention* (antidiuresis).

Sodium, potassium, and chloride deficiencies are common in the presence of some conditions such as vomiting, diarrhea, or malnutrition. A magnesium deficiency also commonly occurs with alcohol abuse. Hypomagnesemia is of particular concern because it results in neural excitability which may precipitate seizure activity (Wolfe and Victor, 1971, p. 105). Respiratory alkalosis, likewise, has been observed during alcohol withdrawal and has been implicated in the development of seizures and delirium tremens (Wolfe and Victor, 1971, p. 198).

HEMATOPOIETIC SYSTEM. Adverse effects of alcohol on hematopoiesis result in abnormalities of red blood cells, white blood cells, and platelets, which give rise to the occurrence of anemias, difficulties in counteracting infections, and interferences in the clotting mechanism. The patient shows symptoms of severe infections and frequently presents with hematomas. Complete blood counts provide evidence as to the existence of anemias and abnormal white blood cell counts. *Vigilance is particularly necessary when an individual is placed on anticoagulant therapy.* Frequent monitoring of prothrombin time is indicated. In addition, protection from infections may be lifesaving, since patients have difficulties fighting such conditions as pneumonia and bronchitis. These abnormalities are reversible with abstinence from alcohol and proper nutrition.

SKELETAL SYSTEM. Alcoholism in the elderly contributes to skeletal complications in at least two ways. It increases osteoporosis and contributes to fractures by increasing the risk of trauma. A syndrome of nontraumatic osteonecrosis of the hip, which may be caused by fat emboli blocking end arteries, is being recognized in chronic alcohol consumers (Lieber, 1977). Impaired coordination as a result of high blood alcohol levels is a contributing factor to falls and consequent injury and fractures. This is of particular concern in the older age group which is already at risk for skeletal injuries.

CANCER. An association between drinking and cancer of the mouth, pharynx, larynx, esophagus, and liver has been observed clinically for many years. The reasons for this association are unclear but among the possibilities are the prolonged effects of alcohol on body tissues and the possible presence of carcinogenic substances in some alcoholic beverages. (U. S. Department of Health, Education, and Welfare, 1974). The incidence of cancer in these sites in the elderly person should serve as clues to the presence of a possible alcohol problem.

Tools for Assessing Alcoholism

A number of screening tools for assessing problem drinking are available and useful. Most of these include criteria relating to a person's job history and so are of less use with the individual over 70 who, in most cases, is retired. For the older person a more applicable tool to identify problem drinking is the MacAndrew and Holmes MMPI Alcoholism Scale for Older Alcoholics and Problem Drinkers (Apfeldorf and Hunley, 1975). This scale is said to effectively discriminate elderly domiciled alcoholics and disciplinary offenders from non-alcoholics (Apfeldorf and Hunley, 1975, p. 651).

In order to establish the extent of impairment in all areas of functioning it is necessary to obtain as complete an assessment as possible. A nursing history and a physical examination should be performed with the elderly person in mind. The guide to a nursing history, developed by Heinemann and Estes (1976, pp. 24–31), is particularly useful in obtaining essential information. This tool has been adapted to aid in identifying the particular needs, problems, and concerns of the aged.

There are two versions of the history. One gives the nurse or other health care providers a full data base on the alcoholism problem. This can be found in Estes and Heinemann, 1977, pp. 224–226. However, there are times when the patient's condition or other circumstances require a more rapid gathering of only high priority data. This assessment instrument, adapted to the elderly, can be found on pages 201 to 203.

Because of the high risk of denial and the effects this has on reporting behavior it is probably of more importance with alcoholics than other patients to gather both validating data and an expanded picture of the situation from those who know the patient best. Information from relatives and/or friends should be elicited whenever possible. In addition to assisting the nurse in understanding the patient's attitudes toward alcohol and aiding the nurse in evaluating the response, interviewing the family adds perspective on family attitudes and relationships.

The history must include a thorough exploration of social, emotional, and physical aspects of the patient's life. It must provide information about past and present drinking habits, including the amount and type of beverage consumed, frequency of use, situations in which alcohol is used, attitude toward alcohol, perception of drinking behavior, and the effects of alcohol on performance.

Beyond taking a history, a physical examination is important because it serves to broaden the base of clues that lead to identification of physiologic problems coexisting with, or consequent to, alcohol abuse. Because of alcohol's effect on the nervous system and the possibility of trauma secondary to alcohol abuse, *neurologic status checks* must be an integral part of any physical assessment process. Particular attention must be given to the assessment of the elderly person's orientation because of the possibility of the presence of organic brain syndrome. Loss of sensation in the hands and feet is suggestive of peripheral neuropathies. In addition, the presence of an enlarged liver with or without ascites and jaundice must be noted in evaluating for liver disease.

Prognosis

Prognosis is related to multiple factors including the time of onset and physical well-being. Suc-

cessful management of alcoholism in the group with early onset is doubtful. Abstinence is essential to regaining a better degree of health, but the outlook for abstinence in this group is not good.

Conversely, the prognosis for improvement in those who began drinking later in life is favorable. It is associated with the ability to effectively deal with the stress that triggered the drinking. When this occurs, chances for recovery are good.

Management

Treatment regimens for the alcoholic problems of elderly patients must take into account the interaction of the status of aging as well as the problem drinking. They must provide for resolution or amelioration of pathophysiologic disturbances in addition to creating an atmosphere conducive to nondrinking.

Rehabilitation of the recovering elderly alcoholic is delayed until physiologic stability is achieved. Heinemann and coworkers (1977) found that major factors related to the termination of treatment include the existence of serious physiologic problems. This points to the importance of meeting the patient's physical needs.

Factors Influencing Treatment Outcomes

TIME OF ONSET. Those elderly problem drinkers who begin drinking late in life, often in response to losses, are usually responsive to treatment. They appear to be better candidates for rehabilitation than those whose alcoholism began earlier and continues into old age (Mayfield, 1974; Zimberg, 1974). The elderly person who has been drinking problematically over a lifetime may not benefit as much from treatment. In general, however, all elderly alcohol abusers are likely to participate in treatment if agencies have programs geared to them.

ATTITUDES AND BELIEFS OF PROVIDERS. Additional factors influencing treatment and clinical progress are the attitudes, beliefs, and values held by those providing care. It is difficult for some providers to effectively treat the aged problem drinker. Both alcoholism and old age are seen by some as irreversible, hopeless conditions offering no possibility of lasting change.

Some professionals believe that the older person has a right to live the last years of life in whatever way he chooses. If this includes excessive alcohol consumption, no one has a right to interfere. They raise the question of why elderly persons should be asked to confront problems of which they may soon be permanently relieved. Other providers feel attention and services should be given to nonalcoholics. Still others are uncomfortable with alcoholics.

These are issues and realities that health care providers who deal with elderly alcoholic persons must confront and resolve before intervention is instituted. Attitudes, beliefs, and values need to be explored not only before but also during the treatment process or their existence may constitute serious obstacles to any success in rehabilitation.

CHARACTERISTICS OF TREATMENT AGENCIES. The difficulty in obtaining treatment for elderly alcoholics is the fact that most alcohol treatment agencies are not organized with the aged in mind. There are, however, some nursing homes that limit admission to those with alcoholism problems. Personnel in nursing homes and other agencies presently working to meet the health and illness needs of the elderly are generally unaware of the extent of alcohol problems among their patients. They are, therefore, neither educated nor organized to meet the needs of this segment of their patient population. It has been suggested that alcoholism services for the aged need to be developed in conjunction with geriatric services. For this population there needs to be a close coordination of treatment of medical and social problems and the management of alcoholism. When the nurse identifies an alcohol problem in a patient she has the option of planning intervention approaches or referring the problem to appropriate treatment personnel. Almost every community has community alcohol centers (CAC) and alcohol treatment facilities. The CACs generally provide information, evaluation, and referral to the proper agency, while many treatment centers accept clients for treatment directly. Obtaining the proper match of patient needs and appropriate treatment facilities is still more of an art than a science and is best accomplished by persons with knowledge of and experience with alcoholism.

One of the important issues to address is that of staff development for nurses who work in nursing homes, doctor's offices, or wherever alcohol problems in the elderly may be confronted. Available resources, though differing between communities, generally are increasing. The two major organizations concerned with prevention and treatment of alcoholism throughout the country are the National Institute of Alcohol Abuse and Alcoholism (NIAAA) and the National Council on Alcoholism (NCA). The NCA has local chapters in all major cities. The chapters have a wealth of information available in the form of audiovisual aids, literature, and human resources. They also have knowledge of local facilities for treatment of alcohol problems.

The National Clearinghouse for Alcohol Information (NCALI), P. O. Box 2345, Rockville, Maryland 20852, (301) 948-4450, and the National Center for Alcohol Education (NCAE), 1601 North Kent Street, Arlington, Virginia 22209, (703) 527-5757, are divisions of NIAAA and provide information upon request.

Alcoholics Anonymous (AA) has branches throughout the country and is another source of assistance for the alcoholic. They are listed in the telephone book and all meetings are open. The individual who is interested can attend any meeting— nurses to learn, patients to receive help. This group, along with Al-Anon (for families of alcoholics) and Al-Ateen (teenagers with alcoholic parents), frequently provides speakers on a variety of alcohol-related subjects.

A Treatment Typology

A simple typology, which can be useful in choosing appropriate approaches to management of the elderly problem drinker, has been developed (Rathbone-McCuan and Bland, 1975). The plan is based on data indicating the presence or absence of symptoms of the following:

1. problem drinking
2. health problems
3. inadequacies in the social network

Data in these major areas then need to be translated into a statement of the patient's specific diagnoses or problem that the nurse proposes to address.

Steps in Treatment

Treatment of alcoholism involves several steps. These include confrontation with and acceptance of the disease, setting of goals, and general management planning.

CONFRONTATION. The first step in treatment of the elderly alcoholic is the same as that for any person who has a problem with alcohol abuse. It is to confront the person with the facts of excessive drinking and what it does to his life. Generally this experience is uncomfortable for the patient and usually arouses anger and hostility. To deal with these feelings the patient may attempt to manipulate the situation in order to make it more comfortable or he may employ a variety of defense mechanisms, the most common of which is denial. Confrontation, therefore, must be a deliberate action based on well-thought out strategies and it must be tailored to the demands of the situation.

Common components that must prevail prior to every confrontation are that the nurse has adequate data about the patient and his situation, her knowledge of alcoholism is broad enough to allow her to arrive at valid judgments, and her attitudes and feelings about alcoholism are in control allowing a nonjudgmental interaction to ensue. With these conditions prevailing, the nurse selects the appropriate time to inform the patient of the facts that she has gathered. In an unemotional way she explains alcoholism, what is likely to occur with continued drinking, and what the options are, as she sees them.

Denial is a response that must be expected since the elderly alcoholic person may tend to protect his drinking behavior in order to be able to continue it. Presentation of facts and avoidance of an argument is one way of dealing with denial. If denial persists, the nurse must continue this confrontation process at some other suitable time, remembering that the course of action ultimately is the patient's decision.

Manipulation is another mechanism frequently used by the elderly alcoholic person to avoid altering his drinking behavior. It is a process whereby the alcoholic controls or uses others to satisfy his own needs without considering the needs, wishes, or values of the other persons involved (Betts, 1976). This often is a frustrating experience for the nurse since she is made to look disorganized and uninformed. If she anticipates manipulation, the nurse is able to note the discrepancies between the patient's words and actions and consistently call them to his attention (Betts, 1976). In addition, it is helpful to limit the focus of the interaction to the topic at hand. Tendencies for the patient to relate tangential information are not tolerated. This conveys to the patient that manipulation is ineffective. As the patient comes to acknowledge his problem, he will begin to deal with his needs directly and find it unnecessary to use manipulation.

TREATMENT GOALS. The overall goal for alcoholics is to stop drinking or at least to decrease alcohol consumption. *Abstinence* is the goal for those elderly persons who have consumed alcohol problematically over an entire lifetime. *Decreased consumption*, which is only recently being considered a possibility, may be an appropriate goal for some of those who are relatively recent abusers. An additional goal is that of developing alternative, more effective, coping responses to deal with the underlying reasons for the dependence on alcohol.

Initially the nurse and patient may have different goals for treatment. It is of utmost importance that each communicate his or her goals clearly to the other. Negotiation toward establishing mutually agreeable goals can then take place. Writing down these proposed goals is a concrete reminder of this agreement. Such a step promotes understanding for an elderly person who might be forgetful and permits both nurse and patient to evaluate progress toward achievement of the defined goals.

A *nutritionally-adequate diet* is important. Alcohol irritates the digestive system and causes a diminished absorption of nutrients. A patient's limited funds have often been spent for alcohol rather than food. Cessation or diminution of drinking will allow for more complete absorption of essential nutrients. The nurse also needs to give some attention to helping the patient begin to eat adequately again. This means gathering data on usual eating patterns (when not drinking), problems perceived in obtaining, preparing, and consuming an adequate diet, and resources or assistance he will accept.

Hand tremors, ataxia, paresthesias, and anesthesias which are frequently seen during withdrawal may persist in an elderly person despite a nutritious diet and vitamin supplements. This indicates irreversible nerve damage and has implications for management of the elderly person's environment. Low tables with sharp corners may be an environmental hazard for a person with lower extremity anesthesia. An injury caused by bumping into a sharp object may not be noticed and go unattended, perhaps leading to infection. Normally the healing process slows down with aging and is further diminished in the presence of nerve damage and blood cell alterations. Thus, a safe environment must be established in order to minimize the risk of injury to an older person.

Of equal concern is smoking, which is frequently seen in alcoholic persons, and/or cooking done by a person with anesthesia of the upper extremities. This person, because of diminished sensation, may minimize heat damage incurred from these or other sources. This, too, has implications for secondary infections and healing. The affected person needs to be taught the inherent hazards and ways of preventing injury. For example, a smoker with hand anesthesia can be taught to put the cigarette out before it burns down to the fingers. Similarly, a cook can be encouraged to protect his hands by using hot pads while cooking.

Another general area for nursing management is that of *mobility and safety*. The unsteadiness of gait and the incidence of increased osteoporosis associated with alcoholism make these individuals a high risk for fractures. Again, reducing alcohol intake decreases some of the risks, but attention to safety features in the environment of these patients is important.

Perhaps most important in the treatment of the elderly alcoholic person is the *consideration of loneliness and alienation*. These are difficult problems to solve with the elderly. To counter the problems of alienation the elderly person must feel a part of a social group, although many have never been part of groups. Part of the assessment that must precede planning in this area is gathering information from the person about past group memberships. Referral to a social or recreational center designed specifically for older persons may be helpful but only if it is compatible with interests or previous patterns. Beyond personal preferences it is important also to assess the aged person's mobility and the location of the facilities, keeping transportation options in mind. For example, many elderly people do not drive but can get around by bus. This process becomes more difficult however if bus transfers are necessary to reach a destination or if traveling at night is involved. Carpools may be feasible alternatives for some. One other approach that has been used is to link the older person with a foster family or friendly visitor program.

Another management approach to the problem of alienation is the *purposeful use of reminiscence*. Having interested, participating listeners as one recalls earlier, perhaps better, times in one's life can serve to enhance the person's self-esteem. It also conveys a sense of worth of at least having had a meaningful existence and being able to share that with persons in one's current environment. Reminiscing groups can be established in senior citizen centers, daycare centers, and retirement or nursing home settings—any place where a group of elderly persons congregates. Such groups can become cohesive because of this sharing (Ebersole, 1976). Functional capacities do not remain at an optimal level but deteriorate unless they are stimulated.

Participation in groups where appropriate functional activities occur can assist in maintenance.

Alcoholism is recognized as a family problem. While many elderly alcoholics may be alone and isolated, some are still very much involved with family members. These people need to be involved in the care and management of alcoholism. Frequently the functioning of the family has been severely affected by the presence of the alcoholic person and often the alcohol problem has become the focus of interaction. In this process each family member may have developed an associated behavioral problem. Thus, in order for the alcoholic person to recover and for the family to begin to function normally, the family dynamic must become a focus for treatment. Individual members may need additional help.

Since alcohol is often consumed in order to alleviate anxiety caused by stress, one of the most effective ways to decrease alcohol consumption is to acquire *alternative coping behaviors*. The elderly person who drinks excessively in response to losses such as death of a spouse or retirement may be particularly suited toward developing new ways to lessen anxiety. Some possibilities are progressive relaxation, biofeedback, assertiveness, and autogenic training. It must be emphasized however, that such efforts at helping the older persons cope with losses must have been preceded by an identification of the emotional stress and a chance to work through the feelings of loss.

Also, all of the interventions described above are to some extent dependent upon monetary resources. The financial plight for many old people is grim. Since the aged are less likely to seek out and utilize community resources they must be made aware of their right to take advantage of what is available to them.

Management of Acute Alcoholic Syndromes

Hangovers occur in any individual, alcoholic or not, who consumes a large amount of alcohol in one timespan. They occur from 12 to 14 hours after the start of drinking and include symptoms of lassitude, thirst and dry mouth, headache, nausea, gastrointestinal disturbances, and general indisposition. There is controversy as to whether this syndrome represents a form of mild withdrawal or the effects of congeners contained in drinks (Kissin and Begleiter, 1974).

Taking the patient's drinking history will allow

the nurse to predict whether this person is likely to develop more severe withdrawal symptoms. The person whose heavy drinking was confined to one episode will recover from a hangover with time, rest, quiet, and adequate nutrition. Such myths as drinking black coffee and taking cold showers to relieve hangovers are of no benefit. On the other hand, the person who has been drinking heavily over a prolonged period of time may need management of impending withdrawal.

Management of the Alcohol Withdrawal Syndrome

Interventions are directed to prevent the occurrence of hallucinations, seizure, and d.t.s and to suppress the severity of those present. This is accomplished by substituting a long-acting central nervous system (CNS) depressant for the short-acting one, alcohol.

It is known that keeping the blood level constant for several days causes gradual return to the preintoxication state of motor and mental function (Johnson, 1961). Any of the drugs having cross tolerance with alcohol will serve as a substitute for alcohol. The benzodiazepine class of sedatives is most frequently used because of their large margin of safety. These include Librium and Valium. Larger than average doses generally are required to achieve a state of sedation (light sleep), since the person's tolerance for alcohol also confers tolerance to these drugs.

However, the elderly person's greater sensitivity to any drug may make him more susceptible to these as well. Smaller initial doses are indicated pending evaluation of response. For this purpose, careful monitoring of vital signs is essential. The pulse, in the absence of other conditions affecting its rate, such as infections and cardiac problems, is a sensitive indicator of therapeutic response. A pulse rate which remains high may be a sign of impending delirum tremens or concurrent illness. As vital signs stabilize the dosage of CNS depressant drugs should be slowly and steadily decreased until the drugs can be discontinued.

Administration of an adequate diet and fruit juices is indicated as soon as the person can tolerate them to maintain hydration and provide nutrition. The amount of protein present in the diet needs to be reduced when liver damage has been diagnosed or is seen as high risk, since interference with protein metabolism may precipitate hepatic coma. Vitamin supplements, particularly of the B complex group, are often prescribed to overcome deficiencies.

PREDICTING INTENSITY AND PROGRESSION. The intensity and advancement of withdrawal symptoms is proportional to the quantity and duration of alcohol consumption (Kissin and Begleiter, 1974, p. 17). If nurses can gather data on the amount of drinking and the number of days, they can make a reasonably accurate prediction of the kind of withdrawal symptoms to expect (Tables 11-2 and 11-3).

TABLE 11-2. Predicting occurrence of withdrawal symptoms if one pint of whiskey per day is consumed.

Symptoms	Length of Drinking Episode
Tremulousness	2–10 days
Hallucinosis	11–22 days
Delirium tremens	22 days

TABLE 11-3. Predicting occurrence of withdrawal symptoms if one fifth of whiskey per day is consumed.

Symptoms	Length of Drinking Episode
Tremulousness	2–3 days
Hallucinosis	4–7 days
Delirium tremens	10 days

PREDICTING ONSET OF SYMPTOMS. Just as it is possible to predict the intensity and progression of withdrawal symptoms, it is possible to predict and be ready for the appearance of these symptoms following cessation of alcohol intake (Table 11-4). Variations in these time spans occur, but these estimations provide a guide to the nurse in anticipating the severity of symptoms and in giving some

TABLE 11-4. Prediction of onset of withdrawal symptoms.

Symptoms	No. of Hours Between Last Drink and Onset of Symptoms
Tremulousness	6–8
Convulsions and hallucinations	10–30
Delirium tremens	40–50

indication for their occurrence. Thus the need to obtain accurate information from the patient or a member of this family as to the quantity of alcohol consumed, the length of *continuous* alcohol intake, and the time the last drink was taken become evident for the planning of interventive care.

The prevention of seizures, especially if they were experienced in prior episodes of detoxification, may necessitate anticonvulsant therapy during the withdrawal period. Data on problems during previous episodes becomes very important. Hypomagnesemia has been implicated in the occurrence of withdrawal seizures (Wolfe and Victor, 1971). When values fall below normal, administration of magnesium is indicated.

Sleep disturbances such as frequent awakening, increased rapid eye movement (REM) sleep, and decreased slow-wave sleep usually are pronounced during withdrawal. They may last from weeks to months. Techniques of relaxation are preferable to drug therapy with elderly persons. An appropriate relaxation technique that has been found effective is progressive relaxation.

During the withdrawal syndrome the central nervous system is aroused. Therefore it becomes very important to maintain an environment that is low in disturbing stimuli. A well-lighted room, free from loud noises and sudden jarring, promotes comfort and minimizes stimuli that may agitate an already-aroused nervous system. Most important is the presence of a sympathetic person. When nursing personnel are not free to take on this role and family members or friends are unavailable, the nurse should think of Alcoholics Anonymous as a resource.

It is recognized that following an acute episode of intoxication the elderly person is more ready than at other times to begin planning for his recovery. The nurse can assist the person in making plans designed to facilitate this recovery process. While this is important, it must be recognized that older alcoholic patients exhibit an appreciable deficit in short term memory following an intoxicated state. In a recent study it was found that performance on short term memory tests of older alcoholics (50 years of age and older) was on a par with alcoholic persons with Korsakoff's syndrome. However, one month later the older patient's performance was comparable to that of other alcoholics. These findings suggest any verbal therapeutic attempts made with older patients ought to extend beyond one month. Prior to that time the elderly alcoholic might not be able to benefit from counseling and other verbal interventions (Cermak and Ryback, 1976).

In summary, the aim of nursing management is to assist the elderly alcoholic person to achieve and maintain a healthy and satisfying pattern of functioning that does not depend on the use of alcohol. In order to accomplish this an environment must be created that permits the person to change his behavior so that his physical and psychosocial needs are met without reliance on alcohol. The nurse who is knowledgeable about the management of acute and chronic phases of alcohol abuse and whose attitude is one of acceptance of this illness will be able to guide the patient toward improved health and eventual recovery. Those who treat and care for alcoholics realize that there will be ups-and-downs during the treatment phases. They must not be disappointed or expect too much from the patient.

Special Problems

Certain biologic and pathophysiologic changes occurring in the elderly require special attention among those with alcohol problems. These are drug interactions and brain syndromes.

Drug Interactions

The drug, alcohol, interacts with such other drugs as antibiotics, anticoagulants, antihistamines, digitalis preparations, barbiturates, diuretics, insulin, and iron preparations (Seixas, 1975). Impairment occurs at all levels: absorption, metabolism, storage, and utilization.

Drug interactions of particular concern in caring for the elderly include both over-the-counter and prescription medications. Table 11-5 lists some common drugs and their interactions with alcohol for which nurses need to maintain a high level of awareness.

In addition, the alcoholic person develops cross tolerance to drugs belonging to the same group as does alcohol, including barbiturates, sedative-hypnotics, and minor tranquilizers. Larger doses of any one of these drugs are required in order to achieve therapeutic effectiveness.

Brain Syndromes

Chronic alcohol abuse, heavy drinking, and alcoholism have already been implicated as primary or related causal factors in many pathologic conditions. Acute and chronic brain syndrome are two conditions that are often superimposed on acute and/or chronic alcoholism. Characteristic signs and symp-

TABLE 11-5. Common drugs and their interactions with alcohol.

Drugs	Interactions
Anticoagulants	Increases risk of bleeding and changes in associated lab values
Antihypertensive agents	Increases risk of hypotension
Aspirin	Increases gastric irritations with high risk of gastric bleeding and ulceration
Monoamine oxidase inhibitors	Increases risk of hypertensive crisis (applies primarily to those alcoholic beverages containing pressor amines such as beer and wine)
Nitroglycerin	Increases risk of hypotension
Sedative drugs	Potentiate each other's CNS depressive actions with risk of fatal consequences

toms of organic brain syndrome includes impairment of orientation for time, place, and person; defects in memory and cognitive function including comprehension, calculation, problem solving, learning, and judgment. Emotional responses are easily elicited and can be inappropriate to the stimulus (Busse and Pfeiffer, 1973, pp. 91–93).

ACUTE BRAIN SYNDROME. The acute brain syndrome is a confusional state of sudden onset, usually associated with acute physical illness such as infection, heart failure, metabolic disturbances, anemia, hepatic failure, alcoholism-drug intoxications, or vitamin deficiencies. Acute brain syndrome is differentiated from chronic brain syndrome in that the former is reversible. Both are descriptive terms that are unrelated to etiologic factors (American Psychiatric Association, *Diagnostic and Statistical Manual of Mental Disorders*, ed. 2, DSM II, 1965). The patient suffers from fluctuating disturbances in memory, orientation, and intellectual functioning. He is fearful and apprehensive. Delusion and hallucinations may be present (Maletta, 1975, p. 217). Distinguishing this phenomenon from that of the alcohol withdrawal syndrome may be difficult. It requires that a careful history of alcohol intake be obtained from a relative or friend. These data should be complemented by a determination of blood alcohol level (see quick form of nursing history for emergency

situation, p. 201). Blood assays for the presence of other drugs and abnormalities also are indicated.

CHRONIC BRAIN SYNDROME. Chronic brain syndrome (organic brain syndrome, OBC) occurs as a result of brain disease, arteriosclerotic brain disease, alcoholic brain disease, and so forth. It is characterized by a gradual onset. The patient demonstrates symptoms of impaired memory and deterioration in level of intellectual functioning, in mood disturbances, in thinking, in perception, and in behavior. The array of disturbances is not necessarily an indication of the severity of brain damage and it is sometimes difficult to make an accurate assessment of the level of intellectual capacity in a depressed, angry, or hostile patient (Maletta, 1975, p. 218).

A brief, objective measure of organic brain syndrome frequently used by medical personnel is the Goldfarb Short Portable Mental Status Questionnaire (Pfeiffer, 1975). Patients are asked to answer questions as to time, place, important political leaders, and so forth. One drawback to this approach is that individuals who see themselves as well-oriented to time, place, and so forth have been known to become insulted at these questions and to answer them facetiously or refuse to answer. A second limitation, in terms of the alcoholic patient, is that there is no evidence as to whether this test could be successfully employed to distinguish impairment of mental processes resulting from alcoholism from other conditions. Nevertheless, it is one approach that, used in a discriminating way with appropriate patients, can be useful.

Some studies have compared status and the clinical course of alcoholic and nonalcoholic patients with organic brain syndrome. In one psychiatric institution the mean age of the alcoholic population was about eight years younger than that of the nonalcoholic group. On personality tests they showed significantly more abnormal responses. They also scored significantly higher on nursing-need summary scores, indicating a higher need for nursing care. The nonalcoholics in this study showed essentially no cognitive impairment and were in relatively good physical status. A thirty-month follow-up study showed that more of the alcoholics (37 percent) died than did the nonalcoholics (12 percent), and the alcoholics were younger (Rosin and Glatt, 1971). There are, on the other hand, studies that report no significant differences between alcoholic and nonalcoholic patients with organic brain syndrome (Simon, et al., 1968).

Special Problem

Some facilities have found that the use of alcohol increases socialization and promotes appetite and relaxation for the residents. These programs of wine/beer are appropriate for people who are not opposed to alcohol and have no alcohol or alcoholism problem. However, an alcoholic cannot drink again. Therefore, personnel responsible for arranging the wine or grape juice should know those people who are to participate and should not tempt those with past/present drinking problems with alcohol.

Evaluation

Ultimately the effectiveness of nursing care in the treatment of the elderly alcoholic person is seen in his abstinence from alcohol accompanied by the restructuring of a lifestyle that is meaningful to him as a recovering person. The recovery process, then, includes withdrawal from alcohol, the resolution of related physiologic and psychosocial problems, and the restructuring of activities and demands of daily living without alcohol.

**NURSING HISTORY FOR USE WITH
PATIENTS WITH ALCOHOL PROBLEM***
(Adapted to the Elderly)

Guidelines for Interviewer

Introduce self

Tell patient: (1) Purpose of the interview.
                (2) Reviewing life circumstances may create some discomfort.
                (3) Refusal to answer specific question(s) is all right.
Obtain verbal permission from the patient to proceed with interview.

Place of interview_____ Date _____

Name of interviewer _____

Patient's name _____Ethnic group _____ Age _____ Sex _____
(Use only first name or initials if agency requests)

Birthplace _____ Past occupation _____

Last grade attended _____ What is the source of your income? _____

What do you consider to be difficulties in your present situation?

What do you most want help with at the present time?

Drinking History

When did you have your last drink?

When did you start your last drinking bout?

What have you been drinking during this last drinking episode?

How much alcohol did you consume each day during your last drinking episode?

---

* Shortened form for rapid data collection of high priority information. For full data base instrument see Estes and Heinemann, 1977, pp. 224–226.

NURSING HISTORY (cont.)

NURSING HISTORY (cont.)

Psychosocial Status

Are you currently taking medication for emotional problems? If yes, describe.

General Medical History

Does (or did) anyone in your family have the following:

Diabetes _____ Heart trouble _____ Mental illness _____

Alcohol problems _____ Epilepsy _____ Cancer _____

Symptoms Related to Gastrointestinal System

Did you eat when you drank?

What is your usual eating pattern?

When not drinking:

When drinking:

Are you nauseated?

Are you vomiting or having dry heaves?

Have you ever vomited blood? If yes, when?

Have you ever had stomach ulcers or other stomach problems?

Has your skin or the white of your eyes ever turned yellow?

Have you ever been told you have problems with your liver?

Do you have diabetes? If yes, what medication do you take?

Symptoms Relating to Neurologic System

What reactions occur when you stop drinking?

Tremors _____ D.T.s _____

Seizures _____ Other _____

Hear or see things _____ _____

Have you ever taken Dilantin or any other drug for seizures?

Have you experienced tingling, pain, or numbness in hands or feet?

Have you experienced muscle pain in your legs or arms?

Are you experiencing any difficulty in keeping your balance?

Are you experiencing any difficulty with your vision?

Symptoms Relating to Cardiovascular and Pulmonary System

Do you have heart trouble? If yes, describe.

Do you have swelling of the hands and feet?

Do you have shortness of breath?

Do you have chest pain?

Are you taking any medication for heart disease?

NURSING HISTORY (cont.)

NURSING HISTORY (cont.)

Drug Taking Other than Alcohol

What drugs do you take that you have not mentioned?

Prescribed drugs _____

Nonprescribed drugs (e.g., Aspirin) _____

Drugs obtained on the street _____

What is your usual manner of taking drugs?

As directed _____

More than directed _____

Less than directed _____

According to what you feel you need _____

According to what you feel you want _____

Are you allergic to any drugs?

Do you have any reactions to the drugs you take? Please describe.

BIBLIOGRAPHY

Apfeldorf, M., and Hunley, P. J.: Application of MMPI alcoholism scales to older alcoholics and problem drinkers. J. Studies on Alcohol 36:645–53, 1975.

Bailey, M. B., Haberman, P. W., and Alksne, H.: The epidemiology of alcoholism in an urban residential area. J. Studies on Alcohol 26:19–40, 1965.

Benensohn, H. S., and Resnick, H. L. P.: A jigger of alcohol, a dash of depression and bitters: a suicidal mix. In Seixas, F. A., Cadoret, R., and Eggleston, (eds.): Ann. New York Acad. Sciences 233:15–21, 1974.

Betts, V. T.: Psychotherapeutic intervention with the addict-client. Nurs. Clin. N. Am. 11:551–8, 1976.

Blane, H. T.: The Personality of the Alcoholic; Guises of Dependency. New York: Harper & Row, 1968.

Busse, E., and Pfeiffer, E.: Mental Illness in Later Life. American Psychiatric Association, 1973, pp. 91–93.

Cahalan, D.: Problem Drinkers. San Francisco: Jossey-Bass Publishers, 1970.

Cahalan, D., and Kissin, I. H.: American drinking practices: summary of findings from a national probability sample I. Extent of drinking by population subgroups. J. Studies on Alcohol 35:856–62, 1974.

Cermak, L. S., and Ryback, R. S.: Recovery of verbal short-term memory in alcoholics. J. Studies on Alcohol 37(1):46–52, 1976.

Characteristics of aged alcoholics studied constitute high proportion of elderly geriatric patients. Geriatrics Anonymous 7:1, 1968.

Cohen, S.: Geriatric drug abuse. Drug Abuse and Alcoholism Newsletter 4(2):1975.

Craik, F. I.: Similarities between the effects of aging and alcoholic intoxication on memory performance, construed within a "level of processing" framework. In Peter, I., and Parker, E. S. (eds.): Alcohol and Human Memory. New York: John Wiley & Sons, 1977.

Criteria for the diagnosis of alcoholism. Criteria Committee, National Council on Alcoholism, Ann. Intern. Med. 77:249–58, 1972.

Diagnostic and Statistical Manual of Mental Disorders, ed. 2. (DSM II). American Psychiatric Association.

Drew, L. R. H.: Alcoholism as a self-limiting disease. J. Studies on Alcohol 29:956–67, 1965.

Ebersole, P.: Reminiscing. Am. J. Nurs. 76:1304–1305, 1976.

Estes, N., and Heinemann, M. E. (eds.): Alcoholism: Development Consequences and Interventions. St. Louis: C. V. Mosby Co., 1977.

Farberow, N. L., and Morivaki, S. Y.: Self-destructive crises in the older person. Gerontologist 15:333–7, 1975.

Fidler, J.: Loneliness—the problems of the elderly and retired. Roy. Soc. Health J. 96:39–41, 1976.

Fitts, W. H.: Manual: Tennessee Self-Concept Scale. Nashville, Tennessee: Counselor Recordings and Tests, 1965.

Forrest, G.: The Diagnosis and Treatment of Alcoholism. Springfield, Ill.: Charles C Thomas, 1975.

Gaitz, C. M.: Characteristics of elderly patients with alcoholism. Arch. General Psychiatry 24:372–8, 1971.

Gitlow, S. E.: The pharmacological approach to alcoholism. Md. State Medical Journal, 19:93–96, 103–106, April, May, 1970.

Goodwin, D. W.: Is Alcoholism Hereditary? New York: Oxford University Press, 1976.

Graux, P., et al., Alcoholism of the elderly. Rev. Alcsme, 15:46–8, 1969.

Heinemann, M. E., and Estes, N. J.: Assessing alcoholic patients. Am. J. Nurs. 76:785–9, 1976.

Heinemann, M. E., Moore, B., and Gurel, M.: Need Patterns Related to the Treatment of Alcoholism. To be published in Communicating Nursing Research, 1977.

Hershenson, D. B.: Stress-induced use of alcohol by problem drinkers as a function of their sense of identity. J. Studies on Alcohol 26:213–16, 1965.

Johnson, R. B.: The alcohol withdrawal syndrome. J. Studies on Alcohol, pp. 66–76, 1961.

Jourard, S. M.: Disclosing Man to Himself. New York: Van Nostrand Reinhold Co., 1968.

Kissin, B., and Begleiter, H.: The biology of alcoholism, Vol. 3: Clinical pathology. New York: Plenum Press, 1974.

Kramer, M.: Patients in State and County General Hospitals. Public Health Service Publication No. 1921, Chevy Chase, Maryland: National Institutes of Health, 1969.

Law, R., and Chalmers, C.: Medicines and elderly people: a general practice survey. Br. Med. J. 1:565–8, 1976.

Lieber, C. S.: Metabolic Aspects of Alcoholism. Baltimore: University Park Press, 1977.

Maletta, G. J.: Survey—Report on the Aging Nervous System. U.S. Department of Health, Education, and Welfare, Washington D.C., 1975.

Mayfield, D. G.: Alcohol problems in the aging patient. In Fann, W. E., and Maddox, G. L. (eds.): Drug Issues in Geropsychiatry. Baltimore: Williams & Wilkins, 1974.

McNichol, R. W.: The Treatment of Delirium Tremens and Related States. Springfield, Ill.: Charles C Thomas, 1970.

Moss, G. E.: Illness, Immunity and Social Interaction, New York: John Wiley & Sons, 1973.

Parker, W. J.: Alcohol-drug interactions. J. Am. Pharmaceutical Assoc. N510(12):664–73, December, 1970.

Pascarelli, E.: Drug dependence: An age-old problem compounded by old age. Geriatrics 109–114. Dec. 1974.

Peplau, H.: A Working Definition of Anxiety. In Burd, S. F., and Marshall, M. A. (eds.): Some Clinical Approaches to Psychiatric Nursing. New York: Macmillan Publishing, 1963.

Pfeiffer, E.: A short portable mental status questionnaire for the assessment of organic brain deficit in elderly patient. J. Am. Geriatric Society 23:433–41, 1975.

Plaut, T. F.: A Report to the National Cooperative Commission on the Study of Alcoholism. New York: Oxford Press, 1967.

Rathbone-McCuan, E., and Bland, J.: A Treatment typology for the elderly alcohol abuser. J. Am. Geriatric Society 23(12):553–7, 1975.

Rathbone-McCuan, E., and Bland, J.: Diagnostic and Referral Considerations for the Geriatric Alcoholic and Aging Problem Drinker. Presented at the Gerontological Society's 27th Annual Meeting, Portland, Oregon, October 28–November 1, 1974.

Rosin, A. J., and Glatt, M. M.: Alcohol excess in the elderly. J. Studies on Alcohol 32:53–9, 1971.

Rotter, J.: Generalized expectancies for internal vs external control of reinforcement. Psychological Monographs: General and Applied 80:1–28, 1966.

Saville, P. D.: Alcohol-related skeletal disorders. In Seixas, F. A., Williams, K., and Eggleston, S. (eds.): Medical Consequences of Alcoholism. New York: Academy of Sciences, 252:287–91, 1975.

Schuckit, M. A.: Family history and half-sibling research in alcoholism. In Sexias, F. A., et al. (eds.): Nature and Nurture in Alcoholism. New York: New York Academy of Sciences 197:121–5, 1972.

Schuckit, M. A., and Cahalan, D.: Evaluation of Alcohol Treatment Programs, Report N74–53, Navy Medical Neuropsychiatric Research Unit, San Diego, 1974.

Schuckit, M. A., and Sunderson, E. K. E.: Deaths among young alcoholics in the U.S. Naval service. J. Studies on Alcohol 35:856–62, 1974.

Schuckit, M. A., Miller, P. L., and Hahlbohm, D.: Unrecognized psychiatric illness in elderly medical-surgical patients. J. Gerontology 30:66–5, 1975.

Seeman, M.: Alienation and engagement. In Campbell, A., and Converse, P. E. (eds.): The Human Meaning of Social Change. New York: Russell Sage Foundation, 1972.

Seixas, F. A.: Alcohol and its drug interactions. Ann. Intern. Med. 83:86–92, 1975.

Simon, A., Epstein, J., and Reynolds, L.: Alcoholism in the geriatrically mentally ill. Geriatrics 23:125–31, 1968.

Smith-DiJulio, K., Heinemann, M. E., and Ogden, L.: Care of the alcoholic patient during acute episodes. In Estes, N. J., and Heinemann, M. E. (eds.): Alcoholism: Development, Consequences and Interventions. St. Louis: C. V. Mosby Co., 1977.

Stotsby, B. A.: Social and clinical issues in geriatric psychiatry. Am. J. Psychiatry 129:117–26, 1972.

Travelbee, J.: Intervention in Psychiatric Nursing. Philadelphia: F. A. Davis Co. 1968.

Ujhely, G. B.: The Nurse and Her "Problem" Patients. New York: Springer Publishing Co., 1967.

U.S. Department of Health, Education, and Welfare, First Special Report to the United States Congress on Alcohol and Health, 1971.

U.S. Department of Health, Education, and Welfare, Second Special Report to the United States Congress on Alcohol and Health, 1974.

Winokur, G., et al.: Alcoholism ill: diagnosis and familial psychiatric illness in 259 alcoholic husbands. Arch. Gen. Psychiatry 23:114–11, 1970.

Wolfe, S., and Victor, M.: The physiological basis of the alcohol withdrawal syndrome. In Mello, N. K., and Mendelsohn, J. (eds.): Recent Advances in Studies of

Alcoholism. Rockville, Maryland: National Institute of Mental Health, 1971.

World Health Organization Expert Committee on Mental Health, Alcoholism Committee. Second Report, WHO Technical Report Series, No. 48, August, 1952.

Worthington, B.: Alcoholism and Malnutrition. In Estes, N. J., and Heinemann, M. E. (eds.): Alcoholism: Development, Consequences and Interventions. St. Louis: C. V. Mosby Co., 1977.

Zimberg, S.: The elderly alcoholic. Gerontologist, 14:221–4, 1974.

Zimberg, S.: The psychiatrist and medical home care: geriatric psychiatry in the Harlem community. Am. J. Psychiatry 27:1062–6, 1971.

12

Cancer

Doris M. Molbo

QUICK REVIEW

CANCER

DESCRIPTION	Chronic systemic diseases characterized by the inability of the patient's repair and immune surveillance systems to control the proliferation of uncoordinated and abnormal cells in all tissues of the body. Such cells may metastasize to other sites and organs. Cancer must be considered as many diseases, not one.
ETIOLOGIC FACTORS	Decreased immune response increases risk of cancer in the elderly. Lifetime of exposure to multiple carcinogens.
HIGH RISK	Over age 60 incidence of cancer: 91% of all prostate, 74% of all digestive tract and of multiple myeloma, 75% of bladder, and 63% of lung. Rate of incidence increases with age because there are fewer people left to be at risk.
DYNAMICS	Primary tumor growth may be the same as in young patients. Metastatic growth sometimes is slower.
SIGNS AND SYMPTOMS	Often difficult to identify since they may be part of previous/concurrent diseases. Important to take a detailed history and establish regular assessment of symptoms for high incidence cancer.
COMPLICATIONS	In addition to complications of cancer of specific sites, treatment causes special problems. Nutritional status, stomatitis, and pain require special attention. Isolation, abandonment, and loneliness are particular risks. Attitudes of nurses, doctors, and family.
PROGNOSIS	Varies with site, stage of illness, and metastasis. Sometimes better than younger person in breast; worse in prostatic, GI, and oral.
NURSING MANAGEMENT	Should be based on latest knowledge of standard treatments (radiation, surgery, chemotherapy), requires keeping up with proliferation and change in modalities. Positive attitude that old people have the right to therapy and rehabilitation. Include patient in decisions on management of disease. Monitoring signs and symptoms to identify early disease. Manage complications of disease and therapy; pain, nausea, stomatitis, alopecia, and isolation.
EVALUATION	Control of pain and isolation. Degree of patient/family participation in ongoing decision making and adjustments in daily living. Effective advocate for patients so they have the same resources, care, and consideration afforded young people with cancer.

Cancer is complex and vast in scope. It can involve every tissue and organ system in the body. Therefore, this chapter does not propose to be a mini-textbook about cancer. General and specific references are given in the bibliography for both basic and advanced reading.

The intent of the chapter is the following:

1. To identify the magnitude of the cancer problem in the aged population as it may be anticipated in the nurse's caseload in hospitals, nursing homes, ambulatory care practices, and community health care.

2. To provide pertinent insights and application of cancer knowledge to the unique status of the elderly person with cancer.

3. To confront the "give up" management perspective with a more rational basis for decision making so that the nurse can assist the elderly cancer patient and his significant others to make decisions with which they will be satisfied.

Age-Related Biases

When cancer literature is reviewed, reference in general is given to the fact of increasing incidence of the disease(s) with age. However, the specific emphases of the literature are directed to the incidence, detection, treatment, and rehabilitation of the child, the young adult, and the middle-aged adult with cancer. Specific reference to the disease(s) in the elderly is sparse.

As cancer and the elderly patient are considered, it is necessary to face a certain general truth: health care professionals have different attitudes about cancer in the young and productive adults than they do about cancer in the elderly. Toward cancer from infancy through age 60, the professionals feel and express anger commensurate with the youth or potential productiveness of the person. Cancer becomes the enemy to be wiped out. Toward cancer in the elderly, the professional feels dismay at its presence, perhaps frustration, but not the directed anger. There tends to be a submissiveness to its presence and a bowing to the inevitable.

EFFECTS OF THE PROFESSIONALS' BIASES. The identification of age-related biases toward triaging and management of cancer has been made early in this chapter because readers must think about its possible presence and its philosophical antecedent in themselves and in those with whom they interact. The effects of values are important. Just as they influence the spearheading of aggressive research and care in childhood cancers, so, too, they influence all facets of cancer programming for the elderly—identifying or ignoring signs and symptoms, ordering or ignoring diagnostic tests, performing or avoiding treatment measures, and considering or neglecting rehabilitation.

EFFECTS OF SOCIETAL BIASES. Health care professionals are not alone in this pervading feeling about cancer in the elderly person. The general public and the family—even the elderly person himself—may feel and display a "give up syndrome" when cancer is suspected: See nothing, expect nothing, do nothing.

VALUES AFFECTING DIAGNOSTIC AND TREATMENT DECISIONS. It is true that persons over 70 have made delicate compensatory adaptations within the physical, psychologic, and social spheres of their being. They have accretions of stressors at the time they encounter cancer. This means complex problems, complex decision making, and complex care.

However, the oft-heard, "He's old, let him be. He's lived his life; he shouldn't have to have more pain or suffer any more," must be counterbalanced with the knowledge necessary to honestly answer the following questions:

Will he suffer more or less in the future if treatment or rehabilitation are denied now?

What are his goals? What tasks of life are left to be completed?

What do his perceived loved ones understand of the answers to the above questions? What can they give? What do they want?

Etiologic Factors

The incidence of cancer increases with age, although the exact etiologic factors of malignancies in any age group are not known. There are theories on causation but there are no definite answers. In terms of specific malignancies there are relationships among environment with its many carcinogens, lifestyles, and malignancies. If you believe what is popularly printed, almost everything you eat, drink, or with which you come in contact is a potential cause of cancer.

Acknowledgment is made to Roger E. Moe, M.D., Associate Professor of Surgery, University of Washington, Seattle, for his contribution in reviewing this chapter.

Of all the various theories of etiology, it seems rational to expect increasing incidence of cancer with increasing age. Elderly persons have been exposed for long periods to the most suspected of carcinogens, radiation and chemicals. They have had years of surges and ebbs of hormone production. They have had a lifetime experience of breaking and repairing cell chromosomes. They have had numerous experiences of loss, depression, and despair. (Even Galen in 200 A.D. observed that more "melancholy" women developed breast cancer than sanguine ones: Schmale and Iker, 1971; Bahnson, 1974.) It is also known that as one gets older the immune response is decreased, a factor which increases the likelihood of malignancy.

Underlying this variety of etiologic factors is a unifying theory, which currently prevails. This theory follows these steps:

1. Chromosomal breakage occurs with infection, carcinogens, genetic factors, and environmental radiation exposure in all persons from birth throughout life.

2. The cells can repair themselves through an enzyme system (Ringborg, 1977). If this fails, the abnormal cells which result are destroyed by a competent immune system of two kinds of lymphocytes—T-cells and B-cells—which are responsible for the quick destruction of all abnormal cells.

3. When this immune system or its parts do not function at optimum, abnormal cells have an opportunity to reproduce themselves, doubling rapidly, and forming a mass of abnormal, uncoordinated, reproducing cells within a few days/weeks time, depending on the site. This is called a cancer.

4. The thymus, an organ of the immune system, begins to progressively age and atrophy by the age 35. The immune system generally is not a competent system in the elderly person (Adler, 1975). There is primarily a decrease in the ability of the cell to repair itself after age 54.

5. Other factors besides aging also affect the competency of the immune system. Some of these are prolonged response to stressors (Solomon, et al., 1974; Fox, 1976), prolonged or frequent circadean rhythm changes (Ehlert, 1965), and/or deficient nutritional status.

Incidence/High Risk Sites

Incidence rates, or number of new cases diagnosed in a specific population within a given time period are most often expressed as numbers within 1000, 10,000, or 100,000 population. Because the numbers of older people are fewer in the general population, incidence figures should also be studied in relation to the specific population of the elderly as well as within the general population.

Because there is no nationwide system in the United States for reporting the incidence of cancer, it is important to know the source of any data, the date, and how representative it is of the total or regional picture.

The incidence of cancer diseases increases with age (Table 12-1). Since the years 70 and over are of interest in this book, Table 12-2 has been compiled from the National Cancer Institute's Third National Cancer Survey, 1969–1971, to show the distribution of the primary site oncologic diseases in the population of 70 and over, in the decade 60 to 69, and in those from birth to age 59. This is expressed in percentage of occurrence or incidence. In Table 12-2, note that 47 percent of all oncologic diseases of digestive organs occur in people over 70 years and that 60 percent of all male genital oncologic diseases occur in those 70 and over, with 64 percent of prostate cancer occurring *after* 70. The summed percentage of people 60 and over show that 91 percent of prostate cancer, 74 percent of multiple myeloma, 74 percent of digestive malignancy, 75 percent of bladder cancer, and 63 percent of lung cancers occur in that group. The frequency of the "silent malignancies" is apparent, i.e., those with insidious onset or mimicking symptoms, i.e., multiple myeloma, bladder, prostate, ovary, gallbladder, and vulva. Sixty-two percent of all reported malignancies occurred over 60 years of age.

TABLE 12-1. Incidence of cancer at various ages.

Age	Incidence by Percent
Birth to 19	2
20–29	2
30–39	4
40–49	10
50–59	20
60–69	26
70+	36
	100

Data from the Third National Cancer Survey, National Cancer Institute, 1975.

TABLE 12-2.   Distribution of primary sites by age groups.

| | Percentage by age | | | | |
Primary Site	Under 59	60–69	70 and over	Total 60+	N
All Sites	38	26	36	62	*181,027
Buccal	45	28	27	55	6,531
Total digestive	26	27	47	74	45,428
Esophagus	34	32	34	66	2,030
Stomach	23	25	52	77	6,248
Colon	25	26	49	75	18,427
Rectal	27	29	44	73	8,171
Liver	33	27	40	67	1,331
Gallbladder	15	24	61	85	1,007
Pancreas	25	28	47	75	5,775
Total female genital	54	24	22	46	18,578
Cervix	67	17	16	33	5,523
Corpus	48	30	22	52	6,629
Ovary	53	23	24	47	4,594
Vulva	32	19	49	68	614
Total male genital	14	26	60	86	16,088
Prostate	9	27	64	91	14,812
Total urinary	30	28	42	70	11,862
Bladder	25	28	47	75	7,840
Renal	41	27	32	59	3,634
Total respiratory	38	33	29	62	27,210
Larynx	45	33	22	55	2,517
Lung	37	33	30	63	24,049
Breast	52	22	26	48	24,676
Lymphomas	54	20	26	46	5,942
Leukemias	39	20	41	61	5,894
CLL	27	19	54	73	1,534
AGL	46	21	33	54	1,401
CGL	39	20	41	61	880
Multiple myeloma	26	29	45	74	2,143

Data from the Third National Cancer Survey, National Cancer Institute, 1975.
* The total N includes the following in addition to those listed above:

Bone—   28% of patients over 60
Eye—   40% ″   ″   ″   ″
Brain—   33% ″   ″   ″   ″
Endocrine— 25% ″   ″   ″   ″
Melanomas—33% ″   ″   ″   ″

Breast

Figure 12-1 shows the incidence of breast cancer in women at the age of diagnosis in the states of Washington and Alaska. This histograph coincides with national data and the often heard statement that breast cancer is most frequent between the years of 45 and 65. What that statements means is, of all the women with reported new breast cancer, 52 percent of them were between the ages of 45 and 65. Table 12-2 and Figure 12-1 give the impression that breast cancer is relatively unimportant in the elderly woman. At least there are other malignancies that seem to be more prevalent in the older age group and are greatest in people over 60.

However, when the number of patients by age group having a certain malignancy during a specific period (incidence) is plotted with the number of

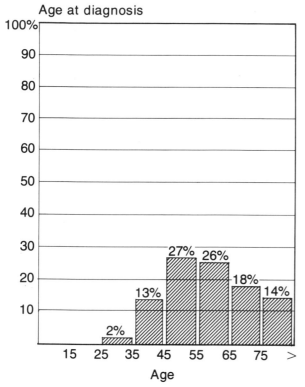

Age at diagnosis

FIGURE 12-1. Incidence of breast cancer in females by percentage at age of diagnosis. (From Cancer in Washington and Alaska by the Washington-Alaska Regional Medical Program, 1973, with permission.)

persons of that group in the population, a different relationship is seen. Figure 12-2 shows the incidence of breast cancer in all women between the ages of 40 and 85 (and over) by 5-year groups. It also shows the specific female population in each of those 5-year groups. The largest number of women in the female population peaks at 45 to 50 and gradually tapers off toward the low at 85 and older. The incidence of breast cancer also peaks at 45 to 50, plateaus, and tapers off after 60 to 65 years. Thus, the peak years of incidence seen in Figure 12-1 are also present in Figure 12-2. Nevertheless, note that at 45 to 50 years when the peak incidence is 3100, the female population (at 45 to 50 years) is 661,500, or one out of every 324. At age 60 to 65, the incidence of breast cancer is 2940 women in a female population of the same age of 442,190, or one out of every 150 women her age has breast cancer. At age 80 to 85, one woman out of every 112 women her age will have breast cancer. As the incidence and the specific population lines draw closer together, the ratio increases. Thus, breast cancer *increases* with age.

A ratio is a more meaningful means of expression when working with small numbers of elderly patients than thinking of percentage of populations of 1000 or 100,000. (Figures 12-3 through 12-9 show this relationship of incidence by age group to population by age group through the expression of a ratio.) Further, incidence by age groups of white persons are plotted against white populations by age

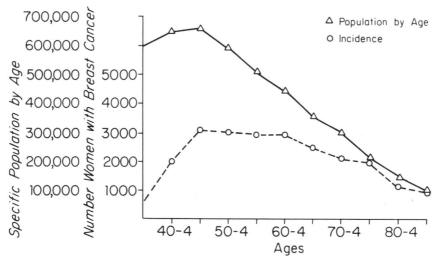

FIGURE 12-2. Incidence of breast cancer in women over age 40, and specific population of all women over age 40. (Third National Cancer Survey, Monograph 41, National Cancer Institute, Bethesda, Md., 1975)

groups; incidence by age groups of black persons are plotted against black populations by age groups. Figure 12-3, therefore, shows a closer relationship of breast cancer in aged black women to white women than is usually acknowledged in the litera-

ture (Holland, 1974). At age 45 to 50, one of every 210 white women and one of every 275 black women has breast cancer. At age 85 and over, 1 of every 108 white women and 1 of every 150 black women has breast cancer.

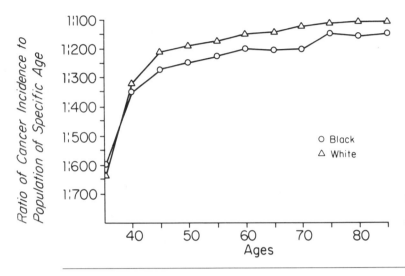

FIGURE 12-3. Ratio of breast cancer incidence to age-specific populations by five-year cohorts. (Based on data from the National Cancer Institute, Bethesda, Md., 1975)

Uterus

CERVIX. Black women have a higher incidence of cervical cancer which rises earlier (35 to 40) than white women. This difference is maintained to age 85 and older (Fig. 12-4). At age 80 to 85, one black woman out of every 267 black women her age will have cervical cancer. It is apparent then that cervical screening is important, especially for the elderly

black female. Table 12-2 shows that cervical cancer occurs more in women 59 and younger. Figure 12-4 shows a steadily increasing incidence when compared with the specific age group involved. Therefore, if pap screening is important for the population under 59, where one white woman of every 1000 (and lower) will have cervical cancer, even more important are screening or regularly scheduled yearly pap tests for the older population where

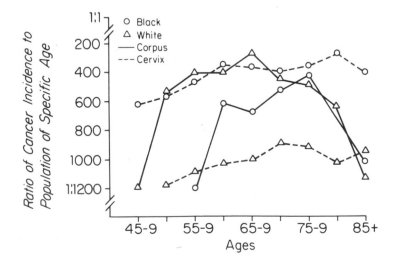

FIGURE 12-4. Ratio of uterine cancer incidence (corpus and cervix) to age-specific populations by five-year cohorts. (Based on data from the National Cancer Institute, Bethesda, Md., 1975)

one out of every 890 women age 70 to 75 will have cervical cancer.

CORPUS. The incidence in cancer of the body of the uterus (corpus) in black women begins and peaks 10 years later than in white women (Fig. 12-4). This cancer peaks in black women at age 75 to 80 (1 out of every 422). At this same age in white women there is a decrease in incidence, having peaked at age 65 to 70 (1 out of every 270). At age 80 in both black and white women, incidence drops. It is unknown whether this means that the

population no longer contains those women who are at risk for uterine cancer or whether it means that women over 80 have silent and unreported uterine cancers or ignored and unreported cancers.

Prostate

Figure 12-5 shows the high incidence of prostatic cancer in the white and black male over 60 (also compare with Table 12-2). The importance of annual digital examinations in this population and earlier is apparent.

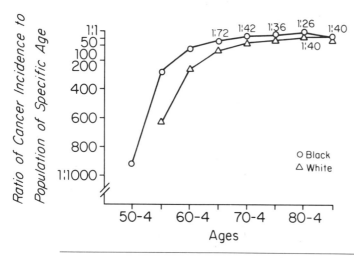

FIGURE 12-5. Ratio of prostate cancer incidence to age-specific populations by five-year cohorts. (Based on Third National Cancer Survey, Monograph 41, National Cancer Institute, Bethesda, Md. 1975)

Lung

There are differences in incidence in black and white males from black and white females in cancer

of the lung (Fig. 12-6). Women develop the disease later in life than men. The drop in incidence ratio at age 80 may, as in Figures 12-4 and 12-5, only reflect lack of case finding and reporting. National

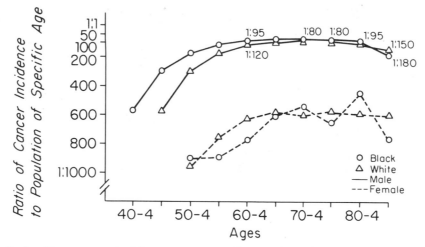

FIGURE 12-6. Ratio of lung cancer incidence to age-specific population by five-year cohorts. (Based on Third National Cancer Survey, Monograph 41, National Cancer Institute, Bethesda, Md., 1975)

Cancer Institute data relied on histologically-verified reports during diagnosis, treatment, or postmortem. Therefore, cancer incidence may indeed be higher in all older persons than presently known.

Colon

Figure 12-7 shows the importance of vigilance for colon and rectal malignancies for men, women,

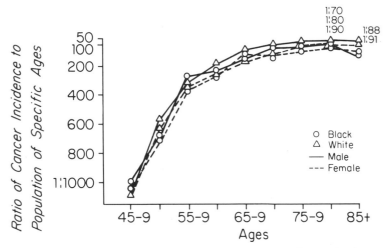

FIGURE 12-7. Ratio of colorectal cancer incidence to age-specific populations by five-year cohorts. (Based on Third National Cancer Survey, Monograph 41, National Cancer Institute, Bethesda, Md., 1975)

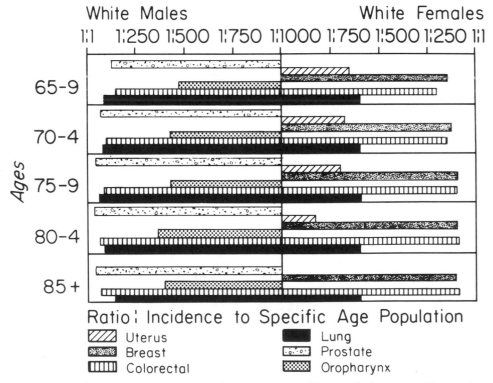

FIGURE 12-8. Ratio of cancer incidence in six sites to age-specific populations over 65 years in white males and females. (Based on Third National Cancer Survey, Monograph 41, National Cancer Institute, Bethesda, Md., 1975)

black, and white from age 50 and older. The extremely high incidence of this malignancy over 75 is startling.

Sex and race

Figure 12-8 compares the incidence of cancer in the six highest incidence sites in white men and women by age group. Of all sites, it is apparent that males of all ages over 65 have a greater incidence of cancer than females. Further, the incidence ratios of all sites increases with age. This is also seen in black males, Figure 12-9. However, oropharynx cancer decreases to less than one in 1000 black males by age 85, whereas one white male in every 390 has oropharyngeal cancer at 85 and over. This site of cancer is not frequent in black or white women.

When the incidence of uterine, breast, colorectal, and lung cancers are compared between white and black women of different ages (Fig. 12-8 and 12-9), the greater incidence in all sites is seen in black women. The dominance of breast and colorectal cancers in black and white women and the domi-

nance of prostatic, colorectal, and lung cancers in black and white males is apparent throughout all ages. At age 80 to 85, one of every 100 males (white) has lung cancer (1:94 in blacks), one in 68 has colorectal cancer (1:61 in blacks), and one in 40 has prostatic cancer (1:26 in blacks).

Dynamics

Cancer is not one disease. It is many diseases that vary in symptoms, growth rate, response to treatment, rapidity of metastasis, and prognosis according to the organ and tissue involved, the sex, age, physical resources. and other numerous patient factors.

Cancer is not a localized disease, involving only the discrete breast node or the visible oral ulceration of malignant cells. It is a systemic disease. Prior to the proliferation of those malignant cells into a tumor mass, or prior to the proliferation of those lymphocytes or granulocytes of leukemia, a systematic immunologic body function failed, permitting the pro-

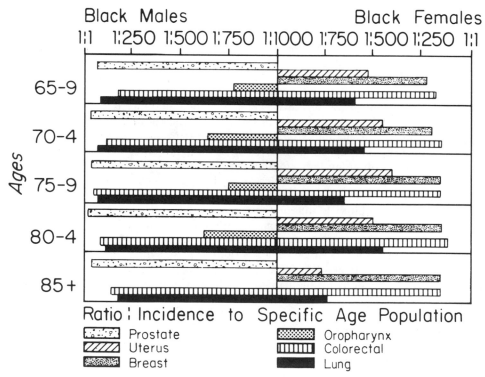

FIGURE 12-9.   Ratio of cancer incidence in six sites to age-specific populations over 65 years in black males and females. (Based on Third National Cancer Survey, Monograph 41, National Cancer Institute, Bethesda, Md. 1975)

liferation of malignant cells and the uncontrolled tumor growth.

Therefore, depending on these specific factors, it is difficult to generalize many dynamics peculiar to cancer in the older person. Generally, cancer has a more silent and insidious early course in the older person. Generally the primary tumor growth *may* possess the same doubling time (proliferation rate) in the older person as in the young person. In some sites (organs and tissues) this may *not* be true since, for example, it is believed that the breast cancer involving glandular tissue (adenocarcinoma) of the premenopausal woman is a *different* disease than the adenocarcinoma of the postmenopausal woman and, therefore, cannot be compared.

Generally the metastatic spread from any site may be slower in the old person. The older person usually is less capable of receiving a maximum dose of radiation or chemotherapy and has increased vulnerability to greater toxicities of the treatment, greater response to the volume of tissue breakdown occasioned by the treatment, with greater destruction of malignant cells and healthy cells to treatment modalities. When the individual's immunocompetence is a required factor for remission or for post-therapy maintenance, the older person generally may be considered disadvantaged since his immune system is the aged system which permitted the primary growth.

Generally the cancer of the older person is "found" at a later stage than a younger person. Often treatment involves *control* of malignant disease rather than cure of primary disease. Many people believe that the elderly need care, not cure. Yet care need not exclude cure (Shouten, 1975). Generally there are as many treatment options available for the older person as for the young and as many modifications of therapy protocol. The oncology team coordinator has a unique responsibility: to interpret to the older patient, to hold visible the many options, and to communicate the implications of those options to both patient and professionals alike. Unless she fulfills these functions of patient advocate they probably will not occur, particularly for the patient with cancer who is old.

Signs and Symptoms

Problems Associated with the Elderly

Patients, their families, and health professionals alike are exposed regularly to the American Cancer Society's messages, "Know Cancer's Seven Warning Signals":

A change in bowel or bladder habits
A sore that does not heal
Unusual bleeding or discharge
A thickening or lump in breast or elsewhere
Indigestion or difficulty swallowing
Obvious change in wart or mole
Nagging cough or hoarseness

The elderly as a group, however, may receive different responses from the health professionals when they present themselves with signs and symptoms in these areas. One individual indicated that she had been trying to find a gynecologist who did not regard the seven danger signals as a sign of her old age. At the point when she was writing about her experiences, she had contacted four physicians who assured her that her condition was nothing more than the result of her advancing age (Cullen, et al., 1976).

It is true that some of the warning signs cannot be used as exclusive signals of malignancy for the elderly. An increasing number of debilitating diseases present in the older person tend to confound or mask the presence of the usual symptoms of malignancy. For example, a person already may have degenerative bone disease, pulmonary disease, and impaired bowel and urinary functions. He may have lived many years with unhealed leg ulcers or with loose uncomfortable dentures with resulting traumatic ulcers. He may have anemia for which he is receiving treatment. Thus it is more difficult to recognize the importance of new signs so similar to his existing ones.

It becomes more than usually important then for the patient and the family to identify to the health care providers *all* of the signs and symptoms present, both old and new, at the time of a physical examination so that the professional can logically study the significance of the combined and newly-presenting symptoms of both progressive and new disease.

The use of ongoing, well-documented problem oriented health records can be of tremendous value in this instance. They allow the health professional to assess the patient's symptoms and signs at present and in relationship to the retrospective combination of previous symptoms and their diagnosis.

The health care provider must be prepared to view the patient with "fresh" eyes and an open mind in order to consider new possible diagnoses and the possibility of a newly-developing malignancy. Does the fatigue, anemia, and gastric discomfort signal another small hemorrhage from the hiatal hernia, or does it portend new disease, malignant disease? The enlarged prostate of the elderly male may be present, and, with no change in symptoms, a malignancy may begin. Leukoplakia might easily be identified in the mouth or on the labia if monilia does not coexist.

There are some signs and symptoms which are definitive of malignancy that are more easily located and defined in the elderly. For example, the atrophy of the mammary or glandular tissue of the breast in the woman over 65 minimizes the amount of palpable normal tissue in the breast. There remains only fat tissue, usually only in the lower quadrants, and supportive tissue. The woman who has had earlier premenopausal benign cystic disease will, if she has not had exogenous estrogen replacement, be completely free of any palpable remnants of the cystic disease by age 65. Therefore, when the breast is examined in older women, *any* palpable lesion that is not normal fat tissue is likely to be a malignant lesion. Further, when hormonal stimulation decreases and vaginal secretions cease, *any* vaginal discharge must be suspect.

Particularly in the elderly, with their problem of coexisting disease, it becomes important to record all signs and symptoms, review them at appropriate intervals (weekly/monthly) and observe for their continued presence, exacerbation, and progression or for new symptoms, which when combined, indicate the increasing probability of malignant lesions. (See Scheduling Screening Programs later in this chapter.)

Specific Signs and Symptoms in High Risk Organs

The elderly are a high risk group for malignancy; therefore, the usual signs and symptoms of malignancy must be considered at all times. In the following section pertinent risk factors for particular target organs that are at highest risk for malignancies in the elderly are considered.

PROSTATE. Prostatic malignancies are the most common tumor in males over 80 years of age (see Figs. 12-5, 12-8, and 12-9). Studies have shown that many unsuspected prostatic malignancies are found at autopsy. Rullis and coworkers (1975) state that, of all patients having surgery for benign disease, one of every four (25 percent) will have unsuspected carcinoma; between ages 70 and 79 this will increase to 40 percent or one out of every three patients; and between the years 80 and older, two of every three

patients will have histologic evidence of prostatic cancer. In view of this high incidence of prostatic malignancy in the over-65-year age group it is important for males over 50 to have at least annual digital rectal examinations for prostatic disease. The prostate with malignant disease will feel hard, nodular, and fixed.

Signs and symptoms of prostate malignancy are similar to those of benign prostatic hyperplasia—frequency, nocturia, narrowed urinary stream and decreased force, difficulty in starting and stopping urinary flow, and chronic retention with overflow frequency. In addition there may be hematuria and hematospermia (see Chapter 17). Urinary infection, unaccompanied by pain and fever may accompany both benign and malignant disease (Bergevin, 1976).

COLON AND RECTUM. Cancer of the colon and rectum are found most often in the elderly, with cancer of the colon more common in women and cancer of the rectum more common in men. Cancer in this site is increasing in the United States.

The symptoms vary with the location. Cancer of the ascending colon may manifest itself only as a dull pain and unexplained anemia. Constipation or diarrhea are more common with cancer of the descending colon and rectum. Blood and mucus in the stools are common.

Changes in bowel habits and character of stool require the older person to be a good observer and historian, as well as one who can remember other coexisting factors such as the following:

1. the amount of water and other fluids taken during the time period.
2. types of foods eaten, e.g., fatty foods, no proteins, high protein, only carbohydrates.
3. changes in activity and exercise patterns.
4. new medications (iron, tranquilizers, large doses of aspirin, etc.—see Chapter 16, pp. 318, 319, 322, and 325).
5. presence of depression

In addition to the discovery of bowel lesions through visits to the private physician, the American Cancer Society also sponsors screening programs as demonstration projects or part of established public health programs. These involve examining stool specimens for occult blood using Hemoccult test. This is a more reliable test than the guaiac and is inexpensive and convenient.

In order to achieve an accurate finding, the persons should refrain from eating red meat for three days prior to the test. When such screening programs are instituted in nursing homes it becomes important that all residents be reminded at each meal the reason for the temporary change in the menu. They also need to know why this routine test is being done. But, after the testing is over, it is equally important to insure that all residents have once again resumed their previous diets, including red meats.

UPPER G.I. The upper G.I., a large congregate of sites (esophagus, stomach, liver, gallbladder, pancreas), includes those of high incidence over age 60 (Table 12-2). Symptoms often are silent or masked by other ongoing situations. Occult G.I. bleeds may alert the patient and nurse dramatically to esophageal or gastric cancer. More subtle symptoms, however, have usually gone unnoticed. Any gradual loss of appetite should be suspect for upper G.I. malignancy. Sudden aversion to meat usually means the presence of a G.I. malignancy. These symptoms, must be differentially checked. Are the symptoms associated with depression? Has the oral status of the patient changed, i.e., broken denture, oral infection, loose dentures, or caries? Have there been changes in food preparation, size of serving, or food preparation for ease of chewing and swallowing? Is the problem no appetite or is it difficulty in swallowing? This may easily be tested by the comparative ease of swallowing solids, versus liquids, versus semisolids such as Jello, custards, or watermelon, which are easiest. The presence of discomfort or pain by site or time relationships to the intake of food may be difficult to ascertain in the elderly by retrospective history. The patient may be willing to keep a diary (when shown) for a two-week period. If incapable of doing it, nursing home staff may keep it for him by focusing specific questions to him at pertinent time intervals to the mealtime of the day. Rapid loss of weight is always suspicious of G.I. malignancy; therefore, accompanying the diary should be a recording of biweekly weights. Dark velvety-appearing skin lesions in groin or axilla may signal gastric or intestinal carcinoma (Bergevin, 1976). Jaundice may be a late sign of pancreatic or liver malignancy.

VULVA. The presence of extreme pruritus, especially at night, is the initial warning of vulvar malignancy. Since vulvar malignancy often occurs in combination with monilial infection and since both cause pruritus, often with monilial infection. In addition, make. Diabetes mellitus also presents with vulvar pruritus, often with monilial infection. In addition, both monilia and malignant leukoplakia show as white lesions; however, the monilia can be carefully removed with a tongue blade while the leukoplakia

cannot. Cancer of the vulva is a very friable lesion which bleeds easily.

The best screening for this malignancy is the annual gynecologic examination and an awareness of the presenting symptoms by older women and all health care providers.

UTERUS. Early gynecologic symptoms of malignancies often are scant and transient. After one or two days of spotting, this early warning of a gynecologic malignancy in the aged woman may cease and only the late symptoms of an enlarging abdomen will betray late ovarian carcinoma. Early spotting followed only later by bleeding, hemorrhage, or foul discharge will signal malignancy of the corpus or cervix respectively.

Where there are coexisting hemorrhoids or an abraded prolapse of the uterus or bladder, spotting on undergarments or toilet tissue may be misinterpreted. All blood spotting should be checked to discover its point of origin *as soon as it is first noticed.* Early gynecologic malignancy is diagnosed by inconsistent spotting. It should not be ignored.

Corpus. Malignancies of the body of the uterus are most frequently seen in obese, white, hypertensive, and diabetic women. Spotting of blood will be the only symptom until a later increase and prolonged flow of blood will occur, accompanied by pain. Screening for endometrial malignancy is by endometrial cytology.

Cervix. Cervical malignancies are less frequently seen in the elderly white woman than those involving the body of the uterus. However, it is frequently seen in older black women (Figs. 12-4 and 12-9).

Annual pap smears are the screening program for cervical lesions. Special consideration must be given in doing pap smears and pelvic examinations on older women. Secretions are scant at this age and the atrophied introitus and vagina (particularly in nulliparous elderly women) makes the examination painful and difficult. Special precautions include using the smallest speculum, generously lubricating both speculum and gloves, giving consideration to restricted mobility in hip and knee joints when positioning the person in stirrups, and giving reassurance and support during the procedure. If a doctor is doing the procedure, this means the nurse is at the head of the table, *not* with the doctor. If the woman has extremely limited motion in the joints or severe pain, a lateral position is sometimes less painful while still allowing sufficient exposure. This position is also less embarrassing. The 70 and 80-plus generation were children at the turn of the century when modesty was firmly imprinted; this modesty still prevails for them. Additionally, this may be the first pelvic examination some women have ever had.

BREAST. There seems to be a relationship between hypothyroidism and breast cancer. It is believed that many old people have undiagnosed hypothyroid disease and that some may even have myxedema. This may be a silent population within the community or nursing home who are at risk for breast cancer.

Breast cancer rises in incidence with age (see Figs. 12-2 and 12-3), yet, as the older woman's breasts change contour because of the atrophied glandular tissue, she has the mistaken idea that she is no longer at risk. "I have nothing there anymore. I'm too old for breast cancer." We as professionals need to get our own thinking turned around (see Table 12-2 and Figs. 12-1, 12-2, and 12-3) and then change this fallacy about breast cancer in the elderly woman.

The atrophy of the mammary or glandular tissue of the breast in women over 65 minimizes the amount of palpable normal tissue in the breast, leaving only fat tissue, predominantly in the lower quadrants. Even women with premenopausal benign cystic disease will, by age 70, have no palpable remnants of the disease if they have not had exogenous estrogen replacement since menopause. Therefore when the breast is examined in the 70-year-old woman or older, *any palpable lesion which is not normal fat tissue is likely to be a malignant lesion.*

In the general population there is a higher incidence of breast cancer in both upper quadrants, but especially the upper outer quadrant (47 percent of all breast cancers). This probably also pertains to breast cancer in the elderly. Nipple and areolar areas may be higher sites of involvement in the elderly woman than in the general female population (Moe, 1978).

It is of note that when breast cancer does occur in the male, it occurs after age 65.

Breast Self-Examination. Breast self-examination (BSE) should be taught to all women so that when they grow older it is a health habit that will be continued. It is unfortunate for the older woman that so much publicity is given to the 40- to

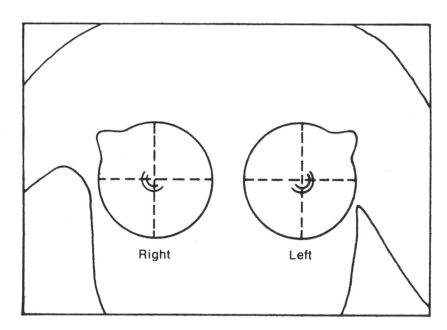

The different "feels" in my two breasts
/// Glandular tissue
⟨⟩ Fatty tissue
∷∷∷ Firmness under Breast (Infra-mammary ridge)
XX Other (locate on your "map" and describe)

FIGURE 12-10. Breast self-examination diagram. (Copyright by D. Molbo, Breast Health Program, Department of Physiological Nursing, University of Washington, Seattle, 1978)

50-year age span in connection with breast cancer frequency (see Figs. 12-2 and 12-3). This approach has led many elderly women to believe they are too old for breast cancer and that, therefore, there is no need for breast self-examination. As reinforcement of this fallacy, no publicity encourages the older woman to practice breast self-examination and there are few programs that are adapted to the needs of the older population.

The elderly have the easiest breast of any age in which to identify normal tissue (fatty tissue) each month. Each woman can develop a personal "map" which will show her the distribution of fat in her breast. Anything else felt should be reported to a health care professional (Fig. 12-10).

Breast self-examination instruction should be given to all residents in retirement homes and nursing homes. Those women who can no longer carry out the examination should have it done by nurses especially educated in BSE. It should be on a monthly examination schedule.

Mammography. Controversy over mammography, diagnostic breast x-ray, arose in 1976 because of reported concerns over the amount of radiation exposure. Since that date, technician competence has been assured, and the technology itself assures that absorbed radiation by the patient is very little, only a few millirads. In addition, the breast tissue of the woman over 70 is not dense, but loose, and, therefore, requires few exposures and only low dosage for quality films. Breast xerography is a diagnostic breast x-ray study differing only by a Xerox Corporation film processing method producing a strikingly detailed blue and white film.

Annual mammography as a diagnostic tool for women over 70 should hold no fears. The radiation exposure will be low, the number of pictures necessary will be few, even for the old patient with pendulous breasts, and the procedure is not uncomfortable or long. *However,* all older patients should be prepared for the x-ray procedure—the appearance of the room, its safety, the proximity of personnel when they are left alone, and especially exposure of the breast only as necessary. Many older women, especially those of the generation over 70, have Victorian modesty which is unchanged by their age or skinny bodies. Their modesty should be respected and preserved by all personnel working with them. The use of paper capes, open in the front but affording cover for the patient's back, seems to give a greater sense of protection and some warmth as well.

LUNGS. Lung cancer shows a rising incidence in the elderly, not only among males but also among females. Cigarette smoking became popular during World War I, with accelerated smoking habits among males thereafter. That generation is now 70- to 80-years old. World War II involved women who went into war assembly line work and associated cigarette smoking. Subsequently, the female incidence of lung cancer has also risen in recent years. Those female generations who have smoked for 30 years are now 50- to 80-years old. They are at high risk (Fig. 12-6).

Cough and hoarseness, particularly combined with a history of cigarette smoking or work in occupations with high air pollution, need to be checked for lung malignancies. The presence of clubbed fingers, unrelated to a cardiopulmonary problem, may be suspect for lung malignancy. This often coexists with symptoms of painful joints and extremity edema (Bergevin, 1976). Screening includes chest x-ray pictures and sputum cytology.

ORAL CAVITY. Individuals with a history of tobacco use (pipe, cigar, or cigarette smoking or chewing of tobacco) are at higher risk of oral cancer, especially when accompanied by a high use of alcohol. It is often present among those with a history of use of cigarettes and alcohol. Males are at highest risk presently and the incidence is increasing in females. Painful ulcerations, often associated with dentures should receive prompt differential diagnosis.

Leukoplakia usually presents in several specific sites: especially the floor of the mouth or the tongue borders, but also the buccal, lips, and vermilion angles. No white lesion of the mouth should be ignored. Leukoplakia is considered the major premalignant lesion.

Any reduction in the range of tongue movement may signal a cancer of the floor of the mouth. This may be an early sign, even before any visible lesion is seen or palpated. Early malignancies of the mouth are *not* painful or tender. This is a differential decision between an early malignancy and early nonmalignant lesion. Systematic and regular oral examinations are important for cancer vigilance.

Oral examination should be a part of the armamentarium of most health care providers. Nurses aides in nursing homes should be capable of examining the oral cavity for abnormalities on a monthly basis. (See Chapter 8 for specifics).

LARYNX. Heavy smoking for over 20 years, and heavy smoking accompanied by high alcohol intake, place the male, white or black, at high risk. Symtoms are obvious in this cancer, and patients often are diagnosed early. The cure rate is correspondingly high.

Coughing, persistent hoarseness, and husky voice associated with progressive phonation difficulties will alert the patient to seek help for a possible laryngeal malignancy. Dysphagia and coughing increase. The patient will especially have early difficulty with consonants g and k. "Keep the goat" may be phonated, "____p the ____t."

CHRONIC LYMPHOCYTIC LEUKEMIA. Chronic lymphocytic leukemia is a leukemia common above age 60, especially in males. The symptoms are insidious—an increase in blood lymphocytes, fever, weight loss, enlargement of spleen and liver, and fatigue.

Prognosis

Cancer is a chronic disease. It does have remissions, and some types of malignancies have been arrested and cured. Since metastasis usually is slower in older people, it is not as fulminating a disease as in younger people. Probably the old person dies as the result of an infection, complication (pneumonia), or another chronic illness rather than directly from the cancer itself.

Results of therapy often are referred to as survival rate. This is the number of patients living at a stated interval (5 to 10 years) after the beginning of the first planned treatment. Survival rate tables reflect the general population and are not broken down by age, especially the over-70 group.

Mortality

Cancer mortality is an inconsistent and unreliable statistic, particularly for the elderly. Ignored symptoms and treatment, and death certificate statements identifying the last obvious disease syndrome, i.e., heart failure or pulmonary edema, distort the accuracy of cancer mortality figures. However, for your interest and cautious interpretation, Figure 12-11 is given. Note that it is based on numbers of deaths per 1000 in a *general population*.

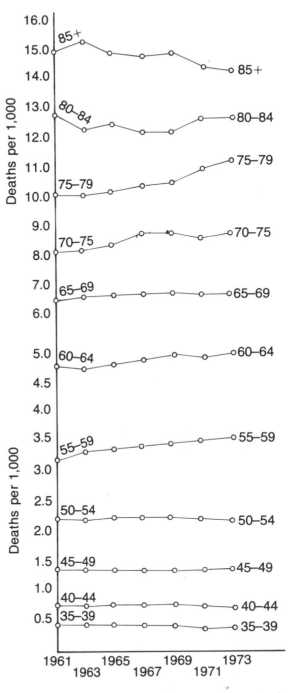

FIGURE 12-11. Cancer death rates, ages 35 to 85 plus (U. S. Public Health Service data) in the United States from 1961 to 1973. (Adapted from Cancer 28:28, 1978).

Scheduling Screening Programs

Screening programs are possible for malignancies of breast, lung, colon, rectum, oral cavity, and uterus (Table 12-3). It is possible to set up appropriately periodic routines for examining the elderly for malignancies, thus assuring the greatest possibility of early detection in a high risk population. Figure 12-12 shows a sample schedule that might be used by retirement homes, ambulatory care clinics, nursing homes, and so forth.

In the absence of monthly examinations, at least the record should be reviewed for reported signs and symptoms. This record review may pick up malignancies that have symptoms of other conditions which have been ignored, resisted treatment, and/or persisted. The record analysis is purposely staggered throughout the year for increased vigilance of all areas.

Blood Tests and Cancer Screening

It would be good if the elderly person could be spared the anxiety and physical discomfort of

TABLE 12-3.   Cancer detection approaches.

Site	Common Warning Signals	Screening Tests	Differential Diagnostic Tests
Breast	Lump or thickening in breast	Breast self-examination monthly (done by nurses in institutions), annual checkup, mammography, thermography	Aspiration of fluid from breast masses, breast biopsy, chest x-ray, study, skeletal survey
Colon and rectum	Change in bowel habits and character of stool, rectal bleeding	Annual checkup, proctosigmoidoscopy (especially persons over 40), occult blood stool exam, digital exam	Colonoscopy with biopsy, barium enema
Kidney and bladder	Change in bladder habits, urinary difficulty, urinary bleeding	Annual checkup with urinalysis, occasionally exfoliative studies	IVP, retrograde pyelography, nephrotomography, selective renal arteriography, venacavography
Lung	Persistent cough or hoarseness, lingering respiratory ailment (history of smoking or proximity of air pollution)	Annual checkup, chest x-ray studies, sputum cytology	Roentgenography, fluoroscopy, tomography, bronchography, angiography, bronchoscopy including bronchial washings and sputum cytology, scalene node biopsy, mediastinoscopy, lung scans
Oral	Sore that does not heal, dysphagia (history of smoking)	Annual checkup by physician or dentist (monthly in nursing homes by aides)	Oral cavity examination includes nasopharynx, oropharynx, and laryngopharynx. X-ray studies include plain films, tomograms, barium swallow, contrast studies of larynx and chest. Biopsy of all suspicious lesions
Prostate	Various urinary difficulties	Annual checkup including digital exam	Needle or open biopsy, serum acid phosphatase, bone scan
Skin	Sore that does not heal, change in wart or mole	Annual checkup	Excisional or incisional biopsy
Stomach	Indigestion, meal intolerance, anorexia	Annual checkup, occult blood stool test	Upper GI series, gastric analysis, exfoliative studies, endoscopy
Uterus	Unusual bleeding or discharge	Annual checkup including pelvic exam and pap smear, exfoliative studies	Schiller's test, tissue biopsy, fractional D & C, one biopsy, lymphangiography, colposcopy

Adapted from Sato, P.: The detection of cancer. In Burkhalter, P., and Donley, D. (eds.): Dynamics of Oncology Nursing. New York: McGraw-Hill Book Co., 1976.

some screening tests and initially could have a blood test to determine the presence or absence of cancer. One such test is available, though it does not indicate the location of the malignancy. This is the CEA (Carcino-Embryonic-Antigen test). It measures the serum tumor antigen. At present it is often used to determine the prognosis of the patient who has been diagnosed as having a malignancy by some other test. Its use at this time for initial screening, however, is limited in the elderly.

Diagnostic Tests

Sometimes diagnostic tests are avoided by both professionals and family. The feeling that, "She can't take any more suffering," often is valid; however, it must be appraised carefully. Most important, the patient should be included in any decision making. It could be that the present suffering could be relieved to some degree in just knowing that someone had recognized it and wanted to do something about it.

Some diagnostic tests are simple and cause no problems other than the anxiety regarding the outcome or the uneasiness of strange interpersonal contacts, the absence of familiar supporting persons, and the strange foreboding environments. Such problems can be mediated by health care professionals.

Other tests may be more difficult for the elderly, either because they entail detailed instructions, energy draining preparation, difficult maneuvers, or pain. They should be assessed and discussed without personal bias with the elderly person on his level of comprehension. The costs of energy, the stressors, pain, anesthesia, and difficult or long positioning (e.g., proctoscopy, tomograms, CAT scanning) must be balanced against the next set of questions: *If it is cancer, what then? What stamina (physical and emotional) does the person have to live with the treatment protocols and effects? Which will cause the least harm—the treatment or allowing the disease to take its course? Which will give the greatest quality of life to the remaining time?*

Take an example of a decision that did not add to the quality of life:

Mrs. A was 82, alert, communicative, and had been a very active person. Now she lay on the examination table in the emergency room gasping for breath. Her eyes dilated with fear, she grasped for suppor-

	Jan	Feb	Mar	Apr	May	Jun	Jul	Aug	Sep	Oct	Nov	Dec
Breast	Y X R	X	X	X	X	X	X R	X	X	X R	X	X
Cervix	Y R						R					
Colon-Rectum	Y		R					R				
Lung		R					Y					R
Oral	X			X	Y R	X		X	R	X	X	R
Prostate	Y	R						R				
Uterus	Y R						R					

Y—Yearly screening or examination by physician, nurse, or other major health care provider
X—Examination by patient or staff
R—Record analysis checking for symptoms that may have accumulated and could be indicative of cancer

FIGURE 12-12. An examination and record assessment schedule for systematic surveillance for malignant disease.

tive hands and clung. Mrs. A had cancer of the thyroid, manifesting itself as a constantly growing mass at the base of her neck. At first her family thought she was developing a goiter. But then they considered the question, "What if it's cancer?" Their response to this question was to ignore the condition. Some months later Mrs. A found breathing increasingly difficult. Because her earlier fears about the obviously enlarging neck mass had received no recognition or help, she began to withdraw from communication about herself with her daughter and son-in-law with whom she lived. She felt neglected, helpless, and isolated from her only perceived loved ones.

This malignancy could have been diagnosed by the use of a radioactive isotope of Iodine, I_{131}. The procedure would have been a very simple one. Her particular cancer could have been successfully treated with a *therapeutic* dosage of the same isotope, with possible adjuvant radiation therapy. In all it would have necessitated drinking the cocktail, a few hospital days, no pain, and a few outpatient trips to the radiation department. Here the balancing of the stress of diagnosis and treatment versus stress of failing to treat the tumor obviously falls on the side of treating the disease.

All patients and their families have the right to make informed decisions. Therefore, nurses should see and assess for themselves what the impact of the various diagnostic and treatment protocols involve, so that they can give accurate neutral information about the options. The relative payoff, the discomforts, ways in which it can be modified, and so forth should be described and considered.

On the other side of the coin, professionals who work regularly in diagnostic treatment areas need to be conversant with the particular needs and problems of the elderly. How can one manage the need for toileting, the coughing, the dry mouth during tomography with its long periods of immobility? The unknown; the isolation; the preparation for the tests; the sensory assault of the environment; the procedure; the awkward, embarrassing, or painful positioning; and the lengthy time involved take their energy toll on the elderly patient. All these things must be taken into consideration when making decisions concerning diagnostic tests.

Elderly patients require food and water (if permitted) prior to any diagnostic test; they also should be taken to the toilet. Elderly patients require *pain relief before* coming to the x-ray department or other

diagnostic area. They require relief of anxiety before being transported to a strange area for a strange examination for perhaps an unknown reason, or a fright-provoking reason. However, the disaster-crisis repertoire of the elderly person can handle fears of knowns better than the anxiety of unknowns. He should know why the test is necessary and be promised continuing communications about the condition. He should know the time dimensions of the examination including the estimated or real waiting times involved. For instance, a bone scan takes 1 hour and 9 minutes, *but* there is a 3-hour wait between injection and scan.

Within a diagnostic department such as the x-ray department, careful positioning consistent with the patient's peculiar anatomy and respiratory or skeletal discomfort should be performed before the examination. This may take time, but it is well spent if the examination can be continued to its completion. Insensitive pre-examination positioning, pain, thirst, and a full bladder mean eventual interruption of an examination, a repeat, more time, more radiation. Certain examinations require a different vigilance before and during the examination: elderly patients scheduled for lymphangiograms should have the assurance of a prior pulmonary function test; all examinations requiring dye preparations should make personnel alert to danger of reactions in the elderly patient.

In the University Hospital at the University of Washington, a full-time professional nurse is employed in diagnostic radiology; she anticipates needs of such patients and supports and cares for them when they are in the x-ray department. Nursing care is needed by patients in diagnostic x-ray departments. The patients' needs are not and cannot be met by x-ray technicians or physicians intent upon their priority task of getting a good film. Regular nursing staff cannot be reassigned for long time periods to stay with patients in the x-ray area. Yet patients' needs continue, even increase, and an x-ray-based nurse is one solution.

The decision to withhold information regarding diagnosis, diagnostic tests, and treatment options is a formidable responsibility for any professional to assume. The right of any individual to make these decisions for another is increasingly being held in question. With the concept of informed consent comes the right to know and to receive information without prejudice. It also exacts the accompanying need of help from one human to another.

One aspect of the decision regarding going

ahead with diagnosis and treatment or allowing the disease to take its course that is often not considered is the question of who will care for the individual when the inevitable metastasis occur. Treated cancer *may* metastasize, untreated cancer *will* metastasize. If the primary disease is so overwhelming to contemplate, certainly the prospect of living with metastatic complications is even more difficult. Will the nursing staff be capable of caring for the patient with neglected cancer of the breast when it erodes? I have found that aides in nursing homes, who become the grandchild or great grandchild to the elderly for whom they care, are unable to cope with the abandonment of the elderly by the professionals. These aides try to serve as surrogates for absent family, but they are angered even further by evidences of withholding treatment. The problems of living with obstruction, with bony metastasis and its pain and immobility, must be considered when the decision is made to avoid diagnosis and treatment.

The decision to ignore initial symptoms, diagnosis, and treatment is no less easy than to proceed with treatment. It may in fact be harder since it carries the harder burdens of responsibility for predictable outcomes. All decisions should be made in the light of currently available oncology knowledge with application to the elderly person. They cannot be made in the realms of biased feelings, attitudes, and personal fears alone.

Treatment

Modern cancer treatment is based on the objective of reducing the mass (or quantity) of cancer cells by the easiest modality (surgery, radiation, or drugs) and then relying on or stimulating the patient's own immune system to get back on the job and destroy the stragglers. Surgical procedures and radiation destroy a cancer mass in one specific site (or several metastasized sites). Chemotherapy has the same ability, but, in addition, it is used systemically to destroy cancer cells far from the primary site. For this reason chemotherapy is particularly effective in the treatment of leukemia. Immunocompetence of the patient is required after these therapies have been discontinued.

Modalities

Treatment modalities appropriate for the elderly patient are numerous. Although surgery previously was the most often used, other primary methods of treatment are now appropriate as well as combinations of treatment and adjunctive forms which augment or support the primary method. For instance, a 70-year-old woman with a localized breast tumor could have simple excision as primary treatment, followed by radiation or chemotherapy. She might have primary radiation treatment or primary hormone treatment. All these decisions can and must be made individually, with consideration for the patient's reserves for treatment and convalescence and *her* life goals and trajectory.

Some procedures can be modified. For the patient with prostatic cancer it may be reassuring to know that various surgical routes may be possible. Thus, for the compromised patient, a perineal approach is often chosen and is less traumatic for the patient.

Such decision points are necessary and possible only by open discussion with the physician about alternative treatment modalities. We must remove ourselves from the fatalistic giving-up attitude when cancer is diagnosed in the old. For the old person who still wants to live, giving-up is interpreted as abandonment and more isolation to bear. Perhaps that is reason enough to consent to die. But then it is the professional who has consigned him to death, not the patient.

Since there are almost daily changes in protocols for chemotherapy, radiation, and surgery, information on specifics of these treatments are not given here. Journal articles and talking with private physicians can provide the most up-to-date information on cancer care in a given area.

SURGERY. The basic principle of cancer surgery has been to excise the tumor completely and to excise through healthy tissue in order to minimize spread of the malignant cells. This has meant that surgical procedures of the past were radical. Surgery of the future probably will utilize other modalities as combinations. For instance, the mass can be reduced prior to surgery (radiation and surgery in cancer of the corpus uterus) or, by using a simpler surgical procedure, radiation or chemotherapy can be used post-surgery to continue to reduce the tumor. Surgery, that necessitates anesthesia, is difficult for the elderly patient.

RADIATION. Radiation therapy is of two types: external and internal. *External radiation* involves a utilization of X rays (i.e., cobalt 60 unit) while the patient is considered either an inpatient or outpatient. The radiation is delivered in measured divided doses over time. *Internal radiation* involves sealed sources of radiation which are placed into body cavities or implanted directly into the tumor as needles. Internal radiation also involves an unsealed source, namely fluid radioactive isotopes. These are selectively absorbed into the tumor mass physiologically. Radium, cesium, $Iodine_{131}$ and $Phosphorus_{32}$ are examples of these internal radioactive elements.

There are fatiguing elements associated with radiation therapy in addition to the patient's feeling of isolation. Such problems are discussed under management later in the chapter.

CHEMOTHERAPY. The optimum drug dose is the critical dosage that produces the maximum therapeutic benefit with the minimum amount of risk or morbidity. Because the selectivity of chemotherapeutic agents for only neoplastic tissue is low, it follows that all therapy will result in some healthy tissue dysfunction. Therefore, there is a therapeutic range before the minimum effective dose (MED) and the maximum tolerance dose (MTD). This margin, or therapeutic index is especially narrow in the older person. This means fewer drug combinations, less flexibility with combination therapy, and potentially greater risks and hazards of dosage if therapeutic effects are to be achieved in the older person. In the child and the young adult, the reticuloendothelial system demonstrates more resiliency and, therefore, more rapid recovery than in the older patient. In the older person, the gastrointestinal tract and the central nervous system are less tolerant of drug toxicities, and the immunologic status of the older person is less favorable for therapy benefits. Therefore, to achieve the therapy goal, there must be a 40 to 50 percent reduction of dosage of most chemotherapeutic agents (the ratio of risk or morbidity to the potential benefits) in patients over 65-years old. For example, reduced dosages of Vincristine and Vinblastine are necessary to protect the aged patient from neuropathies.

For the old person, effective and safe dosage cannot alone be determined by body surface/weight. It must be determined individually by vulnerability of the older person to the anticipated toxicity of drugs. This requires pretreatment assessment of his medical risk status, that is, the critical systems of brain, heart, kidney, lungs, and liver to the expected effects of the drugs. For example,

Adriamycin is known to affect cardiac status.
Adriamycin also can compromise glomerular filtration and, thus, renal function.

Bleomycin increases the risk of subacute pneumonitis and pulmonary fibrosis.
Vincristine increases risk of ileus and secondary obstruction.

Where the status of the individual may be compromised already through previous pathology, the toxicity risks increase significantly. Thus, in chemotherapy, the nurse as well as the physician and the patient need to be alert to clinical changes in order to make in-course corrections so that the dosage can be both safe and effective.

The use of steroids and hormones has improved individuals' drug status, particularly that of older females.

Immunotherapy. Immunotherapy is the newest area of therapy. It is seldom used with older people at the present. The reason this treatment is not effective in this age group is the fact that older people already have a compromised immune system.

Factors that Influence Treatment Decisions

There are areas of assessment to be made for any patient prior to planning a cancer treatment program. This is especially necessary for the elderly patient. All patients should be assessed in conjunction with the results of the diagnostic examinations for the type of the cancer and its extent. This is called staging, or classification. The patient also needs to be assessed for his physical and metabolic capabilities for various kinds of treatment. Last, the patient needs to be assessed for his nutritional status because of current recognition that nutrition is important adjunctive treatment to the primary or combination treatment being planned.

STAGING OR CLASSIFICATION. An evaluation of the patient should be done to classify the disease. This will be used in determining a therapy plan and, later, to assess the response to therapy and the nature of any future adjunctive therapy. Classification of the disease should be done particularly with the elderly patient in order to fully examine the alternative courses of treatment available and to plan the most advantageous cure-care regimen.

Classification provides a means of expressing in internationally understood language the type of tumor, its rate of growth, and its size and extent.

The international TNM system involves an assessment of the primary Tumor (T), the presence of Nodes (N) and Metastases (M) by judging the presence or absence of T, N, M into three or four set categories. Therefore, T_0, T_1, T_2, T_3, T_4 indicates the increasing size of tumor from 0 to 4; N_0, N_1, N_2, N_3 indicates qualities or locations of nodes; and M_0, M_1, M_2, M_3 indicates no metastases (M_0) or increasing presence of metastasis (M_1 to M_3).

Because each site and histologic tissue has a different behavior in malignancy as in health, the TNM expression will be different. The shorthand expression of a breast tumor which is $T_2N_1M_0$ precisely says

T_2 = tumor more than 2 cm and less than 5 cm
N_1 = axillary and movable nodes
M_0 = no evidence of distant metastasis

If the nurse is to be an accurate interpreter to the patient, and is a patient's advocate, it is important for her to know this language and its significance for treatment considerations. The reader is referred to a small paperbound handbook of 100 pages, the *TNM, Classification of Malignant Tumours* (see references).

METABOLIC CHANGES. Three other major areas of capability impinge on the decisions regarding treatment. These are the status of the brain, heart, and kidneys. Based on an assessment of the functional status of these three organs, treatment protocols are modified to adjust to the person's vulnerability. Modifications are made in protocols which might offer optimum management of the tumor in terms of the person's recognized restorative capabilities. Simple surgical procedures may be combined with radiation to save heart and brain. Drug changes or drug selectivity can be planned to spare liver and/or renal inadequacies.

Both the effects of the treatment and the disease itself result in metabolic shifts, occasioned by the resultant tissue destruction and negative nitrogen balance. For more extensive treatment of this important subject the reader is referred to the writings of Francis Moore (1965). With the elderly, one must add the metabolic changes associated with aging. This total field requires more research.

NUTRITION. There is an increasing recognition that patients who are malnourished prior to radiation and chemotherapy respond less well to these modalities. They exhibit earlier and more frequent toxicities. To increase the efficacy of all therapy, nutrition is considered supplementary. A nutritional assessment is made prior to establishing the particular therapy to be used (see sample of one method of nutritional assessment, p. 228). High protein, high caloric diets are begun before any treatment. Hyperalimentation is being used increasingly to assure proper nutrition throughout the course of the treatment (Lanzotti, 1975; Schein, 1975).

IMMUNOCOMPETENCY. Immunocompetency is one body function in which age-related diminution has occurred. This plays an important part in decisions on treatment for the elderly. In treating cancer, the combination treatment is aimed at removing as much of the existent tumor as possible with the assumption that the immunocompetence of the person will then exert its potential for destruction of the remaining tumor cells and against further malignant cell proliferation. The immunocompetence of the elderly person is very precarious and the assistance the elderly person receives from his own protective system is variable. Therefore, when any therapy protocol requires immunocompetence, the patient's immune status should be determined. For example, it has been found that marrow transplant has not been successful for patients over the age of 60. Thus, rather than depend on the person's immunocompetence, chemotherapy alone is used in these leukemias.

Nursing Management of Complications of Cancer Therapy

At this time, many of the complications associated with radiation or chemotherapy such as skin breakdown, nausea, vomiting, diarrhea, or stomatitis seem no more common in the elderly than in other age groups. However, when they occur, their effect on the nutritional status of the patient may be more devastating than in the younger person.

Nutritional Status

The nutritional status of the older person is often less than ideal at the initiation of therapy, and so the shift to negative nitrogen balance may be more rapid and severe. Therefore, nutritional assessment of cancer patients is very important. It is calculated according to age by figuring relationship of muscle mass (caliper measured) to height and weight (Cancer Research, 1977).

The patient who is malnourished prior to chemotherapy (and probably also radiation) suffers more toxicities of therapy than those with nutritional reserves of fat and protein muscle mass; therefore,

NUTRITIONAL ASSESSMENT SUMMARY

Patient _____ Room _____ Physician _____ Date _____

Service _____ Diagnosis _____

Admission Weight _____ Height _____ Ideal Weight _____

PARAMETERS	PATIENT VALUES	ASSESSMENT		
		>90% Standard Not Depleted	60–90% Standard Moderately Depleted	<60% Standard Severely Depleted
Weight/height	kg cm			
Triceps Skin-fold (TSF)	mm			
Mid-Arm Circumference (MAC)	cm			
Mid-Arm Muscle Circumference (MAMC) MAMC (cm) = MAC (cm) − [3.14 × TSF (cm)]*	cm			
Lymphocytes, total count	mm^3			
Albumin, serum	g/100 ml			
Total Iron Binding Capacity (TIBC)	mcg/100 ml			
Transferrin Serum transferrin = (0.8 × TIBC) − 42*	mg/100 ml			
Urinary Creatinine	mg			
Creatinine Height Index (CHI) CHI = $\frac{\text{Actual Urinary Creatinine}}{\text{Ideal Urinary Creatinine}} \times 100$*				

Hematocrit _____%   Hemoglobin _____g/100 ml   Cellular Immunity: ☐ Positive   ☐ Negative

Dietary Intake Evaluation: Calories _____Cal/24 hr   Protein _____g/24 hr

Protein Status: Nitrogen Balance = $\frac{\text{Protein Intake}}{6.25}$ − (Urinary Urea Nitrogen + 4)*   ☐ Positive   ☐ Negative

Nutritional Status: ☐ Marasmus (M)   ☐ Kwashiorkor (K)   ☐ Combination M-K   ☐ Normal

Proposed Nutritional Therapy: _____

_____

_____

_____

_____

Presented as a service to the medical profession by Ross Laboratories, Columbus, Ohio 43216, Div. of Abbott Laboratories, USA.
* Blackburn, G. L., et al.: Nutritional & metabolic assessment of the hospitalized patient. J. Parent. Enteral Nutr. 1:11, 1977.

the maintenance of nutrition becomes imperative (Copeland, 1975).

The nurse needs to assess the patient's usual food preferences and eating patterns. Using these data, she must ensure that each mouthful of food the patient takes is high calorie and high protein. The best assistance for this diet (semi-soft, tasteful, and nutritionally sound) is to be found in a small diet manual by Aker and Tilmont, *A Guide to Good Nutrition During and After Chemotherapy and Radiation,* 1979.

Dehydration

Dehydration is another problem in the elderly, particularly for the person receiving chemotherapy. Dependent on optimally-functioning renal and hepatic systems, many chemotherapeutic drugs are given at toxic dosage levels for therapeutic benefit. Methotrexate, for instance, is excreted by the kidneys within 48 hours after administration. To minimize toxicities that will require dose adjustment, the patient is required to drink 3 to 4 L of fluids prior to and during the first few days of drug administration. Such quantities are difficult to ingest unless divided into half-hour to one-hour intervals for the patient so he can see progress in drinking such an ocean. Further difficulties are incurred when this patient also has swallowing difficulties with or without association to stomatitis. Watermelon is often effective as a supplement to IV fluids in these patients. Watermelon is more easily swallowed than fluids and keeps the mouth soothed and moist.

Nausea

Nausea may be present as a symptom prior to treatment. It, thereby, increases the anxiety-depression level and decreases the nutritional status of the patient when his treatment is begun. All are negative influences on optimum treatment outcome. Nausea may also be a sequela to treatment protocol, especially during radiation (see Taste Distortions) and chemotherapies. Nausea may also be the constant attendant with pain in the advancing metastatic stages of disease.

It should be recalled that any autonomic nervous system stimulus can trigger nausea. Therefore, environmental factors can accentuate nausea or modify nausea, though never eliminate it when it is caused by malignancy or its treatment. Food odors, institutional odors, and industrial odors may increase the nausea of this patient (who may also have distorted perceptions of odors as a result of the disease). Of all the commercial deodorizers, the most unobtrusive and effective for this kind of patient is a few *drops* of Natron 40 (Rosemont, IL) placed on clothing, bed, or food tray. It will absorb and completely eliminate odors. A fragrant, burning candle is also pleasing and effective *if* it can be monitored for safety. All other deodorizers provide their own conflicting odor to the one they attempt to mask and add an irritating sound when it has a vaporizing unit.

Gastric motility can increase nausea. After a successfully accomplished small meal, some skilled nurses suggest a slow, short walk to modify the gastric motility and possibly decrease the nausea.

The sight of food and the very thought of food (especially when accompanied by perceived putrifying meat odors) will accentuate nausea. Small attractive portions, given frequently, may be advantageous.

It should also be remembered that certain emotions (anxiety, fear, and depression) potentiate nausea. Pain accentuates nausea. Therefore, the nauseated patient should be kept pain-free (or pain-controlled) and, in addition to the management of all previously-mentioned factors, the patient should receive specific medication for nausea relief. For some younger cancer patients undergoing chemotherapy today, little seems to afford relief. Some patients have experienced relief of nausea, retching, and vomiting by eating marijuana (Rosenberg, 1972). This is unrecognized professionally and not prescribed (though condoned). It is not known whether this is necessary for the elderly patient's relief or what its effects are on the elderly patient.

Taste Distortions

The usually-diminishing taste perceptions of the elderly, their confusion of bitter and salty, and accompanying burning sensations are further complicated by cancer and the therapies of cancer. Decrease in taste discrimination or threshold doses not seem to be related to any specific site of cancer; it does seem to be related to the extent of the disease. Patients with advancing metastatic disease have a high sucrose threshold, i.e., they have an increasing lack of recognition of this substance (DeWys and Walters, 1975). They also have an aversion to meat, which is presented by a lowered threshold recognition of urea. Patients who have certain types of radiation therapy will also complain of a "foul or putrid meat taste," rendering them nauseated and anorexic. Patients receiving radiation and chemotherapy often describe their "blah" food. This is due to a taste elevated perception threshold of sweet and lowered thresholds of bitter. These thresholds will return to previous state approximately 80 days after radiation stops (Conger, 1969).

A complete supplement which includes protein, can be used in all foods in the form of *Sustogen* (powder) or *Sustocal* (liquid) by Mead Johnson, or *Ensure* (liquid with soybean base) by Ross Laboratories. *Instant Breakfast* can also be added to food, so that large quantities of food are not necessary.

Patients with meat aversion often can tolerate fowl and fish (if the concentrated odor which accumulates under a hot plate protector is released before serving the plate to the patient). He may also tolerate eggs, milk, or cheese in prepared dishes rather than in their natural state. Coffee, cocoa, chocolate, or coke may not be enjoyed because they are "too bitter." All patients may be able to tolerate their "blah" foods by adding seasoning and sugar.

The attractiveness of the plate with small portions, color variety, and a tray or table decoration is very important for these patients. One oncology unit decorates petite sandwiches and all beverages.

Stomatitis

There is no evidence cited in the literature that the stomatitis induced by chemotherapy or radiation therapy in the elderly patient is different, more severe, or requires a longer period for healing than in younger patients. In general, however, this would be expected since the effects of aging are more pronounced in the oral tissues than anywhere else (Franks and Hedegard, 1973). Irreparable damages to atrophic oral tissues over a period of time make the elderly patient especially vulnerable to additional trauma and infection. The aged mucosa lacks the protective layer of keratinized cells. Further, the thinning of the epithelial layer of the oral tissues, the reduced blood supply, and reduced micronutrition generally result in a reduced capacity of the oral tissues of the elderly to recover from any new insults.

Oral tissue changes owing to aging and pathology as well as those of no specific importance are to be found in the oral tissues of all elderly people. Therefore, a carefully recorded oral assessment should be done pre-radiation or pre-chemotherapy

(see Chapter 8). Particular attention should be given to the soft tissues. Because most practicing dentists' concerns focus primarily on hard tissues, their graphic worksheets are difficult to adapt to this use. An assessment sheet for soft tissues has been designed by Schum, Hardin, and Lindquist. This graphic display of buccal, gingival, and palatal areas, the floor of the mouth, tongue (anterior and ventral), and lips can be used to indicate the location and size of any lesion. Lesions are defined according to their dental or dermatologic significance. This permits the nurse to carry out a professional oral examination, to document her findings, and to be capable of communicating findings to dentists with expected reliability and clarity. The oral assessment and recording should be continued every five to seven days throughout the therapy, and whenever the patient complains of burning or oral pain. A scoring system has been devised for easier periodic evaluation of the oral status of such patients.

Stomatitis appears to begin its course with burning sensations, signs of erythematous mucosa, and eventual mucosal breaks and ulcerations. These are usually complicated by coexistent infection, usually monilial or viral (Hardin, 1976; Schum, 1977).

Salivary changes also occur during or as a part of radiation/chemotherapy induced stomatitis. The volume of saliva already is reduced (xerostomia) and its viscosity is increased in the elderly. Volume and viscosity of saliva also undergo further major changes after chemotherapy and radiation therapy. The saliva becomes ropy and tenacious after exposure to an accumulated 5000 rads or to a total body exposure of 1000 rads (Hardin, 1976; Lindquist, 1978). Saliva changes become apparent after the fifth day post-chemotherapy. The pH, proteins, and electrolytes of saliva, already altered because of age, always undergo further change because of cancer therapies. As they change the oral environment, the oral flora changes. Thus monilial infections (Candida albicans) are particularly troublesome, as are herpes simplex infections. Therefore, patients with dentures or partial restorations should cleanse them thoroughly of debris and secretions at least four times daily and permit the mucosal areas to be bathed by the saliva at night. The denture should be placed in a Nystatin solution at night. Cleanliness of dentures is important during this period when the infection increases rapidly, particularly in the presence of pooled secretions (the patient can't swallow them) and especially in the warm moist environment created by an upper plate or a snug fitting lower (Davenport, 1970). Since there may be soft tissue edema as stomatitis develops, the elderly person should be alerted to dentures that may begin to feel tight and which, in themselves, may provide further irritation and ulceration by friction or pressure.

A decrease of saliva results in a loss of its cleansing and lubricating qualities for the oral tissues. There is a decrease in oral tissue protection, both soft and hard (salivary calcium bathes the teeth), and this makes the wearing of dentures, mastication of food, and swallowing very difficult. Nutrition, hydration, and communication are seriously affected when reduced saliva is accompanied by stomatitis.

The patient with stomatitis often requires analgesic relief administered parenterally and locally. The local use of Chloraseptic or Xylocaine Viscous which has a very disagreeable taste, has given way to the more effective-in-every-way oral medication Dyclone (Dow Pharmaceuticals), which is a liquid.

Oral hygiene is important. It is possible that, if good hydration and oral hygiene are maintained prior to chemotherapy and radiation therapy, stomatitis may be minimized. This is yet to be documented. However, oral hygiene during stomatitis provides the only relief by removal of debris, plaque, and tenacious secretions. For severe stomatitis, toothbrushing may be too rigorous; use *Toothettes*. Though the literature has prescribed for over 50 years the use of hydrogen peroxide (an irritant to mucosal tissue) and glycerine mixtures (drying to mucosal tissues), it is my belief and my colleagues' belief that an irrigation of 500 cc to 1000 cc normal saline is most effective. It is physiologic, nonirritating, and refreshing to the patient. Some find a tepid solution to be comfortable; others find that a room-temperature solution is cooling to painful tissues. Such an irrigation should be given by gravity flow: a can or plastic bag with tubing hung from a pole or door (Hardin, 1976). It should *not* be given by water-pic or other high pressure method. The amount of such pressure is capable of driving the organisms deep into the tissue. In an immunocompromised patient, a locally-controlled flora (or a locally-contained infection) can become the nightmare of septicemia.

The literature does have some early but scant advice about which dentifrices and mouthwashes to use and not use (Allen, 1975; Kowitz, 1976). The elderly patient undergoing cancer therapy should carefully avoid those which are mucosal-irritating,

i.e., those with an alcohol base and those that contain chloroform and "whitening" abrasives. The reader is referred to the few references available on the subject (Allen, 1975; Davenport, 1970; Kowitz, 1976).

One of the complications of radiation to the hard tissue of the mouth is dental caries and alveolar bone necrosis. The nurse should ensure that the patient has seen a dentist *before* radiation cancer therapy begins. Teeth should be cleaned, gingivitis noted and treated, caries filled, extractions done, and a clean socket assured. The day before radiation therapy, fitted mouth molds are filled with a fluoride preparation and set in place over the upper and lower teeth. This pretreatment has been found to reduce caries substantially.

Skin Problems

Though there are major skin changes with aging, there seems no corresponding increase in radiation-trauma to the aging skin when compared with younger patients. Instructions to all elderly patients undergoing radiation therapy are:

1. Keep the irradiated skin clean and dry at all times. Use only mild soap, rinse well, and pat dry. Remove perspiration and secretions.
2. Avoid clothing friction. Wear loose clothing. Allow air to dry skin fold areas of breast, groin, gluteal fold, and axillae.
3. Cornstarch in skin folds or baby oil may be used. No Vaseline or other ointments that will macerate the skin.
4. If redness and irritation occur, the previously-mentioned measures may be used. When there is skin breakdown, Burrows Solution still seems to do the job.
5. Previously irradiated skin should always be protected from the sun. The patient should be reminded about protective clothing at all times, during treatment and after.

Refractory excoriated skin areas from stomal excretions or as a result of immobility and enforced bed care are devastating to the patient, family, and staff.

Pruritus often is an irritating symptom for the elderly person, but the pruritus of vulvar or vaginal cancer, of attendant monilial infections, or of the Hodgkins or liver cancer is intolerable. Pruritus or itching, like pain, is influenced by many factors. Like pain, it has both an input component involving the C fiber nerve endings and a processing component which is handled in the cortex. C fibers are stimulated by metabolic cellular changes or by tissue enzymes from actual tissue injury. The response to scratch or not is modified by its significance, cultural implications, fatigue, pain that is coexistent, or anxiety. After excessive scratching, rubbing, and so forth, the superficial C fiber ending will be damaged and bright burning pain will be experienced as A pain fibers are stimulated. Itching cannot be stimulated again until regrowth of the C fibers. When major epithelial damage from scratching occurs, pain may be experienced for a long period.

Patients with pruritus, as with nausea, experience greater pain. Therefore, all management should be aimed at minimizing any further "itch" stimulus. Cool and cold reduces the activity of C fibers; therefore, a cold dry local application to the part (labia) may abate the sensation. (The reverse action of cold applications should be recalled; therefore, these are short applications only.) Cold and pressure will inactivate C fibers. Reduction of warm clothing may minimize pruritus. Reduction of fatigue, worry, anxiety, or embarrassment will also influence this symptom (Brewer, 1966). Sometimes local or parenteral medication is used. Often patients will control this problem themselves if they know the principles.

Infection

While it is generally accepted by health care clinicians that the aged are more prone to develop infections and that infection is a major cause of death, it is surprising that there is little specific information on immune responses of the aged to infection. Hijmans and Hollander (1977) cite this as a major task for immunogerontology. The frequency of infection in the cancer patient and particularly in the aged patient with cancer is also recognized by clinicians. In general, its frequency in the cancer patient is attributed to a deficient immuno status, neutropenia, and decreased immune globulins. Specific research and published literature is necessary in this clinical area for the aged cancer patient. The following, therefore, is pertinent to cancer patients in general, unless specifically cited for the aged patient.

The frequency of infection in cancer patients in influenced by the type of neoplasm: solid tumor, lymphoma or myeloma, or the leukemias. Approximately 75 to 80 percent of leukemia and lymphoma patients have infections during the course of the disease, usually with multiple episodes. Septicemia is 20 times higher for leukemia patients than for patients with solid tumor metastatic disease. Septicemia occurs in 60 percent of patients with leukemia, 50 percent of patients with lymphoma, and 5 percent of patients with solid tumor metastasis (Bodey, 1974). Thus, it is noted that infection is most frequent in those malignancies which in themselves unfavorably alter to a maximal degree the immune system's ability to stimulate an inflammatory and phagocytic response. One may wonder, therefore, if these quoted figures may not be even higher among the aged population with cancer who, in addition to their malignancy, have a concomitant alteration of the immune system to unfavorably respond to inflammatory and phagocytic response.

While fever usually is associated with cancer, a consistent fever in a cancer patient usually is attributed to a coexistent infection. It must also be noted that fulminating infection in cancer patients can be present with little fever detected. The significance of this can be seen in Table 12-4 where autopsy has verified the existence of infection. Be-

TABLE 12-4. Infection in cancer patients.

	Acute Leukemia	Chronic Leukemia	Lymphoma	Solid Tumor
Febrile episodes*	5	1	2	1
Febrile days	48	14	23	11
% infected at Autopsy	70	80	75	15–40

Reprinted from Bodey, G. P.: Infections in patients with cancer. In Holland, J. F., and Frei, E. (eds.): Cancer Medicine. Philadelphia: Lea and Febiger, 1974, with permission.

* per 100 hospital days

cause of the general lack of inflammatory response, pneumonia can be present in these patients without clinical recognition; urinary tract infections can be present without pyurea. Other common sites of infection are the oral cavity, the GI tract, and the skin.

The pathogens most common in the cancer patient are the gram-negative bacilli (particularly Pseudomonas aeruginosa and Clostridium perfringens), fungi (particularly Candida albicans and Aspergillus fumigatus), viruses (particularly herpesvirus which causes herpes zoster and herpes simplex), and protozoa (Pneumocystis carinii).

Because the exact locale of the infection in these patients may be unknown and difficult to determine, a working diagnosis is made by the primary presence of a febrile state. Subsequent evaluation should be made through urinalysis, chest x-ray study, and cultures of blood, urine, sputum, skin, and oral lesions, and any other suspected site. Specific antibiotic therapy and antibiotics and leukocyte transfusions as combined therapy are started as early as possible. An immediate increase in caloric intake should be started and maintained, including an increase in total protein. If this is inadequately provided by mouth, a hyperalimentation line should be placed. This is very important. Protective environments for the patient with infection and the vulnerable patient before infection include the usual isolation techniques and also special laminar air flow rooms. The effects of this isolation on the psychologic health of the patient creates another important nursing management concern.

In general, the prophylactic and treatment response to the bacterial infections for the cancer patient show greater promise than treatment of viral and fungal infections. In the latter, both the diagnosis and treatment is difficult. Infection must be considered a major complication for the cancer patient, and particularly the older patient who has cancer.

Exposure to Unintended Radiation

It has long been considered an acceptable admission procedure to allow persons with radium or cesium implants to be placed in a two-bed unit. Often two patients, each with implants, have been placed in the same room. This practice is decreasing, however, with the recognition of increased risk to the staff owing to the increased radiation exposure. However, it is still common practice to have the patient with an implant share the two-bed unit

with an older patient, one who is seen as no longer being in the reproductive years. In light of what is known about the increasing incidence of malignancies in the older person and the possible influences of cumulative exposures to cancerogenic factors over a long lifetime, the wisdom of such a two-bed admission should be carefully considered. When it must occur, assess the safety measures necessary.

Figure 12-13 shows the decreasing areas of radiation exposure as the distance increases from the bedside of a patient with cesium implant in the vagina. It should be remembered that, since the half life of radium and cesium is hundreds of years, there will be no change in this exposure rate from day to day. It is a working constant. The exposure (expressed in millirads or absorbed body units), decreases by each square foot distance from the bed. The inverse square law applies: Each foot away from the source reduces the radiation exposure by each foot squared. For example: increase the distance from the source by 2 feet and the exposure decreases by a factor of 4 (two squared). Thus in Figure 12-13 the millirad readings on the right side of the bed are:

Distance from the bed	Millirads
Up to 1 foot	100
2 feet	50
3 feet	25
4 feet	12, etc.

The Joint Commission of Hospitals Accreditation Manual indicates that beds in a two-bed room can be 3 feet apart, but no less. Note, therefore, that a bed positioned to the right at 3 feet places that bed in the range of 10 to 20 millirads per hour. Given that the patient with the cesium implant has 52 hours of therapy, the roommate will absorb 728 millirads in those 52 hours to the total body. This is considerable exposure, especially to a person in an age group that has already accumulated years of other intermittent radiation absorbed through diagnostic tests, environment, and television.

By contrast, if the bed is placed to the shielded side of the bed the patient will receive only 300 millirads in the same 52 hours. Therefore, the placement of lead shields between beds is necessary. Distance between beds can be increased also, with resultant decrease in millirads. Nurses are urged to monitor such rooms at interval distances with dossimeters as was done to obtain the readings

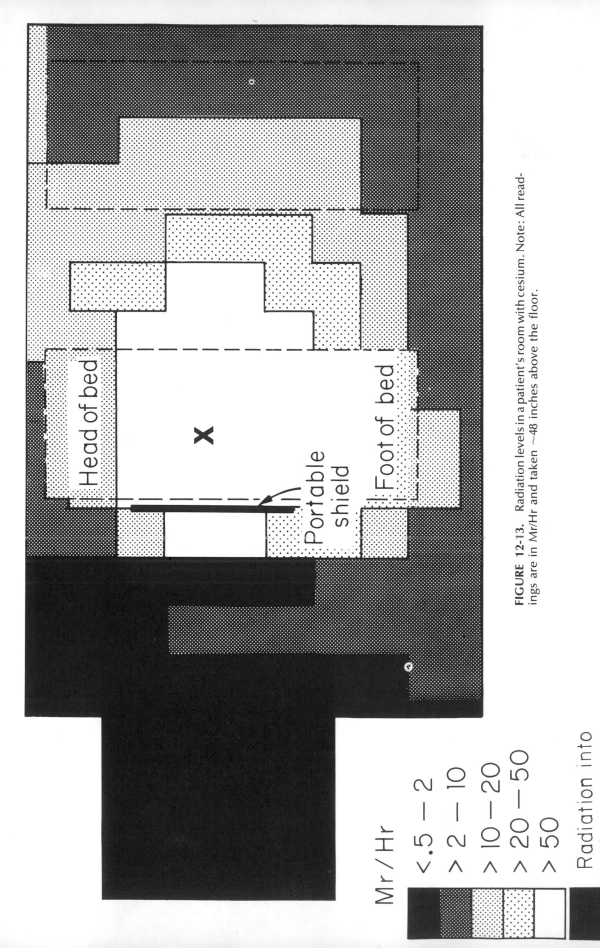

FIGURE 12-13. Radiation levels in a patient's room with cesium. Note: All readings are in Mr/Hr and taken ~48 inches above the floor.

Head of bed

Foot of bed

Portable shield

X

Mr / Hr

< .5 — 2
> 2 — 10
> 10 — 20
> 20 — 50
> 50

Radiation into adjacent room

shown in Figure 12-13. The radiation safety or occupational safety officer in your organization is obliged to help you. When such measurements are taken, the wall in the adjacent room should also be monitored. In Figure 12-13 you will note that there was radiation leakage through the wall from the foot of the bed. A bed patient whose head was at that part of the room would have received 1.0 millirads per hour for the 52 hours or 52 millirads to the head. Elderly or young nurses must be extremely vigilant about controlling patient hazards that may affect their own future health.

Isolation and Sensory Deprivation

During the treatment period, patients who receive implant therapy can experience isolation and sensory deprivation that signals to them the closing off of meaningful contacts. They may see this as only the beginning of isolation and loneliness associated with their disease and potential prognosis. Such fears, realistic or not, may coincide with the patient's or relatives' attitudes toward cancer. As a result of the isolation during treatment the patient may emerge from the hospital a more introverted, seclusive, lonely person, not by choice, but by perceived circumstances.

To minimize or prevent this complication, nurses need to be involved actively in helping the patient to retain an adequate sensory environment and appropriate social contacts, despite the presence of radiation hazards.

In order to maintain low exposures, persons entering the room should position themselves so as to receive minimal radiation. For example, with the vaginal implant, the positioning would be at the head of the bed. From this vantage point, patients can be assisted with their meals, they can be comforted. Urinary tubing and collection bags can be extended as far to the end of the bed as possible. Family (nonpregnant) members can safely sit 2 or more feet away from the patient at the head of the bed and interact in a way that gives comfort and caring to the patient. This is a safer, more rational approach than the fear-motivated procedure of saying "Hello" from the doorway and throwing in the washcloth.

Hope or hopelessness is sown during this period of time. Because of the amount of tissue destruction (protein) desired by the treatment, the patients' ensuing negative nitrogen balance predisposes to a physiologically-based depression (Moore, 1968). All

efforts of the staff and family, therefore, should be directed to minimizing additional daily potentials for increasing this natural depression. Every effort should be made to avoid interpersonal disputes, environmental irritations, social isolation, and the "leper complex."

When therapeutic radioisotopes are used, the same risks of isolation exist. The patient is again in an isolated room. However, using the hospital regulations in effect in any institution, and the necessary safeguards of gowning and sometimes gloving, these patients need not spend endless hours alone.

Because the sense of personal isolation begun in the hospital does not end there, but only portends the future, it becomes important for nurses in institutions to maintain contact with those who follow-up on these patients in ambulatory or home care settings. Hospital nurses on cancer treatment units need to know whether their efforts to create a sharing of the illness experience and to minimize isolation is being effective or not. Feedback from discharged patients, from families, and from health care providers is important.

For reading on loneliness, its diagnosis, and management, see Chapter 25.

Pain

It has been said that pain is always linked with cancer and that it is the pain that the patient fears and dreads. Older persons have had a lifetime of pains: pains of loss, of failure, of hardship, of physical injury. They have coped with pain of many kinds and intensities. Therefore, their pain language is different as they compare and their affect is different from the young (unless very ill) because their energy reserve is knowledgeably limited. "Pain itself passes, and is quickly forgotten (acute pain). Suffering passes, but the fact of having suffered never passes. A man acquainted with the terror of pain is irrevocably changed." (Buytendijk, 1962, p. 28)

Suffering is personal; it is the manner in which a person responds to his experience. Therefore pain relief is very personal and a private language. Lasagna (1968) responds that his patients consider any relief from severe to moderate pain most important to them. This is called "patient gratitude." Least gratitude was expressed for the relief of slight pain or relief of "very severe" to pain when it remained "severe." If patients believe nurses incapable of relieving very severe pain, do they feel it unnecessarily energy-draining to continue communicating the presence of that pain?

The fear of pain and suffering of pain of cancer should be alleviated as much as possible by the regular administration of a pain medication. A routine administration without his request for a drug maintains the patient in comfort, spares him the necessity of proving or justifying his pain, and assures the professional's reliability to care for him.

Too often nurses withhold narcotics from cancer patients because they don't want to make the patient "an addict." This kind of judgment is misplaced responsibility. The goal of the nurse should be to to keep the patient comfortable and alert so that he can use his limited energies as he wishes. If the patient needs medication more frequently and in increasing amounts, give it to him. Doses of narcotics that are increased gradually to otherwise lethal amounts for other patients may be tolerated by the one with cancer. For the terminal patient this is not to be avoided.

Tranquilizers can be used with narcotics. Narcotics can be attenuated. Demerol reduces blood pressure in the elderly and isn't that effective an analgesic for cancer. Therefore it should be avoided. Methadone is used. Marijuana and heroin are being studied for their use in control of pain. An alcohol nerve block may relieve intractable pain.

Loss of Hair

Attendant with some chemotherapeutic drugs, (complete) loss of hair must be expected. A shocking development, it will begin to occur soon after the drug administration and progresses rapidly. The patient should be prepared for the eventuality and given time for a wig, cap, or other head covering arrangement. The American Cancer Society (ACS) can be a resource for wigs. Hair will begin to grow back 6 to 8 months after treatment. It may not be the same texture or color, however.

Crisis

Cancer has many implications. Pain, isolation, disfigurement, and death are no less feared by the older patient. Cancer is capable of precipitating a crisis in the life of every patient and family (Oppenheimer, 1967).

Crises often are handled differently by the older person. Familiar enemies over many years of living, crises are not categorized as with the young into physical, interpersonal, financial, and so forth. The older person knows that, whatever the precipitant that threatens his precarious shell, his coping, whether it's good or bad, will be energy-demanding where energy resources are wanting. Conservation of energy is essential to the old. Therefore, William Thackeray's picture of old Charlotte is typical, who

> Seeing his body borne by on a shutter,
> Went on cutting bread and butter.

The response of the older patient to the diagnosis and treatment of cancer can be unresponsive and seemingly inappropriate in the face of threat, pain, and death. The response *is* appropriate to the perceived need for energy conservation for the long haul, often the lonely journey without loved and committed ones to help. Crises in the old, as in the younger person, reopen life's box of previous trials and testings and losses. He is assaulted anew by them all. The older person meeting one more crisis requires:

1. Dependability and commitment by at least one person to help at regularly expected intervals.

2. Concrete and definite statement of the physical problem(s) so that he can formulate concrete thoughts and statements of its effect on him.

3. Feelings of order and control in those helping him so he can reorder and recontrol his life. (Ambiguities, whispered or inaudible conversations, and nonverbal communications that shut out the patient are very detrimental.) The physical setting, too, should show order and control when the individual feels the disequilibriums of crisis surrounding him. This is why the patient's attempts at order and control through routines should be accepted by the professional.

4. Help to state his problems and plan solutions according to his life needs.

5. An evolving respect of interdependence with another person no matter how weak or frail he feels.

Many who are elderly still maintain strong values of independence. These and others who in the past might have been willing to claim some help have been alone and responsible for many years. Such old do not expect help; they will not *exact* help, i.e., they will not ask. When the values of the social worker or the young nurse expect that need must be expressed and help requested before anything is extended, then this patient population will remain without help until extreme need forces crisis behavior. Bereft of their own strength and ability, such independent old are forced into relationships of dependence because they have exhausted themselves without help. Most crises can be averted and energies conserved. To be able to offer help so that the other does not lose confidence is a great ability. To be able to recognize the weakening stride and the need of support is essential.

Suicide

The question of suicide and the cancer patient is under-investigated and under-reported. There is a higher incidence of both male and female suicides with cancer than the general population. Danto (1972) and Dorpat (1968) reported that cancer is common among elderly suicides.

The classic study of Farberow and coworkers (1970) has reported unusually high suicide potential in men over 65 with cancer of the throat. This occurred when they had low pain tolerance and perceived no emotional support systems since their own physical and psychologic reserves were exhausted. A higher degree of sensory losses was present in patients with voice loss, deafness, and blindness. They also observed that, even when suicidal intent was present in those terminally ill who were weak and practically unable to move, the patients still used a variety of methods to suicide, all requiring vital energies for planning and implementing that plan. Suicide can occur in the most reduced physical state of terminal illness.

Patients seem to assess their own conditions. When the deficits of life outweigh the positive factors, a suicidal decision may result. Thus Schneidman concludes that the evidence of additional supports (providing help through helpers) may be the decisive factor that influences terminal patients over 65 to live out their lives. Prevention is seen as the professional's responsibility:

1. Patients should not be alienated from human contacts. In this study (Farberow and coworkers, 1970), transfer to a private room to "await death" was detrimental.

2. No matter how many others support them, patients should not be written off by doctors who avoid the terminally ill for "those more in need of" his skills. His loss of interest and involvement is interpreted by the terminal patient as one more rejection, the last avenue of hope blocked. Suicidal

decision is precipitated in the isolating disquiet of helplessness and hopelessness. These suicidal old cancer patients were called "implementers" (Farberow, 1970). They had an active need to be in control; they refused and demanded and the busy staff responded by reactions of irritability. Their distrust of his requests was evident by their charting:

Patient *appears* to exaggerate pain.
Insists he is cold; *refused* blankets and *insists* on heating pad instead.
The patients controlled their lives to the end in the only way they perceived possible without help.

3. Interpersonal resources of any institution should be capable of being mobilized to show support to the terminal patient.

4. Exercise in physical care and comfort should be evident and available. Among these should be pain alleviation without fear of addiction.

Suicide potential is highest in older-aged males with head and neck malignancies. It is high if the following factors are present in any stage of disease (Farberow, 1970):

1. Emotional stress
2. Depression, agitation, anxiety, or mood swings
3. Low pain tolerance
4. Excessive demanding and complaining behavior
5. Controlling and directing activity
6. Alert and oriented
7. Exhausted physical and emotional resources including perceived lack of support of staff and family (Farberow, 1970).

For specific crisis intervention and suicide literature, the reader is directed to the references. No cancer patient in crisis or contemplating suicide should be thrown into restraints. Such a person is crying out for human help. Staff or specially trained community crisis workers can supply that lifeline and dignity (Seligman, 1975).

Rehabilitation

Even as diagnostic methods and specific treatment modalities are appropriate and available for the elderly person, so, too, is rehabilitation. Rehabilitation for the elderly must be realistic and attainable. Neither age nor cancer is a deterrent to consideration, planning, and operationalizing a rehabilitation protocol for the patient.

Since the modality of some rehabilitation efforts seems physically oriented, e.g., exercise therapy for the women with mastectomy, it is important to remember that the goals and outcome of that kind of rehabilitation far exceed the range of motion achieved. Rehabilitation affects a patient's physical/psychologic/social and spiritual being. It can potentiate the treatment. It can provide integration at a time a patient needs it most.

> Henri was an interpreter, articulate in four languages. Retired, he "helped out the company" and volunteered a 50 percent work week. He was 74 when he sought dental assistance for a painful mouth lesion. Radical neck dissection for Stage III squamous cell carcinoma of the floor of the mouth was performed in September. Determined and full of trust in his professional care, Henri weathered the pain and the mutilating surgery, just as he endured the effects his surgery had on others. He wanted to live.
>
> Winter was late that year and he had only enough convalescent energy to integrate himself into the seasonal changes of the fall: fading brilliance, nostalgic sounds and smells, measured days, less and less energy, assessment of the harvest. Slowly and carefully he put his garden to bed for the long harsh midwestern winter ahead—for the last time. It was a sad parting.
>
> He had radiation therapy. The incision began to break down, his pain increased, and winter settled in.
>
> During one return clinic visit, a dentist measured him for a temporary prosthesis. Henri returned jubilant and full of hope. "They wouldn't go to all that work and expense if they didn't think I'd make it to spring. I'll see spring again." Strength returned.
>
> Henri lived out his winter. He worked on relationships important to him. He lived till the dawning of capricious spring days. On his window sill, pepper seedlings stood in a row.

Rehabilitation assessment with the elderly patient involves the following:

1. What does he *want* to be able to do (goal)? Henri wanted time for his final integrating tasks of life. (Erikson's stage of age: integration or despair)

2. What is attainable with help? Hope was attainable for Henri; it extended his limited time.

3. What does that help entail? Help with energy-draining activities of dressing change, shaving, and so forth. Help with waning appetite. Support for the

daily vicissitudes, losses, and disappointments that stole energy and hope Henri required for his goal.

Rehabilitation in cancer is a new concept. People are surviving longer following therapy and now resume parts of their previous lives. This makes rehabilitation necessary to insure quality to life. If he does have cancer, what will he do after treatment is given? Or, what will he be like after treatment? For the cancer patient, both disease and treatment create posttreatment problems. Rehabilitation is the answer.

Prostheses

Facial defects created by radiation and/or surgery require long and rigorous surgical procedures during which the patient is unsightly, often voiceless, and certainly isolated and alone. This patient must draw strength and courage from another—family, friend, or staff. He will not be able to make it alone.

Permanent stomal care guidance is needed by patients who have had GI, GU, and Gyn malignancies and surgery. Those with laryngeal stomata also require help. The most functional prosthesis for the individual should be sought as soon as possible. Before that time, the options should be discussed: what types are available, their various advantages, and cost. Rehabilitation is operating with a continuing bank account in contrast to a closed account.

The United Ostomy Association and the International Association of Laryngectomees (IAL) provide information and volunteers to assist with rehabilitation for such patients. The volunteer members of the IAL are elderly themselves and, therefore, can knowledgeably talk to a peer about the difficulties and needs of the age group. The Ostomy group has younger volunteers; an older volunteer should be requested, as well as one who has a stoma as a result of cancer.

Permanent prosthesis for the woman who has had a mastectomy should not be neglected. Though she is old, she will still care how she looks. A prosthesis is also necessary for balanced weight and contour. The Reach to Recovery volunteer, an ACS program, will assist the older woman as she asks for and selects a prosthesis in her store for the first time. They will also reinforce the importance of arm exercising, arm protection (from sun, axillary shaving, blood pressure measurement, blood drawing) and specific wearing apparel.

Voice Retraining

Voice retraining sources usually are identified by the oncology team of professionals. When such arrangements have not been made, the nurse can contact the IAL office in New York for an authorized listing of speech pathologists for the retraining of laryngectomy patients (some specialize only for the stroke patient) and for trained volunteers in their community. The Lost Chord Club, a social club of laryngectomized patients and their spouses, may be helpful. Members of this group also make hospital visits if requested. Local contact can be made through the area American Cancer Society.

Gesturing, writing, whispering, and buccal speech are temporary communication systems, and are to be avoided as poor substitutes for esophageal speech. Unfortunately, the laryngectomized patient often has intermittent follow-through when he re-enters the community, i.e., his own home or a nursing home. His problems are many, isolation may be overwhelming, depression usual, suicide temptations frequent. Both daily and weekly assessments should be made. As one means of restoring relationships, it has been suggested that grandchildren or great-grandchildren visit as often as possible since the ambulatory grandparent will be expected by them to assist as before, show them things as before, and join in fun as before. Happy is the grandparent-patient who has this resource available to him or her.

The most skilled physical therapist and the most functional prosthesis are doomed to failure if rehabilitation does not also help the elderly person to maintain and sustain active involvement with at least one person (hopefully more) who cares about him, and he for that person(s). Without that person, the elderly cancer patient cannot fulfill his basic need to love and be loved and to feel that he is worthwhile to himself and to others. Without at least one person he cannot interpret his life and integrate his life; without that one person he cannot live.

Evaluation

Evaluation of the nursing management for the elderly oncology patient begins with the attitude of the nurse. She must accept that old people with cancer can be treated successfully, that they have the right to participate in decision making about their disease/care/therapy, and that to do so they need to be fully informed. Since cancer is frequently not as fulminating in people over 70 as it is in younger-aged people a slower pace but no less aggressive attack can be mounted. Alternate plans should be outlined listing all the options, other health problems, costs in energy and money—these should be discussed with the patient and his family. The nurse will then support the decision and actions of the patient even though they may not agree with her own values.

Patients who are old and have cancer are not always afraid of dying. They do fear pain and being alone. Both of these can be prevented and may be the cornerstone to effective management for the cancer patient.

BIBLIOGRAPHY

Adler, W. H.: Aging and immune function. Bio Science 25:652–657, 1975, pp. 652–657.

Aker, S., and Tilmont G.: A Guide to Good Nutrition During and After Chemotherapy and Radiation. Seattle: University of Washington, 1979, ed. 2.

Allen, A., et al.: An investigation of the clinical and histological effects of selected dentifrices on human palatal mucosa. J. Periodontics 46:102–112, 1975.

Bahnson, C. B.: Epistemological perspectives of physical disease from the psychodynamic point of view. Am. J. Public Health 64:1034–1040, 1974.

Banerjee, A. K.: Geriatric medicine. In Israels, M. C., and Delamore, I. W. (eds.): Haematological Aspects of Systemic Disease. Philadelphia: W. B. Saunders Co., 1976, pp. 408–419.

Bergevin, P.: The increasing problem of malignancy in the elderly. Med. Clin. N. Am., 60:1241–1251, 1976.

Bistrian, B., et al.: Prevalence of malnutrition in general medical patients. J.A.M.A. 235:1567–1570, 1976.

Bodey, G. P.: Infections in patients with cancer. In Holland, J. and Frei, E. (eds.): Cancer Medicine. Philadelphia: Lea and Feibiger, 1974.

Brewer, J. I., Molbo, D., and Gerbie, A.: Gynecologic Nursing. St. Louis: C. V. Mosby Co., 1966.

Buytendijk, F. J. J.: Pain, Its Modes and Functions. Chicago: University of Chicago Press, 1952.

Cancer in Washington and Alaska. Seattle: Washington-Alaska Regional Medical Program, 1973.

Conger, A., and Wells, M.: Radiation and aging effect on taste structure and function. Radiation Res. 37:31–49, 1969.

Copeland, E. M. and Dudrick, S.: Cancer: Nutritional concepts. Seminars in Oncology 2:4, 329–335, 1975.

Cullen, J. W., Fox, B. H, and Isom, R. N.: Cancer: The Behavioral Dimensions. New York: Raven Press, 1976.

Danto, B.: The Cancer Patient and Suicide. J. Thanatol. 2: 596–600, 1972.

Davenport, J. C.: The oral distribution of Candida in denture stomatitis. Br. Dental Journal, 129:151–156, 1970.

DeWys, W. D., and Walters, K.: Abnormalities of taste sensation in cancer patients. Cancer 36:1888–1896, 1975.

Dorpat, T., Anderson, W., and Ripley, H.: The relationship of physical illness to suicide. In Resnik, H. (ed.): Suicide Behaviors. Boston: Little, Brown & Co., 1968, pp. 209–219.

Ehret, C. F.: Significance of circadian rhythms. In Bruce, A., and Sacher, G. (eds.): Aging and Levels of Biological Organization. Chicago: University of Chicago Press, 1965, pp. 209–217.

Fernandez, G., and Schwartz, J.: Immune responsiveness and hematologic malignancy in the elderly. Med. Clin. N. Am. 60:1253–1271, 1976.

Fox, B.: Premorbid psychological factors as related to incidence of cancer. Field Study and Statistics Program. Bethesda, Md.: National Institutes of Health, National Cancer Institute, 1976.

Franks, A. S. T., and Bjorn, H.: Geriatric Dentistry. Oxford: Blackwell Scientific Pub., 1973.

Hardin, B. K.: A Description of Oral Health Using a Prescribed Protocol of Oral Hygiene in Young Oncology Patients Receiving Bone Marrow Transplantation. Unpublished Master's thesis. University of Washington School of Nursing, Seattle, 1976.

Hijmans, W., and Hollander, C. F.: The pathogenic role of age-related immune dysfunctions. In Makinodan, T. (ed.): Immunology and Aging. N. Y., Plenum Medical Book Co., 1977.

Johnson, T. (ed.): The Complete Poems of Emily Dickinson. Boston: Little, Brown & Co., 1960, p. 323.

Kowitz, G. M., Lucatoro, F. M., Cherrick, H. M.: Effects of Mouth Wash on the Oral Soft Tissues, J. Oral Med., 31:2, 1976, pp. 47–50.

Lanzotti, V., et al.: Cancer chemotherapeutic response and intravenous hyperalimentation. Cancer Chemotherapy Reports, Part I. 59, 437–439, 1975.

Lasagna, L.: The clinical measurement of pain. Ann. N. Y. Acad. Sci. 86:28–37, 1968.

Lindquist, V.: A Descriptive Study of the Effects of Radiation Therapy on Saliva and Oral Mucosa in Cancer Patients. Unpublished Master's thesis, University of Washington School of Nursing, Seattle, 1978.

Mackay, I. R.: Aging and immunological function in man. Gerontologia 18:285–304, 1972.

Moe, R.: Personal Communication, 1978.

Moore, F. D.: Metabolic Care of the Surgical Patient. Philadelphia: W. B. Saunders Co., 1968. (This is an excellent reference even though it was published several years ago.)

Moos, R.: Coping With Physical Illness. New York: Plenum Medical Book Co., 1977.

Oppenheimer, J.: Use of crisis intervention in casework with the cancer patient and his family. Social Work 12:50, 1967.

Ringborg, U, Lambert, B., Swanbeck, G.: DNA repair in conditions associated with malignancy. In Nieburgs, H. (ed.): Prevention and Detection of Cancer, Vol. I. New York: Marcel Dekker, 1977.

Rosenberg, T.: "How Can I Not Be Among You," Grenwich, Connecticut: Eccentric Circle Cinema, 1972. 16mm film.

Rullis, I., Schaeffer, J. A., Lilien, O.: Incidence of prostatic carcinoma in the elderly. Urology 6:295–297, 1975.

Schein, P., et al.: Nutritional complications of cancer and its treatment. Seminars in Oncology 2:337–341, 1975.

Schmale, A. H., and Iker H.: Hopelessness as a predictor of cervical cancer. Soc. Sci. Med. 5:95–100, 1971.

Schum, Cynthia: A Description of Oral Health in Patients Receiving Chemotherapy for Treatment of Cancer. Unpublished Master's thesis, University of Washington School of Nursing, Seattle, 1977.

Seligman, M. E.: Helplessness. San Francisco: W. H. Freeman Co., 1975.

Shouten, J.: Important factors in the examination and care of old patients. J. Am. Geriatrics Soc. 23:180–183, 1975.

Solomon, G. F., Amkraut, A. A., and Kasper, L.: Immunity, emotions and stress, with special reference of stress effects on immunity system. Ann. Clin. Res. 6:313–322, 1974.

Theologides, A.: Why cancer patients have anorexia. Geriatrics 31:69–71, 1976.

Third National Cancer Survey: Incidence Data. Monograph 41, DHEW Publication 75–787. National Institutes of Health, National Cancer Institute, Bethesda, Md., 1975, pp. 100–135; 450–451.

TNM, Classification of Malignant Tumours. International Union Against Cancer, Geneva, Switzerland. 1974.

Wood, N. K, and Goaz, P.: Differential Diagnosis of Oral Lesions. St. Louis: C. V. Mosby Co., 1975, pp. 198–211.

General References

Burkhalter, P., and Donley, D.: Dynamics of Oncology Nursing. New York: McGraw-Hill Book Co., 1978.

Clark, R. L., and Howe, C.: Cancer Patient Care. Chicago: Year Book Medical Publishers, 1976. (Though not written for specific problems of the elderly, it provides rationale for interventions necessary before, during, and after surgery, radiation, chemotherapy, and immunotherapy, as well as combination. It is not a nursing text; implications for nursing can be drawn from the text.)

Clinical Oncology, A. Manual for Students and Doctors. Committee on Professional Education of UICC (eds.). New York: Springer-Verlag, 1973. (Readable, reliable, easy-to-find information handbook, outlining malignancies of all sites by risk factors, epidemiology, diagnoses, treatment, and prognosis. 89 figures. Recommended.)

Davidoff, A., Winkler, S., and Lee, M. (eds.): Dentistry for the Special Patient, the Aged, Chronically Ill and Handicapped. Philadelphia: W. B. Saunders Co., 1972.

Donovan, M., and Pierce, S.: Cancer Care Nursing. New York: Appleton-Century-Crofts, 1976.

Franks, A. S., and Hedegard, B.: Geriatric Dentistry. Oxford: Blackwell Scientific Publications, 1973.

Holland, J. F., and Frei, E. (eds.): Cancer Medicine. Philadelphia: Lea and Febiger, 1974. (Very complete, all aspects. A large book. Ask your medical staff to purchase and use their copy.)

Rubin, P. (ed.): Clinical Oncology for Students and Physicians, A Multidisciplinary Approach, ed. 5. Rochester, New York: University of Rochester, 1978. (Published by American Cancer Society, paperbound, outlined, references.)

Sutnick, A., and Engstrom, P. (eds.): Oncologic Medicine, Clinical Topics, and Practical Management. Baltimore: University Park Press, 1976.

TNM: Classification of Malignant Tumours, ed. 2. International Union Against Cancer, Geneva, Switzerland, 1974. $1.00. (Indispensible guide for the individual or nursing unit library. It clarifies all complexities of staging, grading into a unified classification.)

Epidemiology and Incidence

Fraumeni, J.: Persons at High Risk of Cancer. New York: Academic Press, 1975.

Holland, J. F., and Frei, E. (eds.): Cancer Medicine. Philadelphia: Lea and Febiger, 1974. (Very complete, all aspects. A large book. Ask your medical staff to purchase and use their copy.)

1978 Facts and Figures. New York: American Cancer Society, 1978.

Old, L.: Cancer Immunology. Scientific American 236:62–79, 1977.

Ringborg, U., Lambert, B., and Swanbeck, G.: DNA repair in conditions associated with malignancy: aging and actenic keratosis. In Nieburgs, H. (ed.): Prevention and Detection of Cancer, Vol. 1. New York: Marcel Dekker, 1977.

Third National Cancer Survey, Incidence Data. DHEW Publication 75–787. National Institutes of Health, National Cancer Institute, 1975.

Waterhouse, J. (ed.): Cancer Handbook of Epidemiology and Prognosis. Edinburgh: Churchill-Livingstone, 1974.

Special Topics

Chemotherapy

Greenspan, E.: Clinical Cancer Chemotherapy. New York: Raven Press, 1975.

Carter, S., and Bakowski, M.: Chemotherapy of Cancer. New York: John Wiley & Sons, 1977. (Useful handbook (paper) of anti-cancer drugs, administration, toxicity, and symptoms. Also an overview of treatment considerations for cancer by location, histology, and combination protocol.)

Crisis Intervention and Suicide

Ebersole, P.: Crisis intervention in the elderly. In Burnside, I. (ed.): Nursing and the Aged. New York: McGraw-Hill Book Co., 1976.

Farberow, N., Schneidman, E., and Leonard, C.: Suicide among patients with malignant neoplasms. In Schneidman, E., Farberow, N. and Litman, R. (eds.): The Psychology of Suicide. New York: Science House, 1970.

Kastenbaum, R., and Schaberg, B.: Hope, survival and the caring environment. In Jeffers, F., and Palmore, E. (eds.): Prediction of Life Span. New York: D. C. Heath, 1975.

Oppenheimer, J.: Use of crisis intervention with the cancer patient. Social Work 12:2, 1967. (An older article, but no one has written it better.)

Parad, H. J. (ed.): Crisis Intervention: Selected Readings. New York: Family Service Association of America, 1965. (If you want only one book on crisis intervention, this must be the book.)

A Guidebook for Local Communities Participating in Operation Independence. Washington D.C.: National Council on the Aging, 1975. (Description and addresses of organizations, councils, and cluster services to assist the elderly person/patient—all states. Bibliography.)

Nutrition

Aker, S., and Tilmont, T.: A Guide to Good Nutrition During and After Chemotherapy and Radiation, ed. 2. Seattle: University of Washington, 1979. (Recipes combat anorexia and nausea. Each spoonful is nutritionally loaded. Spiral. Recommended for staff and patients.)

Caird, F. J., Gudge, G. T., and Macleod, C.: Pointers to possible malnutrition in the elderly at home. Gerontology Clinic 1:47–54, 1975.

Conference on nutrition and cancer therapy. Cancer Research 37:7 Part II, 1977. (Selected content: Anorexia and cachexia in neoplastic disease; nutritional problems associated with GI, GU, endocrine cancers. Nutritional consequences of radiation, chemotherapy. Determination of nutritional needs. Nutritional management [oral enteral feeding, parenteral]. Excellent and important. Nutrition is placed in primary role for successful cancer management. Consider it a cancer nutrition book.)

Conger, A., and Wells, M.: Radiation and aging effect on taste structure and function. Radiation Research 37:31–49, 1969.

Copeland, E., and Dudnick, S.: Nutritional aspects of cancer. Current Problems in Cancer 1:5–47, 1976. (Good exposure of issues cited for Conference on Nutrition and Cancer Therapy [mentioned previously].)

DeWys, W., and Walters, K.: Abnormalities of taste sensation in cancer patients. Cancer 36:1888–1896, 1975.

Oral Problems

Pindborg, J.: Atlas of Diseases of Oral Mucosa, ed. 2. Philadelphia: W. B. Saunders Co., 1973. (Excellent descriptions accompanied by true color illustrations of oral conditions of malnutrition, trauma, infection, and malignancy. A necessary resource book wherever elderly patients are cared for.)

Ostomy Care

Mahoney, J.: Guide to Ostomy Nursing Care. Boston: Little, Brown & Co., 1976.

Radiation

Radiation Oncology.—Special issue. Cancer 26:5, September–October, 1976. (Eight articles describe present and future status of radiology in primary and combination therapy. Glossary and diagrams.)

Specific Sites

Bergevin, P.: The increasing problem of malignancy in the elderly—New concepts in diagnosis and management. Med. Clin. N. Am. 60:1241–1251, 1976.

Cope, O.: The Breast: Its Problems. Benign and Malignant and How to Deal with Them. Boston: Houghton-Mifflin Co., 1977.

Fernandez, G. and Schwartz, J.: Immune responsiveness and hematologic malignancy in the elderly. Med. Clin. N. Am. 60:6, 1976, pp. 1253–1269.

Kragelund, E.: Resectability, operative mortality and survival of patients in old age with carcinoma of the colon and rectum, Dis. Colon and Rectum 2:617–621, 1974.

Leis, H. P.: The diagnosis of breast cancer. New York: American Cancer Society, 1977. (Illustrated 26-page booklet. Bibliography. Very good synopsis and illustrations of signs.)

Pierson, R.: Surgery for gynecologic malignancy in the aged. Obstet. Gynecol. 5:523–527, 1975.

Shedd, D. P., et al.: The nurses role in rehabilitation of cancer patients with facial defects. American Cancer Society, 1974. (Illustrated)

Patient Readings

Aker, S., Tilmont, G., and Harrison, V.: A Guide to Good Nutrition During and After Chemotherapy and Radiation, ed. 2. Seattle: University of Washington, 1979. (Spiral. Distributed by Dietary Department, Fred Hutchinson Cancer Research Center, 1124 Columbia Street, Seattle, WA 98104.)

Cope, O.: The Breast: Its Problems, Benign and Malignant, and How to Deal with Them. Boston: Houghton-Mifflin, 1976.

Keith, R. L., and Shane, H.: Looking forward—A guidebook for the Laryngectomee. Rochester, MN: Mayo Foundation, 1977. (Line drawings show anatomy, anatomic change by surgery, stoma care. Text includes preparations for surgery and after, sexuality, rehabilitation, how to make stoma bibs, recipes, glossary.

Strax, Phillip. Early Detection: Breast Cancer is Curable. New York: Signet Books, 1974.

Facts on Breast Cancer. American Cancer Society, 1978.

Facts on Uterine Cancer. American Cancer Society, 1978.

Facts on Colorectal Cancer. American Cancer Society, 1978.

Facts on Lung Cancer. American Cancer Society, 1978.

Unproven Methods of Cancer Management. American Cancer Society, 1976.

Also—Always call local American Cancer Society for new or additional patient pamphlets/literature available without charge. Nurses should request placement on the mailing list to receive Ca, an excellent journal on cancer, by contacting the local ACS Division.

APPENDIX 12-1
ORAL EXAMINATION RECORDING FORM

The Oral Examination Recording Form, which follows, has been designed diagrammatically for ease in documenting abnormalities of color, texture, tenderness, and/or lesions in the many specific areas of the soft tissues of the oral cavity. Recorded descriptions lack precise location, size, and changing characteristics without such a tool. This tool, which emphasizes soft tissues rather than the hard tissues, e.g., teeth, can be used whenever oral assessments are performed.

This tool can be used advantageously at the initial assessment of the cancer patient. It is a permanent documentation of the pre-therapy condition of the mouth and can be compared with all sequential examinations, which will also be documented on the tool. No data now exists regarding specific oral changes and their extent in the old cancer patient's mouth. Careful documentation should be made and maintained by all health providers to older patients. The form shown here is a simplified version; a copy of the form for use with computer feed-in is available from the author of this chapter (Doris M. Molbo, University of Washington, Seattle WA 98195).

The diagrams of the soft tissues follow the sequence of the oral examination, i.e., lips; left and right buccal mucosa, anterior midline to posterior fossa; soft and hard palate; pharyngeal arches and pharynx; tongue, superior aspect; tongue, inferior aspect and floor of mouth; maxillary and mandibular gingiva. A solid filled outline of the lesion is drawn within the specific location, giving the shape and approximate size within the territorial subdivisions of the tissues provided by the drawings. By using dental and medical descriptive terminology, observations can be communicated with reliability and authenticity. In the absence of the computerized format, these descriptions can be abbreviated so that description accompanies the outlined shape, approximate size, and locale of each lesion or site of bleeding. An example is shown on page 245, where vesicles and ulceration are identified and described in lips and buccal mucosa.

ORAL EXAMINATION RECORDING FORM ©

Lips:

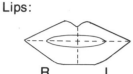

R   L

Buccal Mucosa:

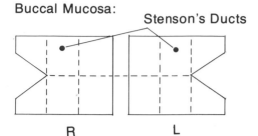

Stenson's Ducts

R   L

Hard and Soft Palate:

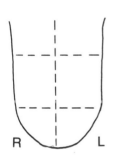

Gumline

R   L

Uvula

Pharyngeal Arches and Pharynx:

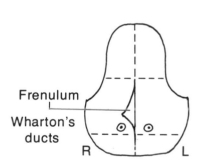

Uvula
Arches

R   L

KEY

Tissue Color

0—Pink (normal)
1—Red (increased)
2—White (decreased)
3—Blue (cyanotic)
4—Yellow
5—Brown
6—Other

Lesions

0—No lesions
1—Inflammation
2—Ulcer
3—Abrasion
4—Bulla
5—Ecchymosis
6—Macule
7—Nodule
8—Patch
9—Petechiae
10—Plaque
11—Tumor
12—Vesicle

Texture

0—Smooth, wet
1—Dry
2—Furry
3—Cracked

Bleeding

0—No bleeding
1—Minimal
2—Moderate
3—Severe

Tenderness

0—No tenderness
1—Minimal
2—Moderate
3—Severe

Tongue and Floor of Mouth:

R   L

Superior aspect

Frenulum

Wharton's ducts

R   L

Inferior aspect

Gingiva:

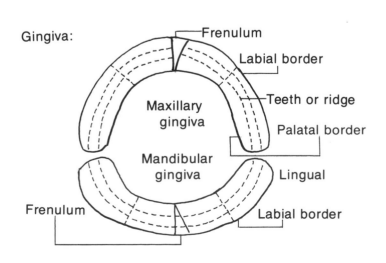

Frenulum

Labial border

Teeth or ridge

Palatal border

Maxillary gingiva

Mandibular gingiva

Lingual

Frenulum

Labial border

An example of how to use an oral examination tool.

Oral Assessment: Patient complains of mouth pain that makes eating difficult. He also has itching and tenderness on left upper lip.

Small vesicles are seen on upper lip at corner and extend into buccal aspect of mouth, upper left. Color surrounding vesicles normal. Small 0.5 cm. (or measured by inch) ulcer noted on upper right buccal mucosa. Inflammation ×3 and very painful to any touch (Pain ×3). Right and left lower buccal mucosa normal color and tissue. Lips, gingivae, tongue, and palate normal.

Assessment: See completed form below.

Plan:

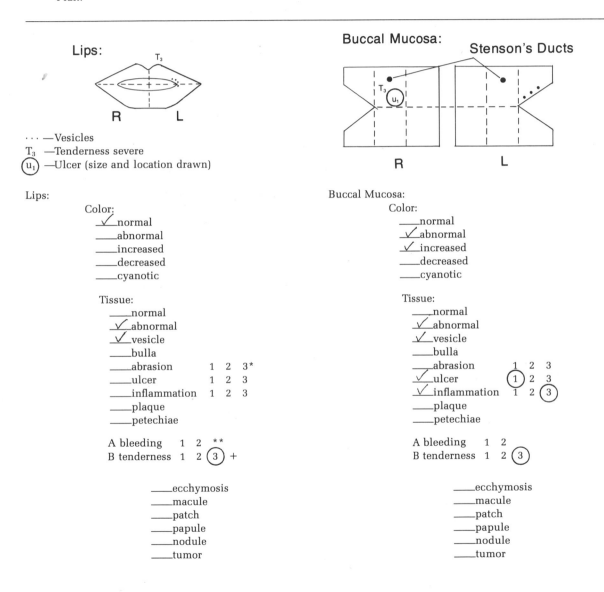

Lips:

Buccal Mucosa:

Stenson's Ducts

R   L

··· —Vesicles
T_3 —Tenderness severe
u_1 —Ulcer (size and location drawn)

Lips:
- Color:
  - ✓ normal
  - ___ abnormal
  - ___ increased
  - ___ decreased
  - ___ cyanotic

- Tissue:
  - ___ normal
  - ✓ abnormal
  - ✓ vesicle
  - ___ bulla
  - ___ abrasion   1 2 3*
  - ___ ulcer   1 2 3
  - ___ inflammation   1 2 3
  - ___ plaque
  - ___ petechiae

- A bleeding   1 2 **
- B tenderness 1 2 (3) +

  - ___ ecchymosis
  - ___ macule
  - ___ patch
  - ___ papule
  - ___ nodule
  - ___ tumor

Buccal Mucosa:
- Color:
  - ___ normal
  - ✓ abnormal
  - ✓ increased
  - ___ decreased
  - ___ cyanotic

- Tissue:
  - ___ normal
  - ✓ abnormal
  - ✓ vesicle
  - ___ bulla
  - ___ abrasion   1 2 3
  - ✓ ulcer   (1) 2 3
  - ✓ inflammation   1 2 (3)
  - ___ plaque
  - ___ petechiae

- A bleeding   1 2
- B tenderness 1 2 (3)

  - ___ ecchymosis
  - ___ macule
  - ___ patch
  - ___ papule
  - ___ nodule
  - ___ tumor

* 1. minimal 2. moderate 3. maximum
** bleeding 1. intermittent 2. continuous
+ tenderness—by patient evaluation

13

Cardiovascular Problems

Judith Atwood

QUICK REVIEW

CONGESTIVE HEART FAILURE (CHF)

DESCRIPTION	A collection of signs and symptoms which together represent decompensation of the heart as a pump in a patient with underlying heart disease.
ETIOLOGIC FACTORS	Heart disease. Precipitating factors can include *diseases* such as cardiac, renal, respiratory, and hepatic; *management failures* including drug toxicity, fluid and electrolyte imbalances, and inappropriate nutrition; *environmental factors* (cardiac risk factor management) such as smoking, poor nutrition (obesity, malnutrition), and stress; *activity* inappropriate to the patient's needs; *psyche* including depression, fear, and denial.
HIGH RISK	CHF risks increase with age owing to prevalence of atherosclerosis in aged.
DYNAMICS	Leads to abnormal retention of water and salt with congestion and changes in function of various organs and tissues (lungs, kidneys, liver, other parts of GI tract, peripheral edema)
SYMPTOMS	Dyspnea on exertion, orthopnea, paroxysmal nocturnal dyspnea, coughing/wheezing, hemoptysis. Anorexia, nausea, and vomiting. Oliguria. Edema. Chronic fatigue, weakness, and changes in mentation.
SIGNS	Cardiac enlargement, abnormal cardiac sounds and precordial activity, fine moist rales, less perfusion at lung bases, distended neck veins.
DIFFERENTIAL DIAGNOSIS	Noncardiac disease with similar signs and symptoms often develops more slowly, CHF more rapidly.
PROGNOSIS	Poor with hypertension, especially women, atrial fibrillation, aortic valve disease, pulmonary heart disease, emboli. In elderly: generally good for normal life span since those with severe cardiac disease generally die earlier. Also related to ability to appropriately alter lifestyle.
NURSING MANAGEMENT	Reduce cardiac workload, increase myocardiac contractility (effective taking of digitalis glycoside), reduce sodium and water retention (diuretics and diet).
EVALUATION	Reduction in edema, dyspnea on exertion, other signs and symptoms. Balancing work load with capability in a way that is satisfying to the individual. Satisfaction with diet, work coping with signs and symptoms, compliance with regimen.

QUICK REVIEW

ACUTE ARTERIAL OBSTRUCTIVE DISEASE

ETIOLOGIC
FACTORS

Usually arteriosclerotic vascular disease and its sequelae.

HIGH RISK

Persons with arteriosclerosis and associated risk factors, e.g., diabetes.

DYNAMICS

Emboli or thrombi suddenly obstruct an artery with rapid tissue ischemia distal to occlusion.

SIGNS AND
SYMPTOMS

Early: Dramatic onset.
    Pain: burning, aching, severe, steady, aggravated by motion
    Color: pale, then cyanotic
    Temperature: cold
    Edema: minimal
    Pulses: absent distal to occlusion
    Function: sensory and muscle decreased
Late: Tenderness decreased, muscles soft, paralysis, swelling, flexion contractures, resistance shifts from some marked to none. Flaccid.

DIFFERENTIAL
DIAGNOSIS

Venous thrombosis.
Prognosis
Untreated: 50% will have gangrene, 40% mortality rate
Treated: Variable, depends in part on promptness of emergency treatment

MEDICAL
MANAGEMENT

Surgical removal of embolus or thrombus, may need amputation, anticoagulant therapy, prescribe coumarins indefinitely

NURSING
MANAGEMENT

Protect limb from trauma and pressure. Keep at room temperature. Keep limb level in relation to body. Monitor effects of anticoagulants—bleeding. Monitor for potential drug interaction. (See Chronic Obstructive Disease for living with ischemia.)

EVALUATION

Individuals at high risk should know signs and symptoms. Should know how to reach appropriate health care resources and have phone or dependable way of contacting another person. Injury to limb is prevented.

QUICK REVIEW

CHRONIC OBSTRUCTIVE VASCULAR DISEASE

DESCRIPTION   Ischemia owing to gradual reduction in blood vessel caliber.

ETIOLOGIC FACTORS   Atherosclerosis, thrombophlebitis.

HIGH RISK   Elderly, diabetics, hypertensives, obese persons, sedentary, hyperlipidemics.

DYNAMICS   *Arterial:* Atheromatous plaques develop on intima of arteries, particularly at joints and bifurcation areas and more commonly in lower extremities. Plaques progressively occlude lumen and/or become site for thrombus formation. Ischemia results with fibrosis and atrophy. Collateral circulation may develop, protecting tissue integrity.

Venous: Development of superficial thrombophlebitis may lead to extension to deep venous system and high risk of pulmonary emboli.

SIGNS AND SYMPTOMS

		Arterial	*Venous*
Skin & tissue of limb		Thin, shiny, atrophic; nails thicken and ridged; hair disappears	Bronzing in ankle area
		Ulcers tend to locate on toes or trauma risk areas on foot	Ulcers tend to locate in ankle area
Color of limb		Pale and grayish on elevation; slowly becoming dusky red on dependency	Normal; may be cyanotic on dependency
		Advanced: bluish gray mottling unchanged by position	
Skin temp.		Cool	Normal
Edema		Rare	Present
Pulses		Decreased or absent distal to obstruction	Present but may be hard to feel 2° fibrosis
Pain		*Exercise:* on walking identifiable distance. Increased by speed and incline; relieved by rest. Symptoms: cramps, aching fatigue, tightness, numbness	None (minimal)
		Rest: (Advanced disease) gnawing, persistent, severe, always in foot. Aggravated by elevation. Coldness, numbness, stocking anesthesia	

PROGNOSIS   *Arterial:* Dependent on development of collateral circulation.
Venous: Depends on severity of disease and careful care.

COMPLICATIONS   *Arterial:* Painful ulcers, immobilization, ischemic neuropathy.
Venous: Pulmonary emboli, stasis ulcers.

NURSING MANAGEMENT   Directed to modify ADL to maintain circulation and prevent complications and to live as effectively as possible with restricted circulation.
Graduated walking program (venous only). Diet for normal weight goal; not prescribed in atherosclerosis. Decreased or ceased smoking. Pain control for satisfying sleep and

Continued on next page.

Quick Review (*Cont.*)

maintenance of ADL and lifestyle (arterial primarily). Meticulous foot care (see Chapter 23). Management of lifestyle with ischemic arterial ulcers: bedrest, pain and infection prescriptions (soaks, antibiotics—based on cultures). Knowledge of and compliance with restriction of hot water and heating appliances to lower extremities.

EVALUATION (NURSING)

Actual adjustment of ADL and lifestyle to include walking regimen, weight reduction diet, changed smoking patterns. Success in control of pain—adequate sleep, data on effect of pain on lifestyle. Effectiveness in coping with decreased mobility in ADL. Knowledge of and skill in foot care; and/or use of support systems; status of footwear. Availability and use of necessary support systems to manage ADL with restrictions as a result of ulcers/gangrene. Skin and tissue integrity. Ulcer healing.

QUICK REVIEW

VARICOSE VEINS

DESCRIPTION

Dilation of superficial leg veins (saphenous system).

ETIOLOGIC FACTORS

Structural weakness in venous valves leading to incompetence and increased hydrostatic pressure plus weakness in venous walls.

HIGH RISK

Elderly, family history of varicosities, parous females, occupations that have required long standing, e.g., barber, surgeon, clerk.

SIGNS AND SYMPTOMS

Enlarged tortuous veins in legs, telangiectases, aching legs, leg fatigue, edema, heavy blood loss.

DIFFERENTIAL DIAGNOSIS

Determination of competence of saphenous and communicating systems.

COMPLICATIONS

Rupture of a vein with heavy blood loss and fear. Superficial venous thrombosis which can lead to chronic venous insufficiency and/or ulcers. May also spread to deep venous system and possibly result in pulmonary emboli.

MEDICAL MANAGEMENT

Vein ligation/stripping. Injection of hypertonic solution. May elect not to treat directly.

NURSING MANAGEMENT

Introducing support hose or TED stockings. Exercise/activity schedule to enhance venous return and minimize stasis by avoiding prolonged sitting or standing. Development of a functional plan with patient/family/neighbors, plus the associated skills to deal with the possibility of a vein rupture.

EVALUATION

Knows actions needed to manage heavy blood loss or complications. Manages ADL and treatment regimen. Knows signs and symptoms of venous thrombosis and seeks therapy. Tender loving care of extremities.

CONGESTIVE HEART FAILURE

Description

Congestive heart failure (CHF) is a collection of signs and symptoms rather than a disease. The signs and symptoms represent a level of failure of the heart as a pump in a patient who has some type of underlying heart disease. None of the manifestations is present only in heart failure; thus it is not possible to point to any particular symptom and make the diagnosis. The findings can roughly be divided into abnormal cardiac signs (these usually occur early and require specialized cardiovascular nursing skills to detect) and the congestive symptoms of other body organs or systems. The usual affected organs include the lungs, kidneys, liver (GI tract), and sometimes, in the elderly, the brain, where dysfunction is manifested by symptoms of poor perfusion such as confusion.

Congestive heart failure is a continuum of conditions varying from mild chronic failure to acute failure. The latter can present suddenly as pulmonary edema or even cardiogenic shock, while the most difficult-to-treat variant of the former is generally refractory heart failure. This is a state in which decompensation continues despite adherence to all of the standard therapeutic measures. These patients need a comprehensive medical workup to determine if the cardiac problem might be amenable to surgery, to identify extra-cardiac diagnoses which need treatment, or to identify and treat other complications which have developed. If no treatable problem can be identified, management will be a particular challenge, calling on all of the resources of the nurse. The prognosis is poor.

Etiologic factors

The first consideration in determining the etiologic factors of congestive heart failure is knowing what type of heart disease the patient has, the signs and symptoms of that disease, and how it precipitates heart failure.

CARDIAC DISEASE. Atherosclerotic and hypertensive heart diseases are responsible for over half of the cases of heart failure in the elderly. Recent myocardial infarction is another important cause of CHF in this age group. Other heart diseases that can precipitate CHF include ischemic disease, rheumatic disease and other valvular problems, congenital disease, and cardiac muscle and tissue diseases of all origins (e.g., pericarditis, myocarditis, endocarditis, cardiomyopathies). Cor pulmonale and other pulmonary diseases as well as an entity called senile heart disease, thought by some clinicians to be related to the involutional process of aging on the heart, can also result in heart failure. (The latter entity is not universally accepted as existing.) Since a discussion of the characteristics of each of these diseases is beyond the scope of this presentation, the nurse wishing more knowledge about them is advised to consult appropriate parts of this book and nursing and medical texts, some of which are cited at the end of this chapter.

NONCARDIAC DISEASE. Noncardiac diseases or conditions can exacerbate or precipitate congestive failure in a susceptible patient. Important among these are renal, liver, and lung diseases. Paget's disease of bones, hyperthyroidism, skin disorders, diabetes mellitus, cerebral thromboses, major infections, surgery, anemia, and prostate problems also can be implicated in some patients.

IATROGENIC DISEASE. Management failures can be precipitated by iatrogenic factors. Drug toxicity, especially from digitalis preparations, serum electrolyte imbalances from a variety of causes, steroid therapy for other problems, and an inappropriately high intake of salt and water—all can cause the patient to do poorly. New arrhythmias (or an increase in existant one) may make the CHF worse. These arrhythmias can be caused by the drug therapy prescribed to treat the failure or by a rapid response to therapeutic modalities. Generally the geriatric patient is less able to compensate as quickly as a younger patient.

ENVIRONMENTAL FACTORS. Failure to modify some of the so-called cardiac risk factors (diet, cigarette smoking, level of activity, stress, obesity, and so forth) can contribute to heart failure. Stress and level of activity can add to existing problems in the elderly. In addition to the propensity to adapt less readily, the elderly often have multiple system diseases or disability and, thus, compensatory mechanisms are readily overwhelmed. Therefore, because of the precarious state of many aged patients, the best management is careful attention to all parameters to prevent the onset of overt failure.

SOCIOECONOMIC FACTORS. The last category of etiologic factors can broadly be termed socioeconomic. Malnutrition, economic constraints, emotional stress, inappropriate physical activity (both too much and too little), and depression or lack of interest in life can contribute to management difficulties.

These factors are a fruitful area for significant nursing assistance to the patient.

Dynamics

The results of congestive heart failure are fairly clear. However, a single satisfactory explanation for the abnormal retention of salt and water and the resultant changes in the functioning of various organs and tissues has not yet been found. This is an area of much current research. The oversimplified theories of "forward failure" and "backward failure" still have some usefulness in understanding congestive heart failure. It is important to remember that neither theory is wholly correct and both are useful only in so far as they assist the clinician to develop a limited understanding of the signs and symptoms of the entity. The *forward theory* postulates that the signs and symptoms are a result of inadequate cardiac output into the systemic circulation. This results in the retention of salt and water because of diminished renal perfusion which, in turn, reduces glomerular filtration rate and stimulates the renin-angiotensin-aldosterone system, resulting in the reabsorption of sodium and water. The *backward theory* postulates that the end diastolic volume of one (or both ventricles) raises when the heart fails. This leads to an increase in the pressure and volume of the atrium and venous system "behind" the failing ventricle. The increased pressure and volume in the venous and, thus, capillary system then leads to sodium and water retention and the transudation of fluid into the interstitial spaces. Currently, as neither theory is totally correct, when the symptoms of venous congestion are most prominent, usually chronic or backward failure is said to be present. When the symptoms of decreased cardiac output are the most prominent, then acute or forward failure is said to be present.

Clinically CHF is often described as either "left sided" or "right sided." Again, this designation is not totally correct since failure of one side of the heart usually results in failure of the other side. Left-sided failure refers to those signs and symptoms of pulmonary congestion resulting from elevated pressure in the pulmonary veins and capillaries. Right-sided failure refers to systemic venous and capillary congestion and the resultant signs and symptoms.

In any event, the theories can help the nurse to recall some basic physiologic concepts, thus enhancing her understanding of the development of the signs and symptoms of CHF. For example, the heart responds to the need for increased cardiac output by increasing the stroke volume and/or the heart rate. Attempts to increase stroke volume can result in hypertrophy of the heart muscle, one of the signs of CHF. Another example is that capillary pressure which is higher than that in the surrounding tissues will result in fluid moving out to the tissues to equalize the pressure. This leads to edema. Once the nurse has a general understanding of the theories about the dynamics of CHF, this information can be applied to analyzing the signs and symptoms of the individual patient together with information about his type of heart disease, other diseases present, the compensatory mechanisms being used, and the total life situation of that individual. From such an analysis, the nurse, patient, and physician (as necessary) find that helping the patient, achieve a plan for coping successfully with the chronicity of his condition frequently is a fruitful endeavor.

Differential Diagnosis

The diagnosis of congestive heart failure is based on a collection of signs and symptoms, none of which is caused only by congestive failure. Moreover, CHF can be precipitated in a patient with heart disease by a wide variety of etiologic agents as discussed previously. Thus a thorough understanding of the total patient is the first step in differentiating CHF from other similar conditions. This is particularly true in the elderly who often have multisystem disease. Other clues in establishing the diagnosis can be gotten from establishing a time course for the development of the symptoms. In general, signs and symptoms of the type similar to those of heart failure but caused by chronic diseases of other organs will have developed slowly and progressively while those related to an worsening of existing failure or the onset of acute failure are often rapid in onset. This is particularly true when trying to differentiate between heart failure and pulmonary diseases.

Allowing the patient to tell his story gives some helpful clues. Ultimately, however, even in the hands of experts, it may be necessary to attempt to treat the presumed congestive failure to see if the patient improves. Failure to improve then usually means that the diagnosis is incorrect.

High-Risk Populations

The nurse should never be surprised to find that the elderly patient has some degree of congestive heart failure. Atherosclerosis, arteriosclerosis, and other types of cardiovascular diseases are extremely common in our society. To identify those patients at especially high risk, the nurse should review the discussion of etiologic factors presented earlier in this chapter.

Manifestations

The classic findings of congestive heart failure include cardiomegaly, dyspnea, rales, and edema. The elderly patient will have the classic findings but may show additional signs or, more frequently, have manifestations not often seen in younger patients. Establishing the diagnosis, as in younger patients, still requires three processes: (1) recognizing the signs and symptoms, (2) specifically identifying the etiologic factors, and (3) identifying the precipitating causes.

Symptoms

Frequently the earliest symptoms of CHF are unrecognized. Nonspecific in nature, they can include muscle weakness, unusual tiredness, or cerebral symptoms such as syncope, mental confusion, or forgetfulness and mild pulmonary complaints.

Pulmonary symptoms include dyspnea on exertion followed by dyspnea at rest, orthopnea, paroxysmal nocturnal dyspnea (PND), cough and wheezing (cardiac asthma), and hemoptysis. It is not always easy to obtain a quick history of these symptoms and, thus, the nurse needs to be alert to any cues the patient may provide about difficulties in breathing. For example, the patient may voluntarily or subconsciously restrict his activities and never complain of dyspnea on exertion. Questions as to what he is able to do and why he does not do more activities may yield a nonspecific answer. In such a patient, careful questioning about his sleeping habits may produce the desired information. Comments about being more comfortable sleeping with several pillows (or any arrangement allowing him to be in a semi Fowler's position) followed up with a question as to what happens when he lies flat for a period of time help to elicit a history of orthopnea. A history of awakening suddenly at night breathless or feeling the need to get fresh air points toward paroxysmal nocturnal dyspnea, a fairly specific symptom.

A history of *Cheyne-Stokes* breathing pattern can be obtained from a concerned family member in many elderly patients. The patient himself may complain of insomnia caused by the breathing pattern. Cheyne-Stokes results from reduced blood flow to the respiratory centers in the medulla.

Coughing and wheezing, while commonly related to pulmonary diseases may be present in congestive failure as the lungs fill with fluid. Usually the cough is not productive.

Hemoptysis, a more ominous symptom, is caused by a variety of problems. It is a common symptom of pulmonary emboli which may precipitate congestive failure. Its presence requires careful investigation.

Another complaint that may be elicited by questioning the patient about sleeping habits is *nocturia.* Careful attention often reveals that the patient's urine output has decreased during the day and is copious at night. Other than the need to get up several times at night, there will be no symptoms leading one to suspect urinary tract problems.

Gastrointestinal symptoms vary from complaints of anorexia, nausea, and vomiting to abdominal distension or fullness and even abdominal pain. The majority of these complaints are thought to be related to increased venous pressure and congestion of the abdominal organs. If the patient is taking a digitalis preparation, these symptoms may be from digitalis intoxication. Moreover, toxicity may cause diarrhea or the patient may complain of constipation from decreased activity. *Gastrointestinal bleeding* and gangrene of the intestine are a serious consequence of CHF resulting from poor perfusion of the involved organs. The onset of these problems usually causes the patient to complain of abdominal pain. *Discomfort* or *pain* (especially with exertion) *over the liver,* related to congestion in that organ may be present. A small number of patients develop jaundice. *Poor nutrition* may develop or be exacerbated because of abnormal glucose and fat absorption and the loss of excess protein. The elderly patient sometimes complain of a *disagreeable taste* in his mouth.

Renal symptoms are primarily those of an upset in the diurinal variation as mentioned above. Decreased output with a high specific gravity is also common.

Signs

The signs of congestive failure can be categorized roughly as those involving the heart, lungs, vascular system, GI tract, and edema. The presence or absence of the various signs depends on the type of congestive failure (the underlying problem/diagnosis causing it), how acute it is, and how early it is discovered.

The cardiac signs tend to be more difficult for nurses untrained in cardiovascular examination skills to appreciate. Basically one looks for abnormal sounds and an increase in the precordial activity which can be seen or felt. Abnormal sounds include the development of a third and/or fourth heart sound, the so-called gallop rhythms because of their similarity to the gallop of a horse. The third heart sound, called an S_3, protodiastolic gallop, or ventricular gallop, is heard just prior to the second heart sound. (Using the bell of the stethoscope, listen at the apex in left ventricular failure, or the lower left sternal border in right ventricular failure, for a low pitched "extra" sound occurring shortly before S_2. The first heart sound can be identified at it occurs at about the time of the fullness [upstroke] of the carotid pulse. If no sound can be heard, have the patient roll into the left lateral decubitus position and listen again.) The fourth heart sound, also called S_4, a presystolic or atrial gallop, is usually best heard between the apex and the lower left sternal border. It occurs just before the first heart sound. The sounds may be easier to palpate than to hear. The S_3 gallop is considered the hallmark of failure. An early diagnostic clue, it is not always present in patients with failure. It may be normal in some individuals, e.g., youngsters. The S_4 gallop is less reliable but in some situations is a reliable early objective finding.

Enlargement of the heart (hypertrophy or dilatation) is present in many conditions, including congestive heart failure at later stages. Look and/or feel for displacement of the apical impulse to the left of the midclavicular line or below the fifth intercostal space. A sternal lift or parasternal heave (both are felt by placing the palm of the hand over the sternum and area adjacent and to the left) may be present. None of these signs is specific to congestive failure.

Sometimes the *murmur of mitral insufficiency* is present in congestive failure. When it is present it is related to incomplete closure of the mitral valve because of stretching of the heart and, thus, development of abnormal relationships in the support structures of the valve. Treatment often abolishes the murmur if it is related to the acute onset of failure.

The *lung signs* include the presence of fine, moist rales in the dependent portions of the lungs (the bases if the patient is not confined flat in bed). These rales do not clear with coughing. Cheyne-Stokes respirations and diffused wheezing may be present. Pulmonary edema can occur with labored respirations, diaphoresis, cyanosis (particularly around the lips, nailbeds), the use of accessory muscles to breathe, and wheezing. The development of this condition requires rapid medical intervention.

The *chest x-ray* picture is more helpful than any of the other tests usually performed to help diagnose heart failure. Generally the heart (one or more chambers) is enlarged and there is an increase in the size of the pulmonary arteries. The perfusion pattern is often changed with a decrease in perfusion to the lower lobes of the lungs and an increase in perfusion to the upper lobes, the opposite of normal. A pleural effusion, hydrothorax, and other signs related to congestion, frequently can be found.

Examination of the arteries and veins is helpful in establishing the diagnosis. Changes in the pulse and blood pressure are not specific and are widely variable, especially in the elderly. *Pulsus alternans,* when present, is detected by taking either the pulse or blood pressure. Its presence indicates poor myocardial function. The blood pressure may be slightly elevated in the elderly with a wider pulse pressure because of the presence of subclinical arteriosclerosis in the legs. *Orthostatic hypotension,* when present, is related to loss of adaptability to position changes in the aged or to hypovolemia, usually because of a rapid diuresis. The pulse may be rapid, but this is difficult to evaluate in the elderly as their baseline pulse varies so widely (50 to 110). Thus a pulse of 90 can represent a significant tachycardia in the patient. An exacerbation of arrhythmias already present or new ones present on the electrocardiogram is suspicious in the right situation but, again, these signs are not specific to the heart failure per se. *Full neck veins,* while not specific to only CHF, is a more common finding. With the patient at a 45-degree angle, the neck veins fill from below and pulsations of the jugular veins may be visible above the clavicle. If the veins are severely distended, the pulsations disappear. Rolling the patient up to 90 degrees may help to elicit the finding. Applying pressure over the liver or abdomen may also help make the pulsations visible again. This is called a positive hepatojugular reflex.

The *liver may be enlarged* and palpable below the ribs. Tenderness over the liver is not uncommon in acute failure. Generally it is not tender in chronic heart failure. A small number of patients (slightly more common in the aged) will develop jaundice. Some may have splenomegaly.

Edema is another sign frequently associated with heart failure. It is a late sign and particular care needs to be taken that it is the so called cardiac edema seen with congestive failure. Aged patients may have edema from a variety of causes including circulatory changes, a high salt intake, varicose veins, and prolonged sitting. Cardiac edema occurs in dependent body parts, is nontender and pitting in nature, and is bilateral. Subcutaneous edema occurs quite late, if at all. Its presence means that the patient has accumulated at least 10 lb. of fluid. Careful monitoring of daily weights and early treatment make this sign less usual.

With the possible exception of the chest x-ray study, the diagnosis of congestive heart failure is often established without using laboratory tests. Various blood studies usually are done to help identify the precipitating causes of the failure and to monitor therapy.

Complications

The complications of congestive heart failure have been presented in the rest of the discussion.

Prognosis

Harris (1970) reviewed several studies and his own experience and pointed out the following observations related to prognosis. The elderly patient who has survived with his heart disease has already increased his chances for a normal life span. Generally those with severe problems have died and the survivors have developed good collateral circulation and adapted their lifestyle to living with their cardiac condition. Patients with senility or a poor general outlook may be less able to cooperate with alterations in lifestyle and, hence, do poorly.

The type of precipitating factors responsible for the development of CHF relate to the prognosis more than does the heart disease itself. Extracardiac stresses that precipitate an episode of acute failure may ultimately cause the patient's demise. However, if the patient survives the acute failure and a recovery period of several months, he may not appreciably affect his life span.

Hypertensive patients (especially women), those with atrial fibrillation, those with aortic incompetence or aortic valve disease, or patients with pulmonary heart disease who develop heart failure tend to do poorly. Elevated blood pressure and atrial fibrillation, the latter often associated with complications such as emboli, correlate with a poorer prognosis. Treatment of basic heart conditions and complications does improve the mortality rates (Harris, 1970, pp. 35, 219).

Overall, the prognosis seems related to assessing the individual as a whole. The ability to medically manage the heart disease, precipitating factors, and diseases of other body organs plays an important part. However, assisting the patient to cope with some alterations in lifestyle and continue to be happy and productive in his own terms is also very important.

Prevention and Management

The most important aspect of management of CHF is prevention of further acute episodes. In the patient who has had previous acute failure, meeting this goal is assisted by understanding the precipitating factors for that episode(s). These factors commonly have a higher probability of precipitating subsequent episodes, and management of the patient should include this consideration. Even without this information, a reasonable prevention plan can be developed by understanding the factors that precipitate failure (see section on etiologic factors), early treatment of other acute illnesses (e.g., acute bronchitis), helping the patient to manage his treatment regimen successfully, and paying attention to all general health promotion measures. Teaching the patient about his health problem, its treatment, and good general health measures, all areas where nurses play an active role, will enhance the probability of successful prevention of CHF.

Management of heart failure is based on three principles: (1) reducing the workload of the heart, (2) increasing the contractility of the myocardium and the cardiac output, and (3) reducing congestion by decreasing salt and water retention. In addition, there are some causes of heart failure that are amenable to surgery. Surgery is no longer unheard of in the aged population, but careful assessment of the total patient must be undertaken by a competent surgical team. Specific data to assist in evaluating the risk to the elderly patient are available.

Reducing the Workload of the Heart

Reduction of the workload of the heart is accomplished by modifying the physical activity of the patient and helping him to achieve a nonstressed emotional state. Achievement of either of these goals requires a careful assessment of the patient and an individualized plan. It is not uncommon to find that measures prescribed to reduce activity are quite stressful emotionally. Many nurses have made helpful contributions by assisting individuals to balance these two needs successfully.

The actual plan for reducing the patient's activity is usually based on common sense. However, an understanding of the Functional Classification and the Therapeutic Classification developed by the New York Heart Association (published in 1964) and an appreciation of the energy cost (in calories per minute or metabolic equivalents) of various activities can enhance one's judgment. Neither tool can be used rigidly since a great many other factors must be taken into account in devising an activity prescription.

The functional classification includes four classes. All patients must have cardiac disease and the symptoms usually include dyspnea, angina, fatigue, palpitations, or other symptoms of cardiac insufficiency. Class I patients are those who can do ordinary activities without the above-named symptoms. Patients fitting into Class II are comfortable at rest but have some limitation of physical activity. Those fitting the criteria of Class III are also comfortable at rest but markedly limited in their tolerance of physical activity. Class IV patients are those who cannot carry on any physical activities without symptoms or those who have symptoms at rest.

The therapeutic classification has five classes, A to E. Class A patients can participate in unlimited activities while Class B patients should avoid severe or competitive activities. Patients in Class C should avoid strenuous activities and moderately restrict ordinary physical activities, while those in Class D must markedly restrict physical activities. Class E patients require complete bed or chair rest. In using the classifications, the nurse should avoid assuming that Class I patients fit Class A activities (New York Heart Association, 1964, pp. 7, 112). It is also important to remember that the patient may have voluntarily restricted his activities, thus making it difficult to accurately assign him to a class.

Tables of energy costs of activities in calories per minute or in METS (metabolic equivalents) are readily available. One good source is a book put out by the Colorado Heart Association, called *Exercise Equivalents*. These data are commonly used in Coronary Care Units to guide post-infarction rehabilitation, although they are equally useful in many other heart conditions. One MET represents the energy spent per kilogram body weight per minute of an average person sitting at rest in a chair. Put another way, this unit gives an approximate idea of the oxygen demands on the body of certain activities. Rest-

ing in bed, sitting, and eating require 1 MET. Activities at 2 METS include washing one's hands and face, while those at 3 METS include using the bedside commode, walking at 2.5 mph, and showering (3.5 METS—water shouldn't be too hot). Using the bedpan requires 4 METS. Many other figures for industrial, recreational, housework, and daily living activities are available. It should be noted that, while these "cost" figures speak to oxygen consumption, they do not include any estimate of the psychologic component of oxygen consumption or to the complications of overactivity or underactivity. Many authors, including Cassem and Hackett (1973), have commented on the psychologic problems accompanying the reduced activity of a post-infarction patient. The loss of ability to do desired activities often causes emotional stress for the elderly (Harris, 1970, pp. 5, 63). Thus severe activity restriction, particularly in an asymptomatic patient, may result in consumption of far more energy than permitting a desired activity whose MET value is slightly higher. Moreover, bedrest is known to increase the demand for cardiac output and myocardial work (Rose, 1972, p. 61). Immobilization also predisposes to deep vein thrombosis, decreased pulmonary ventilation (with an increased risk of pulmonary complications), muscle wasting, loss of postural vasomotor reflexes, further stasis of fluids with skin breakdown and infection, and constipation. Chair rest in a comfortable chair, elastic stockings, stool softeners, and, at times, anticoagulants are some of the measures used to help avoid these complications. Passive range of motion exercises, followed by active exercises, may also be done.

One problem, commonly seen in the elderly, deserves special mention. This is insomnia. It can be produced by several factors including nocturia, Cheyne-Stokes respirations, or confusion and disorientation. The Cheyne-Stokes pattern can often be relieved by aggressive diuretic therapy or aminophylline. Cautious sedation may be tried. Limiting fluid intake late in the day and therapy of the CHF may help relieve nocturia. The confusion at night frequently is related to the use of sedatives, which should be changed or eliminated.

Each patient will require a careful activity prescription with attention to his individual emotional and physical needs. Good nursing and/or team planning can assist most patients with uncomplicated CHF to regain a lifestyle meaningful to that individual.

Increasing Myocardial Contractility

Increasing myocardial contractility and, hence, cardiac output is done by various drugs, the most important being the cardiac glycosides. There are a number of drugs in this category including digitalis leaf (now used less frequently), digoxin, and digitoxin. The latter two are most commonly used. The following discussion focuses on them.

The response of CHF to the use of cardiac glycosides varies with the disease responsible for causing the CHF and/or the complicating factors to be treated. At times the risks of using these agents in patients with heart disease known to be poorly responsive will outweigh the potential benefits. Because this is an area of controversy, nurses will encounter varying philosophies and uses. It is important to understand why the drug is used in any given patient and what the expected and toxic outcomes are. In any event, the vast majority of patients will be receiving some glycoside to treat their CHF.

The incidence of toxicity is alarmingly high. A number of factors seem to be related to this problem, including the following: (1) the diagnosis of CHF is more frequently made on the basis of subtle signs and symptoms, (2) glycosides and diuretics commonly are used together, and (3) early symptoms of toxicity such as anorexia, nausea, and vomiting are not seen as frequently with chemically pure glycosides (digitoxin, digoxin) as they were with digitalis leaf (Hurst, et al., 1974, p. 471). The elderly are particularly vulnerable to developing toxicity to these drugs and when they do are more likely to suffer serious consequences, including death, from their toxicity.

Hurst and coworkers (1974, pp. 470–478) and Spann and his coworkers (1970) have discussed some of the general guidelines for the administration of cardiac glycosides. Their approach is one of several commonly employed.

Cardiac glycosides are used to strengthen and slow cardiac contractions. Usually cardiac output is improved in patients with CHF. The heart rate is slowed by depressing conduction through the atrioventricular junction and by stimulation of the vagal fibers. (Not all types of rhythms are slowed). As the circulation improves a diuresis may ensue. The heart size decreases.

Varying products and dosage schedules are used. The most frequently used preparations are digoxin and digitoxin. They differ in the duration of effect, the efficiency of absorption of oral doses, and the speed of action. In general, digitoxin is longer acting (onset is later too) than is digoxin. The half life is longer and so the time that it takes to reach a steady state is greater. It is completely absorbed orally while figures for the amount of oral absorption of digoxin vary. However, oral absorption of digoxin is incomplete except in the elixir form. Digoxin is excreted unchanged in the urine; thus the maintenance dose for patients with renal failure is lowered. Some clinicians use digitoxin in such a situation. It is metabolized primarily in the liver. Clinicians also vary in (1) whether or not they digitalize a patient and on what basis, (2) the use of loading doses and on what basis, and (3) indications for increasing the glycoside dosage. With reference to the latter point, it is not uncommon to avoid raising the dose of glycosides when treating CHF until optimal therapy with diuretics and other measures has been achieved.

Therapy with the cardiac glycosides is monitored various ways. First it is important to know the expected outcomes and likelihood of developing ontoward reactions. (This is exceptionally important if one of the outcomes is control of tachyarrhythmias and higher doses are used to achieve this effect). A plan is developed and modified as necessary. Changes in vital signs, especially pulse rate and character, in weight, and in urinary pattern are commonly watched for by nurses. Changes in pulse may include the development of bradycardia but can also be more subtle. It is important to note the following changes: (1) an irregular to regular pulse (this can be good, as in the change of irregular atrial fibrillation to regular sinus rhythm, or bad, as in the change from irregular atrial fibrillation to a regular junctional rhythm), (2) a regular rhythm to an irregular rhythm (the latter could be premature ventricular beats), or (3) speeding up of the rate rather than slowing (this could be atrioventricular dissociation).

Laboratory monitoring can include the use of digoxin serum assay levels, serum potassium levels, acid-base studies, and others. Serum drug assay levels are a recent development. Unfortunately there is an overlap in therapeutic levels and toxic levels so they cannot be used as a single measure in determining toxicity. They are useful, however, and commonly done. Monitoring serum potassium is done because low intracellular potassium levels make the myocardium more sensitive to digitalis preparations. The body serum levels of the various electrolytes are dependent on a number of factors. Therefore, a normal serum potassium is not always reflective of intracellular potassium concentration. This is particularly true in the face of acid-base disorders or with rapid changes in the patient. For example, the nurse recognizing that the patient on digoxin and a diuretic is having a massive diuresis will need to check on the potassium status of the patient.

Monitoring of the rhythm status can be done by hooking the patient up to a continuous monitor, by obtaining a rhythm strip periodically, by obtaining a 12 lead ECG at intervals, or by combining several of these measures. Moreover, it is important for the nurse to obtain an ECG if the patient develops pulse changes.

Beller and coworkers (1971, p. 996), in a prospective study of toxicity, reported not only a high incidence of toxicity but also an ominous prognosis. The elderly with advanced heart disease (NYHA Class III or IV), underlying atrial fibrillation, pulmonary disease, and renal function abnormalities seemed to be at greatest risk for developing toxicity with normal maintenance doses of digitalis products.

Not infrequently, cardiac arrhythmias are the first sign of toxicity (Hurst, 1974, p. 471). This is especially true when digoxin or digitoxin are being used, when hypokalemia is present, or when cardiac glycosides and diuretics are being used together. Virtually all arrhythmias or ECG abnormalities can potentially be associated with toxicity. Atrial, junctional, and ventricular ectopic beats, idioventricular conduction defects, and varying degrees of sinoatrial or atrioventricular block are commonly cited manifestations of toxicity. More specifically, frequent premature ventricular beats, often multifocal in origin, atrial tachycardia with atrioventricular block, atrial flutter and fibrillation, atrioventricular dissociation, and various types of blocks, including (infrequently) complete heart block, are rhythms that may need treatment urgently. It is also possible for ventricular tachycardia or fibrillation to occur. Serious rhythm problems often mandate stopping the glycoside. Oral or intravenous potassium may be used if there is an associated potassium deficit. It should be administered with caution to patients with conduction defects. Atropine may help to increase the heart rate in some situations. A pacemaker may be necessary. Antiarrhythmic agents including diphenylhydantoin are used. Other drugs, such as reserpine or Ismelin, can compound the problem and may need to be discontinued. Should the patient require calcium or cardioversion therapy, the risk of fatal arrhythmias is increased.

Gastrointestinal signs and symptoms are common and not easily associated only with glycoside toxicity. Anorexia, nausea, vomiting, and diarrhea are the usual problems. Hemorrhagic nercrosis of the intestines can also occur (Hurst, 1974, p. 476).

Central nervous system symptoms and those related to vision may also be reported by the patient. The former include weakness, fatigue delirium, and, rarely, toxic psychosis. The latter include yellow or bluish vision and scotomas.

Reducing Congestion by Decreasing Salt and Water Retention

Reduction of salt and water retention is accomplished by using diuretics and dietary restrictions. The usual diet has between 8 to 14 gm of salt. Reduction of this amount to 4 to 5 gm may be adequate. If not, or if the diet is unacceptable (unpalatable), diuretics are added to the regimen.

The most important complications of the diuretics occur to some degree with all of the agents discussed. They include problems with potassium balance (generally with hypokalemia although hyperkalemia can occur) and hypovolemia.

Monitoring of diuretic therapy is done in a similar fashion for any diuretic(s) used. Daily weights (or less frequent in some patients) help to monitor progress toward maintaining the patient's "dry" weight if he can tolerate this volume status. It is done both acutely and chronically when the patient can use weight patterns as a valuable tool to assist in regulating therapy. Blood values, especially potassium and renal studies are used frequently during acute therapy and less often during chronic treatment. Measuring intake and output during an acute diuretic phase is helpful. Finally, pulse and blood pressure changes can be helpful, particularly during acute therapy. Signs of an increased pulse and low blood pressure, especially an orthostatic drop in blood pressure, help to detect the onset of hypovolemia.

The thiazide diuretics and related compounds include agents such as chlorothiazide (Diuril), hydrochlorothiazide (Hydrodiuril), and chlorthalidone (Hygroton). They are most useful in chronic congestive failure. Absorbed from the GI tract, they promote increased excretion of sodium, potassium, chloride, and water. Their duration of action varies from 12 hours to 3 days depending on the agent. Their onset of action is about 1 hour. Toxicity includes thrombocytopenia, agranulocytosis, pancreatitis, skin rashes, and hyperuricemia, which may precipitate gout. They may affect renal function adversely and cause azotemia. Hepatic coma can occur in patients with cirrhosis. Therefore, the use of these drugs is contraindicated in patients with these problems. Hyponatremia, hypokalemia, and hypochloremic alkalosis are serious problems in some patients, particularly those also on cardiac glycosides. Potassium supplementation may be required. Chloride should also be given in this situation. Liquid potassium chloride or a potassium-retaining diuretic is frequently prescribed. A word of caution about enteric coated KCL; it can cause ulceration of the small bowel as can some of the newer slow-release tablets (Goodman and Gilman, 1975, p. 819).

Both spironolactone (Aldactone) and triamterene (Dyrenium) promote potassium retention. They also cause some diuresis, but this effect is mild and slow to develop. They are rarely used as primary diuretic agents but may be used as a second agent. Both can cause hyperkalemia and are not used in patients with renal problems. Combination agents such as Aldactazide (spironolactone and hydrochlorothiazide) are commonly used with outpatients for maintenance therapy. The agents generally are more expensive than liquid potassium and may aggravate financial problems in some elderly patients.

Potent diuretics are relatively new. Included are the drugs furosemide (Lasix) and ethacrynic acid (Edecrin). Orally, they act within 30 minutes to 1 hour and last about 6 to 8 hours. Their intravenous action is much quicker, thus making them a valuable tool in urgent situations. Used to treat resistant types of failure, they may require very high doses to accomplish their purpose. Both agents work by inhibiting sodium (and chloride) reabsorption with a concomitant loss of potassium and hydrogen ions. They are effective treatment for renal failure unless the patient is anuric or unless azotemia (and/or oliguria) is present. In such situations they are used with caution, if at all. The dangers of hyponatremia, hypokalemia, and hypochloremia with alkalosis are present. Excessive diuresis with excess potassium loss and metabolic alkalosis, especially if the patient is also taking a cardiac glycoside, still occur, even in experienced hands, and can be catastrophic. Careful monitoring of the result of therapy is essen-

tial. Other toxic effects can include vascular embolism and thrombosis with excess diuresis, hyperuricemia, agranulocytosis, and acute hearing loss (Goodman and Gilman, 1975, pp. 817–848).

Manipulation of the diet of the aged patient may prove difficult at best. Habits of a lifetime are difficult to break. Moroever, the elderly tend to have a higher need for protein (Harris recommends 1.4 gm of protein/kg body weight; p. 66) and, therefore, a relative hypoproteinemia with its consequences on body fluid regulation. Other areas of difference can include poorer tolerance to fats, poor absorption of calcium, and vitamin deficiencies from increased vitamin excretion. Obesity, despite a diet deficient in some of the essential elements, is a frequent problem. The tissue and muscle changes that occur with aging make its diagnosis more difficult. It contributes to both pressure and volume overload on the heart. Finally, those who are chronicially ill often have a poor appetite. Thus, before undertaking any dietary modifications, the nurse will need to assess the entire area of nutrition in the patient (Harris, 1970, pp. 63–68).

Because of the difficulties in severely restricting salt intake, the majority of patients will be placed on a mild-to-moderate restriction and given the appropriate diuretic therapy. A mild restriction (usually about 5 gm sodium) can be achieved by having the patient avoid table salt and foods that are obviously salty. Some salting of food during cooking is permitted. A moderate restriction (usually 2 to 5 gm) includes avoiding naturally salty foods, using salt while cooking, and table salt (Hurst, 1974, pp. 479–480). In order to severely restrict sodium, resources such as those available from the readers local Heart Association usually need to be used (AHA, 500 mg, Sodium Diet).

Many of the animal protein foods are relatively high in sodium. Meat, poultry, and fish can be processed by boiling it several times. Milk, cheese, and eggs may need to be slightly restricted. Some vegetables including artichokes, beets and their greens, carrots, spinach, and celery are also high in sodium. Food processing and preservation often results in the addition of sodium. Labels must be read carefully before a product is purchased. Water is high in sodium in some areas and its addition to beverages and foods during the manufacturing process results in high sodium products. Finally, medications and dental products may be high in sodium. This list is not comprehensive, and so the reader with an interest in this topic is advised to consult the local Heart Association. Bookstores are also an excellent resource as cookbooks, and other books related to nutrition are currently popular (Snively, 1974, pp. 72–75).

The judicious use of spices and herbs in cooking can enhance the palatability of the diet. Generally salt substitutes are permitted unless excess potassium is expected to be a problem.

Other areas of nutrition deserve brief mention. Frequent, small feedings may be necessary for the acutely ill cardiac patient to avoid fatigue. The use of alcohol, coffee, and tea is controversial. Many clinicians permit patients to use alcohol in small amounts, decaffeinated coffee, and some tea. The use of vitamins may be necessary if relative malnutrition is a problem. Vitamins with calcium generally should be avoided. Hurst recommends B-complex vitamins (Hurst 1974, p. 480). The intermittent use of a large amount of high potassium food and potassium supplements can cause problems. Therefore the patient and/or nurse should be knowledgeable about foods high in potassium. Some examples are bananas, dates, figs, prunes, some juices including prune and orange, many of the meats and vegetables, and peanuts.

Arriving at a nutritious, palatable diet prescription which the patient will enjoy is a challenging task for the nurse. Active collaboration with the patient and others is essential in reaching this goal.

Evaluation

The evaluation criteria for judging the effectiveness of management need to be designed with the individual person. The criteria should include both long and short term objectives by which intervention can be measured. The criteria must be realistic and it is desirable if outcomes are those that the person can appreciate. One example is as follows: The long term goal is to modify the dietary intake of sodium in a home patient. One of several short term goals could be to place the patient on moderately restricted sodium diet for one week. Have him follow verbal instructions and guidelines as spelled out in the Heart Association booklet appropriate to his sodium restriction. Have him keep a diary of his food intake and problems he encounters. Review and adjust after one week. Then contract with the patient for a trial period and reevaluation. Early establishment of evaluation criteria that the patient can help to establish and assess helps to achieve a work-able plan for managing the patient with congestive heart failure.

PERIPHERAL VASCULAR DISEASE

This discussion focuses on commonly-occurring peripheral vascular diseases and conditions of the elderly. It is confined to the areas below the diaphragm because the frequency of vascular diseases is greater in the lower extremities than in the upper extremities. Chronic and acute occlusive arterial disease and occlusive venous disease (thrombophlebitis), both in the lower extremities, are discussed in detail. Also included are some references to aneurysms of the abdominal aorta and lower extremity arteries. These are less common than occlusive diseases but are important in the aged population.

Assisting the elderly patient to live with chronic arterial and venous occlusive diseases is a challenging task for the nurse.

Description

Peripheral vascular disease is a term used to categorize a variety of conditions affecting the veins, arteries, and lymphatic vessels of the extremities.

"Arteriosclerosis of the aorta and of the peripheral arteries is the most important vascular disease in old age . . ." (Harris, 1970, p. 269). The term "arteriosclerosis" means thickening, hardening, and loss of elasticity in the arteries. Often it is used interchangeably with the term "atherosclerosis." However, the latter is characterized specifically by the accumulation of lipid substances, frequently called atheroma or atheromatous plaques, on the inner (intimal) layer of the arteries with associated changes in the middle (medial) layer.

"Most disorders of veins are the result of thrombosis of blood within them. . . ." (Holling, 1972, p. 203.) Thus, this discussion focuses on thrombophlebitis and problems of chronic venous insufficiency, one of the potential sequelae of the former.

Etiologic Factors

Atherosclerosis of the aorta and its branch arteries is by far the most common cause of chronic occlusive arterial disease. In the branch arteries the process is called "arterosclerosis obliterans." When found in the aorta and branch arteries, atherosclerosis frequently is also present in the coronary arteries and in the arteries supplying the brain.

The distribution of artherosclerosis tends to be patchy. It is prominent at joints and at areas of bifurcation of branch vessels. It is more common in the lower extremities than in the upper ones, and in the distal rather than proximal aorta. Atheromas are more likely to develop in larger arteries than in small ones. They develop where the stretch or tension within the wall is the greatest or where the artery is subjected to repeated bending, such as at the joints.

The progress of the disease is accelerated by diabetes mellitus, hypertension, obesity, hyperlipidemia, and other cardiovascular conditions. A sedentary life style, associated with poor collateral circulation, can worsen the manifestations of the disease.

The onset of symptoms usually is in the late middle years in men and after menopause in women. Diabetics tend to develop symptoms some ten years earlier than their nondiabetic counterparts.

Chronic occlusion of arteries usually results from atherosclerosis and local thrombosis, generally occurring at the site of a plaque. The most common causes of sudden occlusion of a peripheral artery are thrombosis and embolism. The presence of atrial fibrillation enhances the likelihood of formation of mural thrombi and, hence, the chance of embolism. These emboli commonly lodge in the bifurcation of the common femoral artery. They arise most frequently in the heart of a patient with a myocardial infarction or chronic congestive heart failure. Microemboli from atheromas may also cause acute arterial occlusion. They usually lodge in the smaller arteries of the legs and feet.

Atherosclerosis of the aorta, coupled with the presence of degenerative changes in the medial layer (thought to be part of the process of aging), can cause aneurysms. The majority of these aneurysms are located below the femoral arteries, although they may be found in the thorax as well. Typically they are found in males 70 years of age or older. They are often asymptomatic until they rupture into the retroperitoneal space (most common), into the free peritoneal cavity, or into the other areas such as the gastrointestinal tract (least common).

Dissecting aortic aneurysms are those in which blood extravasates into the medial coat of the aorta. The separation of the coats often extends the length of the vessel but not usually all the way around the lumen. Occlusion of one of the major arterial branches or hemorrhage are the potential catastrophic outcomes. Hypertension exacerbates the progress of aneurysms.

Most of the peripheral arterial aneurysms are caused by atherosclerosis. They are found more commonly in men over 50 years of age and are often multiple. The popliteal arteries are the most common site, but they may be present in other arteries such as the femoral and iliac arteries.

Venous thrombosis (thrombophlebitis) usually occurs in a susceptible person during the course of another illness. The actual cause is obscure. It is known to be associated with venous stasis, hypercoagulability of the blood, and changes in the intimal lining of the vein. Venous stasis may develop from prolonged immobilization. Hypercoagulability may play a role in disease states such as malignancy and blood dyscrasias. Injury may be implicated in the development of thrombophlebitis under conditions of direct trauma, septic thrombophlebitis, and the like.

There are two types of venous thrombosis: superficial and deep. The superficial type usually involves the calf veins and is clinically less important than the deep vein thrombosis. The latter commonly originates in the venous sinuses of the calf. From there it extends to the deep veins of the calf, including the posterior tibial and peroneal veins. Further extension is to the proximal veins including the popliteal, femoral, and iliac veins. The untoward sequelae of pulmonary embolism results from deep vein thrombosis, especially of the proximal veins.

Other diseases may cause peripheral vascular disease in the elderly. However, atherosclerosis and thrombophlebitis account for the vast majority of conditions that cause morbidity in this age group, and they may cause mortality in some instances.

High Risk Populations

The high risk population for the development of atherosclerotic disease is the elderly. Thrombophlebitis is also much more common in the elderly than in any other group. In the section discussing etiologic factors, the associated factors related to atherosclerosis are discussed, as are the major factors in the production of thrombophlebitis and its sequelae.

Thrombophlebitis and pulmonary embolism, the major complication, should be actively sought and actively prevented (when possible) in all patients with conditions favoring increased venous stasis, changes in the coagulability of the blood, and injury to the walls of the veins. Examples include surgery, fractured hips, chronic debilitating diseases (congestive heart failure is of great importance), the postoperative state, prolonged bedrest, prolonged sitting in a chair, past history of venous thrombosis, varicose veins, obesity, and medications (especially hormones). The diagnosis of thrombophlebitis and pulmonary embolism is difficult to make because the signs and symptoms are often vague. The actual incidence of either problem is unknown. However, both are known to be very common among the elderly. Death from a pulmonary embolism in a patient with an otherwise treatable condition is an avoidable tragedy. Unfortunately, it is not uncommon among the elderly.

Dynamics

In both chronic and acute arterial occlusive disease, the signs and symptoms are the results of ischemia of the tissues served by the affected artery. Chronic occlusive disease is characterized by symptoms of arterial insufficiency and signs of reduced arterial blood flow, which are progressive in nature. Acute occlusion is characterized by the same types of changes, but the changes are rapid in onset and progression.

The manifestations of the ischemia depend on the severity of the disease (site and amount), the rapidity of onset, the extent of collateral circulation, and the ability to meet the metabolic demands of the tissues.

Chronic prolonged ischemia produces fibrosis and atrophy of tissues. Necrosis and gangrene can occur in the face of severe ischemia of either chronic or acute onset. This can lead to loss of the affected limb. The fate of an acutely ischemic limb will depend to a large extent on the adequacy of existing collateral circulation. The ischemia ultimately may be less severe when its slow progression allows time for the development of collateral circulation. With acute insult, the collateral circulation may not be as well developed, and definitive therapy should be undertaken rapidly to preserve the limb. Even if the limb is preserved, residual damage may be present, with compromise of the function of the limb. Ischemic neuropathy or intermittent claudication are relatively common sequelae. Necrosis of selected muscles and ischemic thrombophlebitis are less common but do occur.

Aneurysms result from the destruction of the integrity of the wall of an artery. They also can lead to ischemia of the tissues served by these arteries.

Atherosclerotic abdominal aneurysms are de-scribed as fusiform (spindle shaped) or saccular (outpouched with narrow neck). They generally have thrombotic tissue in their lumen. Rupture of an aneurysm may occur eventually from the pressure on the compromised wall. Peripheral arterial aneurysms can rupture also, but this is a less common outcome because of the support of the surrounding tissues. Such aneurysms usually lead to an ischemic process because of sudden occlusion of the artery from thrombosis. Distal emboli also may be produced.

Dissecting aneurysms, with the presence of an intimal tear and fragmentation of the wall of the artery by blood, lead to occlusion of a major branch artery and ischemia of the underlying tissues. They can also cause hemorrhage.

Thrombophlebitis of a major venous trunk leads to passive congestion with elevation of venous pressure and, thus, to transudation of fluid into the extravascular spaces, causing edema. There is usually no compromise of the arterial tree unless the venous tree is completely obstructed. Because there are abundant venous channels, major venous trunks must be occluded before there is a functional disturbance.

Manifestations

Chronic peripheral arterial occlusive disease, commonly referred to as atherosclerosis obliterans (ASO), is basically an ischemic disease. It causes symptoms of arterial insufficiency and signs of diminished blood flow. The most common symptom is intermittent claudication. The most important sign is absent or diminished pulses distal to the occluded artery. The former usually is the presenting symptom and may be the only one.

The development of symptoms is related to the adequacy of collateral circulation. Generally the collateral circulation is adequate to keep the tissues viable but inadequate to prevent claudication when tissue demands with exercise exceed arterial supply.

Intermittent claudication occurs in working muscles and is a result of progressive muscle ischemia. The pain occurs with a given amount of walking, is relieved by resting, and reoccurs when the same distance is walked again. Thus the examiner can assess the progress of the patient by exercising him each time he is seen and comparing the results. Walking rapidly or uphill usually produces the symptom earlier. Usually the pain is described as cramping, fatigue, numbness, and aching or tightness. It may be accompanied by a tendency to limp. The site of claudication and the location of arterial occlusion often closely correlate.

Claudication of the calf muscles (the most common site) and absence of the dorsalis pedis, posterior tibial, and popliteal pulses (Figs. 13-1 and 13-2) correlate with femoropopliteal occlusion. Aortoiliac segmental occlusion causes claudication of the hips, buttocks, and back. This condition is also called Leriche disease. The claudication may be manifested as general tiredness or weakness in the legs. Absence of all pulses except perhaps a faint femoral (resulting from collateral circulation) helps to prevent misdiagnosis of the claudication. Moreover, impotence often is present. (It is not always corrected by surgery.) Claudication of the foot muscles with or without foot lesions and/or calf claudication, results from occlusion of the arteries below the knees. It may be present also in combined occlusion of several leg arteries, e.g., thigh and leg.

Rest pain may occur as the disease progresses and the collateral vessels become occluded or other-wise ineffective. It is a sign of tissue ischemia and may be accompanied by sensations of coldness and numbness. The pain always is present in the foot and frequently is gnawing, persistent, and severe. It is aggravated by elevation of the leg and relieved by the dependent position. Dependency may cause edema with further compromise of the circulation. The development of rest pain should cue the nurse to watch for ischemic ulcers and gangrene.

The absence of pulses is characteristic of ASO. The sites and correlation with segmental diseases has been discussed. In assessing pulses it is important to remember that a small segment of the population will have a normal absence of the dorsalis pedis. The dorsalis pedis and the popliteal pulses are difficult to find, the former because of an inconsistent location. The popliteal pulse requires practice to gain skill in finding it. (With the patient lying with his knees at right angles, the examiner uses the fingertips of both hands and palpates the middle of the popliteal fossa.)

When evaluating the pulses, it is important to keep some basic physiologic facts in mind. The pres-

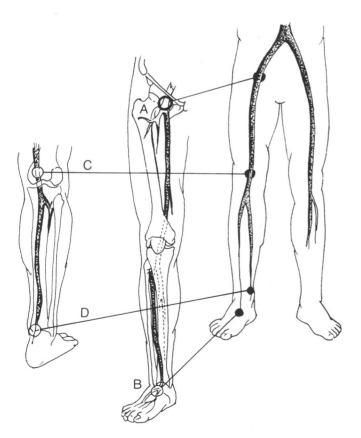

FIGURE 13-1. Pulse sites to check for femoropopliteal occlusion: *A*, femoral; *B*, dorsalis pedis; *C*, popliteal; and *D*, posterior tibial.

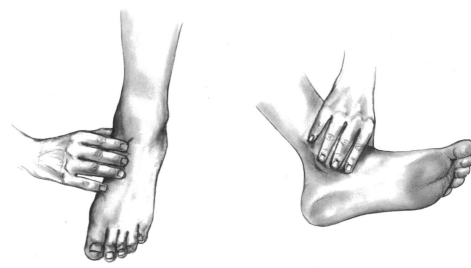

FIGURE 13-2.   Checking the foot for the absence of pulses. (Both pulses may be congenitally absent.) *Left,* Dorsalis pedis pulse. Place three fingers on the dorsum of the foot (not the ankle), usually just lateral to the extensor tendon of the great toe. *Right,* Posterior tibial pulse. Curve your fingers behind and slightly below the medial malleolus of the ankle. (From Bates, B.: A Guide to Physical Examination. Philadelphia: J. B. Lippincott Co., 1979)

sure (pulse) wave is generated by the ventricle and transmitted through the blood, not with it. Thus, it should arrive at the periphery almost simultaneously with the apical beat. Delay is obvious evidence of obstruction. Blood flow is much slower than the pressure wave. Thus, the flow will not arrive as quickly, not always go by the same route, nor be there when there is a pressure wave. It is possible to have relatively normal pressure, a pulse and no flow, or no pulse and plenty of flow. This is true because flow is related to resistance. If resistance is low, flow will be high. For example, a patient with occlusion of the superficial femoral artery may have foot pulses at rest. With exercise, the small vessels open, the pulse disappears, and he begins to claudicate.

Examination of the arteries by palpation also yields important clues. With practice it is sometimes possible to feel a plaque in the femoral artery. It is also possible to hear a bruit (murmur). It is caused by more than about 50 percent obstruction of a major artery. As the high pressure blood flow attempts to pass through the obstruction, vibration of the wall of the artery produces the noise. Once the artery is fully occluded, the bruit disappears.

Color changes in the affected limb are confirmatory signs of arterial insufficiency. Absence of these changes usually means that the patient has good collateral circulation. Pallor is produced by elevating the leg high above the head for one minute. When the

leg is returned to a dependent position, hyperemia occurs and the foot becomes ruborous.

Trophic changes may occur if the ischemia is prolonged and/or severe. The feet and legs feel cold to the touch. The feet have thin, shiny skin which appears atrophic. The nails thicken and opacify. Hair may cease to grow. The development of ischemic ulcers, often on the toes, and gangrene, is a much feared complication. The ulcers are extremely painful. The pain is well localized. Dependency provides some relief, but narcotics often are required.

Diabetic ulcers are differentiated from ischemic ulcers because the former are not painful.

Ischemic neuropathy is characterized by severe burning or shooting pain which begins in the foot and radiates proximally. It is a late sign. The pain occurs in paroxysms. Usually narcotics are required to relieve it.

Numerous tests have been developed in the last decade to aid in diagnosis. These include oscillometric examination, plethysmography, Doppler flowmeter examination, comparison of the arterial pressures with that in the upper limbs, radiography, blood studies to look for elevated lipids and manifestations of other diseases such as diabetes, and angiography (particularly if surgery is contemplated). Angiography (aortography and femoral angiography) locates the site of the occlusion, indicates its extent, and assesses the state of the collateral circulation. Frequently it is the only study done, as the diagnosis is established readily without any additional special laboratory studies.

Acute arterial occlusion, causing symptoms of ischemia and loss of pulses distal to the occlusion, is far more common in the lower extremities. Generally it is caused by embolism or thrombosis. Looking for a source for the former (e.g., atrial fibrillation) helps to differentiate between the two.

The typical clinical picture is dramatic with a sudden onset of symptoms. The suddenness of onset helps to differentiate acute occlusion from the chronic variety. The typical first symptom is burning or aching pain in the tissues distal to the occlusion. It is followed rapidly by coldness and numbness, pallor, and collapse of the superficial veins. Pulses are absent or severely compromised (if there is good collateral circulation). The pain is aggravated by moving the limb, and muscle power is reduced. Paraesthesia may be present. Cyanosis occurs. As the affected tissues begin to die, the tenderness diminishes, the muscles become soft, paralysis develops, joints develop flexion contractures and finally become lax, and slight resistance to extension changes to marked resistance and then to no resistance. There is no early swelling/edema such as exists later when the limb is dead, thus helping to differentiate this problem from venous thrombosis.

Although this is the typical picture, wide variations are possible. This makes the discovery of acute occlusion more difficult before irreparable harm is done. In any event, the presence of several ischemic signs and symptoms with absent pulses presenting acutely should make the nurse suspicious. Because early intervention is necessary to preserve the limb, the patient should be transferred to a medical center where vascular surgery can be performed.

Abdominal aortic aneurysms and peripheral arterial aneurysms usually are asymptomatic. The patient may be aware of a "bulge" over the aneurysm or a pulsatile mass. Frequently the examiner can feel the mass, which may or may not be pulsatile. If the aneurysm is filled with thrombi or other debris, pulses may not be transmitted. Peripheral arterial aneurysms may cause symptoms such as pain, edema, and venous distention if they encroach on adjacent nerves or veins. Aneurysms may also cause arterial occlusion and are subject to rupture. Hemorrhage in the abdomen may lead to rapid death if it discharges to the free peritoneal cavity. Rupture into the retroperitoneal space or other locations presents vague abdominal symptoms. Pain, often severe in the abdomen, lumbar, or pelvic areas, and findings of hemorrhage shock are the usual findings. Peripheral aneurysms rupture less frequently. Rather, signs and symptoms of ischemia from arterial occlusion are more common.

Dissecting aneurysms also rupture. Severe pain in the abdomen or lumbar area may be the only symptom. Others can include a ripping or tearing type of pain, signs and symptoms of ischemia because of circulatory occlusion, and paresis or paralysis.

Superficial thrombophlebitis is of less clinical importance than deep vein thrombosis. Rarely does it give rise to any serious consequences unless the process extends to the deep veins. It is characterized by the spontaneous onset of pain, the skin over the vein is warm and red, edema may be present, pain may occur on using the adjacent muscles, and the vein feels like a hard string. It is sensitive to pressure. A fever may be present or the temperature may be subnormal.

Deep vein thrombophlebitis occurs in the deep calf veins and the proximal deep veins (the femoral, the iliac, and the popliteal). Although this latter type is less frequent, pulmonary emboli, the most life-threatening consequence, usually originate in the proximal veins.

Early symptoms of deep vein thrombosis can include a sensation of heaviness and cramps in the leg, pain in the sole of the foot or a pulling pain along the vein, restlessness, anxiety, and increased heart rate.

Local signs and symptoms such as edema, cyanosis with standing, and a positive Homans' maneuver (forceful dorsiflexion of foot produces pain) may be present.

The presence of these signs and symptoms is helpful in diagnosis. However, Madden and Hume (1976, p. 183) state that with clinical examination alone more than 50 percent of venous thromboses are missed. Because the incidence of fatal pulmonary embolism is high in the elderly and many of these deaths occur to people without otherwise life-threatening illnesses, a high index of suspicion should be maintained, particularly when dealing with high risk elderly patients (see page 261). Moreover, many patients have silent pulmonary emboli.

There are a number of tests for venous thrombosis which can be done at centers having the appropriate equipment. These include venography (definitive test but not readily repeatable), fibrinogen leg scanning (can be used over several days in high risk patients), plethysmography (good for proximal veins), and Doppler flowmeter examination (good for proximal veins).

The most important complication is pulmonary embolism, the diagnosis of which is not always reached easily. Madden and Hume summarized the findings of the national cooperative study stating that the following symptoms, if present, were helpful: dyspnea, pleuritic pain, apprehension, cough, wheezing, hemoptysis, syncope, and perspiration. Signs included rales, increase in the pulmonary component of the second heart sound, phlebitis, gallop (S_3S_4) heart rhythm, and cyanosis. Only one third of the patients participating in this large study had clinical evidence of thrombophlebitis.

The two most useful tests in establishing the diagnosis are lung scans and selective pulmonary angiography. The electrocardiogram, chest x-ray studies, blood studies, and arterial oxygen may show changes but are less reliable (Madden and Hume, 1976, pp. 92–93).

There are two other important complications of venous thrombosis. These are chronic venous obstruction and stasis and the post-phlebitic syndrome. The latter may occur after acute venous thrombosis. The major complaints are aching, tiredness, and a burning pain in the affected leg.

Chronic venous obstruction and stasis is one result of acute thrombosis. The venous valves are destroyed, collateral vessels open up, and the veins become incompetent. Swelling, cyanosis, and dilatation of the small veins result. When the venous incompetence is long term, the skin may break down and venous stasis ulcers can result (see p. 269). They are located usually in the malleolar region. Cellulitis may be present. Other manifestations of stasis include brown pigmented skin, chronic edema, inflammation, atrophy, induration, and dermatitis of the lower third of the leg.

Differential Diagnosis

The conditions discussed herein are misdiagnosed frequently if orthopedic disorders, neurologic disorders, or venous and arterial disorders are not differentiated properly from each other. It is important that all patients receive a thorough venous and arterial examination because concurrent disorders of both systems are common in the elderly. Acute arterial obstruction and venous thrombosis are prone to be confused with each other.

Frequently an acute arterial embolus will occur from the heart of a patient with atrial fibrillation, a recent heart attack, or chronic congestive failure. The pain will be severe and steady, and the limb will appear cold and pallid but will not be swollen. The veins will be collapsed and distal pulses absent. Sensory and motor function will be decreased.

Venous thrombosis causes steady pain and the limb will be warm, cyanotic, and swollen. The veins will be full and distal arterial pulses present. Sensory and motor functions are unimpaired.

Venous stasis ulcers and ischemic (arterial) ulcers also are not always differentiated from one another; this error can lead to improper treatment.

Osteoarthritis of the hip, degenerative disk diseases, ischemic vascular disease of the brain or spinal cord, and mechanical encroachment on the central nervous system may all cause symptoms similar to those of chronic arterial insufficiency to the limbs. Claudication, the typical pain of the latter, is a reproducible pain that occurs after a given amount of exercise in muscles supplied by the affected arteries. It is relieved rapidly by rest. Nonischemic pain, e.g., arthritic, may be worse at the start of the exercise, not relieved rapidly by rest, and has no definite pattern. Pain such as that caused by degenerative disk disease (dermatome) has a pattern. Mechanical pain on the central nervous system may be relieved by changing position. Other neurologic changes are often present, e.g., urinary problems, changes in reflexes, and sensory and motor changes. Neuropathy, characterized by numbness, tingling, burning, and constant pain, may be caused by neurologic problems, diabetes, or advanced arterial insufficiency. Treating the diabetes can help reduce the problem. Thus, it is important to identify the cause of neuropathy.

Finally, foot problems such as intermittent claudication of the foot muscles and tissue wasting of the sole of the foot, caused by arterial insufficiency, are often misdiagnosed as orthopedic in nature.

Thrombophlebitis of the proximal deep veins may be misdiagnosed as cellulitis, lymphangitis, or lymphedema. The presence of inflammation, venous distention, and discoloration favor thrombophlebitis; high temperature and systemic reaction favor cellulitis or lymphangitis.

Probably the most important factor to keep in mind in helping to differentiate arterial disease from other problems is the high incidence of arterial disease being caused by local manifestations of a generalized disease, atherosclerosis. With venous thrombosis it is important to remember the three factors involved in producing it: hypercoagulability, venous stasis, and damage to the vein wall. A high index of suspicion will help to guide the nurse toward the clues that aid in establishing the diagnosis.

Prognosis

". . . peripheral arterial disease is considered to be a maiming disease" (rather than a killing one) (Holling, 1972, p. 68). The same statement could be made for thrombophlebitis if the complication of pulmonary embolism is avoided.

The prognosis of chronic arterial occlusive disease is related to the presence of atherosclerosis in other areas. The occlusive disease contributes little to the mortality rate. Rather, the presence of diabetes or cerebral or coronary atherosclerosis to a large extent determines the outcome for the patient. Arthrosclerosis obliterans also is not always progressive. Therefore, estimating the seriousness of projected morbidity must be done by understanding the manifestations of the condition in the individual patient.

"Without treatment, acute arterial occlusion (embolism and thrombosis) results in gangrene in about 50 percent of cases. . . . Approximately 40 percent of patients with untreated sudden arterial occlusion die, because most of them are elderly and have serious cardiovascular disease." (Hurst, 1974, p. 1612). Embolism to the distal aorta, one of the most serious conditions, threatens the viability of the lower extremities and causes a high mortality rate.

Abdominal aneurysms may rupture into the peritoneal cavity, leading to the rapid demise of the patient. More frequently they rupture into the retroperitoneal cavity and, although the risk of death is still high, treatment in a major medical center can be successful. Dissecting aneurysms also have a high mortality rate. Although medical and surgical treatment has improved, it is still a serious problem.

Prevention and Management

The definitive therapy for patients with chronic arterial occlusive disease is surgery. Usually patients are not referred for surgery until their claudication is severe enough to limit daily activities. The surgeon will decide if the patient meets the appropriate criteria. If surgery is done, it usually involves an endarterectomy and/or a bypass graft. Sympathectomy may be done to relieve the circulation in a chronically ischemic foot. Amputation of gangrenous areas may be necessary.

There are several drugs that may be used occasionally in the treatment of peripheral arterial disease. They include anticoagulants, vasodilators, and drugs that lower serum cholesterol. Anticoagulants are thought not to be useful in preventing arterial thrombosis and are not generally used without additional indications. Vasodilators, while they affect normal vessels, appear not to affect diseased ones. They are still used occasionally. Alcohol, a vasodilator, also appears to help some patients. Because there is no clear evidence that special diets or drugs to lower serum cholesterol alter the course of atherosclerosis, these are seldom prescribed for elderly patients. Knowledge of the side effects of all these drugs is essential if they are used.

Other measures used in treatment are designed principally to prevent complications or to improve the patient's ability to live comfortably with the problem.

A graduated walking program may assist in the development of collateral circulation. Obese patients should be encouraged to lose weight, but generally no dietary modifications designed to prevent artherosclerosis are undertaken, as stated previously. If the patient is a diabetic, strict diabetic dietary control may help. Smoking, which causes vasoconstriction, should be stopped. Doing so may improve claudication. Analgesics, including narcotics, may be necessary for the patient with severe chronic ischemia.

Meticulous foot care is essential for these patients. Feet should be washed daily in warm (not hot) water, dried gently and thoroughly, and covered with clean nonirritating socks. Lubricants are often necessary to keep the skin soft. Shoes and slippers should fit well and be worn at all times. Constricting garters, foundation garments, and other such items should be avoided. Bed socks may be necessary in bed. Infections must be treated early by a professional. Toenails, corns, and so forth require professional care. Local applications of heat must be avoided. Warm socks, leg warmers, body suits, or other such measures may help to keep the extremities from feeling cold. Compulsive care is mandatory to avoid the feared complications of ischemic ulcers and gangrene.

Treatment of ischemic ulcers and gangrene involves four areas: bedrest, pain relief, control of infection, and improvement of blood supply. Infection control may involve the use of boric acid soaks (or other agents such as 1:10,000 solution of potassium permanganate soaks) and antibiotics either systemically or directly with ointments or solutions.

The organisms should be cultured before the anti-biotics are chosen. Removal of eschar or necrotic tissues with an agent such as Elase is preferable to surgical debridement in many situations.

The first decision that needs to be made when acute occlusion of an artery occurs is whether or not surgery to remove the embolus or thrombus should be performed. If indicated, such surgery should be done as soon as possible before the viability of the limb is in serious question. It is possible to do the surgery under local anesthesia. The limb must be protected from trauma and pressure and kept at room temperature prior to surgery. Usually the limb is kept flat but there is controversy about the appropriate position. If surgery is to be delayed or not to be under-taken, anticoagulant therapy (generally with the coumarins) is continued indefinitely if a definite source of embolism can be found. Thrombolytic agents, such as streptokinase have been used experi-mentally but are costly, complex to administer, and not readily available.

Aneurysms generally are treated by resection of the aneurysm and replacement with a prosthetic or autogenous vein graft. Occlusive disease, produced by the aneurysms is treated in the same manner as other occlusive disorders. Treatment of underlying hypertension, with care to avoid making the blood pressure too low, may be done if the patient cannot withstand surgery.

Prevention of the development of venous throm-bosis and, hence, pulmonary emboli, has been the focus of considerable study recently. The identifica-tion of people at high risk and various methods of reducing the risk have been tested. Conventional methods such as early ambulation (after surgery or acute illness), active or passive leg exercises for those confined to bed, wrapping and elevating the legs of those who are immobilized, and various drug regi-mens have all met with varying success. Several mechanical devices providing intermittent calf com-pression have proven quite successful in patients undergoing surgery. It has been demonstrated that the use of elastic stockings which do not fit well (tighter at the ankles with the pressure decreasing progressively up the leg) is not effective and is often dangerous. Drug regimens including the use of low dose heparin, regular dose heparin, aspirin, aspirin and Persantine, coumarin therapy, and others have been tested. Each appears to have a place and the nurse will encounter the use of each in a variety of circumstances.

The principle problem with elastic stockings is improper fit. The mechanical devices may malfunc-tion and are expensive. They can also cause break-down of the skin and discomfort and are not practical for long term use outside of medical centers. Low dose heparin causes less complications than higher doses but may not be effective. Aspirin and aspirin and persantin may also be ineffective and can cause bleeding. Regular doses of heparin and the cou-marins carry a significant risk of bleeding and re-quire monitoring, not always possible outside an acute care setting. Moreover, heparin must be given by injection or drip.

It has become common practice to undertake a major program of prophylaxis in the patient at high risk (see page 261) who is experiencing prolonged immobilization. Therapy generally includes the use of drugs. The patient at high risk who is not immo-bilized may receive drug prophylaxis and should follow other precautions discussed below in relation to patients with chronic venous stasis.

Superficial venous thrombosis generally is treated by wrapping the legs (preferably with well-fitting commercial elastic stockings). The patient may or may not be allowed to be up. While the patient is in bed, the affected leg is elevated and warm applications may be used. If the foot of the bed can be elevated so that the patient is in Trendelen-berg position, venous return is enhanced more readily. The site of pain is marked and if it moves, especially toward the groin, additional measures may be taken, including anticoagulation.

The treatment of deep vein thrombosis is de-signed to prevent the formation of new thrombi and embolism. Bedrest for several days to a week is designed to allow the thrombi present to adhere to the vein wall, thus preventing embolization. Eleva-tion of the legs above the level of the heart increases venous return and decreases venous stasis, thus help-ing to prevent the formation of new thrombi. It also helps to decrease pain and edema. Elastic support hose used while the patient is up, may or may not be used while the patient is in bed. They also assist in promoting venous return. If the patient is allowed out of bed, sitting and standing should be discour-aged since both activities increase the hydrostatic pressure in the veins leading to further edema forma-tion. Contraction of the muscles (which compresses the veins) by walking and bed exercise should be encouraged once the danger of emboli has passed.

Deep vein thrombosis is treated with anticoagulants unless there is a reason to avoid this type of treatment. The usual treatment is with heparin followed by coumarin, both being administered for varying lengths of time. Heparin dosage may also vary. Heparin-related complications may include arterial emboli and bleeding. The bleeding is often seen first in the urine or in fresh wounds including injection sites. Protamine sulfate is the antidote to heparin. It may prolong the clotting time sufficiently to cause additional problems if high doses are used. The use of aspirin in a patient receiving heparin may cause bleeding and should be avoided if possible. The use of heparin is monitored by assessing the clotting time. Various laboratory tests are available to do this.

There are several coumarin products available. They are oral preparations that take longer to be effective and have longer-lasting effects. Initially the dosage is monitored daily by assessing the prothrombin time (other tests are also used). Laboratory monitoring of the dosage is also required at intervals for long term therapy, since the coumarins interact with a large variety of other agents including drugs and foods. The antidote for coumarin derivatives is vitamin K (e.g., Mephyton, Synkayvite). The most serious complication is bleeding, which may require that the drug be stopped. Because the action of the drugs is long acting, bleeding may be more difficult to control than that seen with heparin. Bleeding from the gums, hematuria, purpura, and bruising are examples of signs to be aware of. Among the numerous drugs that the coumarins interact with are phenylbutazone, diphenylhydantoin, salicylates, barbiturates, chloral hydrate, meprobamate, quinidine, and others. The mechanism of interaction is to either inhibit coumarin action or potentiate it. Patients who are responsible for their own drug therapy should be warned to avoid any medication, including those sold over the counter, without checking first with the professional responsible for care. In some situations it is possible to prescribe drugs that interact with coumarin and adjust the dosage accordingly. In that situation the patient needs to understand that failure to take the drug as prescribed may cause untoward effects.

Thrombolytic agents and dextran may be prescribed for some of these patients instead of anticoagulants. The use of these agents is principally experimental in nature.

The primary goal of care for the patient with chronic venous insufficiency is to avoid the complications of venous ulcers or pulmonary emboli. The various preventive measures discussed above are used to accomplish this goal.

Should venous ulcers occur, they are treated in much the same manner as ischemic ulcers with several exceptions. Compromise of venous return by having the legs dependent may cause sufficient edema to compromise arterial flow. (The patient with ischemic ulcers may be unable to tolerate any position where his legs are not dependent because he needs maximal arterial flow.) Therefore, elevation of the legs with subsequent reduction of edema allowing good arterial flow helps to make venous ulcers heal more readily than ischemic ones. Moreover, warm packs (contraindication in the ischemic ulcer patient) help to reduce the inflammation and pain resulting from the usually sterile cellulitis caused by stasis ulcers. The need to debride stasis ulcers is less frequent. Rather, they may need surgical grafting to enhance healing. Occasionally, applications such as Unna's paste boots may be applied after the edema has been reduced to promote healing.

Definitive therapy of pulmonary emboli sometimes is done surgically by performing an embolectomy. However, the results from this procedure have been poor, probably because the underlying condition of the patient usually is poor. Thrombolytic agents have also been used experimentally; good results have been reported with their use in a small population.

Other types of therapy include long term anticoagulation, the use of measures to prevent further thrombi and emboli from forming, treatment of shock if it is present, and the treatment of the respiratory embarrassment. Anticoagulation and preventive measures have been discussed previously. Shock is treated with the conventional measures including the use of vasoconstrictors. Respiratory embarrassment is treated with oxygen and elevation of the head of the bed.

Recurrent pulmonary emboli are treated using a variety of measures. These can include long term anticoagulation, all of the preventive measures discussed above, and two other surgical procedures, venous interruption by ligation and plication or insertion of an umbrella device to trap the emboli.

The need to actively help individuals prevent the complications of the various chronic diseases presented is a very important one. Thus, the teaching role of the nurse is a high priority one in treating these patients.

Evaluation

The evaluation criteria for monitoring self-care by the patient and nursing care can best be established in close collaboration with the patient. The problems caused by the diagnosis, the goals of the treatment plan, the possible outcomes of deviating from the treatment plan, and how the plan will alter the lifestyle of the patient need to be discussed first. From there a goal and specific, measurable objectives for each form of treatment can be derived and used by both the nurse and patient to monitor progress. For example, if the goal is to use antigravity measures to treat chronic venous insufficiency, one objective could be, "Elevates legs for one third of waking hours." A plan to accomplish this would include assessment of daily activities and planning around these to allow time for leg elevation.

BIBLIOGRAPHY

Am. J. Nurs. 77:602–613, April, 1977. (A collection of articles about sex. Included are: (1) sex after a coronary, (2) exercise, sex, and cardiovascular health, (3) the use of stair-climbing ability as a test of readiness to resume sexual relationships, (4) counseling the cardiac patient, and (5) sex after middle age.)

Arbeit, S., et al.: Recognizing digitalis toxicity. Am. J. Nurs. 77:1936–1945, December, 1977. (The action of digitalis preparations, factors increasing risk of toxicity, signs and symptoms, and management strategies. Useful for nurses functioning in ambulatory care settings and teaching patients for more effective self-care, as well as those in acute care settings.)

Atkinson, A. J.: Clinical use of blood levels of cardiac drugs. Modern Concepts Cardiovascular Dis. 42:1–4, 1973. A review of the current state of the art of using blood levels to help determine therapeutic doses of cardiac drugs.)

Beller, G. A., et al.: Digitalis intoxication: a prospective clinical study with serum level correlation. New Engl. J. Med. 284:989–997, 1971. (An excellent article to help nurses understand the manifestations of digitalis toxicity.)

Brest, A. N., and Moyer, J. A.: Atherosclerotic Vascular Disease. New York: Appleton-Century-Crofts, 1967. (Although some of the material is not completely current, this book has excellent sections to enhance understanding of the disease process of atherosclerosis. Conditions caused by atherosclerosis are also discussed.)

Brest, A. N. (ed.): Congestive Heart Failure. New York: Medcom Inc., 1975. (A comprehensive review of congestive heart failure including chapters on the entity itself,

how it affects the heart, lungs, kidneys, and hormone balance; digitalis and diuretics; unusual problems and surgery.)

Caprini, J. A., Zoellner, J. L., and Weisman, M.: Heparin therapy. Cardiovasc. Nurs. Part I, 3:13–16, 1977; Part II, 4, 17–20, 1977. (American Heart Association Publication. The first article discusses hemostasis, historical perspective on heparin use, and the use of continuous infusion therapy. Part II reviews use of minidose heparin therapy and guidelines for intravenous and subcutaneous heparin administration.)

Cassem, N. H., and Hackett, T. P.: Psychological rehabilitation of myocardial infarction patient in the acute phase. Heart and Lung 2:382–388, 1973. (Discussion of the post-infarction psychologic sequelae and practical suggestions for managing them. Presented by two well-recognized authorities in the field.)

Cobey, J. C., and Cobey, J. H.: Chronic leg ulcers. Am. J. Nurs. 74:258–259, 1974. (A discussion of the differences between arterial ulcers and venous ulcers. Included are both the diagnostic manifestations and treatment rationale.)

Conners, P.: Treating leg ulcers. Nursing 77, p. 66–67, May, 1977. (An excellent article covering pathophysiology and treatment of venous stasis ulcers.)

Coon, W. W.: Operative therapy of venous thromboembolism. Modern Concepts of Cardiovasc. Dis. 43:71–75, 1974. (An excellent review of the various operative therapies used in treating thromboembolism.)

Daly, C. R., and Kelly, E. A.: Prevention of pulmonary embolism: intracaval devices. Am. J. Nurs. 72:2004–2006, 1972. (An overview of pulmonary embolism is presented and then the discussion focuses on the use of intracaval devices.)

del Greco, F.: The kidney in congestive heart failure. Modern Concepts Cardiovasc. Dis. 44:47–52, 1975. (The various aspects of renal function in congestive heart failure are explained.)

de Wolfe, V. G.: Assessment of the circulation in occlusive arterial disease of the lower extremities. Modern Concepts Cardiovasc. Dis. 45:91–95, 1976. (This is an excellent article which presents arterial occlusive disease systematically and logically.)

Diseases of the Heart and Blood Vessels: Nomenclature and Criteria for Diagnosis, ed. 6. Boston: Little, Brown & Co., 1964. (New York Heart Association. The therapeutic and functional classifications of heart disease are presented.)

Exercise Equivalents. Colorado Heart Association, 4521 East Virginia Avenue, Denver, Colorado. (Compilation of materials from authorities in rehabilitating the patient with heart disease. Contains information about energy consumption of various activities, an outline of a rehabilitation program, guidelines for evaluating successful rehabilitation, and so forth.)

Feldman, E. B. (ed.): Nutrition and Cardiovascular Disease. New York: Appleton-Century-Crofts, 1976. (A recent comprehensive review of the state of knowledge regarding various diets used in the treatment of cardiovascular disease. Also included are discussions of epidemiology, obesity, vitamin, and trace element intake.)

Fournet, Sr. K. M.: Patients discharged on diuretics: prime candidates for individualized teaching by the nurse. Heat and Lung: Journal of Critical Care, 3:108–116, January–February, 1974. (A helpful article describing a study of three methods of instructing patients about diuretic therapy. Included also are an overview of diuretic therapy and a patient-directed goal program to help in the teaching process.)

Fox, S. M., Naughton, J. P., and Gorman, P. A.: Physical activity and cardiovascular health, Parts I and II. Modern Concepts Cardiovasc. Dis. 41:17–26, 1972. (This is a series of two excellent review articles. The first one focuses on mechanisms by which increased activity may produce beneficial results and the second on an approach to prescribing appropriate physical activity.)

Friedberg, C. K. (ed.): Congestive Heart Failure. New York: Grune and Stratton, 1970. (This book presents congestive heart failure from several approaches. It is written by a well-known cardiologist.)

Gazes, P. C.: Diagnostic clues in cardiovascular disease. Postgrad. Med. 47:71–76, 1970. (The use of the eyes and fingertips is discussed in diagnosing cardiovascular disease. There are several excellent "tips" presented.)

Goodman, L., and Gilman, A. (eds.): The Pharmacological Basis of Therapeutics. New York: Macmillan Publishing Co., 1975. (This text is commonly used as the standard reference book for drug-related data.)

Harris, R.: The Management of Geriatric Cardiovascular Disease, Philadelphia: J. B. Lippincott Co., 1970. (This book addresses the problems of cardiovascular diseases in the elderly. General sections include normal cardiovascular parameters of aging, specific diseases of the heart, and special problems in old age, e.g., CHF.)

Hazzard, W. R.: Aging and atherosclerosis: interactions with diet, heredity, and associated risk factors. In Nutrition, Longevity and Aging. New York: Academic Press, 1976, p. 143–195. (An excellent review of research including that done by the author and his associates. It helps to illustrate the complexity of atherosclerosis and its interaction with disease states.)

Hazzard, W. R.: A pathophysiologic approach to managing hyperlipemia. Am. Family Physician 14:78–87, 1976. (This article describes a rationale approach to treating and diagnosing hyperlipemia. The data presented are part of the data from a multicenter study of this area.)

Hecht, A. B.: Improving medication compliance by teaching outpatients. Nursing Forum 13:112–129, 1974. (This is a report of a study done by the author to demonstrate fewer medication error in patients who have been instructed about their medications.)

Holling, H. E.: Peripheral Vascular Disease: Diagnosis and Management. Philadelphia: J. B. Lippincott Co., 1972.

(An excellent reference about most of the peripheral vascular diseases. Includes (1) a general section including concepts of peripheral circulation and interviewing and examining the patient with arterial disease, (2) disorders of large arteries, (3) disorders of small vessels, and (4) disorders of veins and lymphatics.)

Houghey, E. J., and Sica, F. M.: Diuretics: how safe can you make them? Nursing 77, p. 34–39, February, 1977. (An excellent article describing diuretics, their actions and side effects, and what to teach the patient taking them.)

Hurst, J. W., et al.: The Heart, Arteries and Veins, ed. 3. New York: McGraw-Hill Book Co., 1974. (This is one of the frequently quoted standard references about cardiac and vascular disease. Congestive heart failure and peripheral vascular disease and the treatment modalities for both are discussed in some detail.)

Kappert, A., and Winsor, T.: Diagnosis of Peripheral Vascular Diseases. Philadelphia: F. A. Davis Co., 1972. (Multiple illustrations characterize this text. The various vascular conditions are discussed and findings illustrated. The book is particularly useful in helping nurses recognize the manifestations of vascular disease.)

Kennedy, J. W.: Myocardial function in coronary artery disease. Cardiovasc. Nurs. 12:23–27, 1976. (This is a review of myocardial function in coronary artery disease, current methods for evaluating myocardial performance, and treatment modalities.)

Koprowicz, D. C.: Drug interactions with coumarin derivatives. Am. J. Nurs. 73:1042–1044, 1973. (A review of the actions, toxic effects, patient teaching, and interaction of coumarin drugs. Included are the mechanisms of the interactions.)

Lewis, E. P. (ed.): Nursing in Cardiovascular Diseases. New York: American Journal of Nursing Co., 1971. (Selected articles from Nursing Outlook, Nursing Research, and the American Journal of Nursing related to cardiac nursing were reprinted. Section V concerns congestive heart failure.)

Luckman, J., and Sorenson, K. C.: Medical-Surgical Nursing: A Psychophysiologic Approach. Philadelphia: W. B. Saunders Co., 1974. (The sections discussing surgery, neurologic function, peripheral vascular functions, cardiovascular function, and musculoskeletal function can assist the nurse in understanding peripheral vascular disease and congestive heart failure.)

Lundbaek, K.: Diabetic angiopathy. Modern Concepts Cardiovasc. Dis. 43:103–107, 1974. (One view of diabetic vascular disease and its treatment.)

Madden, J. L., and Hume, M. (eds.): Venous Thromboembolism, Prevention and Treatment. New York: Appleton-Century-Crofts, 1976. (The emphasis of this presentation is prevention of pulmonary embolism and venous thrombosis. Many research studies of techniques for accomplishing this goal are discussed as are current modalities of treatment. There is also an excellent discussion of the prevalence of the problems caused by these entities.)

Miller, R. A.: How to Live with a Heart Attack. Radnor, Pa.: Chilton Book Co., 1973. (This book is done in simple terminology designed to appeal to patients. Many topics and myths are discussed.)

Moylan, J., and Flye, M. W.: Peripheral vascular disease in the geriatric patient. In Reichel, W. (ed.): Clinical Aspects of Aging. Baltimore: Williams & Wilkins, 1978. (Excellent concise discussion of management.)

O'Brien, J. R.: The mechanisms of venous thrombosis, anticoagulants, aspirin and heparin. Modern Concepts Cardiovasc. Dis. 42:11–15, 1973. (An excellent discussion of the factors related to the formation of thrombi and treatment modalities.)

Pinneo, R.: Symposium on concepts in cardiac nursing. Nurs. Clin. N. Am. 7:411–585, 1972. (The entire issue is devoted to a discussion of factors related to coronary heart disease, its treatment, and associated problems. Included is a chapter on pump failure.)

Rasmussen, S., Noble, R. J., and Fisch, C.: The pharmacology and clinical use of digitalis. Cardiovasc. Nurs. 2:23–28, 1975. (The clinical actions, pharmacokinetics, toxicity, and nursing implications of digitalis are presented. The data discussed are based partly on a study by the authors.)

Redman, B.: Client education therapy in treatment and prevention of cardiovascular diseases. Cardiovasc. Nurs. 10:1–6, 1974. (A discussion of the principles of education with application to the cardiac patient. This article is written by a well-known nursing leader.)

Richards, R. L.: Peripheral Arterial Disease. London: E. and S. Livingstone, 1970. (This text discusses peripheral arterial disease by stressing an organized framework for understanding. Chapters include (1) historical introduction, (2) normal peripheral circulation, (3) classification and nomenclature, (4) signs and symptoms, (5) intermittent claudication, (6) acute arterial occlusion, (7) the chronic ischemic limb, (8) the Raynaud syndrome and (9) other vascular syndromes.)

Roberts, B.: The acutely ischemic limb. Heart and Lung: J. Critical Care 5:273–276, 1976. (An excellent review of the basic concepts and facts used in diagnosis and management of acute limb ischemia.)

Roberts, S. L.: Skin assessment for color and temperature. Am. J. Nursing 75:610–613, 1975. (This article can be of great assistance in helping nurses to learn to assess some of the subtle changes associated with peripheral vascular disease or severe congestive heart failure.)

Roberts, W. C.: Relationship between coronary thrombosis and myocardial infarction. Modern Concepts Cardiovasc. Dis. 16:7–10, 1972. (This article, by a pathologist, discusses the examination of coronary arteries after death in patients with a history of an M.I.)

Rose, G.: Early mobilization and discharge after myocardial infarction. Modern Concepts Cardiovasc. Dis. 41:59–63, 1972. (Discussion of the relative merits of rapid mobilization of past M.I. patients. Good presentation of the two viewpoints (early mobilization and longer rest periods before mobilization) for rehabilitating the cardiac patient.)

Rose, M. A.: Home care after peripheral vascular surgery. Am. J. Nurs. 74:260–262, 1974. (This is a basic discussion of the extremity care required after vascular surgery. The emphasis is on helping patients and families do this type care. Several practical hints are included.)

Rubenstein, E.: The high incidence of thromboembolism: prevention and action. Geriatrics 28:116–121, 1973. (An excellent article which discusses the elderly population in particular, and general areas of the diagnosis, treatment, and prevention of venous thrombosis and pulmonary embolism.)

Schwartz, S., et al. (eds.): Principles of Surgery, ed. 2. New York: McGraw-Hill Book Co., 1974. (This is a comprehensive surgical textbook. There are excellent chapters on peripheral arterial disease and venous, and lymphatic disease. Other chapters can also contribute to the nurse's understanding of these problems and their treatment.)

Sexton, D.: Symposium on patients with peripheral vascular disease. Nurs. Clin. N. Am. 12:87–171, 1977. (Devoted to discussing the patient with arterial disease. Articles by contributors include discussion of arterial occlusive disease, atherosclerosis, physical assessment, emotional adjustment, surgery, postoperative care, patient teaching, and rehabilitation.)

Shapiro, R. M.: Anticoagulant therapy. Am. J. Nurs. 74:439–443, 1974. (This article presents the mechanisms of action of heparin and warfarin. She also discusses in some detail the recognition, prevention, and treatment of complications of therapy.)

Snively, W. D., Beshaer, D. R., and Roberts, K. T.: Sodium-restricted diets: review and current status. Nursing Forum 13:59–86, 1974. (This presentation includes an excellent overview of the historical use of salt in the diet, history of low salt diets, salt restriction in treating hypertension, CHF, etc., specifics about low sodium diets and foods, and report of a study conducted by the authors. The discussion of low- and high-salt-containing substances is particularly valuable.)

Spann, J. F., Mason, D. T., and Zelis, R. F.: Recent advances in the understanding of congestive heart failure, Parts I and II. Modern Concepts Cardiovasc. Dis. 39:73–84, 1970. (An excellent two-part article which discusses the influences of contractility, biochemical abnormalities, the autonomic nervous system, peripheral circulation, and compensatory mechanisms on the development of congestive heart failure.)

Sparks, C.: Peripheral pulses. Am. J. Nurs. 75:1132–1133, 1975. (An excellent description of the location of peripheral pulses.)

Syme, S. L.: Social and psychological risk factors in coronary heart disease. Modern Concepts Cardiovasc.

Dis. 44:17–21, 1975. (The risk factors discussed are categorized as sociocultural mobility factors, behavior patterns, and life events. The mechanisms of these factors' effect on the heart and vessels are presented.)

Symposium: pulmonary embolism. Heart and Lung: J. Critical Care 3:207–246, 1974. (A series of six articles discussing implications for nursing practice, radiologic diagnosis, radioisotopic diagnosis, therapy, and overview of pulmonary embolism and massive pulmonary embolism.)

Tanner, G.: Heart failure in the M.I. patient. Am. J. Nurs. 77:230–234, 1977. (A discussion of the cues which may be present in the patient who is developing heart failure. Each cue is explained in relation to its meaning in heart failure.)

Thorn, G. W., et al.: Harrison's Principles of Internal Medicine, ed. 8. New York: McGraw-Hill Book Co., 1977. (Various signs and symptoms, such as dyspnea and cyanosis, are discussed. Also there are sections on disorders of the heart (chapters on CHF and drugs) and vascular system disorders (chapters on atherosclerosis and extremity disease). This is one of the standard medical texts.)

Tikoff, G., and Kuida, H.: Pathophysiology of heart failure in congenital heart disease. Modern Concepts Cardiovasc. Dis. 41:1–6, 1972. (This article focuses primarily on the pathophysiology of heart failure in atrial septal defects, ventricular septal defects, and patent ductus arteriosus.)

Wessler, S.: Prevention of venous thromboembolism by low-dose heparin. Modern Concepts Cardiovasc. Dis. 45:105–109, 1976. (An excellent review of the epidemiology of the problem and the uses of low-dose heparin. Situations in which this therapy is not as helpful are also discussed.)

White, P. D., and Donovan, H.: Hearts: Their Long Term Follow-Up. Philadelphia: W. B. Saunders Co., 1967. (A fascinating book which discusses the natural history of various cardiac disorders in patients whom this "father" of modern cardiology cared for over many years.)

Wissler, R. W., and Vesselinovitch, D.: Regression of atherosclerosis in experimental animals and man. Modern Concepts Cardiovasc. Dis. 46:27–32, 1977. (An excellent review of recent work in this field by pathologists.)

Young, C.: Exercise. Nursing 75, pp. 81–82, March, 1975. (A discussion of the use of an exercise program to prevent the complications of immobility.)

Pamphlets

The following are examples of pamphlets available from local Heart Association chapter affiliates. A complete list can be obtained from the local chapter. Questions not answered by local affiliates should be addressed to: The American Heart Association, Inc., 7320 Greenville Avenue, Dallas, TX 75231.

"Reduce Your Risk of Heart Attack"—an overview of cardiac risk factors

"Anticoagulants, Your Physician and You"—patient oriented information

"Facts About Congestive Heart Failure"—for patients

"PACE, After Your Heart Attack"—adapted from a book by a physician to discuss cardiac rehabilitation from the patient's point of view

"Your Heart Has Nine Lives"—by a physician to discuss rehabilitation and prevention with patients

"Your 500 milligram Sodium Diet"—one of a series for patients about sodium restricted diets

"Examination of the Heart"

"Part One—Data Collection: The Clinical History"

"Part Two—Inspection and Palpation of the Anterior Chest"

"Part Three—Inspection and Palpation of Venous and Arterial Pulses"

"Part Four—Auscultation"

"Part Five—The Electrocardiogram"

An excellent series written for professionals. Can be useful to nurses desiring to learn these skills.

Paperback Books*

Birocher, R., M.D. (ed.): Bircher-Benner Salt-Free Nutrition Plan, Los Angeles: Nash Publications, 1972. ($2.75)

Brunswick, J. P., Love, D., Weinberg, A., M.D.: How to Live 365 Days a Year the Salt Free Way, New York: Bantam Books, 1977. ($1.95)

Bugg, E. W.: Cooking Without a Grain of Salt. New York: Bantam Books, 1972. ($1.95)

Eshleman, R., and Winston, M.: The American Heart Association Cookbook. New York: Ballantine Books, 1973. ($2.75)

Jones, J.: Diet for a Happy Heart. San Francisco: 101 Productions, 1975. ($1.95)

Thorburn, A. H., and Turner, P.: Live Salt Free and Easy. New York: Signet, 1975. ($1.50)

* The prices reflect those charged at the author's local bookstore in 1977. Prices may vary.

14

Cerebrovascular Accidents

Maria Linde

QUICK REVIEW

TRANSIENT ISCHEMIC ATTACKS (TIA)

DESCRIPTION	A temporary deficit in central neurologic function secondary to ischemia caused by decreased or interrupted blood flow to a portion of the brain.
ETIOLOGIC FACTORS	Atherosclerosis, emboli, plaques, spasms of blood vessels.
HIGH RISK	Hypertensive individuals, persons over 65, diabetics, coronary artery disease.
	High risk times: Positional changes that alter the blood pressure.
SIGNS AND SYMPTOMS	Usually disappear within a day. Unable to express or understand. Double vision, blindness in one eye. Loss of function or sensation of an extremity. Temporary amnesia, falling, failure to recognize persons/objects.
PROGNOSIS	If involving carotid territories, 76% risk of major CVA after one or two TIAs.
NURSING MANAGEMENT	Prompt medical evaluation of carotid-area TIA. Post emergency phone number on phone. Teach to change positions more slowly. Have reliable personal contact every day. Encourage to report signs and symptoms, but also be alert for casual reference to signs and symptoms, since they may be ignored or forgotten.
EVALUATION	Backup and emergency resources in place. Understanding of experience and action to take.

QUICK REVIEW

STROKES

DESCRIPTION	Sensory, perceptual, communication, and/or motor dysfunction, secondary impaired blood flow and tissue damage to a particular part of the brain.
ETIOLOGIC FACTORS	Hypertension, atherosclerosis, cardiac disorders, impaired glucose tolerance, anemia.
HIGH RISK	Elderly, blacks, smokers, cardiac patients, diabetics, and those with family history of strokes.
DYNAMICS	Obstruction of blood vessels in brain or extravasation of blood sufficient to cause interruption of blood flow and residual damage.
SIGNS AND SYMPTOMS	May be sudden and dramatic or subtle. Hemiplegia/quadriplegia. Visual field loss, incontinence, sensory losses, alterations in consciousness. Defects in speech, language, swallowing.
COMPLICATIONS	*Physical:* Joint contracture, shoulder separations, constipation, atonic bladder, trauma in areas of decreased sensation, edema of dependent flaccid extremities. *Psychosocial:* Body image change, social isolation, sensory deprivation, depression, fear of another stroke, dependence.
PROGNOSIS	Rehabilitation is more complicated when there is motor and sensory loss. Gains continue long beyond the immediate post-CVA period. Right-sided hemiplegic persons have better chance of living, independently post-stroke. Overall death rate (not age related) 19.5%.
NURSING MANAGEMENT	Build protective systems and environment to compensate for deficits in sensation, visual fields, failure to "own" a body part, loss of judgment, and spatial perception deficit. Maintain joint mobility and strength. Build endurance. Assist patient's family providers to build a working communication system. Build in support—knowledge, respite, encouragement for support persons. Give prompt, realistic feedback to patient.
EVALUATION	Collect data on progress and give concrete feedback to patient regularly. Create flow sheets with variables appropriate to patient's presenting situation to highlight progress or maintenance. Prevention of trauma, satisfaction with adjustments in ADL or lifestyle. Maintenance of support systems over time. Physical status. Participation in events, ADL, other activities.

The risk of strokes increases concurrently with advancing age. In the over-75 age group the estimated prevalence is 95 per 1000. No means has been found to alter these risks since strokes presumably result from the age-related, progressive changes in blood vessels. Because strokes in the elderly frequently result in prolonged adjustment in daily living, nursing management is a significant component of post-stroke health care.

There are two phenomena related to cerebrovascular incidents in the over-70 age group which the nurse must be prepared to recognize and manage: transient ischemic attack and stroke.

TRANSIENT ISCHEMIC ATTACKS

Description

Transient ischemic attack (TIA) is a central neurologic deficit lasting no more than 24 hours, caused by ischemia secondary to interruption of blood flow to a portion of the brain.

Etiologic Factors

The temporary ischemia occurs as a result of atherosclerotic plaques or of spasm of blood vessels. Total or partial occlusion may be caused by emboli and interruption or diminished circulation to a segment of the brain.

High Risk Populations

Persons at high risk of TIAs include those over 65 with hypertension (160/90), with diabetes, and/or with clinical evidence of coronary artery disease. Both sexes are equally at risk among the elderly. This is in contrast to the younger age group where males have higher risk.

Times of higher risk of TIA occur when the individual changes position in such a way as to suddenly change the blood pressure, e.g., supine to standing. Even sudden changes in positions may constitute a danger time for some individuals. Monitoring of blood pressure levels in different positions may give the nurse important clues as to risk.

Dynamics

As a result of a temporary failure to receive an adequate blood supply and, therefore, insufficient perfusion, the affected neurons fail to function or function at a lower level for a period of time.

Signs and Symptoms

Signs and symptoms given here (Table 14-1) for TIAs are localized to the carotid or vertebrobasilar system or a combination of the two. As the label suggests, these signs and symptoms are transient, tending to disappear within a day.

TABLE 14-1. Signs and symptoms of transient ischemic attacks.

Disturbance	Result
Communication disturbance	Unable to express or comprehend written or spoken language
Visual disturbance	Has double vision or temporary blindness in one eye
Loss of muscle control	Unable to use the leg and arm on one side of the body
Amnesia	Cannot recall brief periods of time
Sensory disturbance	Has lost sensation of pain or temperature on one side of the body
Numbness	Lacks feeling in face, arms, legs, and side, especially if only one side is involved
Loss of balance	Falls for no apparent reason, either with a blackout that goes away promptly or without any loss of consciousness
Lack of comprehension	Fails to recognize familiar objects or persons, even those that are quite familiar

Prognosis

TIAs involving the carotid territory carry a worse prognosis for occurrence of a major vascular accident than those in the vertebrobasilar area (Fig. 14-1). The appearance of TIAs in the carotid territory is a serious matter. One study showed that 76 percent of the persons who suffered TIAs of the carotid territory had only one or two of these transient prodromal

FIGURE 14-1. Carotid and vertebrobasilar vascular systems.

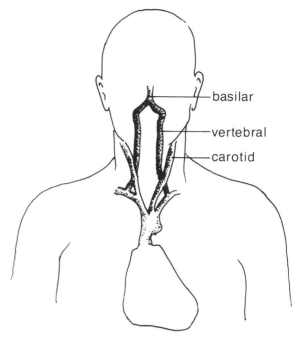

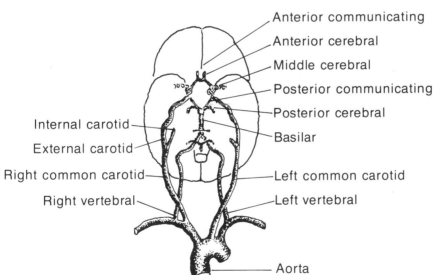

warning attacks before their major episode. This is in contrast to 52 percent of patients with TIAs in the vertebrobasilar territory. Therefore the decision as to what diagnostic tests to make and the treatment to be initiated is a matter of some urgency.

The nursing prognosis in terms of coping with repeated TIAs is very much inherent in the individual. Factors such as available support systems,

ego strength, willingness to take risks to maintain a lifestyle, and general acceptance of the aging process will all contribute to the individual's self-preservation.

If the individual is given a chance to verbalize his fears and understand what is happening as well as participate in the decision making related to his body, his chances for being able to put the experience behind him are greatly improved. Without this the patient is likely to live in fear of the next TIA or the major cerebrovascular accident.

Management

Any person with suspected TIAs should have medical evaluation. However, some individuals who have TIAs may deny their occurrence or do not wish to bother people since the symptoms disappear in a short time. Therefore, the nurse who is aware of the signs and symptoms often will be able to accurately assess and pinpoint the occurrence of TIA from a casual conversation with the patient.

Since TIAs often are warnings of impending stroke, it is important to deal with them. The person, particularly the one who lives alone, needs to have some sense of control—what to do and how to manage if there is a recurrence. The following management measures are important.

1. Post the telephone numbers of the doctor/ nurse or hospital on the telephone.
2. Obtain a long telephone cord and/or locate phone at the bedside.
3. Obtain and use antiembolic stockings if the individual has postural hypotension.
4. Change positions slowly from lying or sitting to standing.
5. Avoid sudden rapid changes of position and movements.
6. Have a family member or neighbor call daily. Check for a community resource—a service of volunteers who phone once every 24 hours with planned backup to check on the person if he does not answer (such as Friendly Phone Visitor).
7. Improve the safety of the environment in the home. (Remove small rugs that act as excellent skating boards; remove furniture in way of passage; add support bars in bathroom and safety strips in the tub.) Some medical supply houses have consultants on the staff who, without a fee, will make a home assessment. An occupational therapist also is an excellent resource.

Nursing management of the person with TIAs also includes contacts with the family and friends. Obtain confidence of the patient to share data on these attacks with nurse. Work with the family on explaining the importance of reporting or what to do when they occur. Their knowledge of the dynamics of the situation and their understanding and support for the person provides immeasurable sustenance.

Medical management consists of surgical intervention as well as pharmaceutical therapy to prevent progression from temporary ischemic episodes to a stroke. The aggressiveness of diagnostic testing and management varies with the number of TIAs that have occurred, the blood vessels involved, and the individual physician's philosophy—and also whether the patient reports the incidents or not. Aggressive diagnosis and immediate surgical intervention is associated with lesions in the carotid system. Bypass of obstructed blood vessels is the most common surgical therapy.

Drug therapy to try to prevent strokes consists of giving platelet inhibitors—aspirin and Persantine in combination. Nursing management in this form of therapy consists of supporting the patient in participating accurately and consistently with the drug therapy. This involves helping the patient to understand why the medication is being given. Timing and dosages vary. One of the side effects of Persantine is headache. For this reason some physicians will suggest that the drug be taken at bedtime where this will not be so noticeable. Others will prescribe the drugs on a T.I.D. or O.I.D. basis.

The use of anticoagulants is common, particularly if there are associated cardiac irregularities. Here, of course, the nurse needs to educate the patient how to observe for bleeding, i.e., easy bleeding, bleeding gums, hematuria, and black or blood-streaked stools.

Drug interactions need to be taught since they are critical. Common drugs such as aspirin, salicylates, quinidine, and thyroid will *potentiate* the drug's effects. Barbiturates, on the other hand, will inhibit the anticoagulant effect. The nurse needs to be aware of this and must make the patient and family aware of these drug interactions.

Hospitalization for TIAs may or may not be used, again depending on the location of the lesion, the physician's preference, and the support systems available to the patient in the home.

STROKES

Description

Strokes are dysfunctions in sensory, perceptual, communication, and/or motor function that result from impaired blood flow to a particular area of the brain. It may have a sudden and massive onset or may be a slowly-developing phenomena over a period of time. The individual may or may not recognize that changes are occurring; this is especially true if the right hemisphere is affected.

Etiologic Factors

Certain other conditions predispose to strokes. These include hypertension, atherosclerosis, mitral stenosis, and any type of cardiac disorder, including ischemic heart disease. Clinical experience indicates an increased risk of cerebral infarction with even modest impairments of glucose tolerance. In the older age group it is well to remember anemia as a cause for cerebral ischemia.

High Risk Populations

Populations at high risk for strokes include the elderly, blacks, smokers, cardiac patients, diabetics, and individuals with a family history of strokes. (There is no difference in risk based on sex in the older age group.)

Dynamics

Blood flow to the brain is interrupted or decreased as a result of gradual narrowing of the lumen, caused by obstruction from local thrombi or atherosclerotic plaques or from emboli from distant parts. Intracerebral extravasations and ruptured aneurysms are less likely to occur in the elderly. However, subdural hematomas resulting from falls do occur.

Signs and Symptoms

The signs and symptoms of stroke may occur as a very obvious critical and massive event or may appear as subtle cues that occur in almost any area of function. The nurse faces a challenge in determining the onset of a stroke.

Subtle Signs and Symptoms

The nurse who encounters the older person in the home, the retirement center, the senior citizen center, or the clinic will want to be alert for the following signs and symptoms that may be indicative of the onset of a stroke:

- The homemaker burns herself when cooking

but doesn't recognize that it has happened. Or the person who has a cigarette burn on the fingers and doesn't notice it. (Sensory stroke)
- The individual who picks up the phone and can't remember a phone number he had been using for many years.
- The person, in getting out of bed, finds himself on the floor but is able to get up.
- The woman who takes out a comb and then forgets how to comb her hair. (Loss of recall in using a familiar object)
- The individual who dials a number and, when the person being called answers, finds himself unable to speak.
- The person who suddenly finds difficulty in swallowing.
- The person who has a sudden numbness in one of the extremities.
- The individual who feels that a curtain has abruptly come across a portion of his visual field. (It usually involves one eye but many do not think to put a hand over each eye to test this.)
- The person riding the bus who suddenly becomes aware that she doesn't know where she is.

The older individual who experiences these small manifestations of a stroke may be unaware of them and, therfore, unable to report them. Another possibility is that he would prefer to ignore them and, therefore, does not report them. If the nurse does not observe the changes or has a hunch but is unable to verify it, she may wish to get information from individuals who have been in contact with the patient—family, neighbors, friends, the mailman, the grocery clerk, and so forth. The history is important, and effort needs to be made to obtain an accurate one.

Major Signs and Symptoms

The signs and symptoms will be drastic and sudden where a large blood vessel is involved. This abrupt onset is one of the most devastating features of a major stroke—the individual is so totally unprepared.

The signs and symptoms in major lesions can be manifestations of unilateral or bilateral involvement, cerebellar involvement, or, where the anterior spinal artery is occluded, a quadriplegic pattern of involvement. The classic signs and symptoms of a stroke include hemiplegia, quadriplegia, hemianopsia, incontinence, sensory losses, alterations, dysarthria, dysphasia, and dysphagia.

SENSORY SYMPTOMS. It is important to obtain specific data on the nature of the losses in the area of sensory loss. Such data are necessary in considering prognosis and planning the management of the immediate environment in such a way as to protect the patient from elements that may cause additional injury. These data may be obtained from the medical data base, or the nurse who has competence may do a sensory examination. (See Bates, 1979, pp. 345–358.) The interpretation of sensory data is difficult and takes practice. Therefore the less-experienced nurse will wish to seek a second opinion until she has gained confidence in her interpretation.

There are times when an older person who has had a minor stroke may not wish to be hospitalized. It is important that an accurate sensory check be made in order to be certain that the individual will not be harmed in areas where he is unable to perceive injurious stimuli. The sensory losses are often so subtle that the patient is not aware of the situation and, thus, may be unable to report it; therefore, it is extremely important that a specific examination for this type of dysfunction be carried out.

COMMUNICATION. Language dysfunctions or deficits also need to be plotted accurately. The deficits can include both comprehension and expression of language, reading, writing, and arithmetic. Again, because these capabilities and functions affect so many dimensions of daily living, it becomes crucial for the nurse to collect accurate data on the areas and nature of the specific deficits in each of the five areas.

COMPREHENSION. The nurse is interested in discovering how much or how little the person can understand, since overestimation or underestimation of a problem leads to poor management. Data on the following areas of comprehension need to be collected.

Does the person respond to a simple request?
"Close your eyes."

Can he respond to a two-step request?
"Close your eyes and touch your nose."

If the person does not respond to verbal commands, will he follow body language?
Demonstrate an activity involving body parts.
Touch your finger to your own nose.

Can he read a newspaper heading? (Be sure he has on his reading glasses)
Or the nurse could print a written request for

him to carry out if he is unable to speak, e.g., "Touch your nose."

Can he carry out simple arithmetic calculations?

Can he make change?
Give him a 50-cent piece and ask him to make change for a 15 or 25-cent purchase. (This is important since some individuals recover all functions except the ability to handle money.)

Can he write a sentence from the nurse's dictation? "He shouted the warning."

EXPRESSION. Another facet in communication deficit is that of expression—speech. Comprehension and expression need to be assessed separately. The person who understands but cannot speak must be both insulted and angered by the behavior of others who assume that the individual who cannot speak understandably cannot possibly understand what is being said to him. However, the two—comprehension and expression—do not necessarily go hand-in-hand. One or the other, or both, may be affected, depending on the location of the lesion.

When the *anterior portion of the frontal lobe* (Brocha's area) is involved, comprehension is intact to varying degrees. However, speech is altered in several ways. In its most severe form the individual may be totally without expressive speech. Or he may retain automatic speech—he can name the days of the week, his own name, and so forth. He may have restricted speech—he tends to leave out verbs, sentences are short, and he points to objects he cannot name (anomia). Such lesions also can cause profanity to become a predominate feature of speech; in fact, sometimes those are the only words an individual can say. This can occur in the vocabulary of someone who has never used profanity before. It may be a manifestation of frustration. It is something the individual cannot control, because of the lesion. Families, friends, and health care personnel need to be counseled to allow the behavior and not to censure someone who does it. The family's and friends' frustration and embarrassment need to be dealt with so that they do not alienate themselves from the individual and cause him even more loneliness.

When the *posterior portion of the frontal lobe* (Wernicke's area) is involved, comprehension is more likely to be lost. This individual's speech is dysfunctional in several ways. He tends to talk a great deal, is difficult to understand because he makes up new words (e.g., pluber or pluver for plumber); says the opposite of what he means; and transposes words in sentences. His sentences do not make sense. Again, the dysfunction occurs in varying degrees.

COGNITIVE FUNCTIONING. Cognitive dysfunction is closely associated with the brain hemisphere involved. Cognitive function among those who survive the acute stage is a crucial determiner of effectiveness in living subsequent to a stroke. Since some of these deficits are subtle, it is important for the nurse to be aware of the risks of cognitive deficits and the location of the associated lesion (Table 14-2).

Some people think that a right-sided hemiplegic person, who has lost language function and who is so aware of his own deficit, is more disabled than the left-sided hemiplegic individual. The latter can speak and usually talks a good game, denying disability. The reality is that the left-sided hemiplegic person rarely is able to regain self-sufficiency. His symptoms of a stroke may be less visible, but, if a major stroke has occurred, he could be devastated in terms of coping ability.

It becomes important for families and health care providers to differentiate the cognitive deficits associated with the location of the lesion. The patient's post-stroke behavior needs to be understood and indeed can be predicted based on the lesion location. Since the behavior of the patient is beyond

his control, knowing what to expect perhaps makes this behavior more acceptable even if it doesn't make it any easier to live with him.

MOTOR FUNCTION AND MOBILITY. Another obvious area for nursing assessment is that of motor function. Strength, endurance, balance, and capability are affected by strokes. Therefore nursing assessments need to be made in all of these areas in order to develop valid plans for management of daily living.

Hand Functioning. The individual whose lesion affects his dominant hand is much more devastated in his daily living than other stroke victims and must learn to cope with usual daily activities in a variety of difficult and awkward ways. The adaptation of previous patterns in utilization of one hand or both in activities is important in the post-stroke period. The devastation of being essentially right handed and losing the function of that hand is a real barrier to independence in a myriad of little daily functions. Where both sensory and motor loss occur the nurse can predict that the functional capacity will be much less, making adjustments more difficult. Therefore it becomes important to incorporate data on both sensory and motor functioning into the management plan. Hand function should be assessed in terms of finger-thumb opposition. If the patient has this, he

TABLE 14-2. Relationship of lesion location to type of cognitive dysfunction.

Left Hemiplegia (Lesion in right hemisphere)	Right Hemiplegia (Lesion in left hemisphere)

Spatial-perceptual deficits
    Loss of depth perception; loss of appreciation of distance, form, and rate of movement of objects
	Impaired language function
	    Reading, writing, speaking, understanding

Judgment problems
    Decrease in concern for personal safety; decreased ability to handle finances
	Perseveration
	    Repetitive speech and motor activities, e.g., washing face repeatedly

Easy distractability	
Short attention span	
Lack of awareness of deficit He talks a good game but performance doesn't match words	Very aware of the deficits
Neglect of involved extremities He forgets the extremities that have been affected with sensory or motor loss	
Unable to transfer learning from one situation to another	
Behavioral style—quick, impulsive	Behavioral style—slow and cautious

can pick up and grip objects to some degree; without it the individual will not have functional use of that hand.

Another consideration in assessment is the care that is taken of the affected hand. Is it ignored? Is it exercised? Is it groomed? Is it allowed to be damaged? Is it owned or disowned? The nurse may begin by asking, "Does this arm and hand feel like it belongs to you?" From this questioning a wealth of data may flow.

The individual's method of adaptation is an expression of his imagination and resourcefulness. One person may use his mouth to grasp or hold articles and to open packages. Another may utilize his functioning hand and increase its usefulness. Others will be devastated by their stroke and increase their dependence on their environment. It becomes important for the nurse to assess not only the dysfunction but also the predicted or actual patterns of adaptation to the dysfunction. For example, ask the patient to open a package of salt or a carton of milk. Assessment of dressing and managing buttons could be made in the office situation by asking the patient to remove his coat or jacket (or observe coping with buttons and zippers). Stockings and shoes are a major problem—again, either ask him how he manages or observe the type of shoes he is wearing and how he removes them and puts them on.

Balance and Coordination. Another feature frequently overlooked by nurses is that of balance. Muscle strength without balance does little for mobility in daily activities. Cerebellar lesions place balance and muscle coordination at high risk. If the patient has adequate speech, he may tell you about problems involving balance. Activities at high risk include any that require the individual to bend over (shoes and stockings, picking up objects, getting in and out of tub or shower, stairs, opening drawers that are low, getting out of bed). The most obvious objective datum is the *gait* of the person. Where the individual uses a wide stance in standing or walking there is a problem with balance. Coordination and balance may also be tested with the finger-to-nose test. Another easy test is to ask the individual to stand and close his eyes; those with balance problems tend to fall to one side.

Where balance and coordination are at risk the individual must work much harder in many seemingly incidental or routine maneuvers. Therefore fatigue becomes a factor to be considered in nursing management.

Strength. Strength involves the capacity to engage in a particular physical demand. For example: Can he come to a sitting or standing position by himself or does he require assistance? How much can he lift? Can he raise his legs enough to climb stairs or get on a bus? Objective data involves observation of the individual in these activities.

Endurance. Endurance involves staying power—the capacity to carry out activities over a period of time. Strokes tend to decrease endurance as well as strength. The individual tires rapidly; this is particularly evident later in the day. The nurse needs to learn how much the individual can accomplish before becoming fatigued. How long a rest period is required before he can engage in activities again? What kinds of activities can he engage in and for how long? How he reacts to constraints on his endurance?

VISION. The most common dysfunctions in vision associated with strokes include loss of visual fields, seeing double and, occasionally, nystagmus.

Loss of Visual Field. Visual field loss may be of several kinds: loss of half of the visual field in each eye; complete loss of vision in one eye; or loss of a quadrant in each eye. A visual field deficit causes many functional risks for the patient. An indication of the types of visual loss and the loss of function is given in Table 14-3.

Data on the patient's visual field are important to patient safety and effective living. The nurse may be able to obtain this data from the medical record. However, these records may not always be available to nurses and, therefore, it becomes important for the nurse to be able to do this testing. The following steps aid in testing visual fields:

1. Stand or sit about 2 ft away from the patient.
2. Have patient cover one eye with hand or piece of paper.
3. Direct the patient to look at the nurse's nose.
4. Move an object (pencil or finger) from outside the visual field toward a point opposite the patient's nose, keeping the object equidistant from patient and nurse.
5. Direct the patient to indicate (verbal or by signal) when he first sees the object and when he loses sight of it.

Figure 14-2 indicates the directions of fields that need to be tested.

Frequently the patient is unaware of the loss of visual fields after a stroke. Without a diagnosis of

TABLE 14-3. Loss of visual fields and resultant functional losses.

Type of Deficit	Loss	Examples of Functional Risk
Homonymous hemianopsia*	*Right:* When looking straight ahead, vision loss is in right half of visual field in each eye	If unaware of visual field loss, fails to compensate by moving the head to see into the blind area
		Ignores objects or persons in the lost visual field—walks into walls, ignores food outside of available visual field, fails to notice people in lost field
	Left: Vision loss is in left half of visual field in each eye	Restricted from driving
		May have visual interpretive defects
Bitemporal hemianopsia	Peripheral half of visual field is lost in each eye	Failure to see objects (stationery or moving) until they reach the central area of vision
		Startle reaction as people or objects "pop" into view
Blindness in one eye		Loss of depth perception and as above

 * If unresolved in two to three weeks, it becomes a permanent disability.

this deficit, the patient may not observe it until he wonders why a paragraph he is reading doesn't make sense (he sees only half of it) or why he runs his wheelchair into a wall when he thinks he is going straight. Even then, the patient may connect these symptoms to some other aspect of his stroke and, therefore, not report it.

The nurse should be on the lookout for these circumstances. Part of nursing assessment involves

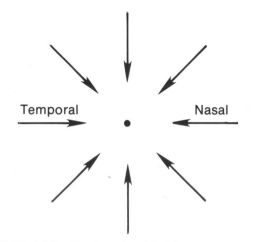

FIGURE 14-2. Testing visual fields.

direct observation of patient activity. Does he ignore objects on the right or left side? Does he bump into door jams or objects on a particular side? Another test situation is to ask him to identify objects on a tray placed before him. He will ignore objects outside his field of vision. It is crucial to record not only the area of loss but also the patient's awareness or lack of it.

Part of patient management is to (1) create a conscious awareness of the deficits that exist in visual fields and (2) help the patient make the accommodations that must be built into their activities.

Diploplia. Double vision usually is reported by the patient. Where there is brain stem lesion it is a predictable symptom. An associated symptom of the diploplia is nausea.

Nystagmus. Nystagmus (irregular jerking movement of the eyeball) can be observed. It can also be elicited by moving an object across the visual field and asking the patient to follow it with his eyes. Some patients are aware of the phenomenon and find it unpleasant. (There are also familial tendencies to nystagmus. In this case there is no stroke-associated pathology.)

EMOTIONAL LABILITY. Emotional lability is an organic problem associated with lesions in the pseudobulbar region, with bilateral hemisphere problem, or with interruption of both corticospinal tracts. However, since both emotional lability and depression frequently are manifested after a stroke, nurses and other health providers often have failed to differentiate between them and with this, management has not been effective.

Emotional lability is a phenomenon characterized by inappropriate ease of laughter and crying, mostly crying. Since crying is also a manifestation of depression, it becomes important to assess the presenting situation. The following pieces of data will help to make an accurate diagnosis of emotional lability:

1. Is the person aware of the behavior?
2. Can the behavior (crying) be interrupted by engaging in another activity such as getting a drink of water or grabbing the back of a chair?
3. Is he embarrassed by the behavior?
4. Does he wish to stop it?

Affirmative answers to these four questions would indicate the presence of emotional lability, rather than, or in addition to, depression. (For signs and symptoms of depression, see Chapter 25 on loneliness.)

Another aspect of assessment regarding emotional lability is the response of the family. Are family members aware that the behavior is an organic phenomenon? Do they have any knowledge about how to control it?

When family and patient understand that the behavior is not an unexpected response but is due to the stroke, the situation may become more tolerable for all concerned.

GRIEVING. The individual who has had a stroke and suffers residual loss of function goes through the grieving process in coping with this loss. It is a normal and necessary response. Because the loss is ongoing, the grieving tends to be recurrent. The stages of denial, anger, bargaining, depression, and acceptance are all seen. However, denial deserves particular consideration with some stroke patients. Those who suffer from left hemiplegia will experience denial as an organic response. It is more properly identified as *neglect* since denial is a defense mechanism and has accrued negative social connotations.

As with the assessment of grieving in any loss situation, the nurse needs data on the stages the individual is currently in and the patterns of coping with the grieving. It is important also to gather data on the response of individuals in the support system with regard to the stroke patient's grieving work. Do they understand what is going on and its necessity? Do they understand the nature of movement from one stage to another? Do they realize it should not/cannot be short circuited or avoided? Can they tolerate the discomfort of the individual's grieving? Do they have respite from it? What help do they wish?

Status of Support Systems

Strokes tend to leave the individual with physical, cognitive, emotional, and communication dysfunctions at some level that remain fairly static for long periods. Many individuals can be quite dependent, but their status does not change. They don't deteriorate and die nor do they get a great deal better after they have achieved the initial major return of function. They present real challenges to those who care for them. Maintenance, and satisfaction with it, is crucial.

Information on the kinds of support systems available and the patient's attitude toward the use of support resources becomes very important. One difficulty is that the person who has had a stroke sees himself as deviant from others, a minority. For some persons this results in an isolation from others, including available support systems. Data on these areas are needed if a useable plan of management of daily living is to be developed.

The family who sees its loved one disabled tends to equate helping with caring. Therefore, it becomes very difficult not to "do for" the person what it is difficult for him to do for himself. The nurse may need to help family members work through the realization that the individual may have to struggle; be frustrated, be angry, and be slow as he does for himself.

The highest form of loving may be that of keeping hands off.

Complications

High Risk Physical Complications

After surviving the acute stage, there are still complications that are a high risk for the person who has had a stroke. These complications are both physical and psychosocial (Table 14-4) and are a result of the residual functional deficit.

TABLE 14-4. High risk physical and psychosocial complications.

Physical Complications	Psychosocial Complications
Joint contractures on the affected side	Body image greatly affected when major portions of the body lack sensation or cease to function normally
Shoulder separation on the affected side	
Constipation—related to less activity, decreased appetite and fiber/fluid ingestion, drugs, and depression	Social isolation at high risk, particularly when the individual has an expressive or comprehension communication deficit; sees himself as deviant or a tremendous burden to others; or when others communicate to him that he is an unwanted burden
Atonic bladder	
Trauma to areas with decreased sensation	
Edema in flaccid extremities that are allowed to dangle for long periods of time in a dependent position	Depression—hopelessness of any improvement in one's status. Sadness at one's state in life.
Sensory deprivation—in terms of the sensations available in the environment, if he becomes more socially isolated (e.g., people don't talk to you if you can't talk with them or don't understand). Whole areas of the body fail to sense stimuli from the environment or proprioceptive impulses	Anxiety over the risk of using up one's social and economic resources as the disability drags on
	Living with fear of another stroke
Fatigue and major increased amounts of time required to accomplish routine activities of daily living	Shifting from independence to dependence—can be catastrophic for individuals who value highly their independence

Prognosis

According to American Heart Association (1975), the incidence of strokes was 1,840,000 with a death rate of 19.5 percent at the time of the stroke. These are national, not age-related, statistics.

In terms of pathology and pathophysiology, those individuals who have only motor losses as a residual tend to do very well. They will have almost complete recovery within a year or so. Those with both sensory and motor losses have a less favorable prognosis. Right-sided hemiplegics, despite their communication difficulties, tend to be able to care for themselves and live independently. They are aware and alert, and a communication system can be developed. Those with left-sided hemiplegia are less likely to be able to maintain an independent lifestyle because of spatial-perceptual deficits in particular.

Nursing Management

The development of a plan for effective management of daily living for the older individual following a stroke is contingent upon accommodating to, substituting for, or supplementing the areas of identified functional deficit. Using the areas noted in the assessment section (Signs and Symptoms), the following components of management need to be considered.

Awareness of Sensory Losses

In order to compensate for loss of sensation, an individual has to become aware of what the specific losses are. A diagram of the body showing the areas of loss of sensation (Fig. 14-3) may be useful in making the ideas more concrete. If the patient and family or caretakers have the information in written form, it allows them to refer to it whenever they wish.

Daily exercises in which he/they touch, rub, handle the part of the body (e.g., hand) that has lost sensation, and name it, may prevent his forgetting that this is a part of his body.

Mechanisms for Compensating for Loss of Sensation

Because the body is not sending messages regarding the position of a part of the body and the forces that are impacting upon it, the *eyes must be used as a compensatory mechanism.* Patients need to be taught to watch the affected extremity—noting the position it is in and anything in the environment that is acting on it, such as heat, sharp surfaces, impact. The patient who has been in a rehabilitation setting before discharge will have been taught to do this. If the individual may not have been exposed to this teaching, it is important for the home health nurse or the nurse in the clinic or senior center to check on whether the individual knows about this and is remembering to do it.

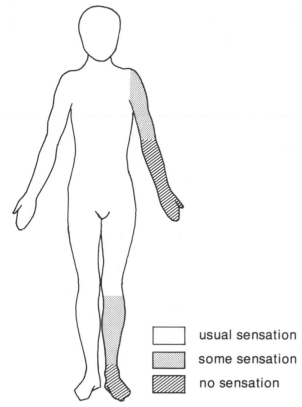

FIGURE 14-3. Body diagram for communicating areas of loss of sensation (see text).

usual sensation

some sensation

no sensation

Where a hand has lost sensation, a bath thermometer, or checking water temperature with the unaffected hand, is important in setting water temperatures for bathing, showering, and hand washing. The use of gloves or protection from the cold would be important in very cold climates.

Motor Function

Nursing management of motor function is concerned with maintaining joint motion, preventing stretching of supporting joint structures, preventing contractures and maintaining or improving muscle strength and endurance.

To maintain joint mobility, it is thought to be sufficient for most people to engage in range of motion activities twice each day, with each joint being put through full range of motion to the point of pain three times per exercise period.

It is important that patients and families understand that the range of motion activities are done in order to prevent loss rather than to restore voluntary muscle function. If they believe that the purpose of the range of motion exercises is to return muscle function, they have been known to quit doing them when voluntary movement fails to return. The result is that the patient develops major contractures that further complicate his life.

POSITIONING. Positioning of affected limbs is important in both daytime and nighttime activities. If a flaccid upper extremity exists, an arm sling should be worn whenever the person ambulates to prevent stretching of the shoulder ligaments with greater risk of shoulder dislocation. A hand splint for maintaining a functional position is important at night. If there is a sensory loss, it is recommended that the individual not sleep more than 20 minutes on the affected side. To prevent turning over to that side during sleep, a pillow may be set behind the patient's back (for those who sleep on the unaffected side). This will avoid injury to affected side where sensory loss exists. For the individual with a flaccid foot, a stack of books wrapped in a towel makes a good foot support in bed.

STRENGTH AND ENDURANCE. Where some function remains, the management plan may be directed toward maintaining and increasing the strength and endurance by activities and exercise. Persons over 70 need some strength for what they *want* to do. They need to learn to judge when they are tired and stop before then. This is very hard to do. The nurse may be helpful in working this through. Many communities have programs of group exercises for stroke patients at the local YMCA or YWCA, senior citizen centers, and Day Care Centers. Nurses in the community should learn about these available resources. For those who enjoy swimming there are sessions for the handicapped in some local community pools. Engaging in activities with others having the same problems may decrease the sense of deviance and social isolation. It may also add incentive to continue to participate in exercises or activities in the home in the interim between sessions.

Booklets indicating exercise and activity programs are listed at the end of this chapter.

One of the problems that stroke patients face as they return to engaging in the activities of daily living is that *they are slower* in all of their physical activities. Everything takes longer and requires more effort. The nurse should plan a sufficient block of time in any encounter to permit patients to accomplish the needed activities at the pace they must set.

Impatience, hurrying them, or stepping in and doing what they should do for themselves is not therapeutic. It is important also for the nurse to help the individual verbalize his problems and to communicate an understanding of what he is experiencing as well as to work with him to develop acceptable plans of a balance of activity and rest that is satisfying to him.

It may be helpful for the nurse to tell the patient and support persons that they will experience frustration in doing things because it takes longer so they need to allow more time for activities and, at least initially, a rest period after an activity.

Older persons who have had strokes have told nurses that venturing out into large gatherings is particularly taxing. Often those who try to reenter into social activities prematurely have a very trying and unsuccessful experience. They then become much more reluctant to try it again and may become more isolated socially. A wiser course may be a deliberately gradual increase in the size of social groups, building up to the larger size ones as tolerance increases. They should arrange with a family member to take them out of the social situation early, before they get tired. If the person knows of this option in advance, he is more likely to be willing to go out.

ASSISTIVE DEVICES. Where motor strength is missing, there are some assistive devices that can make it possible for individuals to engage more successfully in daily activities. Short leg braces, tripod canes, hemiwalkers, and walkers can add to the individual's capacity for mobility.

A wheelchair is contraindicated if an individual has the potential for walking. It has been found to be a real barrier for regaining the ability to walk. The patient becomes dependent on it and it inhibits learning to walk. However, for going out to places where substantial walking is required, a wheelchair can be used, e.g., airports or shopping. Then the wheelchair increases endurance and provides social outlets.

MANAGING FALLING. Persons who have had strokes can expect to fall more often. It becomes a practical issue to give them some control over falls in knowing the best way to fall and how to get up. The individual should be taught to fall toward the unaffected side whenever possible. This allows him to edge himself across the floor using his elbow, hip, and knee (resting as needed) until he comes to a heavy piece of furniture—a sofa or bed. Usually he can use this to brace himself and work up to a standing position.

BALANCE BETWEEN REST AND ACTIVITIES. Patients and their families can be alerted to the increased need to balance activities with rest. With each activity being more demanding because of the dysfunction, it becomes more work and endurance is reduced. Most elderly people find they have greater energy earlier in the day, so those activities that require greater concentration of energy should be scheduled during late morning and early afternoon hours, e.g., visits to the doctor's office.

Vision Deficits

Since the individual usually is not aware of the visual field deficits, the first step is to make him aware of the blind area and the implications this has for daily living. Once he knows where the losses are, he can be taught to turn his head to compensate for loss of vision. In addition, it is important to teach the family and friends about the limitations of visual field. Then they can anticipate that they and objects in the environment will not be seen in certain positions, and they will place themselves within the patient's visual field when they wish to be noticed. A diagram of the blind areas will help both the patient and family see what the problem is and be more active in accommodating to it.

To teach a person with field deficits how to accommodate, the nurse may show him how to deliberately set up an obstacle course using furniture. As he learns to navigate it in the privacy and safety of his own home he learns what he must do to scan the situation to move about more freely.

Reading presents particular problems to the individual with field deficits. He tends to lose his place. A ruler placed immediately beneath the line he is reading, or the use of the finger moving along the line, assists in keeping their place.

The balancing of figures as in checking accounts also is a problem, again because of the inability to keep one's place in the book. He may need the assistance of another person to balance his accounts.

Driving privileges are revoked in many states for individuals with visual field deficits. The individual may have to be helped to readjust to life without the usual form of transportation.

Diploplia is managed by covering one eye. The patch is changed from one eye to the other every two to four hours to keep eye muscles active.

Dysfunction in Communication

Several hazards exist for individuals who experience a residual deficit in communication. Their self-concept can change. They may see themselves as stupid or feel they are losing their minds because they cannot either understand or speak. The nurse needs to be reassuring to the patient that there is no decrease in intellectual powers, nor is the individual out of touch with reality, but that she understands why he may feel that way. Families and other health care providers also need to be included in this preparation (see boxes).

In speaking to the patient it is important to realize that he does not have a hearing deficit; speaking loudly is inappropriate.

ALTERNATIVES TO SPEECH FOR LONG TERM APHASICS. Some patients never recover the ability to speak. Realization of this brings a strong reactive depression and grieving. A high risk time is the point when the high intensity speech therapy or rehabilitative efforts are terminated and the realization comes

---

**GUIDELINES FOR COMMUNICATING
TO THE INDIVIDUAL WITH POST-STROKE
COMMUNICATION DEFICITS**

Talk to him.
Use normal volume—don't shout.
Get the patient's attention before speaking.
Face the patient and be sure the light is on your face.
Have only one person talk at a time.
Use short sentences.
Use concrete language.
Ask questions that require a yes-or-no response.
Avoid double questions (is it this or that?).
Don't change subject matter quickly.
Allow plenty of time for answers (schedule enough time for each encounter and don't give cues of impatience).
Engage only in conversations you have time to finish.
Do not correct his mistakes.
Ignore profanity.
Express your pleasure when he communicates but don't praise in a patronizing way.
Don't attempt mixed messages where your words say one thing and your body says another—nonverbal language is well understood by the patient.
Be honest. Don't pretend you understand if you don't. Share his frustration. "It's very frustrating to try to talk and not be understood."

**GUIDELINES FOR HELPING
THE PATIENT COMMUNICATE**

Do not persist if he becomes frustrated in attempts to communicate.
Ask him to point if he is unable to name what he wants.
Use a series of flash cards or list of words or pictures to reduce frustration.
Communication is easier when he is not tired.
Touching is helpful for a frustrated person.
"No" does not always mean no; it may also mean yes.
Help him to use gestures, pantomime, or other signals if there is a major language deficit. Do not mix speech with a nonverbal communication system.
Keep trying; improvements in speech can occur months and even years after the stroke.
Explore his ability to sing (part of automatic speech). Some persons who can't speak can regain communication skills through singing and records. Use familiar songs, ones he knows well and enjoys. First languages are more easily used than those acquired later.
Express for the patient your understanding of the difficulty of his being unable to speak for himself. Indicate that being angry and frustrated "is okay."
Include the aphasic in decision making in the home as much as possible. (One wife indicated that in 10 years she never made a decision without "discussing" it with her aphasic husband.)
Letters from distant relatives or friends may take the form of tape recordings.

---

that others have given up on him. It becomes crucial that the transition to nonspeech-oriented communication systems be in full use to minimize the shock of loss. Alternatives include (1) pointing, gestures, and pantomime; (2) cards with common requests or words; (3) encouraging nonverbal activities with others so that they can feel self-worth and companionship without words.

It is important to continue expectations for functioning. A person cannot retain his integrity and feeling of self-worth if there is no obligation or responsibility.

The use of speech pathologists and speech therapists can be very helpful. However, it still may fall to the nurse to determine how the speech exercises and activities can be incorporated into daily living and can involve other people in the environment. It also will be incumbent upon the nurse to help to create situations and environments in which the individual can learn from others with the same problems and continue to practice speaking over long periods of time—groups in Senior Citizen Centers, visitors into the home or nursing home, and so forth.

Deficits Peculiar to Left-Sided Hemiplegia

Management of daily living for the left-sided hemiplegic individual must overcome perceptual spatial deficits, insufficient judgment in decision making, and inability to follow through and must meet the need to learn each behavior in every required context since often he is unable to transfer learning. Additionally, his failure to "own" the affected parts of the body creates difficulties. He tends to overestimate his abilities—volunteering to cook the dinner at the Senior Citizen party when his disability obviously makes this impossible.

SPATIAL-PERCEPTUAL DEFICITS. Deficits in the spatial-perceptual area involve distance, depth perception, balance, form, and movement. Focusing on vertical lines in environment (e.g., a doorway or window) will help those who have difficulty maintaining an upright position to correct the imbalance. For depth perception, the patient can be taught to feel the edge of surfaces with the unaffected hand or forearm as a basis for placing objects on them. He tends to relearn movement and forms by experience.

In general, the nurse, the family, and friends should be careful to:

1. Minimize the number of stimuli operating at one time to overcome easy distractability, e.g., no television or background noise while teaching or talking, no extra people—teach alone.
2. Break down all teaching into small steps.
3. Teach the behavior in each of the presenting situations without expecting the individual to be able to transfer learning from one situation to another.

Comprehension is not affected; oversimplification may be seen as a put down. *Performance is affected;* careful critical practice of the steps in the skills is required. Overteaching, overpracticing, and overlearning become important in the performance area. It makes for safer, more predictable performance.

One general device that utilizes comprehension is the placement of written reminders or instructions in strategic places in the environment, e.g., on the shower door post transfer instructions broken into steps:

1. Lock the brake of the wheelchair.
2. Look at your affected foot as you assume standing position.
3. Grasp safety bar with unaffected hand.
4. Pull to standing position.

FORGETTING THE AFFECTED SIDE. The left-sided hemiplegic person needs to reintegrate the affected side as a very conscious experience. He needs to look at it regularly, touch it, and name the parts. It is important to use the functioning arm to do range of motion and passive exercises on the affected side. In order to minimize trauma it is necessary to get into a pattern of visually checking the position of affected limbs, particularly in high risk areas such as the kitchen. In colder climates attention needs to be paid to preventing exposure—mittens may be easier than gloves. Or, where coat pockets are available, pulling the affected hand into the pocket not only affords protection but also may contribute to maintaining balance.

Neglect may be compounded also by loss of visual fields. It is helpful here to place objects, furniture, clothing in the closet, food, and so forth on the side where it is most likely to be seen and noticed. This can reduce neglect to some degree. On the other hand, contractures of the neck toward the unimpaired side are at greater risk in left hemiplegic persons, particularly those with neglect, where they tend to keep the head turned away from the affected side. Teaching them to deliberately turn their heads to the point where they can see areas on the impaired side will do two things: reduce risk of contracture and maintain awareness of their body and environment.

JUDGMENT DEFICITS. The left-sided hemiplegic patient has poor judgment and, thus, disregard for personal safety. The nurse should check to see that performance matches what the patient says he can do. Very often it does not. The nurse needs to be sensitive to the readiness of the patient to accept disabilities in the judgment area—there are times when a patient can take in this knowledge and times when it would be too devastating. Once out of the acute care environment he needs to come to grips with the profile of his abilities and participate in management plans. For example, a person with substantial financial resources may need an executor to help in the use of the money. While the patient may be offended at being faced with this loss of former ability, some examples may enable him to understand the need for a backup.

Another threat to self-concept is in the use of the car. The person will expect to continue to drive and may even take the car out. Many states require passing of a driver's test following a stroke. Family and friends need to be aware of the risk that the person may take the car out because he honestly does not realize the extent of his deficits.

Prompt feedback of a positive nature is important. Where visual neglect is noticed, avoid an approach such as, "Why don't you turn your head so you can see?" Instead, say, "Mary, turn your head (right/left) and you'll see the grandchildren coming." Give positive feedback as the steps are proceeding during an activity. Don't wait till the end. If something is not going well, ask a question that calls attention to the problem, e.g., "Carl, are you matching the button hole to the right button?" Praise is important: "You do well."

Deficits Peculiar to Right-Sided Hemiplegia

The person with right-sided hemiplegia is troubled by language difficulties and the sensorimotor involvement but does not have the degree of spatial-perceptual deficits of the left-sided hemiplegic person. For this reason he is much more likely to be able to resume more independent functioning. His awareness of his disability, while discouraging, is an asset in enabling him to cope with the demands of daily living.

For the few individuals with motor and sensory perseveration (persistent repetition of the same verbal or motor response to varied stimuli), management involves calling it to their attention when it occurs and interrupting the activity, e.g., "Mrs. Johnson, you already washed your face." While the motor perseveration tends to have disappeared by the time the individual reaches convalescent or home care settings, it can recur. The sensory component (repetitive speech) continues longer. It is well for provider and family to be aware of this behavior. An example of this might be:

Nurse: Good morning, Mrs. Johnson.
Mrs. J.: Good morning.
Nurse: What did you have for breakfast today?

Mrs. J.: Good morning.
Nurse: It's good to see you all dressed today.
Mrs. J.: Good morning.

It may or may not be possible to interrupt this pattern immediately. Sometimes changing the motor behavior will serve to change it. These episodes of sensory perseveration tend to be isolated blocks of behavior rather than ongoing.

Support Persons

One of the most difficult tasks in long term management is helping the person who lives with the stroke victim. Living with profound, or even moderate, cognitive sensorimotor deficit 24 hours a day, 7 days a week for months and years taxes the emotional and physical stamina of any human being.

Nurses need to play a role in trying to recruit others to provide regularly scheduled "time off" from each other for these two people. Both persons need it; however, it may be difficult for each to accept. The patient may be embarrassed to have other persons see his disability and he may feel comfortable only with his accustomed companion. On the other hand, the spouse or other care person may experience guilt at leaving the patient and may worry that a "stranger" won't know how to manage.

One approach that has worked to the benefit of both individuals is encountering different people. Where mobility permits, Day Care Centers offer a useful service and therapeutic environment. Home health care aides, volunteer visitors from church groups or clubs, retired persons, neighbors—all could be tapped to visit a few hours occasionally. Often the nurse is the catalyst who sets this in motion.

Try leaving the patient with others. When the visiting nurse comes to do care, the spouse leaves. When visitors come, the spouse leaves. If the spouse can manage a vacation or trip of several days, checks can be made regularly to give reassurance that things at home are going well.

There is no question that the spouse needs to get out to regroup and revitalize. Respite is critical to maintaining the strength to manage long term chronic disability on a round-the-clock basis. Nursing plans of management need to address as much attention to the needs of the support persons as to the one who has had the stroke. For the best outcome, neither can be neglected, even though their needs are quite different.

Evaluation

The person who recovers from a major stroke faces a long rehabilitation period. He may become discouraged frequently by the very gradual recovery he experiences. Recovery does take place and this is important to keep in mind. It is helpful to document the changes that occur. The nurse may suggest and implement a flow sheet whereby the stroke person and his family can follow the progress. The record keeping may be designed according to the person's functional limitations on day one following the stroke. The accompanying Evaluation Flow Sheet is an example of what can be used. These are sample items. The increments could be smaller or greater, depending on the need to see progress with limited or major recovery. The deficits also will determine the variables. The nurse, the patient, and the family should identify the variables that are important to them at a point in time. The items can be updated and new examples added according to the status of the situation.

Rationale for use of the Evaluation Flow Sheet is the following:

1. To assess the improvements of functions.
2. To give evidence that changes occur.
3. To allow patient and his family responsibilities and an active role in management.
4. To enhance self-esteem and body image.

EVALUATION FLOW SHEET

Activity	Date	Comments
Turn self in bed		
Control bowel/bladder function		
Swallow without choking		
Handle oral secretions		
Feed self		
Transfer onto chair/commode wheelchair		
Bathe self		
Take shower/tub bath		
Dress in street clothes		
Apply short leg brace		
Do ROM exercises for upper extremity		
Walk aided/unaided		
Write letters		
Read a newspaper		
Handle checking account		
Take own medications		
Operate a motor vehicle		
Attend a concert/public event		
Go out to visit		
Use a bus (if done premorbidly)		
Use a satisfactory communication system		
Develop lifestyle and support systems that allow for satisfactory time apart and together with caretaker		

5. To recall how much progress has been made since the onset of disability.
6. To have a data base for short term goal setting.

The Nursing Challenge

The nursing management of the older person who experiences a stroke presents a real challenge to nursing. Obviously skilled nursing is important in the acute phase and early convalescence—ultimate progress is affected by the quality of nursing care given in this stage. But probably more demanding nursing occurs as the long road of living with the residual deficits of stroke and aging is encountered (Hodgins, 1964). To be effective the nurse must remain alert to small and slow changes, must consider creative options for dealing with continuing or new problems, and must maintain a professional, positive attitude that, in turn, helps the patient and those who surround him. All these require a special kind of nursing.

The areas to be addressed in nursing diagnosis and management are broad. They touch on almost every aspect of daily living and on coping resources that may be diminished in so many dimensions—physical, communication, sensory, and emotional. The long, unabated stress on support systems demands that they, too, receive critical nursing attention. The nursing expertise requires a working knowledge, not only of the pathophysiology, complications, and rehabilitation phenomena but also of the resources in the community that may be used by the patient and family to share the experience and to gain support.

Satisfaction for the patient, family, and nurse often must be found in slow, tiny gains or, perhaps, in holding one's own. It becomes critical for the nurse to notice and interpret data indicating even small changes so that each participant (including the nurse) has realistic data to document the results of their efforts. It is a major achievement if the nurse is genuinely satisfied with these rewards and helps patients and families find a comparable sense of accomplishment.

All in all, it takes a broad, skilled, perceptive, creative, persistent and positive nursing approach, one that realistically buoys up and maintains those involved as long as necessary. Such a demanding task over a long period of time logically suggests that even the best and strongest of nurses will need to have their well-springs renewed and their perspec-tive freshened. It suggests that the nurses should as carefully document their own ongoing professional and personal resources and arrange for the personal and professional support systems that will enable them to maintain the kind of an approach with the stroke patient and family that will be most effective. Currently there are nurses who are delivering this high quality nursing care to stroke patients; there are more who can.

REFERENCES

Bates, B.: A Guide to Physical Examination, ed. 2. Philadelphia: J. B. Lippincott, 1979.

Burt, M.: Perceptual deficits in hemiplegia. Am. J. Nurs. 70:26–29, 1970.

Geschwind, N.: Aphasia. New Engl. J. Med. 284:654–656, 1971.

Guidelines for Stroke Care. Department of Health, Education and Welfare. U.S. Government Printing Office, Washington D.C., 1976.

Hodgins, E.: Episode: Report on the Accident in My Skull. New York: Atheneum Publishers, 1964. (Hodgins, former editor of Fortune magazine, with remarkable insight and honesty relates the day-to-day experiences of living with a stroke and its residual deficits. His first-hand accounts of his struggles with all the little activities of daily living, the frustration, and the strategies he developed should enable nurses, families, and patients to participate more sensitively and creatively with the experience of living with a stroke.)

Language and the brain. Scientific American, 226:76–83, 1972. (An excellent resource.)

Merritt, H. H.: A Textbook of Neurology, ed. 5. Philadelphia: Lea and Febiger, 1974.

Simenon: The Bells of Bicêtre. New York: Harcourt, Brace and World, 1963. (Fiction. A book written from the perspective of the aphasic patient—what he is thinking and feeling but can't communicate to those around him.)

Toole, J. F., and Patel, A. N.: Cerebrovascular Disorders, ed. 2. New York: McGraw-Hill Book Co., 1974. (Comprehensive, informative, many additional references. Well worth the price.)

Ullman, M.: Disorders of body image after stroke. Am. J. Nurs. 64:84–91, 1964.

Teaching Material for Families

Aphasia and the Family, American Heart Association, Publication #EM 359.*

Body Language. (51-003-A), American Heart Association, Publication #51-003-A.* (Warning signs and stroke.)

---

* Copies available from your local Heart Association.

Do it Yourself Again: Self-Help Devices for the Stroke Patient, American Heart Association.*

Hodgins, E.: Episode: Report on the Accident in My Skull. New York: Atheneum Publishers, 1964.

Kamenetz, H.: Exercises for the Elderly. Armous Pharmaceutical Co., 1971.

Sarno, J., and Sarno, M.: Stroke: The Condition and the Patient. New York: McGraw-Hill Book Co., 1969. (Written in question-answer form, appreciated by families.)

Strike Back at Stroke, U.S. Public Health Service Publication #596.*

Stroke: Why do They Behave That Way? American Heart Association, 1974.* (A very useful booklet that aids in understanding the behavior of persons who have had strokes.)

Strokes: A Guide for the Family, American Heart Association, Publication #EM 204.

Up and Around, American Heart Association.*

15

Diabetes Mellitus

Carol Blainey

QUICK REVIEW

DIABETES MELLITUS

DESCRIPTION

Syndrome of hyperglycemia, large vessel disease, microvascular disease, and neuropathy. Two types—*Juvenile:* rapid onset, no insulin production, ketotic; *Adult:* some insulin production, often asymptomatic, rarely ketotic.

ETIOLOGIC FACTORS

Juvenile: family history, viruses, autoimmune response. *Adult:* family history, obesity, infection, stress.

HIGH RISK

Elderly—risk doubles with every decade. Income (less than $5000 (3:1). Nonwhites (20 percent greater risk); females (2:1). Obesity—risk doubles/every 20 percent excess weight.

SIGNS AND SYMPTOMS

Polyphagia, polydipsia, polyuria, fatigue, weight loss. Skin lesions that are slow to heal, urinary tract or vaginal infection. Obesity; history of myocardial infarction or cerebrovascular accident.

PROGNOSIS

Duration of life is decreased.

COMPLICATIONS

Blood vessel disease (myocardial infarction, retinopathy); blindness; peripheral vascular disease, gangrene; hypertension and renal failure; infections, neuropathy.

NURSING MANAGEMENT

Help the person to be capable of self-management. Skills needed: urine testing, insulin, oral hypoglycemic drug administration, management of diet in a way compatible to lifestyle/finances. Help in attaining and maintaining ideal weight. Aid in recognition and management of hypoglycemia; understanding relationship of hypoglycemia to ADL/lifestyle, current health status; management of risk of hyperglycemia with illness, e.g., gastrointestinal flu, fever; planning consistent appropriate physical exercise; and care of feet.

EVALUATION

Satisfaction with diet and ability to adhere to it in social situations. Sense of competence in identifying changes in physical/emotional status and blood sugar/insulin. Integrity of feet. Appropriate, comfortable use of health care system for consultation. Movement toward normal weight and consistent in appropriate physical exercise. Resources for purchasing medications. Regularity in self-administration of prescribed drugs. Skills.

In the strict sense diabetes mellitus is a syndrome rather than a disease since there is no clear cut definable pathogeneses, etiologic factors, or consistent clinical findings or laboratory tests. The abnormalities of endocrine secretions of the pancreas result in alterations in the metabolism of carbohydrates, fats, and proteins. Eventually there are structural abnormalities in a number of different body tissues. The four general components of the syndrome are hyperglycemia, large vessel disease, microvascular disease, and neuropathy.

Attempts to define diabetes mellitus are further complicated by lack of agreement on standards of normal limits of hyperglycemia, which is the most simple-to-measure component of the condition. Blood glucose level is age related with a gradual increase occurring with increasing age. Fasting blood sugar levels increased by only 2 mg percent per decade after age 30. However, blood glucose 1 hour after glucose loading has been reported to increase by 6 to 14 mg per decade, the variation caused by differences in results, a reflection of various authors using a variety of test doses of glucose and conditions.

Etiologic Factors

The cause of diabetes is not known. There seems to be a component of inheritance in diabetes; currently, however, there is no firm data to explain mechanisms of genetic transmission. Some authorities believe that it is improbable that diabetes is simply a genetic disease (Sussman, 1975). Clearly there are two major forms of the condition: juvenile onset diabetes mellitus (JODM) and adult onset diabetes mellitus (AODM) (Table 15-1). These labels are somewhat misleading because *either can occur at any age.*

Juvenile Onset Diabetes Mellitus

JODM is characterized by a rapid onset, usually affecting individuals under 25 years of age. The individual has essentially no insulin production, is ketosis prone, and is of normal body weight. Current

theories of causation in JODM are (1) genetic, (2) viral, and (3) autoimmune. The theories, greatly simplified here, stem from observation of humans but primarily from mouse studies. Some genetic types seem more prone than others to develop diabetes mellitus. Evidence further indicates that these genetic types seem more prone to attack by specific viruses. The coxsackie viruses A and B and mumps virus are examples of viruses that produce specific lesions of the pancreatic islets of mice. The damage results in an inability to produce insulin. Investigators have also noted changes in the insulin-producing cells of the pancreas that could be due to autoimmune disease (Steinke, 1974). In autoimmune disease the body responds as if some of its own cells were actually foreign tissue and inflammation of the cells under attack alters normal function; in this case the attack on the pancreas renders the beta cells of the islets of Langerhans unable to secrete insulin.

Adult Onset Diabetes Mellitus

A character of adult onset diabetes mellitus is that it usually affects individuals over 40 years of age. These people are obese, rarely become ketotic, and have some ability to produce insulin. Indeed, there is evidence that some of these individuals actually have circulating insulin levels higher than lean people who do not have diabetes. This would indicate some resistance to the effects of insulin since the amount of insulin present is adequate to control blood sugar in thin nondiabetic people. Delayed secretion of insulin may also be implicated in AODM. Maturity onset diabetes of the young (MODY) is being identified with increasing frequency and seems to have the same characteristics as AODM except that it occurs in individuals under 25.

Obesity is a significant factor in the onset of hyperglycemia in AODM. Infection or other stresses, i.e., myocardial infarction, cerebral vascular accident, frequently precede or aggravate the hyperglycemia. Inheritance also seems to be a strong element in AODM.

High Risk Populations or Situations*

Prevalence of diabetes in the United States has increased by more than 50 percent in the decade between 1965 and 1975 and now affects 5 percent of

TABLE 15-1. Comparison of characteristics of types of diabetes mellitus.

	Age	Weight	Ketosis Prone	Insulin Production
JODM	<25	Lean	+	−
AODM	>40	Obese	−	+
MODY	<25	Obese	−	+

* The statements regarding incidence of diabetes are from the National Commission on Diabetes Report to Congress in December 1975 (American Diabetes Association, 1975).

the population. No doubt the ̲   ̲ ̲ ̲cidence is related to improved detection, increasing incidence of obesity, and better care of people with diabetes. The chance of becoming diabetic *doubles* with every decade of life. People with incomes less than $5000 per year are three times as likely as middle-income and wealthy people to have diabetes. Nonwhites are one fifth more likely than whites to have diabetes. Women are 50 percent more likely than men to have diabetes.

Dynamics

Maintenance of adequate glucose levels in blood flow to the brain is a prerequisite of life. Throughout the life of a normal healthy individual the extracellular glucose concentration is confined within narrow limits. Fasting blood glucose is normally between 70 to 100 mg/100 ml plasma and in normal young adults never exceeds 150 mg/100 ml plasma even after the largest carbohydrate meal.

Normal Function

The ability to maintain glucose concentration within this very narrow limit is due to the unique biologic opposition of the two hormones of glucagon and insulin. Varying circumstances such as exercise, stress, or high carbohydrate meals work to change the level of glucose in the extracellular fluid. In the normal basal state the action of glucagon serves to mobilize fuel from cell stores (glycogenolysis), from newly-formed glucose from the liver, and from free fatty acids and glycerol from fat tissue (gluconeogenesis). These function to elevate the blood glucose. Insulin, in contrast to the catabolic function of glucagon, has an anabolic action and serves to store food materials in muscle, liver, and adipose tissue. The amount of glucose entering the extracellular fluid from the liver is balanced by the amount going to the brain and to the liver, fat, and muscle in the basal state.

Exercise. During exercise the balance between glucagon and insulin changes. Increased secretion of glucagon results in a greater amount of glucose in the extracellular fluid. This, in turn, is delivered to the muscle to meet the increased need resulting from exercise.

Food. A high carbohydrate meal with increased exogenous glucose causes the extracellular glucose level to rise, glucagon secretion ceases, and the insulin secretion rises to cause the storage of food materials in liver, muscle, and fat tissue.

Stress. Stress situations, either physical injury or psychological stress, result in the system striving to maintain cerebral glucose levels in circumstances that threaten to decrease blood flow to the area. Hence, the extracellular level of glucose is elevated through the glucagon-insulin balance. The action of glucagon continues to cause the liver to deliver glucose to the ECF while insulin secretion decreases to keep the glucose in the ECF at elevated levels (Joslin, 1971). Stress points up the direct influence that hormones from the anterior pituitary have on the secretion of insulin. Specifically (1) growth hormone; (2) corticotropin controlling the secretion of some of the adrenocortical hormones, which in turn affect the glucose, proteins, and fats; and (3) thyrotropin which controls the rate of secretion of thyroxine by the thyroid gland which determines the rate of most of the chemical reactions in the body.

Abnormal Functioning

JUVENILE ONSET DIABETES MELLITUS. In juvenile onset diabetes mellitus the lack of insulin secretion usually occurs abruptly with a sudden onset of symptoms of polyuria, polydipsia, polyphagia, and weight loss. Owing to lack of insulin to facilitate the movement of glucose into cells blood glucose rises. When the blood glucose reaches levels above 180 mg/100 ml, which is considered the renal threshold for glucose, the glucose is spilled out into the urine, taking water and electrolytes along. In an attempt to meet the cellular need for glucose for producing energy the body begins to break down fat and muscle tissue. Adipose tissue breaks down into free fatty acids, resulting in the formation of ketone bodies that, unchecked, produce ketoacidosis, a medical emergency requiring the attention of an astute physician. Breakdown of protein stores raises the plasma concentration of amino acids and speeds gluconeogenesis. In order to survive, people with JODM require treatment with insulin. To date few individuals with JODM are surviving to advanced age, 70, but the nurse may be involved with some ketosis-prone people.

ADULT ONSET DIABETES MELLITUS. In adult onset diabetes essentially the same process as in JODM occurs but to a lesser extent, dependent on the degree of insulin insufficiency, since there is some secretion by the islets of Langerhans. The advent of the radioimmunoassay in the 1960s has shown that obese people with AODM have higher levels of circulating insulin when compared to lean people who do not have diabetes. Apparently the insulin lack in AODM is a relative rather than the absolute deficiency in JODM. Resistance to the effects of the available insulin is also implicated in the hyperglycemia of AODM. In AODM the hyperglycemia is noted sometimes in routine examination of blood or during a search for causation of other problems such as visual disturbances, slow healing of skin lesions, or urinary or vaginal infections. Often the person is not symptomatic. Obesity, infection, or other body stresses such as myocardial infarction increase the body's need for insulin to balance the blood sugar and the beta cells are unable to produce enough insulin to meet the increased demand. At this time the individual with AODM may become symptomatic with polyuria, polyphagia, polydipsia, fatigue, and weight loss.

Differential Diagnosis

The diagnosis of diabetes mellitus is a situation fraught with problems caused primarily by disagreement in what constitutes an abnormal blood glucose. Consideration of blood glucose must include whether the blood specimen is fasting or after a meal. If a glucose tolerance test (OGTT) is done to establish diagnosis, the patient must undergo three days of 300 mg carbohydrate diet prior to the OGTT in order to secure a valid test. If the individual has elevated fasting blood sugars, OGTT testing confirms the diagnosis but does not provide any additional information. As mentioned before, postprandial glucose concentration levels rise with increasing age. Andres offers the criteria, shown in Table 15-2, for age-adjusted glucose tolerance (Andres, 1971).

The difficulty in diabetes mellitus is not so much one of differentiating it from another condition but rather one of deciding at what point rising blood sugar is due to diabetes mellitus and not solely the aging process. Caution in this is warranted when one considers the impact the labeling of diabetes may have on individuals. It may be an additional disease

TABLE 15-2. Criteria for age-adjusted glucose tolerance.

Age	Fasting	1 hr.	2 hr.	Summary OGTT/2 hr.
50–60	116	203	195	*514
60–70	118	209	205	*532
70–80	120	215	215	*550

Adapted from Andres, R.: Aging and diabetes. Med. Clin. N. Amer. 55:835–846, 1971.

* Values above these levels would be considered in the range of abnormal blood glucose.

piled on top of other diseases with which the individual is coping. It may carry considerable stigma to the individual; it may interfere with his right to drive a car; it may affect his health insurance. The person may feel guilt for possibly passing on a pathologic condition to descendants and, for certain individuals, it constitutes a death warrant. If the patient is symptomatic, i.e., polyuric, polydypsic, with recurring urinary and or vaginal infections, and/or has elevated cholesterol and/or triglycerides he should be treated for diabetes.

Manifestations

The most easily measured manifestation of diabetes mellitus is elevated blood sugar. If an elevated fasting blood sugar (FBS, a specimen drawn after nothing by mouth but water for 10 hours) is elevated, an oral glucose tolerance test (OGTT) is unnecessary. If the person has a normal FBS but diabetes is suspected, an OGTT will provide data on the person's ability to maintain a normal blood sugar after three days of a high (300 mg) carbohydrate diet followed by a 10-hour fast, then a glucose challenge. Twenty-four-hour urine glucose determinations provide useful baseline data. Other relevant baseline data are shown in Table 15-3.

TABLE 15-3. Baseline data.

Cardiovascular	Renal Function	Eyes	Skin	Blood Glucose
Fasting cholesterol/ triglycerides	Urine culture and sensitivity	Blurring of vision	Breaks in skin	FBS
ECG	Blood urea nitrogen	Evaluation of presence of cataracts	Callus formation	24-hour urine glucose
Evaluation of pulses bilaterally	24-hour urine protein	Microaneurysms of proliferative retinopathy		
Lying and standing B.P.	Creatinine clearance			

Prognosis

Actual death rate from diabetes is difficult to obtain since mortality statistics generally do not specify contributing causes of death. Data that are available indicate that 38,000 deaths in the United States in 1974 were directly attributable to diabetes. Diabetes is the fifth leading cause of death from disease. The report from the National Commission on Diabetes suggests that diabetes and its complications are responsible for more than 300,000 deaths annually, raising diabetes to the third ranking-cause of death—behind cardiovascular disease and cancer. The most frequent cause of death for people with diabetes is myocardial infarction. Statistics vary greatly in statements of life expectancy in people with diabetes; however, all agree that duration of life is decreased.

Management

There is considerable controversy about the management of the person with diabetes. The main issue is "tight" versus "loose" control. This controversy is particularly confusing to patients and nurses confronted with changing treatment regimens.

Current medical literature is filled with opinions supporting both views. The primary argument for tight control is that maintaining blood glucose at near normal values may prevent some complications of the condition, particularly the renal problems. The research data are not conclusive. Supporters of tight control argue that time may bear them out and they will have prevented the advent of some complications.

Advocates of loose control propose that the data do not indicate control of complications. They cannot justify risking serious hypoglycemia with possible injury and possible decreased intellectual function. In addition, those advocating loose control point out that there is stress associated with stringent dietary stipulations that seriously alter customary life styles. Nurses helping people cope with diabetes need to be prepared to assist these individuals in understanding the main points of each view.

The nature of diabetes requires that the individual *be well versed in self-management* and, hence, the final judge as to tight or loose control. Main concerns of the nurse clinician are (1) assessing level of understanding, (2) ascertaining learning readiness, (3) determining learning goals, (4) implementing an effective teaching program, and (5) repeated evaluation of learning. It should be empha-

sized that the evaluation needs to be based on actual *unprompted statements* as well as demonstration of required motor skills in urine testing and insulin administration. The North Carolina Diabetes Association publishes an excellent guide for assessment, teaching, and evaluation.

Knowledge required for sound self-management includes urine testing, diet, insulin administration, oral hypoglycemic agents, hypoglycemic reactions, care during intercurrent illness, and foot care.

Urine Testing

People with diabetes need to understand enough about the pathology to appreciate how blood glucose is reflected in urine testing. A person whose understanding goes only as far as knowing their blood glucose is elevated may see little value in testing urine.

Emptying of the bladder and then collecting the next-voided urine specimen within 30 minutes improves the validity of urine reflecting the blood sugar. However, it is recognized that, owing to renal and neurologic changes, results of the urine testing may not correlate closely with blood glucose. For example, patients may have an atonic bladder which does not empty completely. The atonic bladder may mask polyuria from hyperglycemia by collecting larger amounts before an urge to void is detected. Asking the person to measure the volume of the first morning specimen can serve to uncover this problem. Renal changes frequently raise and occasionally lower the renal threshold for glucose, resulting in the urine's testing not reflecting current blood glucose.

Various methods of urine testing have merits and drawbacks. For most purposes dipsticks usually provide a balance between convenience and accuracy. Recording of results is useful as a rough guide to control (see Urine Testing Record).

Timing during actual testing is crucial to accurate results, that is, if instructions state the dipstick is to be inserted into urine for 2 seconds and the color compared to the color chart after 30 seconds, the timing should be done with a watch with a second hand. It should be pointed out that on plastic dipsticks the chemically impregnated paper is on only one side of the plastic strip. If read through the plastic no color change will be noted. Testing paper should not be touched to avoid changing results. Larger forms of dipstick are available for the visually handicapped and arthritics.

Tablets used for testing, Clinitest and Acetest, should be poured into the lid of the bottle and from

Date	7 AM		11 AM		4 PM		8 PM		Comments
	Glucose	Acetone	Glucose	Acetone	Glucose	Acetone	Glucose	Acetone	
January 4, 1979	Neg		½%		Neg		Neg		
January 5, 1979	Neg		Neg		Neg		½%		
January 6, 1979	Neg		1%		2%		2%	Neg	Nausea and vomiting
January 7, 1979	2%	Neg	2%	Neg	1%	Neg	½%	Neg	
January 8, 1979	Neg	Neg	½%		Neg		Neg		

URINE TESTING RECORD

Time

there to the paper or test tube. This will avoid changing test results and skin damage if fingers are wet. Testing for the presence of acetone should be done every 4 hours when the person is ill, or when urines test 2 percent or greater if tests are not usually 2 percent.

Emphasizing the importance of trends of urine results as well as what the test measures, i.e., blood glucose, is useful in avoiding negative connotations from patients using the terms "bad" or "good" tests. Collection of a 24-hour urine specimen is useful in determining control over a day. This is coupled with results of second voided specimens during the day, and aids in determining timing and extent of glucosuria.

Diet

The cornerstone of treatment of diabetes mellitus is diet. In fact, diet was the only treatment prior to 1921 and the discovery of insulin.

GOALS OF DIET MANAGEMENT. The goals of diet treatment are:

1. Achievement and maintenance of ideal body weight
2. Avoidance of wide swings of blood sugar
3. Avoidance of concentrated carbohydrates
4. Normal blood fats
5. Nutritional balance

Consultation by a dietician is of merit, particularly if frequent follow-up is available. If a dietician is not available, dietary management is of such importance that the nurse needs to develop expertise in this area. The reader is referred to Chapter 9, Nutrition, for useful references.

DIET PLANS. General dietary approaches are as follows. The so-called *free diet,* i.e., no restrictions so long as the person has no overweight or underweight problems, no elevated blood fats, or excessive elevations in blood glucose. Next in order is a diet plan called *sugar free* with the only restriction being omission of concentrated refined sugar and items that contain concentrated sugar.

The *exchange system* provides a useful means of attaining the goals of diet treatment. Local chapters of the American Diabetes Association can provide material about the exchange system. Time is required to explain the concept of:

1. The six food groups: milk, vegetable A and B, fruit, breads, fats, and meat.
2. The portions of specific food within the groups.
3. How the set portions of foods within a group can be exchanged for another item within the same food group.

This system provides flexibility in diet by allowing the individual variety and ease in eating away from home. The actual diet prescription requires an evaluation of the following: carbohydrate, protein, and fat distribution; body weight; and need for saturated fat restriction and/or sodium restriction.

The most stringent diet requires actual *weighing or measuring of all food and fluid consumed.* This prevents any error of estimation of portion and calls attention to the importance of diet. It does, however, restrict flexibility in eating.

OBESITY. Obesity is the primary management problem in AODM. The problem is complex and requires an investment of time on the part of the nurse/dietician to gain insight into each individual's problem. Establishing an acceptance of the patient that is not contingent on his size is paramount. Investigation has shown that obese people may be caught in a cycle of feeling of low personal worth because of obesity. This feeling leads to depression which results in overeating which leads to obesity.

Following establishment of acceptance, an accurate dietary assessment can be obtained to determine eating patterns as well as diet components that help to reveal behavior modification needs. For example, once it has been established that the patient is accepted regardless of size, the question, "When and on what foods do you overeat?", may be asked.

After current patterns and eating styles are documented, plans can be made for teaching calorie and nutritional content of various foods. Involving the person in the analysis of the weight problem as well as plans for weight loss works toward greater compliance.

Frequent dietary consultation emphasizes weight loss as treatment. Measurement or weighing of food in the beginning of treatment to teach correct size of portions is useful. Involvement in organizations with the goal of weight control has shown positive results in achieving and maintaining ideal body weight.

Insulin Administration

Basic to safe administration of insulin is the understanding that exogenous or injected insulin is absorbed at a predetermined rate (Table 15-4) as opposed to the action of endogenous insulin, i.e., that produced by the body, which is secreted on a second-to-second basis as determined by the fluctuating blood glucose. Knowledge of onset, peak, and duration of actions of the particular insulin underlines the requirement of daily injection and regularly spaced meals and snacks.

Site Rotation. Areas to include in teaching administration of insulin are possible injection sites and the importance of regular rotation of sites with the goals of (1) giving every injection 1-inch from the other injection sites and (2) reusing a specific injection site only once every 6 weeks. One convenient system is illustrated in Figure 15-1.

Depth of Injection. The angle of the needle during injection is important in order to place the insulin the subcutaneous area. Various methods of pinching up tissue are advanced, but the important point is determination of depth of fat layer. For obese individuals, abdominal sites require longer needles than are provided on disposable insulin syringes. Injecting into the subcutaneous tissue can be facilitated by teaching to pull up the tissue to separate the subcutaneous portion from the muscle. Next, the soft portion of the pinched-up tissue is located and the needle inserted at 90 degree to the angle of the pinch (Fig. 15-2). Sterile technique and careful measurement of insulin require emphasis and practice.

Teaching Insulin Administration. Needing to learn self-injection of insulin can constitute a seemingly overwhelming obstacle to anyone. Helping people understand the need for insulin and teaching injection technique on an outpatient basis has the advantage of minimizing the complexity of the situation as well as having the individual in a more typical situation. It is the author's experience that after an initial session of about one hour, most people can safely manage self-injection with the nurse conducting follow-up by telephone, daily if necessary, until the insulin dose is established. This is coupled with seeing the patient frequently and/or

TABLE 15-4. Approximate action of various types of insulin.

Type	Onset	Peak	Duration
Rapid Action			
Crystalline Zinc (Regular)	30–60 min	2–4 hr	6–9 hr
Semilente	30–60 min	2–4 hr	12–16 hr
Intermediate Action			
Lente	1–2 hr	6–12 hr	18–28 hr
NPH	1–2 hr	6–12 hr	18–28 hr
Slow or Prolonged Action			
Protamine Zinc (PZI)	4–6 hr	12–24 hr	36+ hr
Ultralente	4–6 hr	18–24 hr	36+ hr

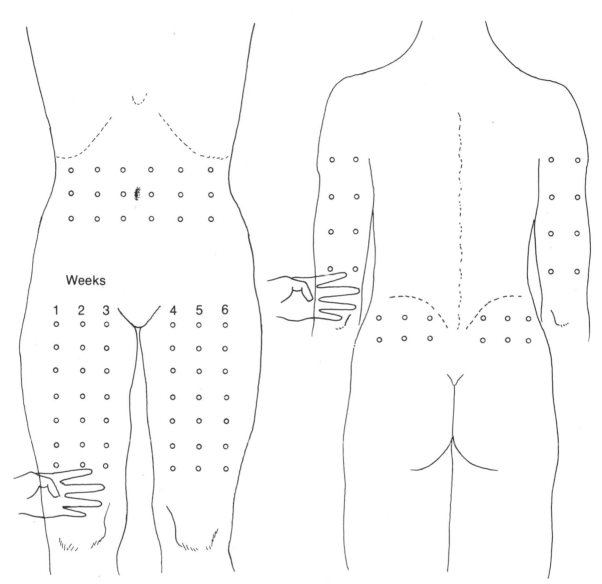

FIGURE 15-1.   Insulin injection sites. Inject one-hand's width from any joint. Make sites 1 inch apart. When using the thighs, begin at the knee and use one row per week. After sites on one leg are used, move to the other leg. If you use this pattern, each site will be used once every 6 weeks.

home supervision for evaluation and further teaching until the person can manage himself safely and confidently.

Oral Hypoglycemic Agents

The University Group Diabetes Study Report has caused concern about oral hypoglycemic agents in relation to increased cardiovascular deaths in patients with mild AODM treated with tolbutamide or phenformin* (Diabetes, 1975). However, some patients are still treated with the sulfonylurea drugs. Hypoglycemia does occur in people taking the sulfonylureas and this necessitates careful explanation to patients. Oral hypoglycemic agents are given in Table 15-5.

_____

* Phenformin was taken from the market by FDA in November 1977.

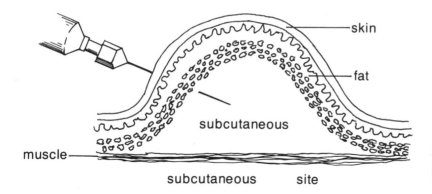

skin

fat

subcutaneous

muscle

subcutaneous   site

FIGURE 15-2. Technique for injecting insulin into subcutaneous site.

Hypoglycemic Reactions

Hypoglycemia from insulin or oral hypoglycemic agents constitutes a potentially serious situation. The geriatric person may have physiologic changes caused by aging and perhaps other illnesses that confuse the interpretation of the signs and symptoms of hypoglycemia. It is imperative that individuals taking drugs that lower the blood sugar know the usual signs and symptoms as well as how to treat the hypoglycemia. There is evidence that frequent hypoglycemic reactions decreases intellectual ability through loss of brain cells.

Exercising skeletal muscles takes up glucose without insulin which results in a decreased need for insulin. People planning exercise should eat some part of their caloric allowance just prior to exercise to avoid hypoglycemia. All persons taking insulin should ingest part of their caloric allowances 6 to 8 hours after taking the medication to avoid hypoglycemia as the peak action of the drug occurs.

Alcohol and Hypoglycemia. Consumption of alcohol by persons taking insulin constitutes a potential problem. Alcohol interferes with the ability of the liver to make new glucose. If a person who has taken insulin ingests alcohol and does not eat he can become hypoglycemic. The injected insulin continues to drive available glucose into cells, and when that glucose supply dwindles the liver normally supplies more. However, with the ingestion of alcohol the liver cannot provide more glucose and the person becomes hypoglycemic. If people who take insulin ingest alcohol they should take some of their daily caloric allowance simultaneously.

Signs and Symptoms. Factors responsible for the symptomatology of hypoglycemia are decreased glucose available to the brain and epinephrine release with a sympathetic nervous system response. The symptoms include tachycardia, weakness, trembling sensations, sweating, pallor, irritability, tremor, and hunger.

Treatment. Treatment of hypoglycemia is intended to increase the blood glucose by oral ingestion of refined carbohydrates, intravenous injection of 50 percent dextrose and water, or intramuscular injection of glucagon. If the person is able to swallow, any of the following will raise the blood sugar: 2 to 3 tablespoons of honey, 10 ounces of

TABLE 15-5. Oral hypoglycemic agents and their reaction time.

Drug	Peak Reaction	Doses Per Day	Usual Total Daily Dose
Tolbutamide (Orinase)	3–5 hr	2–3	1.0 gm
Acetohexamide (Dymelor)	3 hr	1–2	0.5 gm
Tolazamide (Tolinase)	15 hr	1	0.25 gm
Chlorpropamide (Diabinese)	3 days	1	0.25 gm

soft drink that contains sugar, 6 ounces of orange juice, or 3 to 6 sugar cubes. If the symptoms do not abate in 10 minutes repeat the source of concentrated sugar. If the person has an emesis, repeat the sugar. Chocolate bars are not as effective in raising the blood glucose because of the fat content that slows absorption. Hard candy, unless thoroughly chewed, takes time to dissolve.

Identification. It is of utmost importance that the patient wear a bracelet or emblem indicating he has diabetes and that he carries sugar cubes with him. The nurse can reinforce the significance by asking at every visit to see the diabetes identification and sugar.

Following a hypoglycemic episode the person should do two things: (1) eat some source of less concentrated carbohydrate, perhaps the upcoming meal early, to avoid the return of the symptoms, and (2) examine the situation to determine a cause for the hypoglycemia.

Care During Intercurrent Illness

The body has increased need for insulin during infections as a result of insulin resistance and hormonal actions that increase blood sugar. The patient's knowledge of this facilitates understanding of care during intercurrent illness.

Guidelines for the patient during any intercurrent illness such as gastrointestinal flu are:

1. Test second-voided urine every 4 hours for glucose and acetone.
2. Continue fluid intake.
3. Take the usual dose of long-acting insulin in a.m.
4. Eat a daily total of 150 gm of carbohydrate in form of broth, crackers, milk. Space the meals evenly through the day, i.e., 8-11-2-5-8.
5. Call health worker if any of the following occur:
   a. urine tests show acetone
   b. all urine tests show 2 percent glucose when urine not usually 2 percent
   c. if unable to continue fluid intake
   d. if unable to take 150 gm carbohydrate
   e. if urinating frequently

Some patients are able to safely manage decisions regarding need for quick-acting insulin based on urine testing.

Hygiene

Careful general hygiene, including oral care, is indicated in preventing skin and oral infections which, once acquired, may be more difficult to manage owing to high blood sugar and curtailed circulation.

FOOT CARE. Daily care of the feet prevents development of serious problems. Therefore, foot care is an area that merits instruction time (Fig. 15-3). The goal of care is to maintain unbroken skin.

At each visit, if the nurse inspects the patient's feet, the importance of good foot care is reinforced. Particular emphasis through demonstration should be given to patients with decreased sensation in their feet. Peripheral neuropathy and arterial insufficiency, coupled with faulty vision and obesity, add up to potentially serious problems in noticing or perceiving early changes in feet.

Care should be taken in selecting shoes with adequate depth as well as width and length.

Long Term Problems

The main physiologic problems associated with diabetes are large vessel disease, small vessel disease, and neuropathy. Since little is known of the

---

GUIDELINES FOR THE PATIENT OR FOR PEOPLE RESPONSIBLE FOR THE DIABETIC PERSON

1. Inspect feet daily for blisters, breaks in skin, callus, and bruises.
2. Wash with mild soap and then soak in water (tested for temperature with wrist) for 15 minutes. Rub callus or soft corns gently with a pumice stone.
3. Lubricate with any lanolin-type cream, giving attention to callus.
4. Inspect the insides of shoes for foreign objects, nails coming through the bottom of the shoe, or wrinkles in soles or lining prior to putting them on.
5. Avoid stockings with holes or mended places.
6. Avoid placement of feet near any heat source, i.e., stove, fireplace, or heating pad.
7. Always wear shoes or slippers to avoid injury.
8. Break in new shoes gradually.
9. Avoid any constricting garments, i.e., garters, tight girdles, and tight shoes. Apply panty hose carefully to insure evenly distributed pressure.
10. Cut toenails straight across—have someone else assist if unable to reach easily or if vision is impaired.

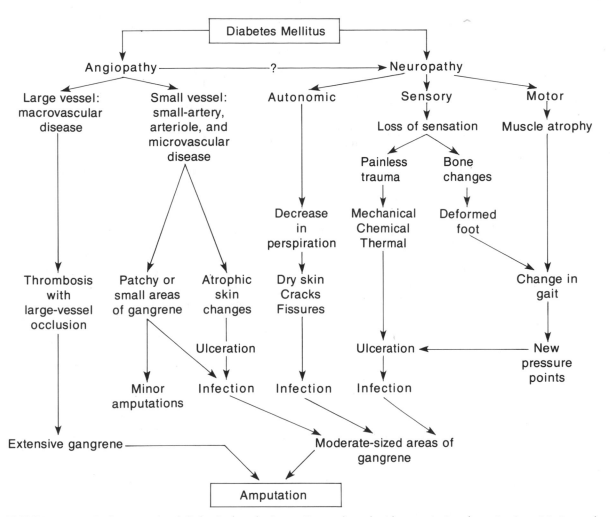

FIGURE 15-3. Pathogenesis of diabetic foot lesions. (Reproduced with permission from Levine, M. E., and O'Neal, L. W. (eds.): The Diabetic Foot. St. Louis: C. V. Mosby Co., 1973)

cause of these changes and care is mainly supportive, the nurse plays an important role in helping people cope.

Management of Large Vessel Disease

Arteriosclerosis and atherosclerosis with result-ant heart disease and hypertension are accelerated in people who have diabetes (see Chapters 13 and 19). As stated earlier, the causes are not clear. Buerger-Allen exercises will maximize the remain-ing circulation of the legs. These should be taught to the patients.

BUERGER-ALLEN EXERCISES

1. Elevate feet above level of heart, i.e., on one pillow until feet blanch—2 minutes.
2. Dangle feet below level of heart until feet turn rubor—3 minutes.
3. Lie with feet level with heart—5 minutes.
4. Repeat these steps five times and do the exer-cises three times daily.

Blood pressure measurements can be taken at each visit. The reader is referred to Chapter 19 for a comprehensive review of accurate blood pressure measurement and management of hypertension. Although the elderly may have long established habits, every effort should be made to encourage abstinence from smoking.

Management of Small Vessel Disease

The primary change in small vessels in people with diabetes is a thickened basement membrane. This change has been seen in capillaries all over the body, but it causes problems primarily in the kidneys and eyes. It has been estimated that Kimmelstiel-Wilson's disease of the kidney, with its accompanying hypertension and decreasing renal function, eventually occurs in 50 percent of people with diabetes. Twenty-four-hour urine collections for measurement of creatinine clearance and protein provide an indication of the severity and progression of the renal disease. At present the research is scanty and the results are inconclusive but it seems control of the blood sugar and hypertension slows progression of the renal disease.

RETINOPATHY. Changes in the vessels of the eyes of people with diabetes can be divided into (1) background retinopthy where changes are in the retina and (2) problems of poliferative retinopathy where eye changes progress through the retina and alter its surface. Figures 15-4, 15-5, and 15-6 illustrate these alterations. The nurse's role is to anticipate or recognize the changes and refer the patient to oph-

thalmology for treatment and to help the person cope with the possibility of decreasing vision (see Chapter 24).

In the nonproliferative form of retinopathy, vision is sometimes spared or minimally affected, depending on the location of the changes on the retina. If the hemorrhages are small they may be absorbed. However, in larger bleeds, as the fibrous bands formed from the hemorrhages contract, they can detach the retina. The vision loss can be slow if it is due to small recurring hemorrhages and exudates, or it may be rapid if it is due to a large hemorrhage and retinal detachment. Protocoagulation, vitrectomy, and pituitary ablation are current treatments, but there is a diversity of opinion as to the effectiveness of these treatments.

LOSS OF VISION. The specter of increasing or sudden loss of vision constitutes a real and serious threat to the older person's independence. A strong component of helping the individual cope is the nurse's provision of current and correct facts pertaining to the nature and treatment of the problem. This eliminates anxiety caused by lack of understanding. Listening and aiding the patient work through plans mentally in the event of decreased independence also eases anxiety.

People with diabetes and serious visual impairment require assistance from someone else. Local offices of Rehabilitation for the Blind offer entry points for assistance. A public health nurse, a friend,

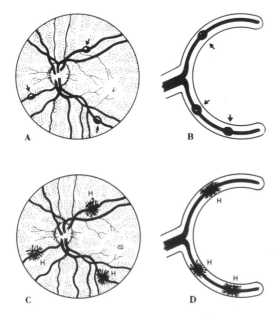

FIGURE 15-4. In the milder or nonproliferative form of diabetic retinopathy, the blood vessel damage is contained within the retina. *A,* Damage first occurs in the walls of the retinal capillaries. Arrows point to areas in the capillary wall which balloon out, forming aneurysms. *B,* Cross section of the eye also shows aneurysms. *C,* The walls of the aneurysms are weak, and blood can easily flow through them. *D,* The cross section shows these hemorrhages contained within the retina. (Reprinted from Blindness Annual, 1969. Washington, D.C., American Association of Workers for the Blind, with permission)

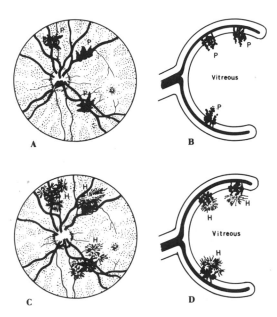

A

B

Vitreous

C

D

Vitreous

FIGURE 15-5. Proliferative retinopathy is the more severe form of the disease. *A,* Vessels (P) have sprouted from the existing ones, proliferating into the vitreous. *B,* Cross section of the eye shows the same new vessels growing into the vitreous. *C,* Hemorrhages which commonly develop surround the new or proliferating vessels. *D,* Cross section shows hemorrhages (H) leaking into the vitreous from proliferating vessels. (Reprinted from Blindness Annual, 1969, Washington, D.C., American Association of Workers for the Blind, with permission)

or a family member is necessary to assist with foot care and insulin injections. A simple adaptation for someone who can inject his own insulin is to have someone draw up a week's supply of the correct dose of insulin in disposable syringes which are then refrigerated. Andros Incorporated of Berkeley, California, manufactures a stiff plastic strip that attaches to a disposable syringe to help indicate when the correct dose has been reached. This and other adaptations of glass and metal syringes deal with the problem of dosage but not sterility or elimination of bubbles. The solution of someone else drawing up the insulin seems more workable.

Management of Neuropathy

The effects of diabetes on neurologic tissue are painful and frustrating. Little is known about the development and treatment of these complications. Problems are manifested in periferal neuropathy with usual involvement of the sensory nerves of the lower extremities. Primary manifestations in the

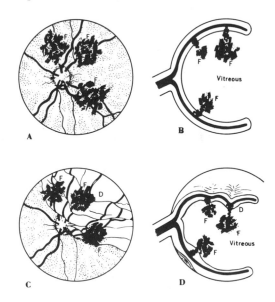

A

B

Vitreous

C

D

Vitreous

FIGURE 15-6. Hemorrhages into the vitreous which accompany proliferative diabetic retinopathy are often replaced by fibrous or scar tissue that forms in the vitreous. *A,* Ophthalmoscopic view shows this fibrous tissue (F). *B,* Cross section depicts the same process with fibrous tissue forming in the vitreous. *C,* Traction from the fibrous tissue has pulled on the retina and caused a detachment (D). *D,* Cross-sectional sketch of the retinal detachment shows the fibrous tissue pulling the retina into the vitreous. (Reprinted from Blindness Annual, 1969, Washington, D.C., American Association of Workers for the Blind, with permission)

lower extremities are decreased sensation with resultant foot problems and painful burning and tingling, especially at night. Neuropathies can affect all body systems, with frequent problems manifested as gastric atony, diarrhea, urinary retention, and impotence.

Careful history and neurologic examination establishes the presence of neuropathies; however, treatment is difficult. Repeated emphasis of the need to look, or if visually impaired have someone else look, at the feet and legs daily is imperative in preventing serious foot lesions. Feeling with hands is not always adequate because of neuropathy in hands and fingers. Dilantin has been used with some success in decreasing the painful burning at night. The treatment is empirical and the side effect of hypertrophy of the gingival margins is common. Older people frequently have dentures, and subsequent problems of ill-fitting dentures occur owing to the hypertrophy. Compromise is achieved by decreasing the dose of Dilantin to reach a middle ground between adequately fitting dentures and some control of the painful burning sensations.

The nurse would do well to have a high suspicion of *urinary retention* and *urinary infection* in people with diabetes. It is useful to encourage voiding every four hours whether or not an urge to void is felt and an attempt should be made to completely empty the bladder at each voiding.

Evaluation

Repeated evaluation of learning with independent verbalization and demonstration of content is emphasized again. Evaluation of control of diabetes is difficult. Stringent objectives of control are advocated by some groups (Metz, 1974; Sussman and Metz, pp. 69–76, 1975).

Helping the older person cope with diabetes is a complex situation. Perhaps the strongest support can be offered by being interested and available—at clinic appointments and by telephone between visits. Asking "What concerns you the most today?" works toward clarifying current personal stresses and short term goals. A realistic look at the elderly person seems to justify adjustment of goals to include:

1. Absence of hypoglycemia
2. Absence of acidosis
3. Attainment and maintenance of ideal body weight

4. Absence of ketonuria
5. Absence of symptoms of polyuria, polyphasia, and polydipsia
6. Absence of infections: urinary, vaginal, and foot lesions
7. Absence of atrophy or scarring of hypertrophy at injection sites

A flowsheet for routine visits aids in evaluating these goals.

CHECKLIST FOR ROUTINE VISIT

Example of data to be evaluated at every routine review of the individual's diabetic status:

polyuria
polydipsia
hunger
hypoglycemic episodes

vagina: burning, itching, drainage
urine: burning, itching, frequency, urgency
vision: blurry, any change
skin: any breaks in skin
feet: callus, breaks in skin, blisters, pain

insulin injection sites: hypertrophy, atrophy

weight
urine test result trends
insulin dose or oral hypoglycemia agent dose
presence of identifying bracelet or emblem
    on person
possession of sugar cube on person

ANNOTATED BIBLIOGRAPHY

Andres, R.: Aging and diabetes. Med. Clin. N. Amer. 55:835–846, 1971.

Andres, R.: Diabetes Forecast. American Diabetes Association, December 1975.

A study of the effect of hypoglycemic agents on vascular complications in patients with adult onset diabetes. The University Group Diabetes Program. Diabetes 24 (Suppl. 1):65–184, 1975. (Part I. Design, methods, and baseline characteristics; Part II. Mortality results [Diabetes, 19 (Suppl. 2):747–830, 1970]; Part V. Evaluation of phenformin therapy.)

Crampton, M., et al.: Diabetes Forecast. American Diabetes Association, December 1975. (Report of the National Commission on Diabetes to the Congress of the United States, December 10, 1975.)

Crampton, M., et al.: Instructions for the Diabetic Patient, ed. 10. The Mason Clinic, Seattle, Washington, 1978. (Available for purchase at the Virginia Mason Hospital Cashier, 925 Seneca Street, Seattle, WA 98101.)

Dye, B., et al.: Starting the person with diabetes on insulin in the outpatient setting: A guide for physicians and nurses. J. Fam. Pract. 5:341–48, 1977. (A detailed guide with desired behaviors, content, and methods outlined to achieve specifically stated goals.)

Flack, R., and Grayer, E. D.: A consciousness raising group for obese women. Social Work, 20:484–487, November 1975.

Marble, A., et al. (ed.): Joslin's Diabetes Mellitus, ed. 11. Philadelphia: Lea and Febiger, 1971. (This book offers classic comprehensive coverage of the treatment of diabetes.)

Metz, R.: Guidelines for managing diabetes mellitus. Bull. Virginia Mason Clin. 28:100–106, 1974.

Levine, M. E., and O'Neal L. W. (eds.): The Diabetic Foot. St. Louis: C. V. Mosby Co., 1973. (Pathogenesis and treatment of foot lesions are explained by this outstanding authority. Plans for preventative care of the feet are carefully outlined.)

Steinke, J., and Taylor, K. W.: Viruses and the etiology of diabetes. Diabetes, 23:631–633, 1974.

Sussman, K., and Metz, R. J. S. (eds.): Diabetes Mellitus, ed. 4. American Diabetes Association, 1975. (Thirty authorities in the field of diabetes present succinct chapters directed to the main areas of concern and major issues in diabetes. Much of the current research on diabetes.)

Watkins, J. D., et al.: Diabetes Mellitus Assessment Guides, 1971. The North Carolina Diabetes Association, 408 North Tryon Street, Charlotte, NC 29202. (Carefully prepared and tested, this provides an effective way of assessing knowledge and motor skills required for sound self-management. Specific content is provided along with a useful interview guide format.)

Williams, R. H.: Textbook of Endocrinology, ed. 5. Philadelphia: W. B. Saunders Co., 1974. (This classic textbook offers detail on the physiology and pathophysiology of diabetes. Interrelationship of other endocrine disorders with diabetes are clearly explained.)

16

Gastrointestinal Problems

Mari Anne Bartol and Margaret Heitkemper

QUICK REVIEW

HIATAL HERNIA

DESCRIPTION	Protrusion of part of the stomach into the thoracic cavity.
ETIOLOGIC FACTORS	Weakening, possibly through degenerative changes, of already flexible attachments between esophagus and diaphragm.
HIGH RISK	*Elderly:* As high as 40 to 60 percent of persons over 60 may have hiatal hernias. *Males:* 50 to 70 percent are at highest risk.
DYNAMICS	*Parahiatal Rolling hernia:* Herniates through the diaphragm near esophageal hiatus. The LES barrier remains intact. *Sliding hernia:* Stomach slides directly through both membranous and muscular openings so that the gastroesophageal junction is above the diaphragm. Sphincter is patulous.
SIGNS AND SYMPTOMS	Frequently no symptoms. Distress mild to severe. Symptoms: heartburn, sour stomach, distress following certain foods, pain or sense of a lump pressure burning at level of xiphoid. Symptoms worse with recumbency, bending, coughing, overeating. Recurrent pneumonia or persistent cough may indicate esophageal reflux with aspiration.
DIFFERENTIAL DIAGNOSIS	Mimics angina, except esophageal pain is associated with eating, angina with exertion, and has no blood pressure or pulse rate changes, pulmonary distress. Difficulty swallowing may be a symptom of cancer of the esophagus.
COMPLICATIONS	Caused by esophageal reflux, esophagitis, or pulmonary aspiration.
PROGNOSIS	Most hiatal hernias are asymptomatic and are managed conservatively.
MANAGEMENT	Antacid therapy—in response to symptoms not at regular intervals. Nutritional—small feedings, low fat, walk or remain in upright position after meals to use force of gravity. Avoid chocolate, cola, coffee. Positioning—elevate head of bed with blocks or bricks and sleep on sides. Be sure dentures fit (to assure good chewing of food and minimize air swallowing). Restrict food and fluids 1 to 2 hours before bedtime.
EVALUATION	Understanding of dynamics of hiatal hernia as a basis for participation in dietary alterations, post-eating routines to minimize reflux, and sleeping strategies to reduce risk of aspiration. Avoidance or management of symptoms, understanding of side effects of ongoing antacid therapy as basis for taking these drugs with least difficulties.

QUICK REVIEW

DIVERTICULOSIS

DESCRIPTION	Diverticuli are sacculations of mucosa through the first layer of the muscularis, predominantly in the sigmoid area of colon.
ETIOLOGIC FACTORS	Age-related atrophy of the musculature, if major factor. Diet of refined foods. Obesity or emotional tension.
HIGH RISK	Elderly (40 percent over 70-years old estimated to have diverticulosis). Persons with problems of obesity, constipation, hiatal hernias, or emotional tension are at higher risk. History of diet high in refined low residue foods.
SIGNS AND SYMPTOMS	Usually asymptomatic. Symptoms are related to increased motor activity of sigmoid—pain in lower abdomen that increases at definite time interval after meals or following emotional disturbance and relieved by bowel movement. Small amounts of rectal bleeding may occur.
DIFFERENTIAL DIAGNOSIS	Rule out other lesions causing rectal bleeding, e.g., tumors.
COMPLICATIONS	Diverticulitis (more common in males) occurs with eating irritating foods or alcohol, severe coughing or straining at stool. Perforation, major gastrointestinal bleeding, peritonitis, abscess, fistulae, and obstruction can occur.
PROGNOSIS	Most individuals remain asymptomatic.
MANAGEMENT	Dietary—minimize spicy foods and alcohol intake. Use high residue diet. Weight control—reduce obesity. Control constipation but avoid harsh laxatives. For hypermotility—anticholinergics may be used.
EVALUATION	Maintain adequate fiber and fluids in diet. Constipation controlled; tension management; and weight control.

There are no clearcut gastrointestinal disease entities that can be attributed directly to the aging process. There are several, however, that show a higher incidence in the elderly. In addition, other gastrointestinal disorders may have a greater impact on the elderly person's general physical and social well-being.

Little research has been done on the effects of aging on the main portions of the gastrointestinal tract. Systemic changes in the functions of digestion and absorption of nutrients seem to be more affected by changes in the cardiovascular and neurologic systems than in the gastrointestinal tract itself. Arteriosclerosis and other circulatory problems may result in reduced splanchnic blood flow and decrease absorption from the small intestine. Degenerative changes in the nervous system may decrease the motility of the esophagus, small intestine, and colon and, thus, increase or decrease transit time through the tract.

ESOPHAGUS

The primary function of the esophagus is the transport of food from the mouth to the stomach. Between the esophagus and the stomach is a physiologic barrier which prevents the backward flow of gastric contents from the stomach into the esophagus. This barrier, approximately 2 to 3 cm in length, is known as the lower esophageal sphincter (LES). It functions as a barrier because of its location below the diaphragm. This location results in a higher pressure than that present in the remainder of the esophagus. The esophagus located above the diaphragm has a resting pressure *below* atmospheric pressure while the lower esophageal sphincter has a resting pressure *above* atmospheric pressure. The pressure in the LES is also higher than the resting pressure of the stomach. The LES, thus, presents a barrier to retrograde movement of food and fluids from the stomach into the esophagus. However, during the process of swallowing, the muscles of the lower esophagus relax, which results in a lowering of the LES pressure, thus allowing the bolus of food to pass into the stomach.

In the elderly person, alterations in both esophageal motility and the LES pressure barrier (primarily as a consequence of hiatal hernia) may result in dysphagia or substernal pain and discomfort.

Esophageal Motility Alterations

With increasing age, changes in esophageal motility begin to occur. In a study of esophageal motility in nonagenarians, esophageal peristalsis was found to follow only 50 percent of swallows, compared to 90 percent in younger persons (Soergel, et al., 1964). These researchers found that, in older persons, there was less efficient deglutition, relaxation of the LES, delay in esophageal emptying, dilation of the esophagus, and an increase in nonpropulsive contractions. This less effective functioning is thought to be related to degenerative changes in the smooth muscle that lines the lower two thirds of the esophagus. Neurogenic, humoral, and vascular changes may also contribute to decreased esophageal motility. Persons with accompanying diabetes mellitus, parkinsonism, or Raynaud's disease are more likely to experience abnormal esophageal motility. Decreased esophageal peristalsis may be partially responsible for the long periods of time necessary for elderly persons to comfortably consume a sizable meal or the necessity of several small meals to equate adequate nutrition in the elderly population.

Many times these changes do not result in symptomatic problems for the elderly person. However, some do experience episodes of substernal pain and difficulty in swallowing. The substernal discomfort produced by altered contractions of the esophagus can be confused with the pain of angina—the substernal area with an occasional person's experiencing pressure and radiation to the left chest wall. The representing symptoms may be confusing to both the patient and the nurse since the patient may have both coronary artery disease and esophageal dysfunction.

Esophageal motility disorders are generally characterized by intermittent rather than progressive symptoms. The person complains of inability to handle liquids as well as solids. Further, certain acidic foods such as citrus juices or tomato paste may cause problems; they are thought to stimulate abnormal esophageal motility.

Hiatal Hernia

The resting pressure of the lower esophageal sphincter has been shown to decrease with advancing age. Hiatal hernia frequently is seen in elderly persons with lowered LES pressure. However, a number of persons also will have symptomatic sphincter incompetence without hiatal hernia.

Description

A hiatal hernia is the protrusion of the stomach into the thoracic cage through an opening in the diaphragm.

Etiologic Factors

Even under normal conditions the esophagus is not rigidly attached to the diaphragm as it enters the hiatal ring. Thus even young individuals can exhibit herniation of the stomach through the hiatal ring of the diaphragm during increased abdominal pressure, such as in forceful vomiting or valsalva maneuvers. Hiatal hernias in the aged may be the result of degenerative changes in the already weak supporting system. As a result the transient herniation may be exaggerated and more frequent.

High Risk Population

The elderly are at high risk of hiatal hernias. The incidence may be as high as 40 to 60 percent in persons over 60. Winsberg (1971, p. 276) suggested that small hiatal hernias are so common as to be considered a normal finding in x-ray studies. Males aged 50 to 70 are at highest risk.

Dynamics

There are two common types of hiatal hernia. The parahiatal *rolling* type is a hernia through the diaphragm near the esophageal hiatus. With this type of hernia, the LES barrier mechanism remains intact. Complications include ulceration of the hernia and stricture.

The second type is the *sliding* hernia. This is the more common type. Here the fundic portion of the stomach slides directly through both the membranous and muscular openings of the diaphragm so that the gastroesophageal junction is above the diaphragm. In the sliding type the cardiac sphincter is patulous, the cardioesophageal junction is incompetent, and reflux esophagitis and esophageal stricture tend to be more common. Pain may be described as a lump, pressure or burning at the level of the xiphoid process, or as a severe viselike pain. It may be referred to the epigastrium, along both costal margins, to the back, upper thorax, or arms. It can be precipitated or made worse by bending, reclining, coughing, overeating, or exertion that increases intra-abdominal pressure. Walking about tends to bring relief, often abruptly (Sodeman, 1974).

Signs and Symptoms

The symptoms of alterations in esophageal motility or LES pressure barriers are extremely variable. Frequently there are no symptoms. Distress, when present can be severe or mild, intermittent or constant. Complaints, when they occur, will be of heartburn, sour stomach, or epigastric distress following the eating of certain types of foods. Symptoms tend to occur with a recumbent position. Recurrent episodes of pneumonia, bronchiectasis, or intractable cough may be indicators of esophageal reflux or obstruction with pulmonary aspiration.

Differential Diagnosis

Not only can esophageal hernias mimic angina and pulmonary distress, large esophageal hernias can also cause difficulty in swallowing. However, difficulty in swallowing may also be a primary symptom of esophageal cancer.

Complications

Esophageal reflux is the primary complication of hiatal hernia and incompetent LES. *Pulmonary problems* result from night-time regurgitation of gastric contents or saliva into the respiratory tract. Elderly persons may be particularly prone to pulmonary aspiration owing to a diminished cough reflex. Also, because of the symptoms of episodic cough which generally interrupt the person's sleep, night-time aspirations may mimic congestive heart failure.

Esophageal reflux of gastric contents can lead to esophagitis. The acidic gastric juice corrodes the mucosal cells that line the esophagus. The esophagitis, in turn, is responsible for the sensations of substernal pain or heartburn. This pain of esophagitis pain may mimic anginal pain. However, esophageal pain is generally associated with eating and with a recumbent position, while angina is related to exertion. Further, with esophagitis there are no blood pressure or heart rate changes. Where the patient has difficulty in differentiating the pain in terms of concurrent activities, the nurse will want to take a careful history of symptoms and associated activities.

Less common complications of hiatal hernia include *ulceration* of the fundic portion of the stomach, stricture and hernia incarceration. These are serious complications in the older person and generally are accompanied by acute pain and/or symptoms of obstruction.

Management

Medical management of hiatal hernias usually is conservative. Surgery does not always correct the situation and relieve the symptoms, so it tends to be reserved for use if medical measures fail and symptoms are severe or when complications such as bleeding or ulceration arise.

Antacids frequently are used for the relief of heartburn or esophagitis. They work through two avenues. First, they neutralize the acidity of the gastric juices and, therefore, decrease the corrosive effect of the reflux. Second, the alkalinization stimulates a release of gastrin (a gastrointestinal hormone) from the stomach; this acts to increase the resting pressure of the LES (Babka, 1973) and blocks or minimizes the reflux of gastric juices. Side effects of prolonged antacid therapy are given in Table 16-1. One way to minimize side effects is to take the antacids in response to symptoms rather than on a regularly scheduled basis. Gaviscon, or other antacids containing sodium bicarbonate, have been found useful for esophageal reflux. These tablets taken after meals help to remove food particles that may be trapped as a result of the herniation. The antacid portion again neutralizes the gastric contents.

Another form of management is to ascertain whether particular foods cause greater difficulties. For example, high fat foods will decrease the LES resting pressure and may predispose to reflux (Babka, 1973). Low fat or skim milk should be used to relieve heartburn rather than high fat whole milk. Chocolate, tea, cola, and coffee have also been found to reduce the LES resting pressure and, therefore, should be limited or avoided. Reducing the amount of animal fat or saturated fats in the diet has been found to be

particularly useful. Smaller, more frequent feedings have been found to be helpful. And the increased risk of reflux in the recumbent position can be decreased by elevating the head of the bed on blocks or bricks for sleep and rest. Walking about after eating effectively utilizes gravity to empty the esophagus and fundus. Lying down after eating is to be avoided.

Table 16-2 summarizes the problems, signs and symptoms, and nursing management in hiatal hernia.

STOMACH

Little is known at this time about the effect of aging on the stomach. The age-related decrease in hydrochloric acid may be the result of gastric cell loss, as in atrophic gastritis. Functionally, relative decrease in stomach acidity could reduce the solubility of acidic drugs such as aspirin (Hanan, 1978, p. 57). It also is thought to hamper the absorption of iron and calcium. Because there is so little evidence of changes in the stomach related to normal aging, it becomes important to view the older person's gastric complaints as presenting the likelihood of pathology. Gastric complaints, therefore, merit investigation as they are likely to be genuine health problems.

Chronic Atrophic Gastritis

Description

Chronic atrophic gastritis, as the name implies, is an inflammatory phenomenon in which the mu-

TABLE 16-1. Side effects of prolonged antacid therapy.

Antacid Ingredient	Possible Problems

Calcium carbonate
    Alkets, Camolox, Alka-2,
    Titralac, Tums, Dicarbosil
	Gastric acid rebound, hypercalcemia, constipation, decreased renal function, safe for low dose occasional relief

Sodium bicarbonate* Soda Mint, Alka-Seltzer	Sodium overload. In large dose may produce systemic alkalosis, increase stomach pH, and increase acid output
Magnesium Milk of Magnesia, Chooz	Diarrhea. Use with caution in those with renal disease
Aluminum Amphojel, Basaljel	Constipation, phosphate depletion

Magnesium-aluminum hydroxide
    Maalox, Mylanta, Gelusil,
    Aludrox, Di-Gel, WinGel
	Phosphate depletion syndrome, low sodium content. Can cause diarrhea or constipation

* Many pharmaceutical firms are reformulating their antacids to reduce the sodium content, so it would be wise to read the labels for sodium content rather than rely on previous information. It must be printed on the label if the antacid contains more than 0.2 mEq per dosage unit.

TABLE 16-2. Summary of hiatal hernia.

Problem	Assessment	Nursing Care
Motility disorder	Episodic substernal discomfort Difficulty swallowing liquids rather than solids Complaints of difficulty taking medications	Feed slowly—never rush the individual Give thick liquids; soak liquids up with bread, toast, crackers, or cookies Increase neural stimulation; give frozen or very cold liquids; mix medication with ice cream or sherbert
Esophageal reflux	Complaints of heartburn; pain or epigastric distress after eating; in very impaired elderly, there is confusion, agitation, increased motor activity, rubbing epigastric or lower abdomen following a meal or during a meal, belching following a meal	Keep head of bed elevated on 4–6 inch blocks after eating; could roll up head of bed 45°; do not lie down following a meal for 45 min to 1 hr, walk about following eating; encourage low fat diet; decrease cholesterol; avoid chocolate, cola, coffee; watch for side effects of antacids and anticolinergics which may be used (see Table 15-1); avoid large meals that result in increased abdominal pressure; discourage eructation and air swallowing; make sure dentures fit
Nocturnal aspiration	Intractable cough, recurrent pneumonia	No eating 1–2 hr before bedtime; no fluids before bedtime; head of bed slightly elevated at 30°; sleep side to side at night
Herniation (sliding or rolling)	May be palpable	Avoid conditions that increase abdominal pressure such as tight fitting clothing, corsets; avoid heavy lifting or straining; weight reduction if obese

cosa becomes thinned, gray or greenish gray, and abnormally smooth, with hemorrhagic patches. It is usually distributed irregularly, but the entire stomach may be involved.

Etiologic Factors

The etiologic factors of chronic gastritis is not known. However, it is associated with aging. It has been found to occur with gastric ulcer, recurrent gastritis, pernicious anemia, and iron deficiency anemia. Dietary patterns, such as use of alcohol, tobacco, coffee, and nutritional deficiencies have been suggested as contributors, but the linkage is inconclusive. Immune reaction is another possibility (Sodeman, 1974). Drugs that cause damage directly to gastric mucosal cells such as aspirin, alcohol, and Butazolidin may also be a factor. Corticosteroids may also be potentially destructive to the gastric mucosal barrier, although the exact mechanism has not been determined.

High Risk Population

Chronic atrophic gastritis has been determined to increase with advancing age. Males are at higher risk than females.

Dynamics

The entire stomach wall is involved in the cellular changes. The mucosa is thin with hemorrhagic patches, the submucosal vessels are visible as red or blue ramifications, and the folds are diminished in size and number. All layers are atrophied. As the severity or degree of atrophic gastritis increases there is a concurrent decrease in chief and parietal (pepsin and HCL acid-secreting) cells. These cells are replaced by goblet cells and fibrous tissue. With the loss of parietal cells there is a decrease in acid output and intrinsic factor secretion. There is disappearance of glandular cells and increase in fibrous tissue. The course is persistent or recurrent with alternate erosions, hemorrhage, and healing.

Signs and Symptoms

The evaluation of symptoms is often difficult. Chronic atrophic gastritis can be demonstrated to exist without symptoms. Symptoms, when they do exist, are varied and vague, nor can their type and severity be correlated with the severity of the gastritis. The most frequent symptoms are loss of appetite, vague epigastric pain, belching, feeling of fullness, nausea, and vomiting.

Complications

Anemia is a potential complication of chronic atrophic gastritis. Achlorhydria decreases the absorption of ferric food iron (Schade, et al., 1968). In addition, the intrinsic factor may be decreased as a result of either cell loss or decreased stomach acidity. Since the intrinsic factor is responsible for absorption of vitamin B_{12} in the terminal ileum, patients with advanced chronic atrophic gastritis may develop a vitamin B_{12} deficiency that may border on pernicious anemia; however, progression to a full-blown state of pernicious anemia is rare. The risk of vitamin deficiency is slightly greater in women than men.

Management

Symptoms may be relieved by use of a bland diet, small feedings, and antispasmodic drugs. This does not treat the underlying pathology but can help the person be more comfortable.

Evaluation

Evaluation criteria concern management of symptoms, control of associated anemia, and the person's ability to manage and obtain satisfaction from the diet.

Ulcers

Recent studies have demonstrated that the prevalence of peptic ulcers increases with persons over 60 (Levral, et al., 1966). Deaths among the elderly from peptic ulcers are increasing, while deaths from stomach malignancies are decreasing.

Etiologic Factors

Ulcers are seen to be related to stress in the elderly—as complications of other diseases and trauma. Drug-induced ulcers are also common among the elderly who take many more drugs than younger persons.

High Risk Population

Any elderly person experiencing a major body insult, whether medical or psychogenic, is at risk of ulcer development, particularly if a preexistent atrophic gastritis is present. Some events known to have precipitated peptic ulcers include fractures, pneumonia, admission to a nursing home—conditions and circumstances that initially may seem quite unrelated to peptic ulcers. Persons who have had strokes or who have chronic obstructive pulmonary disease are at greater risk of peptic ulcers because of attendant rehabilitation/social stresses associated with these illnesses.

Those on ulcerogenic drugs such as aspirin, reserpine, tolbutamide, phenylbutazone, colchicine, corticotropin, or adrenal corticol steroids also need to be observed for incidence of peptic ulcers.

Signs and Symptoms

Peptic ulcer disease in the elderly presents itself differently from the symptoms in younger patients. Epigastric pain is not a prominent feature. More frequently the outstanding symptoms the elderly person exhibits include poorly localized pain, decreased appetite, decreased general energy level, weight loss, vomiting, and anemia.

The usual symptom of bleeding is not a cardinal symptom of ulcer or gastric disease in the elderly. It is more common to see sudden onset of hemorrhagic bleeding resulting from the perforation of an ulcer rather than minor or occult bleeding episodes. Ulcer development in the elderly is an insidious process which may be diagnosed only by upper gastrointestinal x-ray studies. Prior to roentgenography, astute and sensitive nursing observations that are attendent to changes in normal eating patterns, energy levels, and body weight status may be the only clues of gastric pathology.

Differential Diagnosis

Duodenal ulcers are ten times more common than gastric ulcers in the general population. However, the incidence of gastric ulcer is not unexpected in the elderly, particularly those with drug-induced ulcer disease. It becomes important, therefore, that differential diagnosis be made between these two lesions. Symptoms will be similar. The malignancies have been known to occur more commonly in males.

Medical philosophies of therapy vary. Some physicians feel that, since the prognosis is so guarded for stomach malignancies, if there is a possibility of the disease being benign, conservative treatment should be tried for a few weeks. Gastric ulcers improve or disappear in 4 to 6 weeks with adequate treatment.

Ulcers, like many other physical illness syndromes in the elderly, may present as depression. A careful history of eating patterns, stress, drugs, ulcer risk factors, and signs and symptoms becomes important.

Complications

Complications accompanying peptic ulcer disease are of particular importance in the elderly person because of the high risk involved in emergency surgical procedures. Bleeding is the most significant complication of peptic ulcers. Other complications include obstruction and perforation, both of which have a high mortality age group.

Fluid dynamics involved in treatment of the complications create risks in themselves. Excessive or overly-rapid flow of blood transfusions may precipitate congestive heart failure in the older person, while sudden loss of blood volume through hemorrhage increases the risk of stroke and/or central nervous system cell deaths resulting from hypoxia.

Medical Management

Conservative management of gastric and peptic ulcer disease in the elderly person is preferred since any type of surgical procedure poses many possible risks. However, surgical procedures are required for those patients who cannot be managed medically and in those where gastric cancer is suspected.

Some of the earlier strategies in conservative management are now open to question. Half-and-half or whole milk, once a standard treatment, has been found to cause a rebound acid output (Dunkerly, 1976). Low fat or skim milk is seen as preferable.

Agents known to increase HCL production should be avoided. These include alcohol; caffeine-containing beverages such as coffee and colas; spices such as curry, pepper, and mustard; and smoking. Antacids play an important role in the symptomatic relief of peptic ulcer pain. They neutralize gastric

juice and, thus, reduce irritation and further ulceration; however, they appear to have little role in the actual healing process. While there is no debate about their usefulness, they can create some problems for the user, particularly the older person. (See Table 16-1 for some of the side effects.) The nurse can consider these in terms of the presenting problem of the patient—low sodium diet, tendency toward diarrhea or constipation, edema or renal disease. Some antacids increase secretion of acids. Besides these problems, aluminum hydroxide gels and antacids with calcium and magnesium have been shown to absorb antibiotics such as tetracycline. It is also thought that corticosteroid absorption may be hampered by antacids (Piper, 1972).

Antacids decrease the absorption of tetracycline and ferrous sulfate as well as some acidic drugs such as isoniazid, pentobarbital, penicillin, sulfonamides, and salicylates. The effect of enteric-coated products and antacids is the increase of the release of the drug in the stomach. Warfarin is the drug of choice for oral anticoagulants in patients taking an antacid. The absorption or the effect of this drug is not altered by antacid (Ambre, 1973; Robinson, 1971).

The Federal Drug Administration requires that indications for use of antacids be limited to conditions related to excess stomach acid, that drug interactions be listed on the label, and that instructions are clear and concise (American Pharmaceutical Association Handbook, 1977).

Frequently, anticholinergics are given to decrease acid output. Anticholinergics (Belap and Pro-Banthine) and synthetic anticholinergics (Bentyl and Valpin) generally are given three to four times per day, before meals and at bedtime. They help to reduce acidity and hypermotility. However, they should be administered cautiously to the older person. Long term anticholinergic administration can result in a variety of serious side effects. The nurse and the patient should be alert to signs and symptoms listed in Table 16-3.

Nursing Management

Nursing management is related to gathering data on usual dietary style and previous adjustments in terms of gastric distress, on medication-taking behavior and its relationship to introducing or changing a regimen, or on bowel patterns and edema. It also is important to assure understanding of the reason for timing of the medications and setting up of schedules where the medications are taken in proper

TABLE 16-3. Side effects of anticholinergic medications.

Mouth	Dryness owing to reduced salivation may make swallowing difficult and increase dental diseases
	Dryness of the respiratory tract is particularly critical for the patient with chronic lung disease
Skin	Dry, hot, red because of decreased sweating and vasodilation
	Interference with normal cooling mechanisms may predispose the elderly to hyperpyrexia with resultant dehydration in warm weather or hot climates
Eyes	Possible photophobia resulting from widely dilated pupils
	Vision blurred owing to paralysis of accommodation
	Crowding of iris and ciliary muscle into angle of eye chamber may raise intraocular pressure by interfering with draining of the aqueous humor
	These drugs are contraindicated in patients with narrow angle glaucoma
	Caution in all elderly patients owing to the increased incidence of acute, and prevalence of chronic, glaucoma
Urinary tract	Urine retention may occur as a result of loss of bladder tone
	Elderly males with prostatic hypertrophy are particularly at risk
Heart	Due to loss of vagal control, side effects of prolonged tachycardia episodes may include coronary insufficiency, chest pain, and cardiac decompensation (CHF) in patients with a history of heart disease
Constipation	Result of reduced tone and motility of GI musculature
	Particularly at risk is the elderly patient with decreased physical exercise, decreased food volume consumption, and low-residue dietary pattern
Central nervous system	Anticholinergic psychosis
	Confusion, disorientation, belligerence, paranoia-type delusions, dizziness, delirum
	Particularly at risk is the elderly patient who may be receiving anticholinergic medication for psychiatric conditions, i.e., depression

relationship to eating schedules. The patient needs to know what symptoms indicate drug side effects. Those symptoms that should trigger a call to the nurse or the physician's office should be written down together with the phone number, if this is appropriate.

Evaluation

Nurse evaluation concerns the way in which the person participates in dietary management, compliance with the medication regimen, and freedom from symptoms. Medical evaluation deals with the size of the ulcer, associated anemia, weight gain, and freedom from symptoms.

Dumping Syndrome

Symptoms of a dumping syndrome may be exhibited late in life, particularly in the elderly person who has a past history of gastrectomy earlier in his life.

Dynamics

Dumping syndrome is a complex of symptoms that occur after the ingestion of a meal. Because of the decreased capacity or size of the stomach there is increased intragastric pressure when food is taken in. As a result, the stomach empties at a faster rate. A hyperosmotic load is delivered to the duodenum and fluid is pulled into the lumen from the mucosa. Persons who have had gastric resection or vagotomy have risk of developing a dumping syndrome. The incidence seems somewhat less in patients who have had selective vagotomy or pyloroplasty.

Signs and Symptoms

The symptoms, which begin immediately or 10 to 30 minutes after eating, include sweating, faintness, lightheadedness, flushing, and dizziness. The rapid emptying of stomach and subsequent diarrhea may also cause symptoms of cramping pain and nausea. Hypoglycemia occurs in these patients when the hyperosmotic load delivered to the duodenum causes stimulation of insulin release from the pancreas. However, rapid intestinal transit does not allow for proper absorption of the meal and, as a result, the patient may exhibit signs of hypoglycemia.

The rapid shift in fluid from the mucosa into the lumen in response to the hyperosmotic solute can also result in a decreased cardiac output. Tachycardia and blood pressure alterations are the clinical signs of this. Such rapid fluid shift can be especially serious in the elderly patient. Long term malabsorption problems have been observed including anemia, osteoporosis, and fat and milk intolerance.

Management

To avoid such symptoms these people should be encouraged to eat small, frequent meals, avoid foods that are hyperosmolar, and rest (particularly in a prone position) following meals. While some general advice regarding diet can be given to those who suffer from dumping syndrome, diet management is usually an individual trial and error process. This period of establishing dietary habits can be extremely frustrating and uncomfortable (not to mention socially limiting) and the patient needs encouragement and reassurance that his diet can be managed so as to avoid symptoms.

COLON

Diverticulosis

Description

Diverticulosis is the herniation or sacculation of the mucosa through the first layer of the muscularis at the point where blood vessels penetrate the muscle. This begins to develop at about age fifty, with sacculations increasing in number and size with age. They are located predominantly in the sigmoid portion of the left colon.

Etiologic Factors

This is a disease of aging, with atrophy of the musculature in the intestinal wall seen as a contributing factor. Because of its geographic distribution in countries of Western civilization where refined foods are used, diet is thought to be a factor. The refined, low residue foods are thought to alter the colonic motility, with higher intralumenal pressures in the colon created as a result of sustained muscular contractions. In time, such abnormally high pressures may lead to the outpouching of the mucosa. For the same reason, constipation is seen as a possible cause. Obesity and emotional tension have also been suggested as contributors.

High Risk Populations

Risk of diverticulosis increases with age (40 percent over 70 are estimated to have diverticulosis); obesity; constipation; presence of hiatal hernia; history of diet high in refined, low residue foods; and emotional tension.

Signs and Symptoms

The majority of persons with diverticulosis are asymptomatic. Symptoms, when they occur, may be due to the increased motor activity of the sigmoid colon and factors which enhance it. They may take the form of pain in the lower abdomen occurring or increasing in severity at a definite time interval after meals or following emotional disturbance, being relieved or temporarily abolished by a bowel movement. Diverticulosis may also result in slight rectal bleeding.

Differential Diagnosis

Careful investigation to rule out other lesions must precede the attributing of rectal bleeding to diverticula. Sigmoidoscopy rarely shows the diverticula; a barium enema is necessary.

Complications

Diverticulitis occurs in a few persons with diverticulosis, more commonly among males. It is precipitated by obesity, eating irritating foods, or alcohol. Severe coughing or straining at stool may also contribute to development of inflammation. A small perforation of a diverticulum and the associated peridiverticulitis causes the symptoms of left lower quadrant pain, chills, fever, constipation or diarrhea, nausea and vomiting, and as gross blood in the feces. Serious complications include major bleeding perforation, peritonitis, abscess formation, fistulae, and obstruction.

Management

Eating is an important part in the life of old people. Much of their lives focus on food and activities around food. It is used as rewards and in social activities. Nurses in their daily questioning of patients ask about food and liquid intake and related areas (bowels), so it should come as no surprise when patients remark about these same areas. An accurate dietary history is the beginning of effective diverticulosis management.

Diverticulosis is managed by use of a nonspicy diet, weight reduction if the individual is obese, management of constipation, and administration of iron supplement if anemia occurs. The low residue diet often suggested in the past as being appropriate for the person with diverticulosis is now thought to be inappropriate (Berman, 1972). Instead a high residue diet may be used to increase the stool bulk and decrease the abnormally high intralumenal pressures. If hypermotility is a problem, anticholinergic drugs may be used. (See Table 16-3 for important side effects in the elderly.) Harsh laxatives should be avoided in managing this type of constipation.

Hemorrhoids

Description

Hemorrhoids are swollen or dilated superior hemorrhoidal plexus veins which can be located internally or externally. Those located externally are covered by skin, while internal hemorrhoids are covered by mucus membrane.

Etiologic Factors

Hemorrhoids are caused or aggravated by factors that increase intraabdominal pressure or partial obstruction of venous return, e.g., constipation and straining to defecate, portal hypertension, congestive failure.

High Risk

Usually hemorrhoids have developed at an earlier time, particularly among persons who have had occupations that required long periods of standing—barbers, dentists, surgeons, scrub nurses. They also tend to occur in women who have had one or more pregnancies. Persons with a history of constipation, congestive heart failure, and portal hypertension also are at higher risk.

Signs and Symptoms

Clinical manifestations include perianal itching and pain. Bleeding may also occur. Typically it is seen as bright streaking on the surface of the stool; however, it may be more extensive than this. Pain is usually the result of thrombosis of external hemorrhoids and increases with defecation.

Complications

Thrombus formation or strangulation of the blood vessels are the most common complications. Both are accompanied by severe pain. Some individuals find that certain foods such as fresh pineapple, mangos, and certain nuts also increase irritation and pain. Anemia is a risk associated with extensive or ongoing bleeding.

Differential Diagnosis

Rectal bleeding should always be taken seriously in the older age group and checked out medically. One source of anemia could be rectal bleeding.

Rectal bleeding is one of the earliest signs of rectal or colonic cancer. Cancer of the colon is common in the older population. Bright bleeding can also occur with rectal polyps.

Management

Management of hemorrhoids usually is conservative. Surgery is used only if there is disabling pain, bleeding sufficient to cause anemia, or severe anal itching. Hemorrhoids may recur following surgery.

Day-to-day management of hemorrhoids involves stool softeners or bulk-forming agents to control constipation and reduce straining. Pain and pruritus usually can be controlled by soaking in warm water in the tub or sitz bath several times a day, washing the area after bowel movements and application of anorectal preparations. These ointments or creams usually contain an anesthetic agent and emollients. Some also include corticosteroids. Topical preparations are more effective than suppositories because the suppository moves into the upper rectum and does not deposit the medication in the area requiring treatment. Prolapsed hemorrhoids sometimes can be pushed manually back into the rectum to provide relief. Symptomatic relief during acutely painful episodes may be provided by decreasing the amount of time spent standing and by elevating the feet and legs when sitting or lying in bed.

Evaluation

Criteria for evaluation of response to management include the person's ability to participate in control of constipation, hygiene measures, and use of the topical medication. Ultimate evaluation is the relief of symptoms and control of associated anemia.

Diarrhea

Diarrhea can be a more serious problem in the person over 70 than it is in the younger-age group. It is a particular risk for those who already have a precarious fluid and electrolyte balance because of other conditions or drug treatment that fosters imbalance in electrolytes and dehydration.

Description

Diarrhea is the frequent passage of unformed stools, a result of increased bowel motility or interference with the normal absorption of water and nutrients from the bowel.

Etiologic Factors

The older person, the same as a younger person, is subject to intestinal infections and food poisoning that cause diarrhea. Diarrhea also is associated with diseases such as diverticulitis. Malignancy, which can be confirmed by doing a guaiac test or hemocult, will change bowel habits, including diarrhea. Emotions and stress, anticipation of an event, or concern about a problem can cause diarrhea. Fecal impaction should be considered a cause of diarrhea when there is history of constipation. This can be checked easily by doing a rectal.

Medication-incurred diarrhea is a more frequent cause of diarrhea in the over-60 group. Drugs that produce diarrhea (in addition to laxatives taken for this purpose) include:

- broad spectrum of antibiotics (by altering the normal bowel flora)—ampicillin, clindamycin, lincomycin, tetracycline, neomycin, and Keflex

- Guanethidine (Ismelin) (can cause profound diarrhea)
- Colchicine
- Ferrous Sulfate
- Antituberculin
- Magnesium-containing antacids—Gelusil-M, Kolantyl Gel, Maalox, Mylanta, Riopan, Amphojel

Drug-induced diarrhea tends to be mild. It may begin acutely or may be chronic. Abdominal cramping and fever usually are not present. The exception is the patient on broad spectrum antibiotics who develops staphylococcal enterocolitis where fever, severe diarrhea, and crampy abdominal pain are present. This situation should be called to the physician's attention promptly.

Dynamics

The mechanism of diarrhea can be classified as osmotic, secretory, or mixed. Under normal conditions the stool content of water and electrolytes (pH, Na, and K) remain relatively constant despite dietary intake. The type of diarrhea that occurs affects the nature of electrolyte imbalance and it is especially important, with the elderly, to predict the nature of losses that are occurring and replace them.

Secretory diarrhea results from an excessive stimulation or irritation of the intestinal mucosa. As a result an excessive secretion of electrolytes occurs —especially sodium. The increased luminal Na content cannot be totally conserved by the colon and, as a result, Na is lost in the feces. Water will follow the Na and move out of the mucosa into the lumen. The result is a high risk of dehydration. The stool pH is usually neutral, approximately 7.

Secretory diarrhea results from either exogenous sources such as enteric infections or endogenous secretogogues such as deconjugated bile salts. Neoplasms may cause secretory diarrhea also. In the elderly person who has undergone gastric or intestinal resection surgery, secretory diarrhea may occur as a result of intestinal stasis with subsequent bacterial overgrowth. Decreased peristalsis of the small intestine associated with diabetic neuropathy may also lead to bacterial overgrowth and secretory diarrhea (Schedl, 1974).

Osmotic diarrhea occurs when unabsorbed intestinal solute draws water into the intestinal lumen. The presence of solute also holds water in the lumen and diarrhea occurs when the solute and water load exceeds the absorptive capacity of the colon.

Gastric surgery can precipitate osmotic diarrhea through rapid gastric emptying. The hyperosmotic chyme dumped into the duodenum draws water into the lumen. Laxatives such as lactulose and sorbitol, which are nonabsorbable, increase the solute content in the lumen, as do antacids that contain magnesium.

Osmotic diarrhea differs from secretory diarrhea in that it causes potassium loss (in excess of sodium). For patients on potassium-losing diuretics this places them at high and early risk of hypokalemia. Also, in contrast to secretory diarrhea, osmotic diarrhea causes the stool to be acidic as a result of fermentation of unabsorbed solute. Both forms of diarrhea cause water loss and dehydration.

Signs and Symptoms

The person will have stools that are more frequent and more liquid than normal. They may or may not be associated with cramping or fever, depending on the cause. Onset may be sudden or slow. Greenish or yellow-green may imply intense diarrhea with very rapid transit through the small intestine. Mucus is an indicator of an inflammatory process in the colon. Bleeding may occur, as in diverticulitis.

Data should be gathered on usual bowel and dietary patterns; onset of diarrhea; frequency and consistency of stools; associated symptoms; stress; what food was eaten; and any changes of eating, activities, or medication taking, including over-the-counter drugs.

Complications

In the elderly person with diarrhea, the complication of highest risk is electrolyte imbalance (Na^+ and K^+) and saline depletion. Symptoms of saline depletion should be noted. They include furrowed brown tongue, sunken cheeks, loss of skin turgor, orthostatic hypotension, increased hematocrit with stable hemoglobin, flat neck veins, and thirst. With electrolyte imbalance, lassitude is an important added feature.

Of particular importance is the risk of hypokalemia. It is very common but may go unrecognized because the symptoms are apathy, malaise, lassitude, cardiac arrhythmias, profound weakness, and even general paralysis. Where the individual is on diuretics, or has a history of low potassium values, the nurse needs to be alert to both the risks and the insidious presenting symptoms. It is validated by a low serum potassium level. Agate (1971) suggests that it is wise to suspect hypokalemia in any older person showing lassitude, weakness, or prostration when there is also doubt about his hydration. The hypokalemia is treatable but, when missed, is quickly fatal.

Management

The management of diarrhea depends on the cause. Discontinuation of medications causing diarrhea usually results in a return to normal within 1 to 3 days. Where there is any indication of possible impaction, a rectal examination should be done before suggesting the use of any antidiarrheal medications. Maintaining fluid intake during and following diarrhea as well as replacing lost fluids/electrolytes lost is crucial. A nonirritating diet is important until the symptoms subside.

If the diarrhea is a response to lactase deficiency, as may occur following gastric resections, the treatment is to avoid milk and milk products.

Categories of drugs used to treat diarrhea are opiates, adsorbents, astringents, electrolytes, nutrients, bulk laxatives, antipectines, digestive enzymes, intestinal flora modifiers, sedatives, tranquilizers, smooth muscle relaxants, and anticholinergic drugs (American Pharmaceutical Association Handbook, 1977, p. 30). Table 16-4 lists actions of various drugs. It is wise to remember, however, that undertreatment is better than overtreatment with drugs.

Risks of additional fluid loss because of the temperature of the environment is important in those who are dehydrated. Heat occurs daily in warm climates or during summer months. Problems can also occur in winter when rooms are kept at high temperatures and low humidity.

Because of the precarious fluid imbalance in the elderly, electrolytes should be drawn to accurately judge the status of the patient. Sodium and potassium may need to be replaced intravenously during the diarrhea. Diarrhea caused by food poisoning will run its course in several days. This may be too long for a patient to go without medical attention. Fluids and calories need to be maintained during the course of the diarrhea.

The nurse should treat diarrhea in an older patient as a potential emergency. This includes carefully monitoring the person, consulting with the

TABLE 16-4. Pharmacologic treatment of diarrhea.

Drugs	Reactions
Opiates	Decrease hyperperistaltic movement. Intestinal contents slow, allowing absorption of water and electrolytes. CNS depressants.

Adsorbents
   Aluminum hydroxide
   Activated charcoal
   Kaolin
   Bismuth subsalts
   Magnesium trisilicate
   Pectin
	Frequently found in over-the-counter drugs. Adsorption is not a specific action, can also adsorb other drugs given at the same time.

Anticholinergics Belladonna	Decrease intestinal tone. Usually requires prescription. *Do not* give to people with glaucoma. Stop if blurred vision, vertigo, rapid pulse, eye pain develop.

physician, and initiating supportive therapies to prevent complications. Return to normal bowel flora is the aim of treatment once diarrhea has stopped and can be achieved by fermented dairy products, i.e., buttermilk or yogurt.

Some people have irritable bowel syndrome, which is characterized by alternating periods of constipation and diarrhea. It is essential for management to begin with identification and elimination of foods that tend to irritate the bowel. Gas producing foods can be particularly irritating.

Constipation

Constipation is one of the most common complaints of older people and a problem nurses spend considerable time resolving. It has been estimated that 15 to 30 percent of people over 60 take one or more laxatives each week. The idea that all old people have or will have constipation as a result of "wearing out" of the gastrointestinal tract in the course of normal aging is not valid.

Description

Constipation is "the condition in which defecation occurs only at prolonged intervals" (Vander, 1975, p. 400). Feces usually are firm and dry and accumulate in the descending colon. Evacuation is difficult.

Not every one has a bowel movement everyday nor should this be expected. People establish their own bowel functioning patterns of frequency and times of day. The results of one study indicate that the range of frequency of bowel movements is from three times a day to three times a week (Connell, 1965).

Normal fecal matter consists mainly of water, bacteria, undigested cellulose, mucus, cell debris from the turnover of the intestinal epithelium, bile pigments, and small amounts of salt (Vander, 1975). Primarily it is the lower bowel that functions in storage and controlling the release of fecal material. It also has secretory and absorption functions that are of primary interest in the aged population. Mucus is secreted primarily by the goblet cells to lubricate the feces. Its volume is increased by drugs or any other condition that stimulates the parasympathetic nerves and decreased by stimulation of the sympathetic nerves. Absorption within the lower bowel is the active transport of sodium with the resultant osmotic reabsorption of water. Fecal material left in the bowel for long periods of time will reabsorb almost all the water, resulting in hard dry pellets of fecal material or constipation. The elderly person is at risk primarily owing to atrophy of mucous glands and a decrease in the elasticity of the collagenous tissue of the bowel (Williams and Dickey, 1969, p. 885).

Etiologic Factors

Contrary to common opinion, constipation in the elderly is not related to the wearing out of the gastrointestinal system, although Palmer coined a phrase "presbycolon" which would indicate age-related changes (Palmer, 1976).

In the elderly the term *presbycolon* has been used to mean constipation and complications of colon gas and impaction. It includes three forms of constipation—hypertonic, hypotonic, and "habit" constipation. All are found in the elderly.

Hypotonic constipation shows soft puttylike stool in the rectum on digital examination. The colon is full of feces and impactions are common in this form of constipation (Palmer, 1976). This type of hypotonic constipation is due to the lack of motility, both the segmental contraction and those that accomplish mass movement. The aim of treatment in this type of constipation is to stimulate motility.

Constipation caused by hypertonicity of the bowel is characterized by hard, dry stools and, in some cases, lower abdominal pain (Williams and Dickey, 1969). The phenomenon is a result of an increase in activity of the segmental-type muscle contractions, which mix bowel contents, but not of the propulsive-type bowel contracts, resulting in decreased transit time and increased reabsorption of water.

Habit constipation is due primarily to eating habits that include a diet devoid of bulk (cellulose) or conscious/or unconsciously ignoring or preventing the urge to defecate.

General factors that contribute to constipation include:

- Neglecting to respond to defecation urge. Irregular bowel habits developed after a long period of time inhibit normal reflexes—if defecation does not occur when these reflexes are excited they become progressively weaker.
- Diet—inadequate bulk and fluids. Excessive ingestion of foods that harden stools, e.g., processed cheese.
- Chronic enema or laxative patterns.
- Environmental changes: Changes in daily biologic patterns—eating, sleeping, time of bowel and bladder evacuation, lack of privacy for bowel movements.
- Atony or hypertonicity of colon, hypertonicity of ileocecal valve.
- Mental stress, depression, feelings of inadequacy or insecurity (Sklar, 1972), short attention span in impaired elderly.
- Drugs: aspirin, anticholinergic drugs, aluminum hydroxide or calcium carbonate antacids, opiates, e.g., Codeine, Morphine, mineral oil, tranquilizers.
- Loss of abdominal muscle tone.

Constipation also can occur with pathology. The possibility of underlying local pathology always exists. Change in bowel movements and bleeding are symptoms of malignancy. In addition, central nervous system pathology such as organic brain diseases, particularly those with frontal lobe deterioration and perceptual motor disturbances, involving body image will also contribute to constipation.

High Risk Populations and Situations

Individuals on bedrest who take medications that are known to cause constipation (anticholinergics, opiates, barbiturates), who reduce fluids or bulk in their diet, who develop central nervous system disease or local lesions causing pain, or who become depressed—all are at risk of developing constipation.

Dynamics

Any factors that increase the dehydration of the stool, slow the transit time, or interfere with the usual pattern of reflexes will contribute to delayed defecation, production of drier stools, and subsequent difficulty in evacuation.

The presence of fecal material in the rectum alone is not sufficient to initiate the defecation reflex. It must be an amount large enough to exceed the individual threshold of the stimulus. Defecation is a special reflex initiated by mass movement of fecal material into the rectum. The defecation reflex is mediated by the internal nerve plexus. It can be inhibited voluntarily by contraction of the external anal sphincter. Defecation occurs by relaxation of the internal and external anal sphincter, increased peristaltic activity of the sigmoid colon, and contraction of the abdominal muscles. This causes an increase in intraabdominal pressure which is transmitted to the contents of the large intestine and assists in the elimination of feces. Distention of the stomach by food, particularly the first meal of the day initiates contractions of the rectum and frequently a desire to defecate (gastrocolic reflex).

The prolonged use of laxatives can produce anatomic changes in the colon. Removal of the colon was indicated in a study of twelve chronic users of laxatives of 30 to 40-years duration (American Pharmaceutical Association Handbook, 1977, p. 38). It was found that there was loss of intrinsic innervation, atrophy of smooth muscle coats, and pigmentation of the colon. The prolonged stimulation of the neurons by the irritant laxatives results in death of the cell.

Signs and Symptoms

The most frequent indication of constipation is the complaint of the person and the attendant concern. The nurse needs data on what the person considers to be normal bowel movement in terms of frequency and consistency, what the usual patterns of defecation are, and any changes in activity, diet, medication, mood, or pain. The stool should also be observed for size, consistency, and blood. Unless the nurse regularly checks on bowel movements in some way, she will be unaware of constipation until symptoms of fecal impaction occur. There is a need to check in a way that does not focus on bowel movements as the expected daily behavior since this leads people into thinking that they are constipated when they may not be.

Assessment areas include decreased appetite, increased restlessness, frequently noted trips to bathroom, complaints of nausea, increased irritability, headache, abdominal cramping, increasingly active gas pattern, abdominal palpation, absence of bowel movement for a longer time period than the individual's usual pattern, abdominal distention, and urinary incontinence.

Differential Diagnosis

It is important for the nurse to differentiate between the types of constipation—hypotonic, hypertonic, and habit. The treatment for each of these types differs. The wrong form of management will precipitate side effects and produce confounding symptoms that will obscure the original problem. Nurses will, in effect, then be treating a condition they produced rather than the primary problem. An elderly person is likely to have several other attendant problems and cannot afford the physiologic/psychic stress in terms of energy expenditure on an iatrogenic condition.

Complications

Aside from the discomfort and accompanying anxiety the individual experiences with constipation, a major complication is fecal impaction following prolonged accumulation of feces. The complications of constipation more frequently are the effect of the treatment rather than the original constipation.

Management

Treatment of constipation should not be taken lightly by nurses. It is a serious problem and older persons themselves take it seriously. As indicated in differential diagnosis, it is important to take a careful history to find out not only the nature of the problem but also what the individual usually does to relieve the problem. Their own strategies may be very simple and something they can tolerate. If what they use has potential dangers, this becomes an opportunity to introduce change, though the likelihood of change being accepted often is small. Successful therapy often involves trial and error.

Palmer (1976) warns that nurses who care primarily for geriatric patients err when their goal for the elderly is a return to normal by overcoming long-standing bad habits through educational programs. He believes that their efforts should be directed toward relieving the constipation by any available tried means.

Anyone who is constipated wants relief as soon as possible. The first things that are considered usually are laxatives, enemas, and suppositories. The ideal laxative is not yet available. It would be one that was nonirritating, nontoxic, acted within a few hours, produced normal stool, and then allowed the bowel to return to normal activity. Currently available laxatives are classified by their action and include bulk formation, emollient, lubrication, stimulant, saline, and hyperosmotic (Table 16-5).

The nurse must know the dosage of the laxative. One tablet for a young person may be too large a dose for an older person. Try different dosage levels for individuals. In the elderly, a nurse cannot just give a laxative and not monitor the effects of this drug or any other.

In selecting or recommending a laxative to older persons it is important to know the type of constipation they have. For example, it would be foolish to recommend a stool softener to an individual who already has soft stools. Nurses need to be familiar, not only with the patient, but with the mechanical and pharmacologic actions of the drugs in terms of both the therapeutic potential and the harm they can cause. Beyond this, nurses need to be aware of their attitudes toward the use of laxatives and enemas and the way it influences their observation and decision making in managing constipation. When this is resolved and any biases detected, it can be easier for both the patient and the nurse.

Enemas are given to clean the bowel for a number of reasons, including constipation relief. The enema, properly done, is the nearest substitute for the ideal laxative. Improperly administered an enema can produce electrolyte and fluid imbalance, hemorrhage, and spasm as well as local trauma if the nozzle is inadequately lubricated or improperly directed.

As with laxatives, the content of the enema pro-

TABLE 16-5. Laxatives.

Mechanism of Action/Examples	Action and Uses

Stimulants
    Castor Oil
    Senokot
    Nature's Remedy
    Carter's Little Liver Pills
    Cascara Sagrada
    Dulcolax (bisacodyl)
    Feen-A-Mint
    Dorbane (danthron)
	Peristaltic action increased by local irritation to the intestine or by selective action on nerve complex of intestine smooth muscle. Used prior to bowel surgery or x-ray examination. Limited to short term use (1 week).

Bulk Forming
    Metamucil
    Serutan
	Increases peristalsis by increasing bulk. Take 12 hours to 3 days to be effective. Should not be used with patients who have intestinal adhesions, stenosis, or difficulty swallowing because of danger of impaction or intestinal obstruction. These drugs interact with salicylates and digitalis and other drugs. Take each dose with full glass of water.

Emollient/Lubricant
    Colace
    Doxinate
    Mineral Oil* (use the emulsion)
    Emulsified mineral oil**
        Agoral
        Petrogalar
	Emollient—Useful with people who should not strain to defecate. Increases the wetting efficiency of intestinal water and forms oil and water emulsions. Prevents development of constipation, does not improve existing constipation. Used in fecal impactions.
	Lubricant—Soften fecal contents by coating. Useful in keeping stool soft to avoid straining. Long use of mineral oil can produce toxicity and side effects. Affects absorption of calcium, phosphates, vitamins A and D. Do not take with meals as they delay gastric emptying.

Saline Laxatives
    Magnesium Sulfate
    Fleets (sodium biphosphate,
        sodium phosphate)
    Phospho-Soda
    Sal Hapatica
Other
    Milk of Magnesium (magnesium
        hydroxide and peppermint oil)
    Haley's Mineral Oil (magnesium
        hydroxide and mineral oil)
	Intestinal wall acts as semipermeable membrane to magnesium, sulfate, tartrate, phosphate, and citrate ions. Water is retained in the intestine causing pressure which increases intestinal motility. In poor renal function, magnesium is retained which can depress CNS. Sodium can be toxic. Dehydration can occur with hypertonic solutions of saline cathartics.

* Do not take mineral oil with other medication or with meals. Take one hour prior to bedtime to avoid reflux aspiration.

** Use of emulsion (Agoral or Petrogalar) is preferred with the elderly.

duces the action. Soapsuds act by irritating the colon; oils lubricate and soften feces. Water, saline, and milk add bulk by osmotic effect.

The enema should be administered with the person lying on the side—preferably the left side. If the person sits on the toilet, only the rectum is cleaned of feces. Fluid should not be administered with force. Frequently 250 cc of solution is all that is necessary to empty the lower bowel.

Water is absorbed through the large bowel; therefore, accuracy of total fluid intake and output is important, particularly when more than one enema is necessary. When more than two enemas are given

with return that is much less than liquid given, accurate measurement should be made to determine the actual discrepancy. When multiple enemas are given, an isotonic saline solution should be used to avoid electrolyte imbalance.

Suppositories are useful in some instances. The two most commonly utilized suppositories are glycerine and Dulcolax. Glycerine suppositories are used with persons who require lubrication and digital stimulation as a means of eliminating stool. Dulcolax suppositories are used in persons who require added neural stimulation to the intestinal wall. Be aware that Dulcolax produces cramping and can cause problems to a debilitated person. (A mild oral agent such as danthron, ½ tablet, or Milk of Magnesia is preferable.) Suppositories are effective only if they are inserted correctly. They must be inserted above the internal sphincter.

Diet, fluids, and exercise are considerations that, hopefully, decrease constipation. Fiber in foods holds water and helps the stool to pass more rapidly. Exercise, particularly isometric type, may improve sphincter and abdominal muscle tone and improve the efficiency with which the abdominal muscles assist in propulsion of stool out of the rectum.

Many people eat and drink things that help them maintain bowel regularity. These include drinking prune juice or a glass of hot water with or without lemon juice upon arising, or eating raw or cooked prunes. Some older people know that certain foods are constipating to them—milk, bananas, chocolate, angel food cake. This probably is not the cause of their problem, but their beliefs should be respected unless the food is essential to their well-being.

Medications should always be considered as a potential cause of constipation. Knowledge of drugs is essential. Each nurse who cares for older persons should have a list available of medications that have constipation as a side effect. In clinics, offices, or institutions it could be posted in a convenient area.

Prevention

The key note to preventive management of constipation in the elderly revolves around consistency, adequate hydration, proper diet, and exercise. It is important to establish an individual's usual consistent pattern of bowel evacuation. Maintaining this consistency is as important a nursing measure as the administration of a medication. This primarily means providing for the time, privacy, and opportunity at the individual's convenience on a consistent basis. Adequate fluid intake is considered in the realm of 2000 to 3000 cc of daily minimum of fluids such as water, juice, milk, Jello, ice cream, and soft drinks. Coffee, tea, grapefruit juice, or other diuretic beverages should *not* be given as they will eliminate total body fluid as opposed to adding body fluid. Fluid balance in the elderly person is a critical factor; there is very little margin between too much and too little before the person is symptomatic. Most elderly persons, particularly those in an institutional setting, are more likely to be underhydrated. The major area of water reabsorption other than the kidneys is the large bowel. The reabsorp-

tion of fluid from the large bowel will leave hard dry fecal matter.

Dietary considerations revolve primarily around a well-balanced diet. The elderly population at risk in this area are those living in the community where the much talked about "tea and toast" phenomena is most likely to be present. Many elderly people live on rigid, small allowances, and they find one area to save money is on the food budget. Expensive items such as raw vegetables and fresh fruit are eliminated and substituted with cheaper easy-to-prepare items, thus effectively eliminating high residue foods from the diet.

Exercise in whatever form is important for total body functioning. Abdominal exercises such as sit-ups are as viable and exercise for the elderly population as in any age group.

Evaluation

A bowel pattern can be established through a bowel program. Criteria for improvement, however, includes not only improvement in bowel patterns but also participation of the older person in improving his fluid, diet, and exercise patterns. Self-satisfaction with his efforts is important.

Impaction

A fecal impaction is a hard, compacted mass of fecal material in the rectum that the individual cannot expel.

Etiologic Factors

Impaction usually presents when the person has constipation.

High Risk

Individuals with hypotonic constipation, particularly those who are debilitated, immobilized, or have central nervous system lesions are at high risk.

Signs and Symptoms

The individual will report or will be known not to have had a normal bowel movement for several days; however, he may have some leakage of liquid stool and fecal incontinence. Rectal examination and a finding of hard stool in the rectum validates the diagnosis.

Management

The treatment of a fecal impaction involves manually removing the stool with or without prior oil enemas to soften it.

1. Explain the procedure. Insure privacy.
2. Position the person on the side (left side) and drape.
3. Ask him to breathe deeply, slowly, and quietly through the mouth during the procedure.
4. Lubricate the gloved finger with water-soluble gel.
5. Gently break up the impaction, being careful not to traumatize the wall of the rectum. Stop if the person complains of excessive pain.
6. Remove whatever fecal material can be freed from the mass.
7. Do not manipulate the impaction beyond the fatigue tolerance of the person. Allow a rest period following and during removal.
8. Administer a warm oil-retention enema. Allow expulsion of oil and feces.
9. Follow with a cleansing soapsuds enema (do not administer more than two enemas in any 8-hour period).

For three days after the removal of the fecal impaction it would be appropriate to give a combination of stool softener and bowel stimulant. (See Table 16-5 for names of appropriate laxatives.)

Once the initial impaction has been eliminated an assessment of why the individual developed an impaction is imperative. Then a program of preventive management needs to be undertaken to avoid or minimize future recurrences.

Fecal Incontinence

Stool incontinence occurs in a small percentage of noninstitutionalized elderly persons. Brocklehurst identified 10 percent of the elderly patients in four general hospitals were incontinent and in a geriatric hospital the incidence rose to 20 percent. One third of the incontinent patients were found to have evidence of organic neurologic changes and another third were mentally confused (Geokas and Haverback, 1969).

Fecal incontinence can occur among those who are aware of it and embarrassed by it as well as among those who are not conscious of it because of confusion, disturbed consciousness, or brain damage. Inability to control audible release of flatus is probably even more common and can cause some individuals to alter their lifestyle.

Fecal incontinence can occur as a result of organic changes in neural innervation of the rectum, including decreased sensation of rectal filling, increased excitability of the rectal external sphincter, decreased anal muscle tone, or loss of cortical control (Geokas and Haverback, 1969). Local causes include inflammation, cancer of the rectum, prolapsed anus, and the semifluid quality of the stool. Some individuals are so debilitated as to be unable to control the sphincter against the defecation reflex. By far the most common cause of fecal incontinence is gross constipation with impaction in the anal canal and subsequent overflow (Agate, 1971).

Management of constipation and elimination of mental confusion where it exists can be an important way of managing fecal incontinence. A rectal examination to determine the presence of impactions is important. Enemas may be needed for several days to give the person a fresh start. Where control is not possible, suppositories or Fleets enemas to time the defecation and reduce risk of accidents may be useful. The use of absorbent pads and waterproof panties may also be reassuring and allow more mobility for women. These should be used following discussion, explanation, and acceptance by the person involved. Careful consideration and attention to the integrity of the skin should be of paramount importance when utilizing protective devices to avoid skin excoriation.

SUMMARY

The gastrointestinal status of the elderly person is based on long-standing eating and elimination patterns. Thus, the nursing care focus must be oriented to helping the individual manage chronic conditions with the objective of maintaining the functional integrity of the system.

Nurses will find themselves working with persons who have gastrointestinal problems that are not curable in the usual sense of the word. Treatment may be effective for a time but often the problem reoccurs.

The central issue is, then, as it is in any other care or service for the elderly, to balance the risk of the treatment with the gain factor. The goal being the establishment and maintenance of the individual at a functional level. In some cases this may involve taking some attendant risks and producing some side effects—that may be tolerable, if the gain factor is great enough. Nurses must, *in advance*, consider the potential risks and gains inherent in any form of management or in decisions not to treat a condition.

Inherent in chronic conditions in the elderly is the possibility of the nurse's becoming insensitive to the problems as they continue to occur or fail to respond to treatment. It is of prime importance that the assessment, treatment, and evaluation be as aggressive and thorough the tenth time the condition occurs as it was the first. The concept of "fresh eyes" in viewing the patient and the data presented is crucial.

BIBLIOGRAPHY

Agate, J.: Common symptoms and complaints. In Rossman, I. (ed.): Clinical Geriatrics. Philadelphia: J. B. Lippincott Co., 1971, pp. 461–471.

Alikhan, T., et al.: Effects of aging on the motor function of the esophagus and lower esophageal sphincter. In van Trappen, G. (ed.): Volume Proceeding of the Fifth International Symposium on Gastro-Intestinal Motility, Leuven, Belgium, September 3–6, 1975. Typoff Press, Ekelstraat, Belgium.

Ambre, J. J., and Fisher, L. J.: Effects of coadministration of aluminum and magnesium hydroxides on absorption of anticoagulants in man. Clin. Pharmacol. Therapeut. 14:231–237, 1973.

American Pharmaceutical Association: Handbook of Non Prescription Drugs, ed. 5. Washington D.C.: American Pharmaceutical Association, 1977.

Babka, J. C., and Castell, D. O.: On the geneses of heartburn: the effect of specific foods on the lower esophageal sphincter. Amer. J. Digestive Dis. 18:391–397, 1973.

Berman, P. and Kirsner, J.: Diverticular disease of the colon in the elderly. Geriatrics, 27:70–75, 1972.

Castell, D. O., and Harris, L. D.: Hormonal control of gastroesophageal sphincter strength. New Engl. J. Med. 282:886–889, 1970.

Christensen, J.: The controls of gastrointestinal movements; some old and new views. New Engl. J. Med. 285:85–98, 1971.

Connell, A. M. C., et al.: Variation of bowel habit in two population samples. Brit. Med. J. 2:1095–1099, 1965.

Dunkerly, R. G., et al.: Gastrointestinal disorders: the role of diet in cause and management. Postgrad. Med. 59:182–187, 1976.

Geokas, M., and Haverback, B.: The aging gastrointestinal tract. Am. J. Surg. 117:881–892, 1969.

Hanan, Z. I.: Geriatric medications—how the aged are hurt by drugs meant to help. RN 41:57–59, 1978.

Levral, M., et al.: Peptic ulcer in patients over 60—experience in 287 cases. Am. J. Digestive Dis. 11:279–285, 1966.

Modell, W.: Drugs of Choice. St. Louis: C. V. Mosby Co., 1976.

Palmer, E. D.: "Presbycolon" problems in the nursing home. J.A.M.A. 235:1150–1151, 1976.

Piper, D. W., and Heap, T. R.: Medical management of peptic ulcer with antacid ulcer agents in other gastro-intestinal diseases. Drugs 3:366–403, 1972.

Robinson, D., Benjamin, D., and McCormack, J.: Interaction of warfarin and nonsystemic gastrointestinal drugs. Clin. Pharmacol. Therapeut. 12:491–495, 1971.

Rodman, M. J., and Smith, D. W.: Clinical Pharmacology in Nursing, Philadelphia: J. B. Lippincott Co., 1974.

Schade, S. G., Cohen, R. J., and Conrad, M. E.: Effect of hydrochloric acid on iron absorption. New Engl. J. Med. 279:672–674, 1968.

Sklar, M.: Functional bowel distress and constipation in the aged. Geriatrics 27:79–85, 1972.

Sklar, M.: Gastrointestinal diseases in the aged. In Working with Older People, Vol. IV. U.S. Government Printing, Washington D.C., 1974, pp. 124–130.

Smith, C. W., and Evans, P.: Bowel motility. Geriatrics, 16:189, 1961.

Sodeman, W. A., Jr., and Sodeman, W.: Pathologic Physiology: Mechanisms of Disease, ed. 5. Philadelphia: W. B. Saunders Co., 1974.

Soergel, K. H., et al.: Presbyesophagus: Cineradiographic manifestations. Radiology 82:463–467, 1964.

Vander, A., Sherman, J., and Luciano, D.: Human Physiology, ed. 2. New York: McGraw-Hill Book Co., 1975.

Williams, R., and Dickey, J.: Physiology of colon and rectum. Am. J. Surg. 117:849–853, 1969.

Winsberg, F.: Roentgenographic aspects of aging. In Rossman, I. (ed.): Clin. Geriatr. Philadelphia: J. B. Lippincott Co., 1971, pp. 267–281.

17

Genitourinary Problems

Janet Specht and Ann Cordes

QUICK REVIEW

PROSTATIC OBSTRUCTION

DESCRIPTION

Enlargement of the prostatic gland secondary to hyperplasia (benign prostatic hypertrophy) or adenocarcinoma.

ETIOLOGIC
FACTORS

Both benign prostatic hypertrophy (BPH) and adenocarcinoma seem to be related to involutional hormonal changes.

HIGH RISK

White males over 50 have 30 percent chance of BPH with a 30 percent chance of urinary obstruction by 80 years. Adenocarcinoma of prostate is third most common male malignancy. Risk increases with age. 95 percent of histologically-examined prostate of males over 80 years showed malignant cells.

DYNAMICS

Hyperplasia of periurethral glands or tumor growth in this area narrows the urethra, producing some degree of urinary obstruction.

SIGNS AND
SYMPTOMS

If hyperplasia or tumor growth is posterior the condition is asymptomatic in early stages.

Obstructive BPH: Urinary frequency, nocturia, reduced size and force of stream, hesitancy and interruption of voiding, dribbling incontinence, hematuria, retention with overflow.

Carcinoma: Obstruction as above, hematuria, hematospermia, anemia, elevated serum acid and alkaline phosphatases, perineal pain. Hard nodular gland.

DIFFERENTIAL
DIAGNOSIS

BPH, prostatic cancer, neurogenic bladder, strictures, prostatitis. Drugs that may predispose marginally obstructive prostatism to obstruct: atropine-like drugs, tranquilizers, antihistamines, diuretics, bronchodilators.

COMPLICATIONS

Uremia and infection secondary to obstruction. Cancer—metastasis.

PROGNOSIS

BPH: Surgical resection relieves obstruction and mortality rate low.

Cancer: 27 percent 5-year survival rate even when early and late cancers are combined (see also Chapter 12, Cancer).

MEDICAL
MANAGEMENT

BPH: Conservative in absence of obstructive symptoms. Surgery: transurethral, perineal, suprapubic, retropubic. Hormones may be used with persons who cannot tolerate surgery. Long term catheters may be needed.

Cancer: Surgery if resectable (10 percent of cases), radiation if confined to pelvis, or orchiectomy; hormone therapy.

Continued on next page.

QUICK REVIEW (cont.)

NURSING
MANAGEMENT

Be alert to symptoms of urinary obstruction and recognize the emergency nature of acute retention. Monitor intake and output—maintain 2500 cc intake unless contraindicated by other conditions. Monitor medications that increase risk of obstruction. See Chapter 12 for management of cancer. Yearly prostatic examination after age 50.

EVALUATION

Episodes of acute retention are minimized (prevention). Urinary tract infection minimized. Fluid intake is adequate. Awareness of medications increasing risk of urinary obstruction.

QUICK REVIEW

URINARY TRACT INFECTION (UTI)

DESCRIPTION	Contamination of urine caused by invasion of urinary tract by pathogens with subsequent colonization and resulting infection.
ETIOLOGIC FACTORS	Organisms (66 percent are gram-negative rods) entering urinary tract from the contaminated urethral meatus or prostate gland, facilitated in colonization by stagnation in urinary flow, low fluid intake, stasis.
HIGH RISK	Aging, males, *institutionalization,* diabetes, renal failure, hypertension, low fluid intake, *catheterization,* prostatic disease, extended bedrest.
DYNAMICS	Reduced urinary flow decreases the effective washing out of bacteria in the urethra. Stasis dilutes the acidic pH of the urine, making colonization easier.
SIGNS AND SYMPTOMS	Nonspecific fever, vomiting or illness without apparent reason. Frequency, urgency, dysuria, nocturia, turbid urine, lower abdominal discomfort, hematuria. It may also be asymptomatic in the elderly.
DIFFERENTIAL DIAGNOSIS	*Quantitative* urine culture (from immediately refrigerated specimens) 10^5 to 10^9 bacteria per ml findings in two consecutive collections. Isolation of single species of bacteria (multiple species suggests contamination). May also use dipslide if culture facilities not available.
COMPLICATIONS	Urinary infections complicated by other pathology (e.g., obstruction of prostate, cystocele) will not respond to antimicrobial treatment until underlying abnormality is treated.
PROGNOSIS	Untreated bacteriuria can lead to bacteremia (30 to 35 percent fatal) or renal failure, dependent on status of host, despite antimicrobial treatment.
MEDICAL MANAGEMENT	Oral suppressant is used for recurrent infections or those with complicating factors. Antimicrobial drugs. Fluid intake 2500 to 3000 cc daily.
NURSING MANAGEMENT	Be alert to insidious signs and symptoms of lower urinary tract infections, particularly in high risk elderly. Do a dipslide test—order urinalysis performed. Record I & O (0 should be ± 1500 with I of 2500 to 3000). Assure fluid intake 2500 to 3000 cc, using person's usual fluid intake pattern and preferences as basis. Maintain acid ash diet during suppressant drugs (check urine pH). Request Gram stain and culture when infection persists. Monitor signs and symptoms of posturinary tract infection patients carefully for recurrence using a preset timetable and flowsheet for recording.
PREVENTION	Avoid catheterization except as last resort. Assist sexually-active females in achieving greatest protection from urinary tract infection. Maintain mobility. Teach correct perineal hygiene. Use gravitational assistance to empty bladder when needed. Avoid soiled underwear, diapering, and lying in a wet bed. Culture urinals and bed pans.
EVALUATION	Urine remains relatively free of organisms. No signs and symptoms of urinary tract infection. Patient, family, and staff understand and use preventive measures in ADL and lifestyle.

QUICK REVIEW

ATROPHIC VAGINITIS

DESCRIPTION
Atrophy of vagina secondary to epithelial lack of estrogen with resulting vulnerability to trauma and secondary infection.

ETIOLOGIC FACTORS
Decrease in ovarian function and production of natural estrogen.

HIGH RISK
Postmenopausal females not receiving estrogen replacement.

DYNAMICS
With decreased estrogen in the system, the vaginal epithelium thins, superficial cells are fewer, and secondary glycogen production is reduced. Enzymatic catabolism decreases, and the acidogenic balance is lost, leading to rising pH (6–7) and loss of protection from bacterial/fungal/yeast colonization.

SIGNS AND SYMPTOMS
Vaginal/vulvar soreness—shiny, pale, pasty mucous membranes. Dyspareunia, thin scant discharge. Superficial ulceration, blood-tinged discharge, vaginal pH of 6–7.

DIFFERENTIAL DIAGNOSIS
Pap smear to rule out malignancy, culture to rule out bacterial infection. Observe for foreign objects.

pH 3.5–4.1 normal flora
4.0–5.0 Candida
5.0–7.0 Trichomonas

COMPLICATIONS
Secondary infections. Disruption of sexual activity patterns. Broad spectrum antibiotics increase risk of Candida.

PROGNOSIS
Since it is an age-related change, the condition will persist and present the attendant risks and vulnerability.

MEDICAL MANAGEMENT
Varies. Includes locally applied estrogen and systemic estrogen. Mild disinfectant, e.g., Betadine. Douching is controversial.

NURSING MANAGEMENT
Assess usual patterns of perineal hygiene to determine risks of autoinfection. Teach or help female to do perineal hygiene correctly, to maintain a clean, dry perineum, and to avoid autoinfection. Obese persons have high risk of maceration and fissures. Use of fan/hair dryer may help. Recommend cotton panties. Dresses and girdles are less risky than slacks and panty girdles or pantyhose. Alert them to laundry methods and use of hot water in preventing autoinfection. *If* douching cannot be stopped because of previous lifestyle, help person do it with least damage (use mildly acid solution, clean tip, careful insertion, low pressure). Potassium sorbate, postcoitus, may decrease risk of Candida. Avoid over-the-counter powders and sprays. Use K-Y jelly to minimize discomfort and trauma in intercourse. Encourage patient to discuss dyspareunia with physician and seek help to overcome it.

EVALUATION
Indications that the older woman understands age-related changes and the need for new carefulness in perineal hygiene. Incorporation of correct perineal cleansing/hygiene in ADL. Understands signs and symptoms to be reported and need for annual pap smear and pelvic examination. Maintains desired level of sexual activity.

Older persons are at high risk for several problems in their genitourinary systems. Both males and females have higher risk of neoplastic disease in their reproductive organs—benign and malignant. Infection continues to be a threat in the genitourinary tracts. In addition, atrophy and loss of strength in supporting structures cause problems.

As with many other health conditions to which the aged are subject, these problems often are chronic. They make an impact on daily living and lifestyle, often for years. Therefore, they are areas for nursing assessment and management as a part of their total health care.

PROSTATIC DISEASES

Benign Prostatic Hypertrophy

Etiologic Factors

The cause of benign prostatic hypertrophy (BPH) is not known but it does tend to appear with involutional, hormonal changes. Race is a factor. Western white males show the highest incidence, while black males are rarely affected (Sturdy, 1974, pp. 19 and 178; Basso, 1974, p. 352).

High Risk Populations

White males over 50 have about a 30 percent risk of benign prostatic hypertrophy. Among those who reach the age of 80, 30 percent will have impaired renal flow from prostatic enlargement (Moore-Smith, 1973, pp. 19 and 687).

Dynamics

Hyperplasia of the periurethral glands leads to prostatic enlargement. Since the gland surrounds the urethra, growth in that area may lead to the symptoms of urinary tract obstruction. If the growth is predominantly in the posterior region, the condition may produce no symptoms.

Acknowledgment is made to Robert P. Gibbons, M.D., Urologist, The Mason Clinic, Seattle, Washington, for his contribution in reviewing this chapter.

Signs and Symptoms

While benign prostatic hypertrophy cannot be prevented, early recognition is important to successful management. There are three general categories of symptoms secondary to benign prostatic hypertrophy (Culp, 1975, pp. 19, 31–32).

SILENT PROSTATISM. The man is asymptomatic in silent prostatism. The enlarged prostate is discovered only on a rectal examination, where the findings are a firm, smooth, symmetric, and slightly-elastic enlargement of the gland beyond its usual 2.5 cm. heart-shaped size. It may bulge more than the normal 1.0 cm. into the rectal lumen. The median sulcus, normally felt between the two lateral lobes, is obliterated by the hypertrophy (Bates, 1974, p. 212).

OBSTRUCTIVE PROSTATISM. In obstructive prostatism, hyperplasia has narrowed the space for the urethra and the local symptoms are associated with restricted urinary flow. The symptoms are those of changed voiding patterns: frequency, reduced size and force of urinary stream, dribbling incontinence, hesitancy and interruption of the stream during voiding, nocturia. Hematuria may also occur.

OBSTRUCTION WITH DISTANT SYMPTOMS. In late states of obstruction the person suffers from urinary stasis and retention with associated infection, back pressure, changed renal function, and uremic conditions. The "sleepy grandfather" may be suffering from unrecognized uremia (Ehrlich, 1976, p. 528). The symptoms include poor appetite, nausea and vomiting, weight loss, apathy, and stupor. Bleeding is more common with benign than with malignant enlargement (Anderson, 1971, p. 202).

Differential Diagnosis

Diagnosis is based on palpable enlargement of the prostate and positive cystoscopy and radiographic findings. Laboratory data do not confirm hyperplasia but are useful for evaluating the effect of the hyperplasia on the urinary system (Culp, 1975, p. 33).

Benign prostatic hypertrophy has some signs and symptoms in common with neurogenic bladder, strictures, inflammatory disease, and prostatic malignancies. If the nurse is involved in a situation where he or she sees the patient more frequently than the physician and, therefore, is having a significant role in case finding, it will be important to take a careful history as a basis for consulting with the physician and/or making a referral.

One other area of differential diagnosis is associated with drug therapy. The male with only marginally obstructive prostatic desease can be thrown into retention with the administration of atropine-like drugs, tranquilizers, antihistamines, diuretics, or bronchodilators. The nurse who knows a patient has BPH should alert the prescribing physician to the situation if drugs of this nature are prescribed. Where a patient is seen who is on these drugs and exhibiting retention symptoms, the drugs should be stopped if possible and voiding and residual urine evaluated (Ehrlich, 1976, pp. 19 and 528).

Complications

There are certain complications associated with the disease itself and others associated with the treatment. The hyperplasia that causes obstruction leads to complications of stasis and retention with attendant risks of infection. Infection may be acute and/or chronic, requiring continuous antimicrobial therapy. Complete obstruction is a possibility.

A common complication of surgery for benign prostatic hypertrophy is retrograde ejaculation, wherein semen is ejected into the bladder instead of flowing out through the urethra. Patients report it as more surprising than painful. Retrograde ejaculation does not interfere with attaining erection or orgasm unless the patient becomes so psychologically disturbed that it upsets the other delicate mechanisms involved. The man's chances for contributing viable sperm to the ova are significantly affected.

Sterility is inevitable if vasectomy is performed with prostatic surgery. Vasectomy is often done with prostatic surgery to reduce the risk of epididymitis after surgery. Excessive bleeding and incontinence may also occur postsurgically with some patients (Ehrlich, 1976, pp. 529–530).

Impotence should not result from prostatic surgery. It is suspected that previous sexual maladjustment was present when this does occur. There should be good information provided before surgery to reduce the chance of this unfortunate circumstance. It is important that clinicians ask about this problem postsurgically and provide counseling when impotence does occur. There are mental health clinicians working specifically with sexual dysfunction that can be utilized if the patient wants this help.

Prognosis

Surgical resection should relieve the symptoms of obstruction. The mortality rate from this surgery is low (Krupp, 1975, p. 547; Culp, 1975, p. 48).

Medical Management

Treatment usually is conservative in the absence of progressive obstructive symptoms. Conservative management includes ascertaining that renal output is adequate and treating secondary symptoms such as infection.

Surgical removal of a portion or all of the gland is indicated with clear symptoms of progressive obstruction, retention, hematuria or recurrent infection. Surgery may be open prostatectomy utilizing a perineal, suprapubic, or retropubic approach. Transurethral surgery is also widely used because open excision is not necessary and postoperative recovery generally is quicker. The choice of surgical technique depends on factors like the age and health of the patient, the size and location of the gland, and the training and skill of the physician (Ehrlich, 1976, pp. 529–530; Culp, 1975, pp. 43–47).

Hormonal therapy has been used in selected instances with individuals considered to be poor surgical risks. Hormonal treatment is primarily investigative at this time (Culp, 1975, pp. 19 and 47–48; Moore-Smith, 1973, pp. 19 and 687). Occasionally, long term catherer use is necessary when surgery is contraindicated (Ehrlich, 1976, p. 528).

Nursing Management

The primary nursing measure with *benign hypertrophy* is to prevent or at least relieve retention. These patients should be counselled about good voiding habits and a regular fluid intake. They should be taught general measures like voiding when the need is first apparent, keeping underwear clean, and avoiding contamination of the urethra with feces. They should understand the role of fluids in keeping the urine free from bacteria and should ascertain that daily intake is adequate (2500 to 3000 ml per 24 hr). They should understand the progressive nature of their disease so that they too may be alert to symptoms of obstruction. Patients with chronic infection related to obstructive disease may be candidates for suppressive therapy (as described on p. 346). An individual patient's medications should be reviewed to determine whether medications that may potentiate the obstructive problem are being given.

Carcinoma of the Prostate

Etiologic Factors

The exact etiologic factor is not known but there is an association with hormonal factors. The tumor growth is enhanced by androgens and inhibited by estrogens (Sturdy, 1974, p. 189; Krupp, 1975, p. 547).

High Risk Populations

Cancer of the prostate is rare before age 50 but the incidence of this tumor in later years is very high. It is said to be present in 95 percent of the prostates of 80-year-old men examined histologically (Moore-Smith, 1973, p. 687) and it ranks as the third most common male malignancy (Sturdy, 1974, p. 188).

Signs and Symptoms

The clinical picture of prostatic carcinoma may be asymptomatic, even with widespread metastasis or there may be symptoms of obstruction. Symptoms associated with advanced cancer and metastasis include hematuria, hematospermia, back and leg pain (the spine and pelvis are sites of frequent metastasis), anemia (may be extreme as bone marrow is replaced by tumor), elevated serum acid phosphatase, elevated serum alkaline phosphatase, and perineal pain (Krupp, 1975, p. 547; Moore-Smith, 1973, p. 687).

Differential Diagnosis

Rectal examination is essential for detecting prostatic carcinoma. It should be done at least yearly for all men over 45. The cancerous gland is stone-hard, nodular, and fixed. Finding a gland of this description is presumptive diagnosis of prostatic carcinoma (Jaffe, 1971, p. 145; Krupp, 1975, p. 547). Positive diagnosis is assured by cytologic examination of the prostatic fluid and radiologic examination of the urinary tract and skeleton, tumor biopsy, bone marrow biopsy, and laboratory studies (Sturdy, 1976, 191).

The serum acid phosphatase is an indicator of the tumor growth. This often rises as the tumor grows beyond the prostate. The serum alkaline phosphatase often rises with bone metastasis (Sturdy, 1976, p. 191; Krupp, 1975, p. 547).

Benign tumor can cause the same symptoms as malignant tumor. The nurse should promote differential diagnosis as soon as prostatic enlargement is detected. Other causes of obstruction as neurogenic bladder, stones, or stricture should also be ruled out.

Complications

The complications from the tumor include obstructive or metastatic pathology. Obstruction can lead to problems like infection or renal failure. Metastasis to the pelvis and spine is evidenced by low back pain and pathologic fractures at the site of metastasis (Krupp, 1975, p. 547).

The problems associated with estrogen therapy are an increased incidence of thrombi and emboli, nausea and vomiting, jaundice, and fluid retention. Mammary enlargement, testicular atrophy, and decreased libido may also occur (Sturdy, 1976, p. 194). If the patient lives long enough, he can also become resistent to estrogen therapy (Anderson, 1971, p. 204). The patient should be informed of the potential side effects before therapy is started.

Surgical castration (orchidectomy) can be emotionally devastating. Sturdy (1976, p. 194) suggests a subcapsular orchidectomy for younger patients, noting that this procedure excises the glandular testes tissue while still leaving some tissue in the scrotum.

Prognosis

Resources vary on the success of treatment for prostatic carcinoma. It appears that mortality figures may be misleading. Basso (1974, p. 353), for example, writes that a 1960 Veterans Administration study including 3432 patients found similar mortality between estrogen-treated patients and those not treated. Patients treated with high doses (5 mgm) of estrogen had a higher mortality from cardiovascular complications, while untreated patients died most often from the carcinoma.

As with any cancer, cure may be obtained by radical surgery before metastasis. However, most prostatic cancers are not recognized and treated during this early stage. Rowan (1973, p. 40) lists more positive statistics. He reports over half the prostatic cancers are discovered at an early stage and that these cancers have a 55 percent survival rate. Furthermore, when early and advanced cancers are combined, there is still a 27 percent 5-year survival rate.

Medical Management

Less than 5 percent of the prostatic carcinomas are suitable for excisional surgery because of the rare case of finding the tumor early enough (Sturdy, 1976, p. 193). It is difficult to generalize treatment with prostatic carcinoma but treatment modalities include radical surgery, radiation, hormonal therapy or nontreatment, depending on the age and health status of the person. Obstruction is relieved by transurethral resection and this may need to be repeated as the tumor progresses. Orchidectomy and estrogen therapy are widely used because estrogens inhibit the tumor growth while androgens stimulate growth. Radiation therapy is commonly used when the tumor is unresectable but still confined to the pelvis.

Some experts currently are recommending that orchidectomy alone should be used, with estrogens reserved for late stages because of the possible cardiovascular complications associated with estrogens (Basso, 1974, p. 353; Cowdry, 1971, pp. 255–256; Sturdy, 1976, pp. 193–195; Drupp, 1975, p. 547; and Anderson, 1971, pp. 203–204).

Nursing Management

Early diagnosis is essential to effective treatment of prostatic carcinoma. When this cancer is not detected early enough for effective surgical control, the nurse's main role becomes that of contributing to quality of life despite progression of disease. The patient and his family may need help in living with cancer. Dr. Kübler-Ross' book *On Death and Dying* (1969) should be mandatory preparation for any nurse working with terminal patients.

Comfort medication should not be withheld from the patient with metastatic prostatic disease. The nurse should be alert for the possibility of fracture if the tumor has metastasized to the spine and pelvis. A patient with a history of cardiopulmonary disease would be a questionable candidate for estrogen therapy as it may pose as great a risk as the cancer. Since retention may also occur

with malignant tumor, nursing care would also include that for benign hypertrophy (p. 336).

Prostatitis

Etiologic Factors

Relapsing urinary infections frequently are traced to chronic prostatitis. There is a higher incidence of gram-negative infections among the elderly and these organisms often are found with chronic prostatitis (Meares, 1975, pp. 3–4; Drach, 1975, p. 505).

High Risk Population

Men of any age group are subject to acute prostatitis. Elderly men with compromised health status are more likely to harbor infectious organisms that are causative for acute or chronic prostatitis.

Dynamics

The means by which bacteria invade the prostate are not certain. It is postulated that invasion may be through the blood, through invasion of rectal bacteria via lymphatics, through ascending urethral infection, or through reflux of infected bladder urine into prostatic ducts. Sexual intercourse may also be a route of transfer of infectious organisms (Meares, 1975, p. 4).

Signs and Symptoms

Symptoms of acute or chronic prostatitis include urgency, frequency, dysuria, decreased libido, low back pain, hematuria, urethral discharge, or perineal pain.

Acute prostatitis is clinically dramatic and evidenced by fever and chills in addition to the previously described symptoms. The gland is very tender with acute prostatitis.

Chronic prostatitis may be asymptomatic or may include the previously listed symptoms. The gland may feel unremarkable or may have bogginess, edema, and asymmetry. Chronic prostatitis sometimes is associated with psychosomatic illness because it is sometimes accompanied by feelings of fatigue, depression, or decreased libido (Stewart, 1976, pp. 530–531; Culp, 1975, p. 41; Drach, 1975, p. 504; and Meares, 1975, pp. 7–9).

Differential Diagnosis

The gland should not be manipulated for diagnosis of acute prostatitis because of pain and because of possible complications from manipulation such as septicemia. The clinical picture is dramatic enough for diagnosis.

Chronic prostatitis, in contrast, is very difficult to diagnose accurately. The procedure for detecting it consists of studying urine collected before or after prostatic massage as well as studying prostatic secretions. When bladder infection is present, this must be suppressed before accurate diagnosis of chronic prostatitis can be made (Meares, 1975, pp. 4–7; Drach, 1975, pp. 504–507; and Stewart, 1976, pp. 531–532).

Complications

Abscess formation and/or septicemia may result with acute prostatitis. Chronic bladder infection often persists with chronic prostatitis. Incontinence and psychologic impotence may occur when radical surgery is used with chronic prostatitis.

Prognosis

Acute prostatitis usually responds to specific antibacterial therapy. Chronic prostatitis often is not cured but can usually be controlled with prolonged treatment.

Medical Management

Antibiotics are given immediately with acute prostatitis, with medication selection based on susceptibility testing. Bedrest, adequate hydration, stool softeners, sitz baths, hot packs, antipyretics, and analgesics are also used. Urethral dilatation or prostatic massage *should not* be done when this condition is suspected. Sexual intercourse is avoided during acute inflammation (Drach, 1975, p. 511; Meares, 1975, p. 8; and Stewart, 1976, p. 531).

Long term or continuous, low-dose suppressive antibiotic therapy is the most general medical treatment with chronic prostatitis. However, antibiotics may not diffuse from the plasma into the prostatic fluid with chronic infection, so even prolonged treatment may not be effective. The management of this condition is controversial and difficult. Total prostatectomy may be a radical treatment in extreme cases but incontinence and impotence usually occur after this surgical procedure, making it rarely justifiable. Transurethral resection is less radical but also less effective (Stewart, 1976, p. 532, and Meares, 1975, p. 10).

Nursing Management

Nursing care of *acute prostatitis* includes maintenance of hydration and relief from pain and fever. This condition should not be hard to diagnose. Nurses should urge sensitivity testing be done to assure appropriate pharmaceutic management. Gram-negative infections often are the culprit and it may be well to consider whether sources of these pathogens can be determined and controlled.

Chronic prostatitis is especially difficult to treat, and the patient should be included in decisions about the management of his condition. For example, he should be advised that surgery may not relieve his distress and he should have knowledge about the risk of incontinence with the surgical procedure. There should be a continual search for comfort measures as sitz baths or perineal compresses. Staff may neglect this patient because of the chronic nature of his condition. Since coitus may help relieve the symptoms of chronic prostatitis, those victims who have a sexual partner should be provided with privacy and encouragement for this natural human response. The possibility of massage may be considered when intercourse is not a viable option. Staff may have trouble accepting massage if they relate it to masturbation. However, they should understand why massage is used and they also should understand that masturbation can be beneficial psychologically. It is essential that massage not be used if there is possibility of abscess or acute infection.

Prostatic massage is sometimes suggested for symptomatic treatment but this therapy is controversial and said to be less effective in draining the gland of retained secretions than coitus. Sexual intercourse may be effective for symptomatic relief (Stewart, 1976, p. 532, and Drach, 1975, p. 516).

Symptomatic relief may also be secured with hot packs, stool softeners and sitz baths. While alcohol and spicy foods are not contraindicated in moderate amounts, they should be used carefully if symptoms increase as they are excreted in the urine (Drach, 1975, 516). Supportive psychological therapy is used in rehabilitation of chronic prostatitis and some men may be simply advised to learn to live with their problem.

Prevention and Management in Prostatic Disease

Urinary problems of aging males frequently are related to prostatic disease. Urinary retention and obstruction may occur because of prostatic enlargement and this also gives rise to persistent urinary infections. Problems of control like frequency and incontinence may occur before or following prostatic surgery.

Nurses should be informed about diagnostic indices of prostatic disease. Rectal examination is important for early recognition of prostatic malignancy and it should be a part of routine examination for all elderly males. The frequency with which rectal examination is performed should be comparable to the frequency of the female pap smear (every 6 months to a year) because aging males face such a high and increasing risk of prostatic malignancy. Since malignancy is often asymptomatic, rectal examination may be the only way this cancer is detected early enough for viable treatment.

Figure 17-1 illustrates palpation of the prostate with rectal examination.

The nurse should not attempt such examination without special instruction such as that offered by clinical specialists. Bates' *Guide to Physical Examination* discusses the male rectal examination.

Any nurse working with chronic care eventually will be faced with the need to do a rectal for the problem of fecal impaction. It is possible a diseased prostate could be palpated by the alert nurse with this procedure. Any suspected deviation should be further evaluated by the physician. The normal prostate is rounded and heart shaped. The median sulcus can be felt between the two lateral lobes. The enlarged prostate (beyond 2.5 cm) could be suspect for hypertrophy, carcinoma or prostatitis. A hard nodular gland is suspect for carcinoma (Bates, 1979).

Rectal examination should not be used in acute prostatitis because of the pain and complications it could inflict. The clinical symptoms of acute prostatitis generally are dramatic enough to suggest this diagnosis without a rectal examination. Rectal examination also is not a good indicator for chronic prostatitis and nurses should question a diagnosis made solely on the basis of clinical symptoms and examination. Accurate diagnosis of chronic prostatitis is dependent on laboratory examination of divided urine specimens and prostatic fluid.

Obstruction is not necessarily related to the amount of prostatic enlargement. Therefore, the nurse should always be alert for the possibility of obstruction with elderly males. The person with

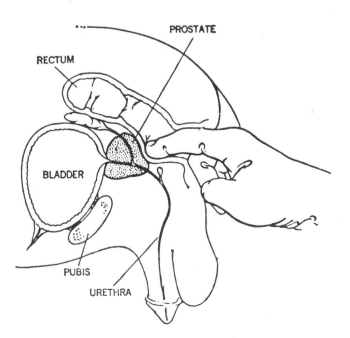

FIGURE 17-1. Rectal examination including palpation of the prostate gland. (Illustration from Your Prostate by R. L. Rowan and P. J. Gillette. Copyright © 1973 by R. L. Rowan. Used by permission of Doubleday & Co., Inc.)

progressive benign hypertrophy or a growing tumor is always suspect for obstruction. A tense bladder can usually be palpated with acute retention except where the patient is obese. The distended bladder appears swollen as the level of the bladder rises above the symphysis pubis. Light pressure on this area reveals a tense, very sensitive area and percussion gives a kettle-drum sound (Mitchell, 1973, p. 301).

If the bladder cannot be palpated because of obesity, acute retention may be diagnosed by suprapubic tenderness and an intense desire to void when pressure is applied over the bladder. Chronic retention is more difficult to detect and percussion above the symphysis pubis may be the only way to feel the large, lax bladder associated with chronic retention (Caird, 1974, pp. 45–46).

Recording intake and output should be a part of the care for prostatic enlargement. Urinary output of 30 to 50 ml/hr usually indicates adequate kidney function, while less than 25 ml/hr (or 500 ml/24 hr) indicates renal shutdown or retention. The bladder normally contains 200 to 500 ml when a person feels the desire to void but, in cases of obstruction, the bladder may stretch to accommodate 1500 ml (Mitchell, 1973, p. 299). Nurses should be able to describe voiding patterns as well as amounts of voiding from the output record.

Alert patients with prostatic enlargement may have learned to control difficult voiding by forcing fluids to a level of more than 3000 ml/day. While this may be helpful in preventing infection from stasis, it could prove dangerous in the event of acute retention. A balance of 2500 to 3000 ml/24 hr intake and 1500 ml/24 hr output is recommended for average hydration and excretion. Intake and output are not expected to be equal since fluid is also excreted through the skin, lungs, and feces. If the intake and output record shows this balance does not exist, the patient with potential obstruction should be advised to limit fluids until the bladder can be drained.

Acute retention can progress into a medical emergency. The initial methods to help relieve retention may include providing privacy, helping the patient stand for voiding, or using a warm water to relax the sphincter. Medications as Urecholine are ordered sometimes. Catheterization is the last of the measures used for acute retention. When it must be done, it is important to remember not to empty the bladder too quickly or shock can result. Generally, no more than 700 to 1000 ml of urine are taken off at one time. Vital signs are monitored closely and are used as an indicator for the amount of volume that can be safely removed (Mitchell, 1973, p. 301).

Surgical intervention may be used with benign hypertrophy and malignancy as well as select instances of chronic prostatitis. The risk of incontinency after surgery varies according to the surgical approach used and the physician's skill. Since this complication is a reality, the nurse needs to be knowledgeable about how to deal with it. It is suggested that all geriatric patients be taught basic perineal control, which consists of voluntary contraction of the anus. This exercise is useful in helping maintain strength of contraction for effective shut-off of both voiding and defecation (Caldwell, 1975, p. 146).

A more stringent, but similar, routine has been reported as useful for treating post-prostatectomy incontinence and/or long-standing incontinence (Krauss, Schoenrock, and Lilien, 1975, p. 534).

Your Prostate by Rowan and Gillette (1973) is an excellent book for teaching the patient about prostatic disease. The author, Rowan, is a urology

---

EXERCISE FOR REDUCING POST-PROSTATECTOMY OR LONG-STANDING INCONTINENCE*

Relax the body entirely.

Squeeze the rectal sphincter as though you are suppressing the urge to defecate.

Relax the hands on abdomen to prevent Valsalva maneuver or intra-abdominal pressure. Fatigue should not occur.

Retraction of the penis should occur.

Perform the exercise 20 to 30 times/hr.

If the patient cannot understand the exercise, the clinician should put a gloved finger in rectum and have the patient contract the sphincter around the finger.

Evaluate the effects of exercise. If incontinence increases rather than decreases as expected, it is probable the patient is not sufficiently relaxed when performing the exercise. Intra-abdominal pressure will increase incontinence.

---

*Adapted from information from Krauss, D., Schoenrock, G., and Lilien, O.: Reeducation of urethral sphincter mechanism in post-prostatectomy incontinence. Urology 5, April 1975, p. 534.

specialist in the field of prostatic disease. Prostatitis, benign prostatic hypertrophy, and carcinoma are discussed with information about their detection and treatment. There is also good explanation of the prostate and the genitourinary system. Drawings illustrate normal anatomy, rectal examination, cystoscopy, surgical procedure, and retrograde ejaculation. A glossary is included.

Evaluation in Prostatic Disease

Surgery is needed with prostatic disease when there is sound evidence of progressive obstruction. The nurse should help the patient obtain detailed information about his surgeon's choice of operative procedure. There is no single "best" approach and the patient's condition may prevent some options. The patient with fixed arthritic hips, for example, would not be a suitable candidate for the lithotomy position required with T U R or perineal prostatectomy (Culp, 1975, p. 44).

Questions that should be answered before surgery are:

1. What is the risk of incontinence with this procedure?
2. What is the risk of other injury (as rectal or urethral sphincter damage) with this procedure?
3. What is the risk of hemorrhage with this procedure?
4. Will vasectomy also be performed?
5. Will sexual function be altered in any way?
6. How does retrograde ejaculation feel?

Relief of obstruction is the expected surgical outcome. When this does not occur, further evaluation is required. Some patients may require a permanent catheter when surgery is not effective or when surgery cannot be performed.

While the preceding guidelines also apply to obstruction secondary to malignancy, there are additional considerations with malignancy. One classification and treatment guideline for prostatic malignancy is given in Table 17-1.

It should be understood that treatment for malignancy is not easily segmented and many measures (as radiation and estrogen therapy) will likely be palliative rather than curative. It is imperative the patient be counselled about expected treatment outcomes and risks and given a treatment choice. The patient's clinical symptoms and periodic laboratory tests of serum alkaline and acid phosphatase are considered measures of the effectiveness of cancer therapy.

Absence of clinical symptoms and negative laboratory tests (negative urine and prostatic secretion) are evaluative criteria for prostatitis. Recurrence of this condition is common and, therefore, patients should be followed at least 6 months after cure and whenever symptoms reoccur (Drach, 1975, pp. 518–519).

URINARY TRACT INFECTION

Urinary tract infections are a common and serious problem of aging men and women. Death from renal failure is often attributed to damage that

TABLE 17-1. A guideline for prostatic malignancy.

Type Tumor	Involvement	Management
Stage A	Clinically unsuspected (tumor discovered during histologic examination)	If tumor is well differentiated, does not need treatment
Stage B	Tumor limited to prostate (few tumors are confined like this)	Radical prostatectomy
Stage C	Tumor extends beyond prostate but no evidence of distant metastasis	Radiation therapy
Stage D	Distant metastasis evident	Hormonal treatment according to symptoms, prognosis limited

Adapted from information from Basso, A.: Genitourinary tract problems of the aged male. J. Amer. Geriatric Soc. 21:353–354, 1974.

occurred to the kidneys as a result of previous urinary infection (Anderson, 1971, p. 126).

High Risk Populations

The incidence of urinary tract infection rises with aging. Women experience a rate of 1 percent increase with each decade of life so that the 60-year-old female has a 6 percent rate of infection. Men are relatively unaffected by urinary infection in early years but this statistic changes after middle age, partially because of the obstructive nature of prostatic disease. Elderly men are said to have equal or even greater rate of urinary tract infection than elderly women (Freeman, 1975, p. 90, and Moore-Smith, 1973, p. 687).

Rates of bateriuria rise in health care facility populations with one municipal hospital survey demonstrating a 30 percent infection rate with women and a 70 percent infection rate with men (Freeman, 1975, p. 91). Rates as high as 65 percent have been quoted with elderly hospitalized patients (Moore-Smith, 1973, p. 687).

Diabetics are at greater risk for urinary tract infection. Their urine serves as a better culture medium with its additional sugar and protein. Renal failure from any previous cause is also associated with increased incidence of infection. Finally, hypertension should be mentioned. Freeman notes, "It is not yet clear whether the bacteria causes renal damage that results in hypertension or vice versa" (Freeman, 1975, p. 101).

The rise of urinary tract infections associated with sexual activity is often documented with younger women. There is little discussion in current literature about this problem among older women. However, an article in a 1975 volume of *Geriatrics* is devoted to this problem. The contention of this article is that older women who are sexually active are especially susceptible to urologic problems. The estrogenic changes of postmenopausal women may predispose them to mechanical irritation and/or urinary tract infection and the extended period of foreplay may encourage the massage of complicating bacteria into the paraurethral glands (Kent, 1975, p. 145).

Instrumentation and catheterization are high risk situations for urinary tract infections and are factors that can be controlled. Freeman writes, "Insertion of a bladder catheter is one of the surest ways to defeat host defenses and create disease where there previously was none" (Freeman, 1975, p. 98). There is an incidence of 1 to 10 percent bacteriuria with any person subjected to instrumentation and a 96 percent chance of bacteriuria with an indwelling catheter connected to straight drainage after 4 days (Freeman, 1975, p. 91). Andriole (1975, pp. 453–454) states conclusively that systemic administration of antibiotics cannot prevent bacteriuria in abacteriuric patients on open drainage or standard indwelling catheter. Susceptible organisms may be eliminated with systemic antibiotic therapy only to permit the entrance of resistant bacteria with the end result being an infection more difficult to treat.

Dynamics

Elderly persons are at high risk for urinary tract infections for many reasons. Obstruction is a major causative factor and it may be clinically manifested by the common problem of urinary retention. The bladder mucosa normally has a low pH which exerts a natural bacteriostatic effect on invading organisms. Urinary retention dilutes the normal acidity of the bladder mucosa, thus reducing its bacteriostatic effect. Furthermore, the urethral meatus (and also the introitus of women) is contaminated normally by some bowel flora. The outward flow of urine serves to prevent the movement of bacteria up from the meatus to the bladder and kidney. When obstruction is present, upward invasion is more likely (Freeman, 1975, pp. 96–97).

It is almost impossible to list the reasons for stasis, retention, and obstruction in the elderly as they are so numerous. Prostatic disease is frequently listed with aging men and cystocele with aging women. However, there is similarity of the sexes with both subject to disorders like meatal stenosis, urethral stricture, urethral and bladder neoplasms, bladder neck contracture, and calculi (Jaffe, 1971, p. 143).

Obstructive neuropathy may be divided into three general groups for classification: (1) obstruction related to prostatic disease, (2) obstruction related to urethral stricture, and (3) neurologic obstruction (Black and Moore, 1969, p. 132). The high incidence of stroke and hemiplegia with the elderly makes the neurologic classification noteworthy.

Immobility, a common problem of elderly, handicapped persons, leads to impaired musculoskeletal function. Body equilibrium is assured in the skeletal system by everyday stress and strain of activity. When mobility is impaired, osteoclastic cells continue to break down living bone substance but osteoblastic replacement function ceases; thus, calcium, phosphorus, and nitrogen are depleted from the bone. Calcium excretion contributes to renal calculi formation. Infection may be related to urinary stasis as well as colonization of this foreign body (Freeman, 1975, p. 100).

Signs and Symptoms

Urinary infection should be suspected when an older person develops symptoms as nonspecific as fever, vomiting, or illness without apparent reason (Black and Moore, 1969, p. 127).

The classic symptoms of lower tract infection are lower abdominal discomfort, frequency, urgency, dysuria, nocturia, and turbid urine. Dramatic (the opposite of insidious) lower tract infection *also* may include fever and chills, hematuria, vomiting, and acute retention (Jaffe, 1971, p. 141). Symptoms suggestive of involvement *beyond* the lower urinary tract are any of the previous symptoms, flank pain, and tenderness. *These symptoms are general and diagnosis should not be made based purely on symptomatology.*

Freeman writes, "The clinician who thinks he has diagnosed urinary tract infections by symptomatology for years must learn new ways" (Freeman, 1975, p. 91). It is entirely possible the patient, and particularly an elderly person, may be asymptomatic, especially in terms of the usual symptoms of lower tract infection (Moore-Smith, 1973, p. 688).

Hematuria deserves special mention. Although it is not uncommon with the elderly, it is always a cause for further investigation. Complications as papilloma, kidney tumor, stones, or hemorrhagic infection are suspect with hematuria. It is more commonly associated with benign than with malignant prostate diseases (Anderson, 1971, pp. 201–202).

Differential Diagnosis

Diagnosis based on localization of symptoms is accurate only 50 percent of the time (Freeman, 1975, p. 91). Quantitative urine culture is used in conjunction with clinical symptoms for accurate diagnosis of lower tract infection. Diagnosis depends on identifying significant bacteriuria.

The concept of significant bacteriuria is based on the notion that a clean-voided urine specimen will necessarily have bacteria that contaminates the specimen as it leaves the urethra. Bacteria would not be expected if urine were collected aseptically from the bladder, but this is not the common collection method. Contamination is a factor to consider especially with elderly or obese women. Fifty-seven percent of the urines collected from elderly women under hospital conditions may show false-positive rates (Moore-Smith, 1973, p. 688). The criteria for separating "true" bacteriuria from contaminated bacturiuria is based on bacterial quantity. Freeman places significance at 10^5 to 10^9 bacteria per ml (100,000 to 1,000,000,000 bacteria per ml). *Medical Diagnosis and Treatment* suggests a value of 100,000 bacteria per ml provided this quantity is found in two consecutive collections (Jawetz, 1975, p. 536). Isolation of a single species of bacteria from a specimen is also criteria for separating "true" bacteriuria. When multiple organisms are isolated, a contaminated specimen is usually suspected.

The single-use female Cath Kit manufactured by Davol is a device that may be used to collect a specimen from the incontinent, totally-dependent female. This catheter is much narrower than an indwelling catheter. Since it is much smaller than the typical 14 French catheter, the risk of mechanical irritation should be considerably less. While catheterization should never be routinely used for specimen collection, this device may be the least traumatic method for catheterizing the female who cannot void into a clean container. The nurse needs to weigh whether laboratory urinalysis justifies the risk of catheterization.

A problem of urinary quantitative culture is the need for immediate refrigeration of the specimen and laboratory facilities for culturing the specimen. Freeman recommends culturing with a urine dipslide when laboratory facilities are limited. The dipslide can be used at home or used in facilities like a rural clinic or nursing home. The dipslide is well described by Kunin who additionally recommends its ease of use, reduced cost, and high reliability (Kunin, 1975, p. 424).

Gram stain which is 80 percent reliable is used for immediate determination of bacterial type (Turck, 1975, p. 444). While 95 percent of urinary tract infections are gram negative, the 5 percent chance of gram-positive rods makes gram stain or culture important prior to antimicrobial therapy (Freeman, 1975, p. 96).

The absence or presence of white blood cells in the urine is useful data but not diagnostic for bacteria. Persistent pyuria without significant bacteriuria is suspect for tuberculosis of the kidney or urolithiasis (Moore-Smith, 1973, p. 688; Freeman, 1975, p. 91; and Kahn, 1971, p. 134).

Complications

Urinary infections complicated by other pathology (as obstruction) will not respond to antimicrobial treatment until the underlying abnormality is recognized and corrected. This illustrates the need for more thorough urologic investigation when bacteriuria persists. This discussion will not describe such procedures as they are beyond the realm of nursing. Suffice to say nursing's responsibility is to ensure that patients receive more complete evaluation when they fail to respond to appropriate antimicrobial therapy. Conversely, nursing also needs to assure that patients are not subjected to instrumentation, which involves risk of bacteriuria, in the absence of basic diagnostic procedure.

Oral suppressant therapy is recommended for treating recurrent infections and/or those with complicating factors. Infection secondary to obstructive disease is an example of such infection. Since treatment options as surgery may not be available for some elderly people, suppressive therapy may be the best choice. Freeman writes, "proper use of suppressants in nursing and custodial homes would probably prevent many hospital admissions every year" (Freeman, 1975, p. 108).

Bacteriuria that persists and is untreated may progress to bacteremia or renal failure. The mortality with either of these complications is great.

Prognosis

Prognosis is limited with debilitated, chronically ill older people. The goal in managing the urinary tract infections is prevention of symptomatic or asymptomatic recurrences and development of dysfunction. While antimicrobial agents are the major form of therapy, the condition of the patient is the most significant factor in the pathogenesis of urinary tract infections (Turck, 1975, p. 443).

The older person who is bedridden with stasis of urine and colonization of a kidney stone has compromised status, as does the incontinent female with stagnant urine pooling in her vagina. Other examples of compromised status are an elderly man with obstruction as a result of benign hypertrophy or an elderly diabetic. The list of compromised status is long with elderly, debilitated persons.

Medical Management

There is some difference in expert opinion regarding therapeutic approach for lower urinary tract infection. While texts agree that acute, symptomatic, significant bacteriuria should be medically treated with antimicrobial drugs, asymptomatic bacteriuria is managed differently. *This is a noteworthy point because asymptomatic bacteriuria is common with both elderly women and men.* Moore-Smith promotes treatment of asymptomatic, significant bacteriuria in the elderly because of the "deleterious effects of urinary infection on renal function which is already likely to be compromised, as well as the known high incidence of chronic pyelonephritis" (Moore-Smith, 1973, p. 688). Turck does not use the term significant bacteriuria. He states, "We believe that, as long as bacteriuria, particularly in the elderly patient, is asymptomatic, vigorous attempts at therapy are not warranted" (Turck, 1975, p. 446). Freeman recommends following high risk persons with culture (dipslide or otherwise) so that significant bacteriuria (symptomatic or asymptomatic) can be treated before bacteremia occurs. He notes that urinary tract infections account for two thirds of the bacteremias with gram-negative rods. Antimicrobial therapy will not significantly alter such infections and bacteremia is 30 to 35 percent fatal (Freeman, 1975, p. 101).

Sulfonamides are widely used with elderly persons with bacteriuria because of the high incidence of gram-negative infections (often Escherichia coli) that are sensitive to sulfonamides. When organisms are not sensitive to sulfonamides, then treatment should follow sensitivities found on culture with appropriate manipulation of urinary pH to match the organisms and antibiotic chosen (Moore-Smith, 1973, p. 688).

An adequate fluid intake and establishment of proper urinary drainage must accompany antimicrobial therapy. Stagnant urine is not rendered sterile by antibiotics. Some sources caution against forcing fluids to the point that antimicrobials are diluted in the urine (Jawetz, 1975, p. 538). Moore-Smith (1973, p. 688), however, believes dilution of antibiotics is a lesser concern compared to the therapeutic effect of decreased bacterial reproduction in diluted urine and the washout effect of high urine flow. (Moore-Smith, 1973, p. 688). Black and Moore (1969, p. 135) promote assessment of renal excretory function to determine the ability of an elder to eliminate the medication. They note dosage may need to be modified to allow for impaired excretory function.

Antimicrobial therapy for urinary tract infection is usually short term. Symptoms that do not subside in a few days should be suspect for complicating factor needing further evaluation. Continuous antibiotic therapy may mask underlying disease or lead to side effects such as Candida vaginitis (Hole, 1976, pp. 219–221).

Oral suppressive therapy often is ordered when long term treatment is needed. These drugs do not replace antibiotics but rather are used to prevent or at least reduce the frequency of acute attacks. These agents have no systemic effect and, thus, have the advantage of not changing the normal flora. Resistance to them rarely develops. The methenamine salts (Mandelamine, Hiprex, and Hexalet) are commonly used suppressants that are safe and effective. They act by breaking the urine down into organic acids and formaldehyde. The formaldehyde effectively suppresses the growth of many urinary organisms. Furadantin and Macrodantin are also used as suppressants. All of these drugs require an acid urine for effectiveness. Additional medication as ascorbic acid may need to be given to assure this acidity (Rodman, 1975, pp. 91–92).

Nursing Management

Urinary infections are so common with the elderly that the nurse needs to guard against complacency about this disease process. It is important that she appreciate that urinary tract infections can and do progress to terminal renal failure or to bacteremia. Debilitated, chronically ill people are high risk for urinary disease and its possible severe complications.

The symptoms of urinary infection can be vague and, therefore, they may be missed without good assessment techniques. General assessment of any patient includes things like evaluating the patient's state of well-being, checking skin turgor and integrity, evaluating cardiopulmonary status, and taking a history of sleep habits. Mental status is an important clue as lethargy may be a symptom of uremia. Distant symptoms like anorexia, vomiting, and restlessness may also herald an infection. It is a good idea to check routinely for urinary infection any time a patient presents symptoms of an altered health status.

Any change in voiding habits signals a need for further investigation. Most nurses are alerted by dys-

uria and will order a urinalysis if their patient has acute symptoms. However, nurses tend to be more complacent about problems like nocturia, dribbling, and incontinence. It may be considered neglect when a concerted effort is not made to identify the cause of such chronic distress. Symptoms such as frequency and dysuria should be recorded to help evaluate the patient's response to infection. However, the nurse should remember that bacteriuria cannot necessarily be localized by symptoms. Furthermore, asymptomatic infection may also be present. Diagnosis is dependent, therefore, on laboratory tests such as urinalysis, dipslide, culture, and Gram stain.

A good record of intake and output (I & O) is one of the most effective assessment tools available to the nurse. There is no excuse for not routinely obtaining an I & O record anytime urinary problems are suspected. Staff may miss a problem of retention without awareness of output. Furthermore, adequate hydration is essential to nursing care for infection. While fluids are one of the most basic care measures, they are also one of the most widely neglected. Urinary output should be at least 1500 ml/24 hr and intake 2500 to 3000 ml/24 hr. The elder who cannot drink this amount may need such fluid replacement therapy as subcutaneous, intravenous, or nasogastric feedings.

Urinalysis is the simplest of tools for laboratory diagnosis but it may not be accurate because of contaminated specimens. When consecutive specimens are obtained with significant bacterial counts, urinalysis is then considered accurate. *Refrigeration of specimens is essential to avoid false counts.* Urinalysis does not identify the pathogenic organism; Gram stain and culture are used for this specificity. While most infections in the elderly are gram negative and will respond to drugs like the sulfonamides, culture should be utilized any time infection persists or is severe.

Freeman (1975, p. 104) suggests a sequence for diagnosis and treatment of urinary tract infections (see box). Nurses should promote the adaptation of such sequence to assure adequacy of treatment for their patient.

Nurses may have a difficult time convincing physicians and other health care professionals that such vigilance is needed for a problem as common as urinary infection. Furthermore, laboratory facilities for diagnosis may not be available in many chronic care settings. Dipslide screening could be utilized as a preliminary test. However, contract

---

**SEQUENCE FOR DIAGNOSIS AND TREATMENT
OF URINARY TRACT INFECTIONS***

Day 1   History, physical, and laboratory examination.
Obtain urine for culture.
Do urine Gram strain if therapy is to be initiated.

Day 2   Repeat urine Gram strain if patient is too seriously ill to gauge effectiveness of therapy. Culture result may be available from laboratory.

Day 3   Check culture result. Sensitivities may be available from laboratory. Adjust therapy if needed. Repeat urine culture if therapeutic outcome is in doubt.

Day 4   Check sensitivities. Adjust therapy on basis of in vitro sensitivities and therapeutic response.

Day 10 Discontinue therapy if result satisfactory. May begin suppressant.

Week 2 Repeat urine culture to document if urine is sterile when patient is not receiving antibiotics. Continue suppressant if indicated.

**Month 3
or 6**   Repeat urine culture to ascertain that bacteriuria has not recurred.

---

laboratory services need to be purchased for more precise diagnosis of bacteriuria. At least one negative culture is considered basic follow-up after treatment for bacteriuria. Patients with recurrent infection need to be placed on routine follow-up for several months.

Nurses can establish the precedence for sequential treatment of bacteriuria by demonstrating this in their own care of the patient. Patients with bacteriuria should have nursing history that will document their response to treatment and follow-up. Follow-up could include establishing a timetable that monitors voiding patterns, general assessment findings, I & O, and dipslide or urinalysis readings. Nurses may want to monitor patients weekly, bi-weekly and then monthly following successful treatment for infection. The frequency of such monitoring could be reduced if dipslide or urinalysis readings remain negative.

The prevalence of urinary infection with catheters is well-documented. The nurse should as-

* From Freeman, J.: Urinary tract infections: prevention, diagnosis and treatment. In Schwartz, A. (ed.): Nephrology for the Practicing Physician, New York: Grune & Stratton, 1975, p. 104, with permission.

certain that catheters are never prescribed for the convenience of the staff. Futhermore, she should attempt to do bladder training and removal of a catheter whenever possible. Exceptions that would probably require a catheter would be neurogenic bladder and obstruction. When a patient must have a catheter, then vigilant aseptic measures must be enforced. Catheter care is described later in this chapter. A penile sheath is preferable to a catheter for male incontinence. Unfortunately, no similar device exists for women; padding with Chux and an absorbant pad are the most likely options.

Sexually-active older women may need nursing assistance in coping with bacteriuria. Some relatively simple measures may prove helpful. The sexually-active patient can "flush" the lower urinary tract by voiding immediately after intercourse and by increasing fluid intake. Bathing before or after intercourse may also help. The male-superior position may be problematic because of the extraurethral stress exerted with this position (Kent, 1975, p. 146). If these simple measures do not provide relief, the nurse should promote gynecologic and urologic consultation. Topical estrogen may be prescribed medically along with procedures like urethral dilitation.

Urinary stasis contributes to infection. Good rehabilitation care that stresses mobility for all patients is basic to preventing stasis. Furthermore, the physical environment should be conducive to good bladder habits. Patients should be assisted with toileting regularly so that they do not hold their urine, thereby contributing to stasis. Provisions should be made to assure that patients can get to the bathroom or a commode during the night without self-injury.

Gravitational assistance is used to empty the bladder and reduce stasis of urine. Patients are taught to lean forwards when evacuating the bladder. The nurse should be aware of the hazards possible with this maneuver. Handrails are a must and the patient may also require a nurse to steady him. Gravitational drainage would probably do little to relieve stasis caused by obstructive disease (Caldwell, 1975, p. 146).

While urinary infections cannot be eradicated by preventive care, hygienic measures may at least reduce the high levels of infection found in hospitals and chronic care facilities. Soiled underwear and lying in a wet bed could give rise to infection. Diapering may make the staff work easier but it may have infection consequences if it means hygiene is less vigilant. Also, it does little to promote patient dignity. Some elderly women use sanitary napkins. Women should be informed about the risks of infection and perineal irritation resulting from their use. Daily routines for perineal care with Betadine wash may help reduce infections. It is possible that improved cleansing rather than Betadine is what actually reduces infections.

Nurses should be alert to items in the patient's environment that may harbor pathogens. Black and Moore wrote, "the metal urinal retained the bacterial flora of a ward in successive layers of calcific incrustation" (Black and Moore, 1969, p. 133). Disposable bedpans and urinals would reduce this transfer of pathogens between patients but the cost of disposable items may be prohibitive and also environmentally wasteful. Care settings should do regular culturing of bedpans, urinals, washbasins, and bathtubs. This should be in addition to maintaining a regular schedule for disinfection and sterilization of equipment.

Pharmacologic treatment of bacteriuria is the responsibility of the physician. However, the nurse needs to be aware of accepted treatment regimen. It is her responsibility to question infection that does not respond to antimicrobial therapy as well as her responsibility to promote Gram stain and culture for specificity in treatment. An additional investigative technique, cystoscopy, is also indicated when infection persists.

Suppressive therapy should be explored as a useful treatment for elderly patients. Effective suppressive therapy depends on an acid urine and the nurse should check the pH of the urine daily when suppressants are ordered. Dietary manipulation can be used to promote acidity of urine. Cranberries, plums, prunes, eggs, meat, and fish produce an acid urine while milk, nuts, other fruits, and most vegetables produce an alkaline urine. These latter foods may need some restriction when the goal is an acidic urine. Dietary manipulation is meaningless without pH readings to monitor dietary effect (Krause and Hunscher, 1972, p. 484). The suppressant Furadantin has the side effect of GI upset and should be given with milk and/or with meals. Macrodantin may be substituted when GI upset persists.

The patient with recurrent urinary tract infection should be considered as possibly harboring infections in other body systems. Low resistance to infection in the elderly may be related to less effective immune systems or immunosuppressive therapy (see Chapter 12). Older patients on immunosuppressive therapy are at unusually high risk for urinary tract and other infections. The goal of nursing management is protection. This may be achieved by:

- spatial separation from others with known infection
- good handwashing technique
- adequate diet

Self-contamination is another source of urinary infection. For example, an elderly diabetic with an open draining stump may harbor gram-negative pseudomonas. Immersing such a patient in bath water will almost guarantee a hard-to-treat pseudomonas urinary tract infection.

Nurses in long term care facilities need to see themselves as infection control agents. They should maintain high awareness of those at risk of infection and high standards for hygiene of personnel and staff. Evaluation of the effectiveness of their endeavors is also critical.

Evaluation

Knowledge of the characteristics of normal urine (see Chapter 7, p. 107) provides the nurse with a rough assessment guide. She knows that if the urine pH rises above 8, organisms can colonize that would not thrive in a more acidic urine. Likewise, she recognizes that dark, strong-smelling urine indicates the need for improved fluid intake. If the urine looks bloody she should automatically pursue urinalysis. Specific gravity measures the ability of the kidneys to dilute and concentrate urine. A low specific gravity is seen with renal damage which can be the consequence of repeated infections. A high specific gravity is found with dehydration with poor fluid intake (Metheny and Snively, 1979, p. 107).

A suggested sequence for medical treatment of urinary tract infections was given on p. 345. Nurses need to establish similar sequence for nursing prescription. The wellness-illness pattern of a patient with recurrent infection and/or a patient who is high risk for infection may be monitored with a nursing flowsheet. The information pinpointed by this flowsheet serves as criteria for evaluation. Nursing prescription is written and revised according to the results of such evaluation.

DATE	URINE CHARACTERISTICS* (Record weekly on Wednesday)	SPECIFIC URINARY SYMPTOMS (Record Daily)	GENERALIZED SYMPTOMS (Record Daily)	URINALYSIS* AND CULTURE RESULTS (Record as ordered)	ANTIBIOTIC THERAPY (Record as ordered)	SUPPRESSIVE THERAPY AND pH (Record as ordered)	INTAKE AND OUTPUT (I & O)* (Record weekly on Wednesday)
Day 1	Record urinary pH, color, and odor	Record symptoms such as burning, frequency and incontinence	Record any deviation from wellness; i.e., fever, nausea, general aching	Obtain urinalysis with initiation of flowsheet	Record dosage and duration of therapy	Record dosage and duration of therapy	Record weekly when no known infection
Day 2				Obtain urinalysis and culture whenever infection is suspected			Record daily with active infection
Day 3	Specific gravity can be done by the nurse or included in lab urinalysis			Repeat urinalysis after antibiotic is finished, 10 days later and then per month			
Day 4				Dipslide can be used for follow-up		Record daily pH with all suppressive therapy	
Day 5							
Day 6							
Day 7	Collect data for a minimum of 3 months						

* Nursing prescription of urine characteristics, I & O, and urinalysis is based on individual patient need. The patient with a good appetite may need I & O only with active infection while the patient with anorexia may need daily I & O.

N U R S I N G   F L O W S H E E T

Catheter Care

It cannot be stressed enough that *catheters present a great risk of bacteriuria to the elderly and should be avoided whenever possible.* They should never be used for staff convenience or for routine urinalysis. However, there are instances such as inoperable obstructive disease or neurogenic bladder when a retention catheter may be a necessity. When one must be used, it behooves nurses to know correct technique.

The catheterization procedure should not be lightly delegated. Some experts recommend it be done only by a specialist such as the urologist. At any rate, it should not be assigned to the least trained personnel as is often the case. Catheterization trauma is reduced by choosing the smallest catheter possible. Catheter diameter in millimeters is determined by dividing the French size by 3. A 14 French catheter is often adequate for women and men. Correct technique includes cleansing the urethral meatus and surrounding area with an antibacterial soap. The technician then regloves and drapes the patient with sterile covers. The organisms that are introduced into the bladder with the catheterization procedure may be significantly reduced if the urethra is then filled with a large quantity of a water soluble lubricant that contains an antibacterial substance (Dale, 1975, p. 475). Daily care includes careful cleansing of the meatus and surrounding area with an antibacterial solution and application of an antibacterial ointment, such as Betadine.

The patient needs to be positioned above the collection container at all times so there is continuous free gravitational drainage of the urine. Taping or pinning the catheter tubing above the level of the container also helps assure this gravitational drainage. Fluid intake should be great enough that urine is produced at the rate of at least 50 ml/hr. This continuous flow should help reduce the rate of upward migration of motile bacteria. The penis is directed headwards with males to prevent erosion of the urethra by the catheter.

A continuous irrigation, three-way catheter or a closed drainage system is advocated when catheterization must occur. The open drainage system where the catheter is simply hooked to the drainage system is not recommended because the incidence of infection with this system is so great. Infection is almost 100 percent within three to four days of catheterization with the open drainage system (Andriole, 1975,

p. 452). This system is the one most commonly used in care facilities or home care and its use should be seriously questioned. It is almost certain bacteriuria will reflux back into the bladder with this system. Air bubbles in the drainage tubing or bacterial motility can enable the organisms to move upstream even when care is taken to maintain good gravitational drainage of the urine.

The three-way catheter with a continuous irrigation system is recommended by some urologists. The bladder is slowly and continuously irrigated with an antibacterial solution with this system. A 0.25 percent solution of acetic acid (2.5 ml of glacial acetic acid in 1 L of sterile water) is an effective irrigating solution providing the pH of the urine is kept at 5 or lower. Use of this solution depends on continual monitoring and adjustment of urinary pH (Andriole, 1975, p. 454). Communicable disease experts, however, recommend against continuous irrigation, citing collapse of bladder walls that in turn prevent complete washing of surfaces. Instead they recommend intermittent clamping for 15 to 20 minutes using the 0.25 acetic acid solution. They also disagree with the use of *any* antibiotic solution because of risks associated with recurrence of drug-resistant organisms that may later reinfect the bladder (Hoffman, 1976).

A prepared rinse that is a mixture of neomycin and polymyxin is also effective as an irrigating solution. The disadvantage of this mixture is the cost and the possible patient reaction to the antibiotics. The continuous irrigation system may be too expensive for routine use but it should at least be considered for the patient with markedly reduced defense mechanisms such as the severe diabetic (Dale, 1975, p. 476).

The closed drainage system is recommended for routine general use. It depends on strict aseptic technique that begins even prior to the insertion of the catheter. This system often breaks down because of staff technique. The catheter is connected to the drainage bag before it is introduced into the bladder and this connection should not be broken. The drainage bag should be emptied at least every eight hours and the bag should be changed at least weekly, using sterile technique. The organisms multiply quickly in standing urine and present a stagnant pool that can colonize the bladder by reflux or capillary action (Garner, 1974, p. 56).

Andriole (1975) states that backflow of urine is a major problem that can be alleviated by purchasing a closed drainage system with a flutter valve to prevent backflow. The flutter valve, however, should not be a substitute for good technique. Raising the collection bag above the level of the bladder would obviously be negligent technique that could not be remedied by a flutter valve. One expert states flutter valves may be disadvantageous because they impede flow of urine (Garner, 1974, p. 56).

While systemic antibiotics are of little use in preventing bacteriuria with the patient on open drainage, they have been effective with closed drainage when their use is based on specific sensitivity testing. Urine is obtained by aspiration through the latex of the catheter (Dale, 1975, p. 477).

The closed system should not be irrigated except with the problem of potential plugging as any irrigation will break technique. When an irrigation must be done, the incidence of infection even with careful technique is high. A catheter change probably involves less risk of infection than an irrigation.

Nurses will be faced with a dilemma when a closed or continuous irrigation system is being maintained and they wish to mobilize their patient. While a patient could feasibly be ambulated a short distance without breaking technique, independence and/or trips away from the care facility or the patient's home would be quite difficult. Nurses need to weigh the problems of the typical open drainage system against the need for activity and social acceptance.

If a decision is made to ambulate with the use of a device like a leg bag, boundaries to reduce patient risk will need to be established.

The suprapubic catheter is an alternative that needs further exploration. It may be the catheter of choice when one must be used. According to Meares (1975, p. 8), there are fewer complications with a suprapubic catheter than a urethral catheter. We do not know why the suprapubic catheter is not more widely used; it may be because the initial instillation requires surgical incision. Minor surgical incision certainly seems preferable if the risk of bacteriuria can be reduced. Suprapubic Foley-type catheters are now available that can be percutaneously placed with local anesthesia.

VAGINITIS

Nurses in clinical geriatric practice will attest to the fact that vaginal irritation and discharge is a frequent problem of elderly women. Interestingly, the problem is described poorly, if at all, in many geriatric texts. Friedrich (1976, p. 1) writes that, although vulvovaginitis is among the top ten problems encountered by family physicians in daily practice, medical school curricula by and large tend to bypass the subject.

Atrophic Vaginitis

Etiologic Factors

Atrophic vaginitis is the most common vaginitis of older women. It may be thought of as a vaginitis resulting from epithelial lack of estrogen nourishment (Friedrich, 1976, p. 17). (Since it may occur also in premenopausal females, authors sometimes use the term *senile atrophic* to make the distinction. The term *senile vaginitis*, however, lacks specificity and generally is considered inaccurate.)

High Risk Populations or Situations

Women who are premenopausal or postmenopausal may suffer from this vaginitis. All geriatric women are considered high risk for atrophic vaginitis unless they are on estrogen replacement.

Dynamics

The female genital area markedly reflects the degenerative changes of aging. External changes of the vulva include a loss of hair and subcutaneous fat with flattening of the labial folds. The vulvar skin is atrophic, appearing thin, shiny, and avascular. The vaginal mucosa shows similar atrophic change and the introitus appears smaller than in reproductive years (Birnbaum, 1971, p. 149).

There is a significant relationship between estrogen levels and vaginal physiology. Friedrich described the vagina as a "complex and sensitive ecosystem (1976, p. 6). He saw it being maintained in balance by several interdependent factors. One can appreciate what Friedrich is describing by a brief comparison of the "vaginal ecosystems" of young and old women. The vaginal epithelium of women in their reproductive years is thick and lined with many protective cells as a result of estrogenic stimulation. There are abundant deposits of glycogen in the superficial layers of the epithelium. Glycogen is important because it functions as a substrate in the enzymatic catabolism of vaginal flora. Lactic acid is produced as a side product of this reaction and it serves to maintain the low vaginal pH typical of young women. This low pH is highly selective for bacterial growth, and so colonization of the vagina generally is discouraged (Friedrich, 1976, pp. 6–8). When ovarian function ceases, the vaginal epithelium returns to a premenarchal state. The epithelium thins and the number of superficial cells are significantly reduced. Since glycogen levels are reduced by this thinning, enzymatic catabolism is also decreased and the acidogenic balance is discouraged. A wide variety of bacteria now thrive as a result of the change in vaginal pH (Friedrich, 1976, pp. 18–19). Bacterial vaginitis is commonly seen when the epithelium is thin, atrophic, and easily traumatized. It tends to be limited to infancy and postmenopausal women (Palmer, 1975, p. 667).

Signs and Symptoms

Symptoms of atrophic vaginitis include vaginal and vulvar soreness, difficult or painful intercourse (dyspareunia); thin, scant discharge; purulent discharge (with bacterial infection); pale, pasty appearance of the vagina; superficial ulceration of the vagina; blood-tinged discharge; and vaginal pH of 6–7 (Henriques, 1976, p. 795; Birnbaum, 1971, p. 150; and Friedrich, 1976, pp. 17–20).

Urinary tract symptoms as dysuria and frequency often occur in conjunction with vaginitis and are often misinterpreted by the patient and medical staff as a urinary tract infection.

Differential Diagnosis

Vaginal discharge is always present, but it becomes significant by increased amount or when there are localized symptoms such as irritation. Speculum examination of atrophic vaginitis may reveal a pasty, pale appearance or inflammation and superficial ulceration (Friedrich, 1976, p. 19, and Birnbaum, 1971, p. 150).

The epithelium of older women is often friable, leading to rupture of surface vessels. Although rupture of surface vessels is common, experts recommend a pap smear to rule out malignancy. Culture is also done to determine whether bacterial infection is present and the causative organism. Bacterial vaginitis may result because of high vaginal pH. There could also be exudate from secondary bacterial infection of a malignant tumor or a foreign object (Friedrich, 1976, p. 19, and Birnbaum, 1975, p. 150).

pH readings are useful for purposes of preliminary identification of the various organisms of vag-

initis. These are taken by placing a small piece of nitrazine paper in the anterior or lateral fornix. Normal flora are expected to predominate when the pH is low (3.5 to 4.1) but pathogens replace these normal flora as the pH rises. Candida, for example, occurs with a pH of 4 to 5, and Trichomonas with a pH of 5 to 7. These infections, which are the cause of much distress with younger women, are not as likely or common in older women in the absence of estrogen replacement. The pH of atrophic vaginitis is typically 6 to 7 and this will support many organisms that cannot thrive in a more acidic environment.

Complications

Oral estrogen replacement can result in cardiopulmonary complications. Broad spectrum antibiotics can promote Candida infection which often is recurring and persistent.

Prognosis

Secondary bacterial infection should respond to specific antibiotic therapy. Long term estrogen replacement may be needed for prevention of secondary bacterial invasion. Topical estrogen therapy should afford the woman relief.

Medical Management

Medical treatment of atrophic vaginitis is described by many experts with some discrepancy in suggested therapies. Some authors recommend estrogen creams, suppositories, and/or oral therapy. Others caution against systemic estrogen because of its possible cardiopulmonary complications. Culture is recommended to determine appropriate antibiotic therapy. Use of broad spectrum antibiotic therapy is problematic because it can give rise to Candida infection. A mild disinfectant as Betadine is suggested by some as preferable to antibiotic therapy (Henriques, 1976, pp. 795–796; Benson, 1975, p. 418; Palmer, 1975, p. 672; Friedrich, 1976, p. 20; and Birnbaum, 1971, p. 150).

There is a difference of opinion regarding the use of douches. Birnbaum (1975, p. 150) suggests consideration of indefinite use of an acid douche such as vinegar in conjunction with topical estrogen. Friedrich, however, states little will alter vaginal pH permanently in the absence of "estrinized glycogen-containing epithelium." He discourages douching during atrophic vaginitis because of the problem of traumatizing delicate membrane with the procedure (Friedrich, 1976, p. 20).

Nursing Management

(See "Prevention and Management of Vaginitis," p. 354.)

Candida Vaginitis

Etiologic Factors

Candida vaginitis (sometimes referred to as fungal or yeast vaginitis) is not typical of older women because it thrives with a more acidic pH. It may occur with diabetes mellitus or with antibiotic therapy (Birnbaum, 1971, p. 150). Experience at the Iowa Veterans Home, Marshalltown, Iowa, seemingly supports this statement. Candida became an almost predictable problem on a female unit following antibiotic therapy.

Candida vaginitis is especially problematic because of its high rate of recurrence. Reinfection from body reservoirs may be among the causes of recurrent infections (Palmer, 1976, p. 670). The mouth, nailbeds, skin, urine, and feces harbor this pathogen and confused, incontinent patients could seemingly be at risk of autoinfections after candidiasis has been established.

Candida albicans is the most common species of this vaginitis but other yeasts have also been isolated (Palmer, 1976, pp. 669–670, and Friedrich, 1976, p. 11).

High Risk Situations or Populations

Candida usually is a vaginitis of younger women but it may occur in the elderly diabetic or after antibiotic therapy.

Dynamics

The altered carbohydrate metabolism of diabetics is a favorable environment for fungal proliferation as is the altered intestinal and vaginal flora following antibiotic therapy.

Signs and Symptoms

Manifestations of Candida vaginitis include vaginal and vulvar soreness; difficult or painful intercourse; secondary symptoms of urinary infections; thick, cheesy vaginal discharge; pruritus (often extreme); and vaginal pH of 4–5 (Henriques, 1976, p. 794, and Friedrich, 1976, p. 11).

Differential Diagnosis

The hyphae and buds of the fungus can be identified by wet smear using potassium hydroxide and by fungal culture. Experts caution against indiscriminate therapy, noting Candida is often "overdiagnosed" because the physician relies on subjective symptoms (Palmer, 1975, p. 668; Friedrich, 1976, p. 11; and Henriques, 1976, p. 794).

Complications

Conceivably the fungi could be transferred to other parts of the body.

Prognosis

Since the vaginal pH of older women is not generally favorable for this fungus, it should not present a difficult clinical problem. However, Candida does have a high rate of recurrence and, once established, it may prove troublesome. The uncontrolled geriatric diabetic could harbor this fungus.

Medical Management

Medical treatment for Candida is the use of fungicidal suppositories and cream such as Nystatin. Gentian violet vaginal painting is also used (Friedrich, 1976, p. 13). Oral Nystatin may be given to eliminate reinfection from the GI tract (Henriques, 1976, p. 794).

Nursing Management

(See "Prevention and Management of Vaginitis," p. 354.)

Trichomoniasis

Etiologic Factors

Trichomoniasis is sexually transmitted. History of sexual activity is pertinent to diagnosis. The trichomonas thrives in a pH of 5–7, so it may occur in elderly women though not as readily (Birnbaum, 1971, p. 150).

High Risk Populations

The sexually-active female may contact this parasite.

Dynamics

A protozoa is the causative organism. It lives quiescently in the paraurethral glands, eventually causing overt infection in the susceptible vagina (Friedrich, 1976, p. 15).

Signs and Symptoms

The main clinical manifestation of trichomoniasis is a copious watery discharge that may be odorous and frothy. Hyperemia of the vagina is characteristic. Pruritus may occur. The vaginal pH is generally between 5–7 (Friedrich, 1976, p. 15).

Differential Diagnosis

Diagnosis is confirmed with a saline wet mount that allows visualization of the causative organism, a motile protozoa (Friedrich, 1976, p. 15, and Henriques, 1976, p. 794).

Complications

The sexual partner, if untreated, may harbor the causative organism. However, there is *generally* spontaneous decolonization of the lower male urinary tract (Friedrich, 1976, p. 16).

Candida growth may be encouraged by metronidazole (Flagyl) therapy given for trichomoniasis (Palmer, 1975, p. 669). Nausea may be a side effect of metronidazole, particularly if alcoholic beverages are also used (Friedrich, 1976, p. 16). Diarrhea and decrease in white blood count are also problems associated with this medication (Rowan, 1973, p. 47).

Prognosis

Trichomonas should be eradicated with proper pharmaceutical treatment. Resistant cases probably are due to reinfection. Treatment may be lengthy (Friedrich, 1976, p. 15, and Krupp, 1975, p. 418).

Medical Management

Metronidazole therapy (Flagyl) is effective. A nightly douche of a 20 to 25 percent saline solution produces a temporarily lethal environment for the protozoa and may be used with resistant or recurrent cases (Friedrich, 1976, p. 16).

Prevention and Management of Vaginitis—Nursing Activities

PERINEAL CARE. A clean, dry perineum is basic to preventing growth of pathogens. The perineum of the obese person may be subject to maceration and fissure and may be impossible to keep dry. A small fan or a portable hair dryer may be helpful in coping with this problem but its use may prove to be an uncompromising task for someone with limited mobility. The need to keep the perineum dry is a strong case against tight-fitting pants or geriatric diapers or sanitary napkins. Cotton lingerie always is advised, as is going without pants when the patient finds this acceptable. It is an advantage that many elderly women prefer dresses and garters instead of synthetic slacks and panty hose that only increase moisture problems. The cause for incontinency or dribbling should be remedied whenever possible or bacterial vaginitis may be inevitable.

Perineal care is often neglected or assigned to the least-trained personnel in care settings. The woman who is doing self-care may neglect it entirely or use incorrect technique. Autoinfection becomes a real possibility. Not all persons are aware of the anatomic relationship of the rectum, vagina, and urethra and a mirror or drawings may help the elder visualize what her nurse is describing. Patients should be taught to wipe and cleanse the perineum from the urethra forward and the rectum back. Without this knowledge, even the most alert patient may suffer from autoinfection.

LAUNDRY. Elders living at home may need help with laundering to effectively rid their clothing of pathogenic organisms. Someone who does her own laundry may rinse her garments by hand, failing to destroy pathogens with the simple measure of hot water laundry.

DOUCHES. Douching is a common habit of many older women and its use probably should be discouraged. However, the nurse may not be able to interrupt a lifetime habit; then her actions may best be directed at altering or modifying the methods of douching. Vinegar and saline douche are supported by several experts as safe and useful for giving a feeling of cleanliness. Overuse of douche, however, dilutes the normal vaginal flora and may increase leukorrheic (abnormal vaginal discharge) symptoms by irritating the thin, atrophic membrane. Soda douche should not be used since it is alkaline and the woman already has the problem of a higher vaginal pH. Technique is problematic, particularly when self-douching is practiced. Delicate vaginal membrane may be damaged, or the unknowing patient may substitute contaminated equipment such as an enema tip. A douche of potassium sorbate is useful after coitus for reducing recurrent Candida infection. Pharmacy can prepare a concentrate of this douche from a stock supply of potassium sorbate powder. The concentrate is prepared in a solution of 10 gm/30 ml. One ounce of this concentrate is then used per quart of water (Friedrich, 1976, p. 14).

OVER-THE-COUNTER TREATMENTS. Over-the-counter sprays and deodorants may be tried by the elderly woman who is attempting to combat problems such as odor or pruritus. She may find it difficult to abandon these remedies unless her nurse can help her find suitable treatment for the underlying cause of her discomfort. Most elderly women are familiar with cornstarch dusting of the perineum and this can follow adequate perineal cleansing. However, medical diagnosis and treatment is necessary for persistent discomfort.

SEXUAL ACTIVITY. Dyspareunia is common with vaginitis. Relief of symptoms (as estrogen for atrophic vaginitis) is paramount to comfort. K-Y jelly may be used as a lubricant with coitus after pathogenic organisms are treated. It is especially important that the woman find relief for her vaginal symptoms or she may abandon sexual intercourse. This is an unfortunate circumstance that need not occur.

Intercourse should be avoided or condoms should be used during active treatment of any infectious vaginitis. The sexual partner should be checked for possible surface infection when an infectious vaginitis persists. Treatment should be matter-of-fact and supportive so the woman does not feel embarrassed and reluctant about seeking help.

PHYSICAL EXAMINATIONS. Breast and abdominal examination should accompany speculum examination of the elderly woman. The speculum needs to be smaller and thin bladed to accommodate the small introitus. Caird and Judge note "in the nulliparous patient, only a single finger examination is possible or humane" (Caird and Judge, 1974, p. 46). They report the cervix rarely is palpable in the absence of polypi or cancer and the uterus usually cannot be felt. Pap smear for malignancy should be done yearly. Culture should be used to identify possible bacterial organisms of atrophic vaginitis. Nursing assessment

will rely heavily on verbal report plus examination of discharge, odor, and appearance of the perineum.

FOREIGN BODIES. Vaginal discharge with a confused patient should be investigated for the possibility of foreign body. After the foreign body is removed, gentle physiologic saline irrigation is useful for washing out any retained particles (as toilet paper) from the vagina.

CHECKING PH. pH readings could be a nursing measure routinely used with vaginal infection. These readings should be helpful in differential diagnosis as well as noting vaginal changes that may support pathogens. For example, pH readings would be beneficial if the patient was being maintained on estrogens; susceptibility to Candida could be projected by a drop in pH from the estrogenic replacement. Susceptibility to bacterial vaginitis could be predicted by a higher pH. Nurses could monitor the effectiveness of acid douches with pH readings. pH could be checked at the completion of douching and an hour or so later. If permanent pH benefit could not be demonstrated, it would seem reasonable to suggest alternate therapy.

LABORATORY TESTS. Nursing should advocate use of correct laboratory procedure for diagnosis of vaginitis. Treatment of candidiasis without potassium hydroxide (KOH) smear or fungal culture should be questioned. Saline smear should be used to diagnose Trichomonas and culture should be used to identify the specific organism of bacterial vaginitis.

MEDICATIONS. Topical sulfonamides are commonly used with atrophic vaginitis and they should be advantageous over systemic, broad spectrum antibiotics that are known to alter normal bowel and vaginal flora. Friedrich (1976, p. 20) writes the effectiveness of topical antibiotics is enhanced by the addition of topical estrogen. The use of disinfectants like Betadine appears to be a safe and recommended practice. However, cultures should be taken to monitor whether this treatment is effective. Betadine ointment should not be substituted for good perineal hygiene.

Supporting Sensitive Women's Health Care Services

Elderly women may not receive adequate health care, particularly with sensitive problems like vaginitis. Alternative health care is an avenue that should be explored. The Emma Goldman Clinic in Iowa City, Iowa, is a feminist clinic that promotes preventive care by involving women as active participants in their own care. The role of patient advocate is used. Each woman who comes to the clinic has an advocate who explains examinations and accompanies the woman to her medical appointment. The clinic has conducted menopause clinics and is interested in serving geriatric women. Only 2 to 4 percent of their patients are currently from the over-65 age group. Common problems of the aged female have not been identified partially because of this small percentage of older patients.

Vaginal Health by Carol Horos (1975) is a book nurses may find useful for patient teaching. It is written in lay terms and includes general information concerning anatomy, gynecologic examination, vaginal health, common vaginal infections, and terminology. Numerous pictures illustrate the narrative. Venereal disease, including herpes genitalis, is discussed simply and effectively. A national listing of feminist clinics is also included.

Evaluation of Vaginitis

Evaluation of vaginitis is dependent on good patient rapport. The woman often needs advice about problems such as dyspareunia or vaginal discharge and yet is reluctant to seek it. The nurse needs to reinforce a positive attitude about sexual response and gently probe to discover whether her patient is experiencing any problems. The patient should appreciate that many of her symptoms could be due to lowered estrogen levels and could be remedied.

When a problem area has been identified, then evaluation would be continent on relief of symptoms (i.e., Does pruritus persist? Is there vaginal and vulvar soreness? Has the excessive discharge been eliminated?). The nurse should base her evaluation on verbal reporting and examination results. Looking at the discharge or taking a pH reading has more merit than simply recording absence of subjective complaint.

Evaluation should also include an assessment of daily hygiene. The nurse should know whether the patient is doing good perineal care, whether douche is used, and the adequacy of procedure. The nurse in a care facility should occasionally assist with the patient's bath and with toileting to assess hygiene. The nurse in the community should be able to get clues from the patient's environment. The public health nurse who establishes good rapport will eventually get an opportunity to assess something as personal as perineal care.

BIBLIOGRAPHY

Anderson, H. C.: Newton's Geriatric Nursing, ed. 5. St. Louis: C. V. Mosby Co., 1971.

Anderson, W. F.: Practical Management of the Elderly. Oxford England, Blackwell Scientific Publications, 1971.

Andriole, V.: Hospital acquired urinary infections and the indwelling catheter. Urologic Clin. N. Amer. 2:451–469, 1975.

Basso, A.: Genitourinary tract problems of the aged male. J. Amer. Geriatric Soc. 21:352–354, 1974.

Bates, B.: A Guide to Physical Exam, ed. 2. Philadelphia: J. B. Lippincott Co., 1979.

Benson R.: Gynecology and obstetrics. In Krupp, M., and Cratton, M. (eds.): Medical Diagnosis and Treatment. Los Altos, Calif.: Lange Medical Publications, 1975.

Birnbaum, S.: The genitourinary system: geriatric gynecology, Part VII. Working with Older People. U.S. Department of Health Education and Welfare, Washington, D.C., 1971.

Black, D., and Moore, T.: Urinary infection in the elderly. Geriatrics 24:126–136, 1969.

Caird, F. I., and Judge, T. G.: Assessment of the Elderly Patient. Great Britain: Alden Press, Pitman Medical, 1974.

Caldwell, K. P. S. (ed.): Urinary Incontinence. New York: Grune and Stratton, 1975.

Carbary, L.: Vaginitis. Nursing Care 7:29–31, 1974.

Cowdry, E. V., and Steinberg, F. U.: The Care of the Geriatric Patient, ed. 4. St. Louis: C. V. Mosby Co., 1971.

Culp, D. A.: Benign prostatic hyperplasia: early recognition and management. Urologic Clin. N. Amer. 2:29–48, 1975.

Dale, G.: Iatrogenic urinary infections. Urologic Clin. N. Amer. 2:471–481, 1975.

Diokno, A. C., and Taub, M.: Ephedrine in treatment of urinary incontinence. Urology 5:624–625, 1975.

Drach, G. W.: Prostatis: Man's hidden infection. Urologic Clin. N. Amer. 2:499–520, 1975.

Ehrlich, R. M.: Benign prostatic hypertrophy. In Conn, H. (ed.): Current Therapy. Philadelphia: W. B. Saunders Co., 1976.

Eton, B.: Gynecologic surgery in elderly women. Geriatrics 28:119–123, 1973.

Exton-Smith, A. N., Norton, D., McLaren, R.: An Investigation of Geriatric Nursing Problems in Hospital. London: The National Corporation for the Care of Old People, 1962.

Feustel, D.: Voiding with an autonomous neurogenic bladder: the role of the rehabilitation nurse specialist. Assoc. Rehabil. Nurses J. 1:5–8, 1976.

Fine, W.: Geriatric ergonomics. Gerontological Clinics. 14: 322–332, 1972.

Freeman, J.: Urinary tract infections: prevention, diagnosis and treatment. In Schwartz, A. (ed.): Nephrology for the Practicing Physician. New York: Grune & Stratton, 1975, Ch. 6.

Friedrich, E.: Vulvar disease, Vol. 9. In the series: Major

Problems in Obstetrics and Gynecology. Philadelphia: W. B. Saunders Co., 1976.

Garner, J.: Better urinary catheter care. Nursing '74, 54–56, February, 1974.

Gleason, D., et al.: Active and passive incontinence: Differential diagnosis. Urology 4:693–694, 1974.

Green, T.: Gynecology. Boston: Little, Brown & Co., 1965.

Hazards of immobility. Am. J. Nurs. 67:779–797, 1967.

Henriques, E.: Vaginitis. In Conn, H. (ed.): Current Therapy. Philadelphia: W. B. Saunders Co., 1976.

Hodkinson, H. M.: An Outline of Geriatrics. New York: Academic Press, 1975.

Hoffman, P.: Urinary Tract Infection and Catheter Care. Lecture at Conference Infection Control for Your Institution. Ft. Dodge, Iowa, May 18–19, 1976.

Hole, R.: Urinary tract infections in women. Nursing Times 72:219–221, 1976.

Horos, C.: Vaginal Health. Coroon, Conn.: Tobey Publishing Co., 1975.

Jaffe, J.: The genitourinary system: common lower urinary tract problems in older persons, Part VII. In Working with Older People. U.S. Department of Health, Education and Welfare, Washington D.C., 1971.

Jawetz, E.: Infections of the urinary tract. In Krupp, M., and Cratton, M. (eds.): Medical Diagnosis and Treatment. Los Altos, Calif.: Lange Medical Publications, 1975.

Kahn, A., and Snapper, I.: The genitourinary system: medical renal diseases in the aged, Part VII. In Working with Older People. U.S. Department of Health, Education, and Welfare, Washington D.C., 1971.

Kent, S.: Urinary tract problems in women are linked to sexual activity. Geriatrics 30:145–146, 1975.

Krause, M. V., and Hunscher, M. A.: Food Nutrition and Diet Therapy, ed. 5. Philadelphia: W. B. Saunders Co., 1972.

Krauss, D., Schoenrock, G., and Lilien, O.: Reeducation of urethral sphincter mechanism in post-prostatectomy incontinence. Urology 5:533–535, 1975.

Kropp, K.: Bacterial infections of the urinary tract (male). In Conn, H. (ed.): Current Therapy. Philadelphia: W. B. Saunders Co., 1976.

Krupp, M. A.: Genitourinary tract. In Krupp, M., and Cratton, M. (eds.): Medical Diagonsis and Treatment. Los Altos, Calif.: Lange Medical Publication, 1975.

Kübler-Ross, E.: On Death and Dying. New York: Macmillan Co., 1969.

Kunin, C.: New methods in detecting urinary tract infections. Urologic Clin. N. Amer. 2:423–424, 1975.

Lauritzen, C., and Pieter, A. (eds.): Estrogen therapy, the benefits and risks. In Frontiers of Hormone Research, Vol. 5. S. Kanger, Basel, Switzerland, 1977.

Lowenthal, M., Metz, D., and Patton, A.: Nobody wants the incontinent. RN 82–101, January, 1958.

Lowthian, P. T.: Portable urinals for women. Nursing Times, 1739–1741, October, 1975.

Maney, J. Y.: A behavioral therapy approach to bladder retraining. Nurs. Clin. N. Amer. 179–188, March, 1976.

McIver, V.: The extended care philosophy: a must for the long-term patient. Canadian Hospital, 34–36, November, 1973.

Meares, E.: Prostatitis: a review. Urologic Clin. N. Amer. 2:3–27, 1975.

Metheny, N., and Snively, W. D., Jr.: Nurses' Handbook of Fluid Balance. ed. 3. Philadelphia: J. B. Lippincott Co., 1979.

Mitchell, P. H.: Concepts Basic to Nursing. New York: McGraw-Hill Book Co., 1973.

Moore-Smith, B.: Medicine in old age: urinary tract disease. Brit. Med. J. 29:686–688, 1973.

Palmer, A.: Vaginitis. The Practitioner 214:666–672, 1975.

Palmer, J.: Bacterial infections of the urinary tract (female). In Conn, H. (ed.): Current Therapy. Philadelphia: W. B. Saunders Co., 1976.

Pollock, D. D., and Liberman, R. P.: Behavior therapy of incontinence in demented inpatients. Gerontologist 14:488–491, 1974.

Rodman, M. J.: Drug therapy today: fighting the second most frequent infections. RN 38:91–95, 1975.

Shuttleworth, K. E. D.: Incontinence. Brit. Med. J. 4:727–729, 1970.

Rowan, R., and Gillette, P.: Your Prostate. New York: Doubleday & Co., 1973.

Sotiropoulos, A.: Urinary incontinence. Urology 6:312–317, 1975.

Specht, J.: research critique of Effect of operant conditioning on modification of incontinence in neuropsychiatric geriatric patients, by Jeanette Grosicki, 1972.

Stewart, B.: Prostatitis. In Conn, H. (ed.): Current Therapy. Philadelphia: W. B. Saunders Co., 1976.

Sturdy, D. E.: Essentials of Urology. Great Britain: John Wright & Sons, 1974.

Turck, M.: Therapeutic guidelines in the management of urinary tract infections and pyelonephritis. Urologic Clin. N. Amer. 2:443–449, 1975.

Willington, F. L.: Problems in the aetiology of urinary incontinence (Incontinence-2). Nursing Times 71: 378–381, 1975.

Willington, F. L.: Psychological and psychogenic aspects (Incontinence-3). Nursing Times 71:422–423, 1975.

Willington, F. L.: The nursing component in diagnosis and treatment (Incontinence-4). Nursing Tines 71:464–467, 1975.

Willington, F. L.: Training and retraining for continence (Incontinence-5). Nursing Times 71:500–503, 1975.

Willington, F. L.: The prevention of soiling (Incontinence-6). Nursing Times 71:545–549, 1975.

Willington, F. L.: Incontinence in the Elderly. New York: Academic Press, 1976.

A film, Recurrent Urinary Tract Infection in Older Patients, available without charge from Burroughs Wellcome Company—16mm. (It discusses recurrent urinary infection in men and women, patients with particular urinary problems, and collecting the urine specimen.)

18

Hearing Loss

George Larsen

QUICK REVIEW

HEARING LOSS

DESCRIPTION	Loss may be sensorineural (hearing becomes less acute) or conduction (interference of sound waves)
ETIOLOGIC FACTORS AND HIGH RISK	Catabolic processes of aging, genetics, toxic drugs, infectious diseases (meningitis, measles, mumps, syphilis), endocrine diseases (diabetes, myxedema), ear drum injury, ear infection, cerumen accumulation, long exposure to noise, or trauma to head.
SIGNS AND SYMPTOMS	Report ability to hear but not understand; increasing sound amplitude does not help. Others say they have "selective" hearing loss. Loss of high tones (consonants).
COMPLICATIONS	Withdrawal from human interaction. Paranoia.
NURSING MANAGEMENT	Screen for hearing problems. Refer to reputable audiologist/otologist and instrument. Assist in making a decision re use or type of hearing aid compatible with life style. Assist in adapting to life with new hearing aid. Assist in cost-effective maintenance of hearing aid. Assist individual family to learn habits of communicating that enhance reception of messages. Assist individual to become appropriately assertive in managing communication of others for most effective reception.
EVALUATION	Degree of comfort and satisfaction with hearing aid. Observed or reported pattern of using the hearing aid. Pattern of participation in usual or desired interpersonal activities. Signs and symptoms of paranoia. Activities to maintain instrument in working condition. Behavior to modify communication patterns of others in terms of own hearing deficit.

Hearing impairments constitute the largest chronic physical disability in the United States. There are at least 17 million elderly persons now and by 1980 the number will approximate 24 million. It is estimated that 13 percent of the elderly will suffer sufficient hearing loss to warrant professional attention.

Hearing loss in the older adult must not be viewed simply as an isolated sensory impairment but as a part of the complex tangle of sensory, perceptual, behavioral, and personality changes that may occur in the elderly.

ANATOMY AND PHYSIOLOGY OF HEARING

A cursory review of anatomy and physiology of hearing is given here in order that the nurse may appreciate the impact of hearing loss in senescence.

Sound

Sounds are actually vibrations of the air moving away from the source, somewhat like the ripples of water when a stone is tossed into a pool. These waves have two major characteristics: one is frequency and the other is intensity.

FREQUENCY. The greater the frequency the higher the pitch, and the greater the intensity the more loudly will sound be interpreted. Frequency can be abbreviated to cycles per second and has been known as Hertz or Hz. It is reported that the human ear can hear from as low as 16 Hz to as high as 30,000 Hz. The normal adult, however, usually will have difficulty with anything over 10,000 or 12,000 Hz.

INTENSITY. The intensity of sound often is expressed in decibels (dB) where 0 dB is the intensity that one can barely hear. Each increase of 10dB indicates 10 times the increase of sound intensity. For examples, 0 dB is at the threshold of hearing; 30dB would be a whisper; 60 dB is classified as normal speech; 80 dB might be likened to the noise of heavy traffic and may result in damage to hearing; 100 dB would be consistent with subway noise; 110 dB would be like that of a nearby passing motorcycle; 120 dB would be like a noise of a jet plane; and 140 dB would be like the sound you would hear standing next to a shotgun blast and would result in pain.

Transmission of Sound

The auricles are designed to concentrate sound waves, especially the high frequencies, and conduct them into the external auditory canal and on to the eardrum. The reason we have two ears is to provide stereophonic hearing so that one may judge the direction from which the sound is emanating.

At the proximal end of the ear canal is the eardrum. At the level of the eardrum, the pressure changes of the sound waves are transformed into mechanical vibrations. The eardrum further acts as a barrier to shelter the delicate contents of the middle ear. It may be considered as a rather opaque window through which certain landmarks of the middle ear can be viewed. Normally the tympanic membrane is slightly cone shaped, something like the diaphragm of a loudspeaker. It is surrounded by a thickened band of fibrous tissue called the annulus. Usually the eardrum is described as pearl gray in color in the normal ear. A particular landmark (Fig. 18-1) in the eardrum is the malleus. The long process and the short process of the malleus are embedded in the eardrum. The short process looks something like a tiny knob at the upper end of the manubrium. The umbo is at the

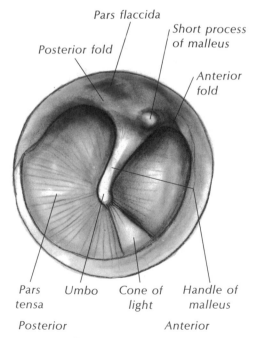

RIGHT EAR DRUM

FIGURE 18-1. Landmarks of the tympanic membrane.

lower end of the malleus, and from the light reflex is directed anteriorly and inferiorly. The significance of the tympanic membrane in diagnosis will be reviewed later.

The three small bones in the middle ear collectively are called the ossicles. Acting as a unit, they conduct vibrations from the eardrum to the oval window, over which lies the footplate of the stapes. These delicate bones not only transmit vibration but they also provide an increase in power that is essential when going from the medium of air to a heavier medium called perilymph in the cochlea. The increase in power is partly accomplished by the leverage relationship of the ossicles. Of greater importance, however, is the fact that the eardrum is much larger than the oval window; thus the vibration of the larger diameter to the smaller is increased by a ratio of about 10 to 1. The vibrations from the oval window set up vibrations in the perilymph which surrounds and bathes the membranous labyrinth containing the end organs of hearing and balance. The cochlea itself is shaped like a snail shell (Fig. 18-2) and, inside of it,

along with numerous other anatomic units, is the organ of Corti. The organ of Corti contains thousands of hair cells, which are the sensory end organs of hearing. The vibration at the oval window is transmitted to the fluid in the cochlea. When the oval window is vibrated or forced inward, the round window "gives" outward. Although there are other anatomic-physiologic aspects in inner hearing, it is sufficient now to say that this fluid movement causes a shearing force on the hair cells, which transforms the sound energy that thus far has been mechanical into electrical impulses. The electrical impulses stimulate the fibers of the 8th cranial nerve to the brain, thus giving rise to the action potentials responsible for nerve transmission. Auditory physiologists generally agree that the hair cells transmit different frequencies, with those responsible for transmitting the higher tones being located at the low end of the cochlea, while those transmitting lower tones are located near the apex.

The hair cells are supplied by nerve fibers, which transmit to the pons in the brainstem. Here the

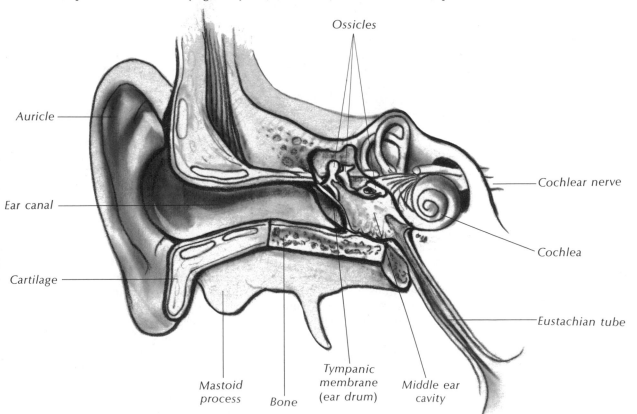

FIGURE 18-2. Anatomy of the ear. (Figures 18-1 and 18-2 are from Bates, 1979)

neural pathways may rise on the same side that they innervate, or they may decussate and cross over to the opposite side. Through a series of synaptic connections, the signal is interpreted in the cortex.

PRESBYCUSIS
(SENSORINEURAL HEARING LOSS)

Hearing loss in the aged may be considered as a catabolic process consistent with other deterioration associated with destructive metabolism. Hearing becomes less acute, usually beginning with high frequencies and progressing toward the low frequencies. In general, this type of hearing loss is referred to as sensorineural, nerve loss, or perceptive deafness.

Etiologic and Risk Factors

Besides the catabolic processes associated with aging, other factors may contribute to the deterioration of hearing. Such diseases as meningitis or viral infections (e.g., measles or mumps), may contribute to hearing loss. High fevers may be a factor in hearing loss, as may diabetes, syphilis, or myxedema. Certain so called ototoxic drugs may contribute to the total hearing loss (e.g., streptomycin, kanamycin, salicylates, and quinine). Although the patient may not remember, it is possible that there has been a contribution to hearing loss from traumatic injuries, such as skull fractures, injury or disease to the eardrum. Exposure to excessive noise also is a factor.

Signs and Symptoms

The person who develops hearing loss is often cast in a distorted world of sound. One may liken this to trying to see through thick fog where the target image is distorted. As the fog increases, the image may be totally absent from view. Individuals who have distorted sound may tend to withdraw from the world and begin to live within themselves, having interference with their primary means of communication. They may begin to appear paranoid as the distortion of sound affects their interpretation of the spoken word. As persons lose the high frequencies of sound, their ability to discriminate speech will become impaired. Frequently they will report that they hear but do not understand. Younger persons around the people suffering presbycusis may blame them for hearing only "when they want to." It is not always

appreciated that the loss of high frequency hearing distorts the high frequency consonant sounds and may leave the low frequency vowels relatively intact. *Understanding of speech depends on the clear perception of the high frequency sounds carried by the consonants* and not on the low frequency sounds of vowels. Individuals with impaired hearing, owing to presbycusis, often hear speech of normal loudness but with impaired clarity.

The first sounds to be lost are some of the *fricative sounds*—f, s, th, ch, and sh.

With greater hearing loss, perception of the *explosive* consonants—b, t, p, k, and d—is also impaired.

If one considers some of the memory impairments described in the other parts of this book and the intellectual changes associated with a stroke, one may quickly see how the additional contribution of presbycusis may accelerate the older person toward what is loosely referred to as senile dementia.

Differential Diagnosis

There is little that can be done medically about presbycusis. However, there is considerable that can be done about conductive hearing loss that may contribute to the total hearing loss, of which presbycusis is only part. As the term implies, conductive hearing loss refers to the interference of the sound wave moving through the ear canal, vibrating the eardrum, and being amplified by the ossicles to vibrate the oval window. In general, disorders interfering with the *mechanics of hearing distal to the oval window may be referred to as conductive hearing loss.*

Assessment

The problems of hearing loss related to aging may be compounded by other hearing problems superimposed upon it. The practitioner needs to know what the hearing loss represents in order to manage or refer it knowledgeably.

Otoscopic Inspection

When examining for hearing loss, a screening otoscopic examination is essential. The relative advantage of the operating versus the diagnostic otoscope is left to the examiner. The speculum placed on the otoscope should be the *largest* that will fit the canal. (The beginning examiner usually makes the mistake of choosing the small speculum when he could use a larger one.)

INSERTION OF SPECULUM. The speculum is inserted to straighten and slightly dilate the cartilage of the ear canal. About halfway to the eardrum, the cartilage ends and the supporting wall becomes bony. Here the speculum pressure is painful. The epithelium lining the bony portion of the canal is very thin and exquisitely sensitive. One must be very gentle when examining this part of the ear canal. In adults the ear canal may be straightened by pulling upward and backward on the auricle. (In young children and infants, it is straightened by pulling the auricle downward.)

HEAD POSITION. The position of the patient's head is most important in aural examination. One might think that with the patient's head perfectly upright, the examiner could look directly through into the ear canal and see the drumhead. This is a common error. Because of the oblique direction of the ear canal, the patient's head must be kept sidewise (toward the opposite shoulder) for easy examination of the canal and drumhead. Students who neglect this step find that they are looking at the wall of the ear canal and not at the drumhead. Usually it is necessary to change the head position several times in order to visualize all parts of the tympanic membrane.

EXAMINING THE TYMPANIC MEMBRANE. When examining the tympanic membrane, attempt to identify the landmarks in the seriatim format (see Fig. 18-1). The landmarks of the normal drumhead vary with differences in the thickness of the drumhead. The malleus is the primary landmark with the short process standing out as a tiny knob and the long process extending inferiorly to about the center of the drumhead. The examiner should attempt to examine the annulus of the eardrum as far as possible, for it is in this area where perforations of the eardrum are most likely to occur. The examiner may see a reflex of light, referred to as the "cone of light," reflecting from the anteroinferior quadrant when the drumhead is in normal position and its epithelium is healthy. Some examiners place a great deal of emphasis on the light reflex and, indeed, its absence may indicate a diseased state. However, too much emphasis should not be placed on the light variation alone.

When examining the drumhead, the color may be of significance in obtaining a clue to the etiologic factors. As mentioned earlier, the healthy drumhead usually is pearly gray and somewhat shiny, although this may all be reduced in the senile eardrum owing to thickening. If the drumhead appears yellow or amber, this may be an indication of serum fluid in the middle ear. If the drumhead appears bluish, and particularly if there is a history of trauma, this may indicate that there is blood behind the eardrum. A white eardrum, like the color of a cottonball, may indicate that there is pus in the middle ear. A red or pink drumhead may indicate an infection of the middle ear called myringitis.

CERUMEN. The most common cause of conductive hearing loss is earwax. Cerumen is a natural protective secretion produced by wax and oil glands located in the ear canal, sometimes with hair follicles in them. Cerumen varies in consistency and amount from person to person because of the relative oil-wax proportion, heredity, coloring of the skin, and exposure to the environment. Excessive wax formation may result from irritating dust or from fungal or bacterial infection in the ear canal, requiring treatment other than removing the cerumen. What appears to be cerumen can actually be hardened discharge from a perforated eardrum or from a diseased canal.

Therefore, besides inspecting the ear canal directly, it is important to inquire about ear disease. If the patient has had otitis media or a perforated eardrum or if you are unsure of what you see through the otoscope, a physician, and preferably an otologist, should remove the material by one or more of several techniques available.

Cerumen Removal. Assuming that there are no contraindications and that the cerumen should be removed, one simple and fast method to use is a dental water pik. If the cerumen is fairly hard or dry, put a few drops of mineral oil or olive oil in the ear canal. Occasionally, the oil takes several hours to soften the cerumen sufficiently. A half-and-half mixture of hydrogen peroxide and mineral oil can be used, but some people find the bubbly noise of the hydrogen peroxide irritating.

The water pik reservoir must be filled with body temperature tap water. If the water is too cold or too warm, it may trigger the vestibular reflex and cause the patient to feel dizzy and nauseated. Turn the pressure of the water jet to its low point and adjust it to greater pressure only as needed. Drape the patient's shoulder with toweling below the ear to be irrigated, and tip his head slightly toward that shoulder. This allows the water to drain more freely. A kidney basin is held below the ear lobe.

It is unlikely that the force of the stream will injure the canal or tympanic membrane, provided space is left around the irrigating tip to let the water escape. One advantage of the water pik tip is that it emits a fine stream allowing ample space for return of water and cerumen. Also, the stream pulsates, which helps break cerumen into small particles and gently but effectively rinses away.

As the cerumen is flushed out, the ear canal should be reexamined with the otoscope. Irrigation stops when the canal is clear. It may be dried by inserting a small length of cotton with a bayonet forceps.

Removal of the wax with a cerumen spoon requires skill. The epithelium, which lines the bony ear canal, is exquisitely sensitive and may bleed when touched. The eardrum itself is less likely to be injured. The cerumen spoon should be smooth edged and must be used under direct vision through an ear speculum. When possible, it is better to insert the spoon and pull the wax forward enmasse rather than pick it out in small pieces. Usually there will be a narrow slit superiorly where the cerumen spoon can be inserted.

Hearing Tests

Only an audiologic study and analysis can provide quantitative information throughout the entire hearing range. An audiologic study is essential before selecting a hearing aid or before deciding on a particular type of otologic surgery. These studies can best be done in combination by an audiologist and an otologist.

It is important to get some information about the type of hearing loss the older patient suffers. Conductive hearing loss should be treated as early as possible to avoid the compounding effects that a conductive hearing loss may have on an already existent sensorineural hearing loss or presbycusis. When a conductive hearing loss is detected, especially after a cerumen plug has been ruled out as the cause, an otlogist should be consulted.

TUNING FORKS. Tuning forks are easy to carry, relatively inexpensive, require little practice in the administration of the test, and are indispensable in a screening examination for hearing loss. The tuning fork tests can differentiate between conductive and perceptive hearing loss. Tuning forks may be purchased in sets ranging from the low to the middle high frequencies, or they may be purchased individually. If only one tuning fork is used, the 500 Hz fork is recommended, because this frequency is less influenced by ambient noise, which one typically finds in a busy institution. If two tuning forks are used, then the next most valuable is the 2000 Hz, because this is a critical frequency in understanding speech. The tuning fork may be best activated by tapping it briskly with a rubber reflex hammer.

Weber Test (Fig. 18-3). Strike the tuning fork with a reflex hammer. Place the vibrating tuning fork on the vortex, forehead, or front tooth (if the person has natural teeth).

Interpretation

Normal hearing or Equal deafness in both ears	will hear in both ears equally
Sensorineural deafness (presbycusis)	will hear tone in *better* ear
Conductive deafness	will hear tone in *worse* ear (because conductive loss masks some environmental noise and cochlea is more efficient in the ear with the conductive loss)

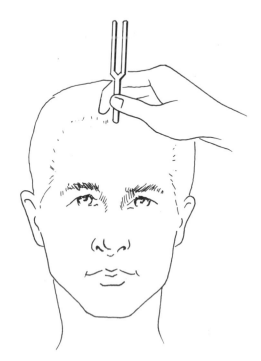

FIGURE 18-3.   Weber test (see text).

Rinne Test. Strike the tuning fork with a reflex hammer and place the handle on the mastoid process (bony prominence behind ear) (Fig. 18-4). Remove the tuning fork from the mastoid process and hold it beside the ear with the tines upward (Fig. 18-5). Ask the person, "Where did you hear the sound better or longer?"

	Interpretation
Normal hearing or Sensorineural deafness	louder beside the ear
Conductive and Sensorineural deafness	equal sound in both places
Conductive deafness	louder on the mastoid process (significantly louder on mastoid process may indicate pure conductive deafness)

SPEECH DISCRIMINATION. Adequate speech discrimination testing cannot be done except with audiometric equipment. However, if a patient reports that he *hears* but does not understand, you may assume that a speech discrimination impairment exists. It may be helpful to stand behind the patient and whisper, or cover your mouth and stand in front of the patient, and ask the patient to repeat the words back to you—sin, fin, thin. The "s," "f," and "th" are high frequency sounds and are easily misunderstood in the patient who has a speech discrimination problem.

Management

Once it has been determined that the older person has a sensorineural hearing loss (presbycusis), one is then faced with the problem of what to do about it. Hearing aids seem to be a natural and logical choice, but a problem is raised immediately. As mentioned previously, the person with a sensorineural hearing loss often does not have a loss of hearing in all frequencies, but rather a reduction in acuity confined to, or more marked at, certain frequencies. Therefore, the hearing is blurred, and if a hearing aid is added to this, the individual's ability to hear is made worse rather than better. This is probably the main reason why so many hearing aids are purchased and then left unused. Another reason for unused hearing aids is that the person may have purchased the hearing aid after becoming accustomed to a certain amount of deafness. When the hearing aid puts people into a world of noises once again, they may find it difficult not only to interpret what is being said because of discrimination impairment but also to

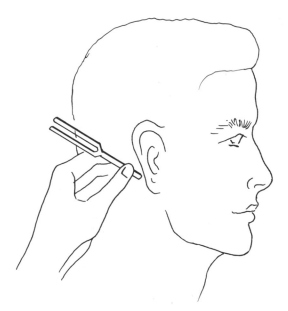

FIGURE 18-4. Rinne test (see text).

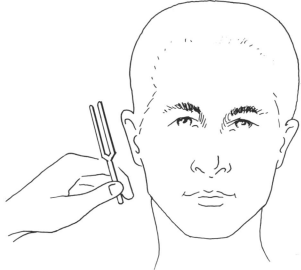

FIGURE 18-5. Second part of Rinne test (see text).

accommodate to the distraction of the noisy world. In cases like this, a hearing aid needs to be selected by a competent dispenser. It should be one that has an amplification curve that helps compensate for the hearing distortion already present.

Although a competent audiologic study and a skilled dispenser of hearing aids will be necessary to properly fit a hearing aid and use it adequately, there are a number of general areas in which the nurse can be of assistance in nearly all cases.

Learning to Live with a Hearing Aid

Understanding the Instrument. Help the person to understand that a hearing aid is a battery-operated, miniature, amplifying system, basically consisting of a microphone, conductive cord, and receiver. It will not cure deafness, nor will it make amplified sounds appear normal. Learning to hear better with the use of the hearing aid requires time and patience. A hearing aid amplifies all of the sounds in our noisy world, not just the sounds we choose to hear. Just as the normal listener, the hearing aid user must learn to ignore the disturbing sounds, and this takes time and practice. If the background noise is overwhelming initially, advise the patient to turn the volume down and watch the speaker's face as he talks.

Wearing the New Hearing Aid. For the new hearing aid user, it is important to wear the aid for short periods of time in the beginning. If the new hearing aid wearer begins to feel nervous or tired, advise the person to turn off the hearing aid and rest for a while. Sometimes it is better to start out with a set period of time, say for about two hours, and add about a half an hour each day until the hearing aid can be worn comfortably from morning until evening.

Volume. A common problem in the use of a hearing aid is to turn the sound too high. This will often distort the sound and blare like a radio when the volume is too great. Another indication of volume being too high, or perhaps a loose-fitting earmold, is a whistling sound or squeal.

Diad and Group Interaction. For the new hearing aid user, it is advisable not to start use of the hearing aid in large groups of people. It is better to start out with one person until the hearing aid wearer is more accustomed to the new sound, and then gradually ease into groups.

Placing the Hearing Aid. Before placing the hearing aid into the person's ear, be sure the switch is off. Straighten the tubing or the cord so that the earmold hangs free with no twist or kinks. For ear level aids, place the hearing aid behind the ear, and then carefully insert the tip of the earmold into the ear canal. Practice before a mirror will help teach the wearer to do this himself, and he should have had some instructions at the time of purchase. For body aids, place the unit where it will be worn, and then proceed to insert the earmold tip. Pull the ear lobe down and, with one hand, gently rotate the mold to conform to the contour of the ear canal. Then push the bottom of the earmold upward and inward. After turning the switch on, adjust the volume to the most comfortable loudness.

Malfunction. If the aid seems not to be working properly, check first to see that the switch is on the "on" position. If the switch is on and the aid still is not working, remove it for closer inspection by first moving the upper portion toward the back of the head. This will disengage the mold from the ear canal, and it can then be removed by simultaneously lifting it up and out. Make sure the cord or tubing is securely fitted into both the aid and the mold since a loose connection may cause a malfunction. Occasionally the channel of the earmold will become blocked by wax. If it is, remove the wax with a toothpick or needle, and then sponge the mold with soap and water and dry it. Sometimes a pipe cleaner run through the channel is needed. Be sure not to get the hearing aid itself wet. If the aid is still not working, open the battery holder and check to see that the battery is inserted correctly. The sign on the battery should be aligned with the sign on the set. When a nonfunctioning aid has a correctly aligned battery, this may indicate that the battery is dead. Remove the old battery and insert a fresh one. You can now test the aid by holding it in your cupped palm with the receiver close to the microphone; turn up the volume. If the aid is working, it will squeal. Turn off the aid and put it on as described previously.

Telephone Use. Some hearing aids, especially the body worn unit, are designed to supply additional amplification that may be needed in special situations, such as telephone. For telephone use, turn the switch marked "T." Then hold the phone upside down with the receiver close to the aid microphone. Sound will then be conducted from the telephone to the aid receiver.

Storage. When the aid is not in use, it should be stored safely away from heat and direct sunlight. It is best to remove the batteries to prevent loss of power. A helpful hint in preserving battery power is to store spare batteries in a refrigerator.

Considerations in Purchasing a Hearing Aid

There is no best hearing aid for all individuals. Aids that test well for one person may not test well for someone else. One should seek professional guidance in obtaining the best aid suited for one's particular problem. There are at least 500 models of hearing aids in the United States market, and they may range in price from as low as $50 to as high as $700 to $800. One would be cautioned to not assume that the more expensive the instrument the better, as many factors go into the pricing of hearing aids, ranging from the details of microelectronics to the profit mark-up.

One of the most significant facts in the multiplicity of available models has to do with the appearance and cosmetics of the hearing aid. Generally speaking, the larger the hearing aid the more capable it is of higher quality sound reproduction. The smaller the hearing aid the more is lost in quality and power.

Types and Power. The body-type hearing aid is the most powerful and probably has the best sound quality, but the cord is cumbersome, and some do not like the appearance. The ear level aid has moderate power and can be worn behind the ear with the tube leading into the ear. It can be hidden by hair. Eyeglass aids are built into the temples of the glasses and are quite expensive, but are hidden. They have moderate power and fair quality. If binaural (both ears) amplification is necessary, glasses are convenient. One problem is that if you take off your glasses, you have no hearing either. This decision needs to be made carefully. The all-in-the-ear model has its only advantage in cosmesis.

Earmold. The earmold is as important as the hearing aid. The earmold must be tailor-made. A soft, plastic, moldable material is first placed in the ear to get a model. This is then prepared in a laboratory, and the full-body model made from this. It is possible to get a semiflex mold for comfort and may be particularly useful for the patient whose ear skin or ear canal is sensitive or subject to skin breakdown. The semiflex mold, however, is more expensive than the hard, acrylic molds. If the earmold does not fit snugly in the ear, then sound will lead around it and back into the microphone, setting up a squeal that is irritating both to the hearing aid user and to those around him who can hear the high pitched squeal. It should be remembered that the cartilage of the ear continues to grow throughout life, and it is possible for the hearing aid user to outgrow the earmold. If the feedback squeal continues, even after the mold has been seated well into the ear canal, then contact with the agency where the aid was purchased should be made again to see if a new mold is needed. One can readily imagine what the squealing interference of noise may do to a person already trying to cope with impaired hearing and adjustment to the hearing aid.

Selection of the Hearing Aid Dealer. Considering the high cost of hearing aids and their upkeep with cords, batteries, cleaning, and adjustments, one would be wise to choose carefully where the aid is purchased. An affirmative answer to a few basic simple questions should help guide one in selecting where to purchase the hearing aid.

1. Does your local Better Business Bureau know of the hearing aid dealer?
2. Does the company offer a rental or trial period before purchase? About a month should be considered adequate. This does not work out well for eyeglass aids or the aid that is built into a tailor-made mold. This can be done only with body aids or ear level aids.
3. Does the company offer training in the use of the aid, that is, help to break it and the purchaser in, how long to wear it at first, where to wear it, and when?
4. How available is service? And how available are batteries?

There has been sufficient controversy about the ethics in use of hearing aids in recent literature that there is serious consideration being given now to selling hearing aids only on the prescription of a physician or written waiver of this requirement.

Research methodology has shown that stereophonic hearing aids, that is, one for each ear, improves the threshold of hearing, increases the ability to discriminate speech, and improves directional hearing. One would think, therefore, that the elderly, if he is going to wear a hearing aid at all, should be fitted with two. However, many report much difficulty adjusting to and using one aid and say that they simply do not want two of them. Even when binaural hearing aids are provided without expense to the person, the disadvantages of using two hearing aids often outweighs the advantages, so that one must be cautious in thinking that two instruments are preferable to one. The practitioner advising the hard-of-hearing elderly person must also take into account how easy it is to manipulate the off-and-on switch and volume dials, as well as to see them.

Communicating with the Hearing Impaired

When communicating with the hard-of-hearing elderly person it is important for nurses, family, and others to remember that there is a deficit in hearing. A hearing loss does not show anything to serve as a reminder of the impairment.

Allow Time to Process Messages. The person with hearing loss uses what hearing is spared but subtly learns also to depend on movement, vision, and tactile sense to get information and maintain contact with the environment. These visual and touch senses take more time to be processed. Thus it is critical to allow for more time in every act of communication.

Get Attention. Before attempting to convey a message, secure the attention of the person. This may be done by speaking their name, pausing, and then conveying the message once the person is looking at your face.

Body Language. Since body language conveys a significant part of your information, be sure not to cover your mouth with your hands or any foreign object. Do not turn your face away in the middle of the message. If you are communicating with two or three persons at a time, be certain to pause at the end of your message to one individual, and then clearly turn the face and look at the recipient of the next message. This will let the hard-of-hearing person know you are finished speaking to him and avoids the embarrassment of having to ask if the conversation is over.

Do not stand in the glare of a bright light or with one's back to a window, but, rather, stand in lighting where your face is easily seen, because facial expression is used. In spite of the importance of the face in communicating, it is important not to exaggerate lip movements. This will distort the facial expressions and the lip reading that the individual may be doing. Likewise, do not shout, because shouting also tends to distort facial muscles, and if the patient is wearing a hearing aid, it will cause a sudden distortion in the amplified sound.

Length of Sentences. It is helpful to use short phrases rather than lengthy sentences. If the person does not understand the first time, then repeat the information, using different words. It is also helpful to use pictures and demonstrations in certain situations.

Intercoms and Telephones. In institutions where communication between staff and patient is done by intercom, a label should be applied at the intercom station warning that a particular patient is "deaf." Convey the message in person to that individual.

Large telephone companies and many who provide reputable services to the hard-of-hearing and deaf can provide amplifying devices to fit telephones. Other devices may be attached to radios and television sets providing personal amplification. Special alarms that use lights rather than sounds are available to awaken the hard-of-hearing or warn them of fire.

Speaking Tubes. For the practitioner specializing in geriatric care, it may be worth purchasing a speaking tube, which is the modern version of the old hearing horn. This device has no electronics or amplifying gear but is simply a means of concentrating sound so that it may be directed to the ear.

Hearing and Memory Impairment. In some instances, you may be coping with a combination of hearing loss and memory impairment. In cases like this, it is useful to establish relationship with the patient where the disorders are recognized and agreement made that you will do your best to cope with them. Having the patient repeat the gist of the message conveyed will assure that it has been heard and helps to reinforce the auditory memory. It goes without saying that paper and pencil should be kept at hand to serve purposes of both memory impairment and hearing loss.

Complications

Relationships are the cornerstones of our existence. Communication is the key to our relationships with people, and hearing is the basis of communication. We are with people in almost everything we do, and we are even with them when we are alone. We fantasize about them in our waking hours, and we dream of them when we are asleep. If our hearing, and thus communication, becomes depleted or impaired, as often happens in the older patient who has impaired sound and sight, one may count on producing hallucinations, imaginary voices, and even visions. This has been proven again and again in experiments where the subjects have been totally isolated from sound and sight. Apparently our need for communication and relationship with other people is so great that, deprived of them, our brain makes facsimiles in an attempt to compensate. This is worth remembering when the practitioner attempts to correlate hearing loss with other factors in understanding the older person.

BIBLIOGRAPHY

DeWeese, D. D., and Saunders, W. H.: Textbook of Otolaryngology, ed. 4. St. Louis: C. B. Mosby Co., 1973.

Dublin, W. B.: Fundamentals of Sensorineural Auditory Pathology. Springfield, Ill.: Charles C Thomas Co., 1976.

Hansen, C. C.: The etiology of perceptive deafness. Acta Otolaryngologica, Supplement 309, Stockholm, Sweden: Almquvist and Wiksell Periodical Co., 1973.

Katz, J.: Handbook of Clinical Audiology. Baltimore: William & Wilkins, 1972.

Knapp, P. H.: Emotional aspects of hearing loss. In Psychological and Psychiatric Aspects of Speech and Hearing. Springfield, Ill.: Charles C Thomas Co., 1960.

Larsen, G. L.: Removing cerumen. Amer. J. Nurs., 76:264–265, February 1976.

Madell, J. R.: The hard of hearing patients. J. Practical Nurs. 23:22–24, 1973.

Otologic diagnosis and treatment of deafness. Clin. Symposia-CIBA, Volume 22, No. 2, 1970.

Schein, J. D.: Deafness in the United States: 1970. Highlights 53:9–11, 1974.

Speaking Tube, 1977. Hal-Hen Company, 36-14 11th Street, Long Island City, N.Y. 11106. (Cost $25,00)

19

Hypertension

Nancy J. Roben

QUICK REVIEW

HYPERTENSION

DESCRIPTION	Sustained elevation of blood pressure above normal for a given age. Criteria vary, but evidence of target organ damage is significant.
ETIOLOGIC FACTORS	Atherosclerotic processes are presumed to contribute to elevated systolic pressure in majority of elderly. Life-long patterns of coping with social and environmental stresses may be important considerations. Renovascular hypertension must be suspected with sudden onset of diastolic hypertension.
HIGH RISK	Majority of persons surviving to 70+ will probably never develop significant hypertension.
DYNAMICS	Arterial pressure is product of cardiac output and peripheral resistance. Increases in peripheral resistance increase diastolic pressure.
SIGNS AND SYMPTOMS	Usually a "silent disease."
DIFFERENTIAL DIAGNOSIS	Accurate diagnosis of hypertension contingent upon obtaining precise, valid blood pressure readings.
PROGNOSIS	No clear indication whether treatment reduces mortality in older-age group.
COMPLICATIONS	Damage to target organs—brain, heart, retina, and kidney. Risks of treatment with overly-aggressive management.
PREVENTION	Emphasis on detection and treatment of adults.
MANAGEMENT	Weight control, sodium restriction, balanced rest and activity levels, relaxation and socialization measures need to be initial priorities. Knowledgeable participation by patient in regimen. Regular supervision/assessment by health care provider.
EVALUATION	Ascertain that the goals of therapy do not seriously impair the quality of life and preferred lifestyle. No clear indicators of results of treatment of hypertension in older persons.

Over the past several decades, health professionals have become aware of the prevalence of hypertension and its significance as a health problem in the adult population. Consequently, there has been a major shift in attitude by health care providers and the community toward detection and treatment programs.

Nurses in a variety of clinical settings are now assuming more of the health care responsibilities in these screening and treatment programs. The Amos Project at Fort Belvoir, Veterans Administration hypertension clinics, and the Ambulatory Care Projects at the Beth Israel Hospital in Boston are but a few of the examples of practice settings where nurses have demonstrated their ability to help patients with hypertension live with a chronic health care problem.

A pattern of responsibility is now developing wherein nurses are being expected to assume growing responsibility for the elderly and their health care problems. When nurses assume these expanded roles, there must be a basic understanding of the health problem of hypertension in the general population. A bibliography is included at the end of this chapter. This will supplement necessary clinical observations and experiences in the care of hypertensive patients before appreciating hypertension in the geriatric setting.

Description

Hypertension (high blood pressure) may be defined as a sustained elevation of blood pressure above that which is considered normal for a given age. Its multifactorial genesis is not well understood. A primary mechanism is presumed to be an increase in the peripheral resistance in the systemic circulation, resulting from vasoconstriction of the very small arterioles. It is thought that some factor is present which contracts the smooth muscle in the arteriolar wall to produce this constriction. These arterioles act much like a nozzle on a garden hose. When the nozzle opening is narrowed, pressure builds up. In the hypertensive patient these arterioles clamp down, thus preventing blood flow to the capillaries. Then the heart must pump harder, increasing the pressure in the arteries.

Acknowledgment is made to Thomas S. Inui, Sci. M, M.D., Assistant Professor of Medicine and Health Services, University of Washington, Seattle, for assistance in review of this chapter.

In most people with high blood pressure the mechanism that causes this marked narrowing of the lumina of the arterioles is obscured. In the geriatric population it may be even more complex since physiologic changes associated with aging must be considered.

The determination of the dividing line between hypertensive and normotensive blood pressure in the aged is somewhat arbitrary. The American Heart Association recommends an age-related definition of hypertension.

Under 40 years of age . . . .140/90 or greater

Over 40 years of age . . . . .140/95 or greater

One commonly held belief in the past was that the systolic blood pressure should be 100 + age. This rule made no reference to diastolic blood pressure level, which we now realize is perhaps most significant. Nonetheless, viewpoints differ among health care providers as to when it should be treated and how the management should progress. Nurses in both institutional and home health care settings will see varying criteria and philosophies of management. In an increasing number of medical facilities, physicians and health care providers are defining an elevated blood pressure greater than 180/100 as abnormal for the elderly patients who have evidence of target organ damage—brain, heart, kidney, and retinal blood vessels.

Etiologic Factors

Usually hypertension is classified arbitrarily as primary or secondary. Primary hypertension has no known or readily identifiable causes. Almost 90 to 95 percent of the hypertensives are classified as having primary or essential hypertension.

It is assumed, in the elderly population, that atherosclerotic processes contribute to this elevated arterial pressure. Consequently, other identifiable causes may be more obscure if hypertension has been of long duration. Frequently, the elevation is predominantly systolic and disproportionate to the diastolic rise. There is loss of elasticity in the aorta so that the intra-aortic systolic pressure rises more abruptly. In addition, the larger muscular vessels lose elasticity and become more rigid. These degenerative changes are accompanied by hyperplasia within the vessel and result in decreasing the caliber of the lumen of the vessel. In some cases these atherosclerotic processes occur in the renal arteries and contribute to a cycle of progressively worsening hypertension.

There are many other postulated causes of primary hypertension, including theories suggesting an over-reactive sympathetic nervous system or change in baroreceptor functioning. Baroreceptors are stretch receptors located in the walls of the heart and blood vessels, particularly the aortic arch. It is thought that they are stimulated by distension of the structures where they are located. Impulses generated by baroreceptors result in vasodilatation, a drop in blood pressure, slowing of the heart rate, and a decrease in cardiac output. One theory suggests that, in hypertension, these baroreceptors may actually be "reset" at a higher level. To what extent this proposed increased sympathetic nervous system activity may be considered a factor in the elderly hypertensive patient is unclear. Certain studies have shown, however, that sympathetic nervous system responsiveness declines with age.

Some observers believe that life-long patterns of coping with social and environmental stresses may contribute to the complex phenomenon of hypertension. However, studies in certain native populations where the pace of life appears to be relaxed, have shown a relatively high prevalence of hypertension. Nor does urban living alone seem to be an important factor, at least in the United States where hypertension is considerably more prevalent among rural Southern blacks than among blacks living in large cities.

The renin-angiotensin-aldosterone system has been studied extensively as a factor in the pathophysiology of essential hypertension. In an interesting study of male hypertensive patients ages 18 to 35 with essential hypertension, a behavioral pattern of suppressed hostility was found in the group of patients who had elevated renin activity. It was proposed that this might be a link with increased sympathetic activity (Esler, et al., 1977). At present there remain many inconsistencies. Renin, a vasoconstrictor substance produced by the kidney, is easily mismeasured and misinterpreted. To what extent it may be of importance in understanding the elderly hypertensive patient is not known. At this time its measurement is not routinely advocated.

It has also been recognized that hypertension and hypertensive cardiovascular complications as well as atherosclerotic complications tend to occur in families. This link with heredity is helpful in establishing the diagnosis of essential hypertension.

A positive correlation between cigarette smoking and sustained hypertension has not been demonstrated. Cigarette smoking is known, however, to aggravate atherosclerosis. In combination with hypertension, it greatly increases the risk of atherosclerotic complications, particularly coronary artery disease. However, in the elderly population its impact on the development of hypertension or its control is considered to be slight.

Certain studies have raised the possibility that regular consumption of alcohol is associated with hypertension. One such study strongly suggests that regular use of three or more drinks of alcohol per day is a risk factor for hypertension (Klatsky, et al., 1977). More data are needed. To what extent alcohol consumption may be of importance in the hypertensive elderly patient is not known.

Hypertension is considered to be secondary if its occurrence can be clearly attributed to an underlying disease or pathophysiologic condition. Secondary causes include adrenal medullary tumor and states of excessive mineralocorticoid secretion such as Cushing's disease or aldosteronoma. These conditions are presumed to be even less common in the elderly than in the younger hypertensive population. They are rare and do not warrant routine extensive laboratory evaluations to exclude.

Renovascular hypertension must be suspected, however, when there is a sudden onset of diastolic hypertension. It may occur in the elderly when an atherosclerotic lesion in a renal artery becomes the site of a thrombotic or embolic process.

Hypertension in the elderly may also be classified as systolic or diastolic or combined systolic and diastolic. Atherosclerotic processes are presumed to be contributory to the elevated systolic pressure in the majority of elderly patients. In addition, however, systolic hypertension in this age group may present itself as a manifestation of severe anemia, Paget's disease of the bone, thyrotoxicosis, and aortic regurgitation, all representing hyperdynamic circulatory states.

Epidemiologic Factors

The consensus of longitudinal studies in population groups indicates the blood pressure rises with age. The prevalence of definite hypertension also seems to rise with age. The National Health Examination Survey of 1962 found that nearly 40 percent of all persons between 75 and 79 years of age had hypertensive disease (National Center for Health Statistics, 1966). This was based on the World Health Organization criterion of a diastolic blood pressure greater than 95 mm Hg. These percentages are of interest when one considers that the survey represented a random sample of the population prior to the advent of detection and treatment programs of the late 1960s and early 1970s.

The Proceedings of the National Conference on High Blood Pressure Education (1973) documents the occurrence of high blood pressure in the adult population of the United States (ages 18 to 79) as follows: approximately 15 percent of whites are afflicted and 28 percent of blacks. The criteria utilized was a systolic ≥ 160 and/or diastolic ≥ 95 mm Hg. We do not currently have accurate data that reflect the dimensions of the problem of hypertension in the over-80 age group.

Certain epidemiologic studies, however, may help us gain some awareness of its prevalence. In 1968, Borhani and coworkers (Borhani, et al., 1975) examined the epidemiologic factors of blood pressure from four population surveys. The age of the population ranged from 15 to 75+ years. The upward trend of average systolic pressure with increasing age was noted. The pattern was similar for males and females in black and white population groups. Two additional insights emerged. Blood pressure tended to be greater in males than in females up to age 55. The reverse appeared to be true after the age of 55, with female blood pressures exceeding those of males. Blacks at any age and of either sex had substantially higher systolic pressures than did whites. The health care provider must keep in mind, however, that the natural history of hypertension is extremely variable in different patients and in the two sexes.

Epidemiologic studies in other cultures, as in the Gilbert Islands and New Guinea, seem to show that hypertension is not prevalent; nor does the blood pressure rise with age. Some investigators believe that a low salt intake may account for this virtual absence of hypertension in these more primitive societies. Additional observations have been made in Japan. In a northeast province, where salt intake approximated 30 gm per day, the incidence of severe hypertension and stroke was found to be very high (Sazaki, 1964).

The evidence for the role of salt in the development of hypertension is indeed controversial. However, in a population where salt is an acquired taste learned at a very early age by flavoring infant foods, one wonders what implications there might be in considering the pathogenesis of hypertension in the aging adults of this society.

Studies of utilization of salt by older persons are not available. It might be predicted, however, that there could be an increase in salting of food as taste buds involved in perceiving sweet and salty flavors are among those that show the greatest decrease with age. It is estimated that almost 64 percent of taste buds have been found to be lost by age 75. Research has also shown that it then requires greater intensity of stimulation to allow the older person with fewer taste buds to experience the taste sensation. It would seem reasonable to think that older adults who have grown up enjoying salt in their food might add more to achieve the same taste experience. Exploration of usual/preferred patterns in salt preference and the intake in the older person would be an important nursing assessment item, particularly in the patient with any degree of renal failure.

High Risk Populations or Situations

Which individuals in the above 65- to 70-age group will develop hypertension? No one knows. Perhaps the majority of elderly persons who have managed to survive to this age group may never develop significant diastolic or systolic hypertension.

Hypertension in the elderly may presume two *common* situations. One represents early onset of hypertension where the patient has managed to progress to older age despite the condition. The second is late onset in which there is a relatively recent elevation occurring at an older age. Aged patients with recent blood pressure elevation may reflect a history of lability during the course of a lifetime, gradually progressing with age to a sustained hypertension. In other patients a sudden onset of elevated blood pressure may be indication of renovascular hypertension secondary to rapidly progressing atherosclerotic disease.

Dynamics

Blood pressure is simply the lateral force exerted against the walls of the arteries as blood flows from the heart. The pressure in the aorta and other large arteries rises to a peak value (systolic pressure) during each heart cycle and falls to a minimum value (diastolic pressure). This arterial pressure is the product of two forces: cardiac output and peripheral resistance. Most of the peripheral resistance occurs in the arterioles and is governed by the contraction of their walls.

The caliber of the arterioles and arteries is under both nervous and chemical control. This is an important concept to have in mind when considering the antihypertensive drugs and how they are presumed to be effective. Nervous impulses from reflex centers in the brain may constrict or dilate the vessels. Chemical substances may alter the size of blood vessels either by acting directly in the vessels or by stimulating sensory receptors and, thus, initiating reflex control.

In general, increases in cardiac output increase the systolic pressure, whereas increases in peripheral resistance increase the diastolic pressure. An important cause of the rise in systolic pressure is decreased distensibility of the arteries (atherosclerotic process) as their walls become increasingly more rigid. At the same level of cardiac output, the systolic pressure is higher in the elderly because there is less increase in the volume of the arterial system during systole to accommodate the same amount of blood because of loss of vascular elasticity.

Health care providers who are assuming major responsibility in the care of elderly hypertensive individuals must have some understanding of these complex interrelationships. They are covered in depth in an excellent programmed instructional text, *Introduction to the Nature and Management of Hypertension* (Freis, 1974).

Differential Diagnosis

An accurate diagnosis of hypertension in itself is contingent upon obtaining a precise and valid blood pressure reading. It is particularly important in the older-age group so that potent and potentially hazardous treatment methods are not recommended needlessly. The American Heart Association (AHA: Recommendations for Human Blood Pressure Determination by Sphygmomanometers) has outlined a method that establishes greater reliability and uniformity in obtaining blood pressure readings. In the elderly special precautions will need consideration when taking the blood pressure:

1. The cuff must fit snugly and provide uniform compression of the extremity. Hemiplegic patients should have the cuff applied to the unaffected extremity.
2. The width of the cuff should be 20 percent greater than the diameter of the limb on which it is used. Use a smaller width cuff on thin or emaciated patients.
3. The lower edge of the cuff should be 1 inch above the bell of the stethoscope.
4. The patient should be positioned quietly for a few minutes prior to taking the recording. The artery over which the blood pressure is being recorded should be located at heart level.
5. The systolic blood pressure should be first determined by the palpatory method. This is done by taking the radial or popliteal pulse if the lower extremity is being used when the cuff is being inflated. The cuff should then be inflated to approximately 20 to 30 mm Hg above the pressure at which the pulse disappears. This will increase the probability of obtaining an accurate systolic pressure—a critical determination in the elderly.
6. When blood pressure sounds are difficult to hear, elevating the extremity above heart level or asking the patient to make a fist and release will frequently increase audibility of the diastolic sound.
7. If successive readings are to be taken, the cuff should be deflated completely between determinations to permit venous return to occur.

Blood pressure reading should be taken in at least two positions—lying or sitting *and* standing. This will enable the nurse to determine any postural changes that can be commonly noted in persons with significant atherosclerotic disease or dehydration. This will also be an important observation when patients are taking antihypertensive agents to minimize potential complications of therapy.

It is important to obtain several base line readings in the older person with newly elevated or recently noted blood pressure elevation. Blood pressure should be taken in both upper extremities with differences noted, particularly if either extremity has sustained injury or incurred disablement from stroke. These base line readings can be done on subsequent clinic visits, or consecutive days in a residence, clinic, or perhaps more accurately at home. Some patients might take their own blood pressure but this ability should be carefully evaluated when blood pressure values may be *critical* to differentiate presence or absence of elevated blood pressure. It is important to remember that the blood pressure often is responsive to emotional and environmental changes. Stress, apprehensions, or uncomfortable sensory environments have a high risk of increasing systolic blood pressure. These factors may be maximized in the medical facility setting.

Elderly patients with irregular heart rates present special problems in obtaining accurate blood pressure readings. In atrial fibrillation, the strength of each beat varies considerably. During early cuff deflation, only a few strong beats are heard, becoming more numerous as the cuff is further deflated. Often an estimate must be made by repeated determinations.

There have been differences of opinion among health care providers regarding the sounds that should be utilized as criteria in determining systolic and particularly diastolic blood pressures. In some settings this has increased the variability in readings. As the cuff pressure decreases there are a series of sounds that are heard. These Korotkoff sounds have five phases (Geddes, 1970).

Phase 1—the first sounds heard as the blood pressure cuff is deflated. It consists of a clear tapping sound which gradually increases in intensity.

Phase 2—during further deflation, a softer muffled sound replaces the clear tapping tone of phase 1.

Phase 3—the reappearance of a sharper tone resembling the first phase but less well marked.

Phase 4—a sudden change when the tapping becomes muffled.

It has been generally agreed that the first sound (Phase 1) can be read as the systolic blood pressure. But there has been no unanimity as to which phase corresponded to the indirect diastolic pressure.

In 1976, however, the Joint National Committee on Detection, Evaluation, and Treatment of High Blood Pressure recommended that the diastolic pressure should be equated to the *disappearance of sound.*

Extensive laboratory testing of the elderly hypertensive patient to differentiate secondary causes of the blood pressure elevation is generally not recommended. In view of the rarity of many of the specific recognizable causes of elevated blood pressure, coupled with both the cost in dollars and the small but real risk to the elderly patient of certain diagnostic procedures, it is recommended that more complex work-up be reserved for the severely elevated blood pressure that perhaps occurs suddenly and is not responsive to the usual treatment modalities.

Manifestations

Despite the wealth of symptoms ascribed to hypertension by many authors and health care providers, there is no characteristic sign, symptom, or syndrome. The blood pressure is simply elevated. It has been referred to as a "silent disease." For exam-ple, headaches frequently do not accompany even severely elevated pressures. Many patients actually feel well and the elevation is casually noted when the patient seeks health care for a minor problem such as an upper respiratory infection.

In the elderly, associated processes of cerebral vascular atherosclerosis may be suggested by unsteady gait, memory deficits, transient ischemic attacks, and strokes. In addition, a history of substernal pain aggravated by exercise or emotion and relieved by rest may suggest coronary artery disease. These signs and symptoms should suggest the possible sequences of ongoing arterial disease known to be aggravated by hypertension.

Complications

In previous sections we have referred to some of the complications of hypertension. One of the major challenges to the geriatric health care provider is to *identify* elderly patients with sustained blood pressure levels in the range of 100+ mm Hg diastolic and/or 180+ mm Hg systolic. Their evaluation should then be directed toward ascertaining damage to target organs (brain, heart, retina, kidney), to estimate the biologic significance of the hypertensions.

Concomitant associated problems such as congestive heart failure must be considered. In the Framingham Study (Kannel, et al., 1972) it was found that in 75 percent of patients with congestive heart failure in the age range from 30 to 62 years, the dominant etiologic precursor was hypertension. At this time there are no similar studies of an older population with which similar conclusions might be drawn.

Another important finding from the Framingham Study (Kannel, et al., 1970) was that increased cardiovascular mortality and/or morbidity was associated with both systolic and diastolic blood pressure elevation. Women with normal diastolic blood pressure but borderline or definitely hypertensive systolic pressure have a risk 50 percent above the standard. With these findings in mind, the disproportionate rise in systolic pressure seen in aging must be looked at with concern. Again, there are no similar studies for people over age 62.

Data from the Framingham Study has recently been analyzed to show that there are certain cardiovascular risk factors that *appear* to be important considerations in the geriatric age group. Little can be done to alter age, sex, or heredity factors. The most controllable of these risk factors was felt to be hypertension (Castelli, 1976).

In the Chicago Stroke Study (Shekelle, et al., 1974) patient characteristics related to stroke in a population of noninstitutionalized persons 65 to 74 years of age were examined. In both black and white persons, it was found that hypertension was significantly associated with increased risk of stroke. Applying the data from this study, these investigators implied that 25 percent or more of the total incidence of stroke in persons 65 to 74 years of age may be attributable to hypertension.

These studies are difficult to ignore when considering the elderly patient with hypertension. It is certain that studies of population will need to be done in the very near future. At present we simply do not clearly know which patients present the greatest risk both to the elevated blood pressure and to the treatment of hypertension.

One cardiac complication may need additional interpretation. When the workload of the heart becomes too great in pumping blood against the elevated peripheral resistance/pressure, the heart (especially the left ventricle) may become enlarged and act as a reservoir for abnormal amounts of blood because it is then an inefficient pump. Pressure backs up into the lungs and symptoms of congestive failure can occur. As the heart muscle increases in size, the blood supply (coronary arteries) to the heart itself becomes inadequate and symptoms of coronary insufficiency with chest pain may occur. Myocardial infarction could become a part of this sequelae or logical consequence. This is a very simplified explanation of a complication of hypertension frequently referred to as hypertensive heart disease. It can occur when sustained hypertension, often in combination with atherosclerosis, is ignored or poorly controlled.

Long term behavioral effects may also be associated with hypertension. There is some suggestion that intellectual change may occur. A study at Duke University Center for the Study of Aging and Human Development (Wilkie and Eisdorfer, 1971) found that diastolic hypertension ($\geq$ 105 mm Hg) was related to significant intellectual loss over a 10-year period among individuals initially examined in their 60s. Antihypertensive drug usage could not be controlled in this study.

In addition to the complications of the elevated blood pressure, there must be concern regarding complications of therapy. Special considerations are crucial when patients on antihypertensive agents are moved along the health care continuum. The following case synopses illustrate some of these potential complications of therapy.

> Mr. B, age 72, was admitted to a hospital surgical unit for a repair of an inguinal hernia. He has had hypertension for several years. He has been taking a diuretic and methyldopa 250 tid. His blood pressure on admission was 170/95 mm Hg. The morning after admission he collapsed on the floor and hit his head while trying to get out of bed.

This particular example illustrates frequent complications of drug treatment when the patient is taken from his home setting. When, in the more organized hospital setting, the patient encounters more or less stress and better dietary sodium observation combined with bedrest and less exercise, the hypotensive episodes can be common. To help prevent these episodes, the blood pressure should be routinely monitored in both lying and sitting positions, even though the patient is both ambulatory and well.

> Mrs. A, age 82, is no longer able to live alone in her home. Her relatives arrange for her to go to a nursing home. Her admission orders include her antihypertensive drugs and a low sodium diet that she had been prescribed but poorly adhered to at home. Five days after admission she collapses after leaving the dining room.

The alert health care provider might have questioned whether the antihypertensive drugs had actually been taken prior to nursing home admission and what the normal dietary patterns have been.

> The Mr. B in our preceding example had a successful hernia repair. His antihypertensive medications were never reinstituted postoperatively because the blood pressure continued to be about 150–160/80–90 mm Hg. Two weeks after the hospital discharge he was seen in the outpatient clinic as a follow-up visit. His incision was well healed. His blood pressure was 200/104 mm Hg.

This is a frequent finding in outpatient settings. Patients do not restart their antihypertensive medicines and the blood pressure goes back up. When patients are discharged from hospitals, health care providers must review the *total* plan of care with the patient and family.

When stroke or myocardial infarction occurs in the hypertensive patient, the blood pressure occasionally returns to normotensive levels post-hospital. Why this occurs in unclear. Care must be taken to follow the blood pressure of these patients. The nurse must be alert to reestablishment of hypertensive levels, if they should recur.

There is an increased potential for drug problems in the geriatric population when multiple drugs are taken or more potent drugs are utilized. If malnutrition and/or liver or kidney impairment are factors, there is even a greater danger. Acute episodic illness, as common to any age group, may pose additional hazards for the elderly patient who is taking antihypertensive agents. Hypotensive episodes should be anticipated then and drug dosages may need to be tapered. Patients, families, and health care providers all need to be alerted to these risks.

The elderly person is also vulnerable to the side effects of the antihypertensive agents that the younger patient experiences. Impotence and increased libido may be of great concern to the sexually-active older person. This is when patient-health care provider rapport is critical. Is sexual activity important to this patient and/or his partner? The health care providers may not wish to alert the patient or partner to these side effects (impotence or decreased libido) if they are concerned about suggesting a side effect that may not occur. It is important, however, to ascertain whether changes in sexual lifestyle have occurred, especially shortly after patients are started on either methyldopa or reserpine.

In addition, reserpine and methyldopa may promote or contribute to an underlying depression. If cerebral vascular atherosclerotic disease is present in the elderly, these and other potent antihypertensive agents may further compromise the psychologic equilibrium by increasing symptoms of depression and decreasing mentation.

Frequently observed side effects of diuretics include hyperglycemia, hypokalemia, hyperuricemia, and/or acute gout and muscle cramps. Older patients who are taking concurrent digitalis preparations will need to have their potassium monitored periodically or hypokalemia can lead to arrhythmias and death. Potassium-rich foods (see Chapter 9, page 149, for list), eaten regularly, may not be adequate, readily available, or economically practical. Potassium salts (substitute salt) may be helpful. There is a recent trend to not replace potassium in all individuals as there is controversy as to whether serum potassium always reflects body potassium levels over a long period of time. Symptoms of hypokalemia include neuromuscular disturbances (weakness and paresthesias) and cardiac abnormalities (arrhythmias, increased sensitivity to digitalis, and ECG changes). Potassium may be depleted severely before symptoms occur.

When potassium replacement drugs or potassium-sparing diuretics are used, hyperkalemia will need to be recognized particularly in patients with renal disease. In these patients even use of salt substitutes will be dangerous as there will be decreased renal excretion of potassium. Symptoms of hyperkalemia include the same neuromuscular manifestations as hypokalemia.

As the health care provider gains more experience in the care of the elderly hypertensive population, it becomes more apparent that each patient situation must be evaluated individually as to the significance of the hypertension. There are no clear guidelines. The risks of treatment may be in fact greater than the goals of therapy.

Prognosis

At this time there are no clear indications of the results of treatment of hypertension in older individuals. While antihypertensive therapy has been shown to reduce mortality in the under-60 age groups, it is difficult to know if there are similar implications for treatment with people who are older. It may be that the risks of treatment, the disaccommodations to lifestyle associated with management, and the side effects of pharmacologic agents may outweigh the goals of therapy by seriously impairing the quality of life in those over age 70 who have mild or moderate hypertension.

Prevention and Management

Hypertension in indeed a common condition in the adult population. One key to the prevention of dangerous hypertension in the elderly is emphasis on treatment and detection at an earlier age. Hypertension is simply and inexpensively determined. It has been recommended by the Joint National Committee on Detection, Evaluation, and Treatment of High Blood Pressure (1977) that all persons older than 50 years of age with a blood pressure between 140/90 and 160/95 mm Hg should be checked every 6 to 9 months.

Criteria for Medical Management Regimes

At this point, however, medical opinion varies as to the treatment indications and subsequent management. Multiple factors need to be considered in every geriatric patient prior to initiating therapy.

1. What is the total health status of the individual?

2. Are there other complicated social and economic problems?
3. Is there a history of congestive heart failure or cerebrovascular attack?
4. Might a major reduction in blood pressure immobilize this patient by reducing cerebral blood flow and decreasing mentation?
5. What alterations in lifestyle will the treatment program imposed on the patient/family?
6. What will be the patient participation in the program?

Management of Life Style

Nurses can assume a major responsibility in the management of the elderly hypertensive patient. In developing the plan of care, the attention should be directed toward gradual reduction in blood pressure to the *individual* patient's goal level by utilizing the least potent therapeutic measures. This goal level needs to be established by the appropriate health care provider *and* the patient/family. Initial efforts should stress and include:

- maintenance of general healthful living
- development of a weight control program when appropriate
- limitation on sodium intake (no table salt)
- promotion of adequate rest and exercise
- generation of interest in activities that increase relaxation and socialization

Diet

There is controversy regarding the value of dietary measures to lower blood lipids. In the elderly, little can be done to remedy a lifetime of dietary intake of lipids. Follow-up observation of persons who were in the Framingham Study may at some point delineate dietary measures, if any may be justified for those already elderly.

It is unreasonable to subject the elderly hypertensive patient to diets that are severely restricted in sodium. Restriction to a 5 gm sodium diet could allow use of a modest amount of salt for cooking purposes. This amount of dietary restriction is well below the estimated range of 8 to 14 gm of sodium a day in the United States. It would reduce use of salt at the table and limit salty foods such as bacon, sausage, and snacks as crackers, pretzels, and potato chips. The availability of modern diuretic drugs has made the strict low sodium diet an archaic form of treatment.

Behavior Modification

There has been an increasing interest in utilizing behavioral treatment in controlled studies with hypertensive subjects. These modalities include traditional psychotherapy, biofeedback, relaxation training and meditation, assertiveness training, and systematic desensitization techniques. Behavioral interventions that elicit the relaxation response may be an important adjunct of drug therapy. So far, none of these studies has been done with a geriatric population.

Patient Education

Nurses must involve patients in the formulation of their treatment programs so that there will be integration into the lifestyle at home or in the institution. What does the patient understand hypertension to be? Why is it being treated? Is it cured or controlled? This clinician believes that patients need simple informative answers to these questions initially. They need to understand that hypertension does not mean being "too nervous." It is to be controlled because of the damage that has been shown to occur to the small blood vessels of the heart, kidneys, brain, and eye. Lastly, they need to understand that hypertension can be controlled by remaining on the treatment program and under regular supervision by their health care provider.

Most patients with hypertension are asymptomatic. It is difficult for asymptomatic patients to take medicines and change lifestyles. Good nurse-patient relationships have been found to facilitate and motivate patients to stay with treatment regimens. The long-term "routine" care of the hypertensive patient offers little challenge to the busy physician who must use his or her time for diagnosis and treatment of complex medical problems.

There is a wealth of excellent educational materials for the hypertensive patient available from the American Heart Association and the National High Blood Pressure Education Program in Bethesda, Maryland. Nurses need to become familiar with these resources so that patient education can be individually tailored. Some sources of patient education materials are listed at the conclusion of this chapter.

Basic information can be given to the patient by use of various media, but my experience has led me to believe that effective patient education requires a person-to-person approach to adapt the basic information to the patient's needs. After that point, it may be appropriate to consider forms of group care/education. In the elderly population this may or may not be an appropriate adjunct to individualized care by a consistent provider or team.

Certain elderly patients will be able to take their own blood pressure. This should be carefully evaluated with thought given to how this may be helpful to the individual patient. Patients can be taught by slipping the already wrapped cuff on the arm. The stethoscope (if not a model that is sewn into the cuff), can be used with two flat elastic bands that hold it in place. The special precautions I have discussed previously will again need to be considered. Spotting inaccurate readings is not usually a problem. For example, you would suspect that the patient who shows you a blood pressure of 140/90 mm Hg at every reading may be making a mistake or making up the numbers! Let him know that nobody has a constant blood pressure and that we better evaluate his procedure or reassess his ability to take the blood pressure. It must be kept in mind that elderly patients may have significant atherosclerotic disease and may, therefore, have wide swings of pressure, depending on the time of the day and the particular lying or sitting position in which the readings are taken.

Basic to the accuracy of the reading is the assumption that the blood pressure equipment is functioning properly. Patients and health care personnel must know how to maintain the equipment. Aneroid manometers should be checked every 6 months with a Y-connector hooked to a mercury manometer of known accuracy. If the difference is greater than +/− 5 mm Hg, it should be recalibrated by the manufacturer or authorized service center.

Mishandling of equipment may produce inaccuracies that are invisible at zero but apparent along the 0 to 300 mm Hg range. Tubing and cuff should be inspected regularly for leaks. This can be done by inflation to 200 mm Hg and closing the valve. Pressure should remain stable.

More expensive mercury manometers require less care, especially if they are wall mounted and are usually considered to be more accurate. The service manuals that come with this equipment should be helpful and referred to for proper maintenance on a yearly basis. This is a frequently ignored item, especially in busy medical care facilities.

Patients may wish to purchase the less expensive aneroid manometers. They should be directed toward purchase of equipment that can be serviced easily. The least expensive stethoscope will be adequate for most situations when the purpose is only for taking

of the blood pressure. The total investment in this equipment would be $20 to $35, an inexpensive adjunct to encourage patient participation.

Pharmacologic Management

When the decision has been made that drug therapy will be instituted in the elderly patient, an oral diuretic agent should be selected as the *cornerstone* of drug therapy. A thiazide-type diuretic as hydrochlorothiazide or chlorothiazide is recommended starting with a minimal dosage given once daily in the morning.

The precise mechanism by which the thiazides and other oral diuretics lower arterial pressure is unclear. It is known that they decrease peripheral resistance by inhibiting reabsorption of Na and water in the kidney tubules, i.e., diuretic effect. They may also have a weak vasodilating effect on the arteries. Because the thiazide diuretics also potentiate the hypotensive action of other antihypertensive agents, they should be left as a part of the drug therapy program when other antihypertensive agents are added.

In circumstances where there is evidence of renal failure or congestive heart failure a diuretic such as furosemide (Lasix) may be the diuretic of choice. When renal function is impaired (serum creatinine above 3.5 mg/100 ml), furosemide is preferred because it does not reduce glomerular filtration rate as do the other diuretics.

Dietary supplements are usually sufficient to prevent hypokalemia. Potassium-rich foods (see Chapter 9) may contain, however, a considerable amount of sodium and calories and, therefore, may need special consideration for each patient situation. As an example, raisins have high amounts of potassium, sodium, and calories. They are also expensive for someone why may have a fixed social security income. Many patients are told to drink a big glass of orange juice every day. Frequently they follow the advice but substitute a big glass of synthetic orange juice that will be lower in potassium and higher in sodium than natural orange juice. If the patient is concurrently taking a digitalis preparation, caution is required because hypokalemia potentiates the toxicity of the digitalis. A potassium supplement may be indicated in this situation.

If the blood pressure does not decrease to the goal level after 4 to 6 weeks of diuretic therapy, a second drug may need to be considered. Other drugs that may be added to the diuretic include reserpine, clonidine, methyldopa, hydralazine, propranolol, or prazosin. In general, these more potent antihypertensive agents are *not recommended* or needed for the majority of patients with geriatric hypertension. In many and most situations, a diuretic given one or two times a day will bring down the blood pressure with a minimum of risk of therapy.

When the second antihypertensive agent is needed, a minimal dose should be started in conjunction with the diuretic. The diuretic then becomes even more important to prevent the compensatory fluid retention frequently caused by other antihypertensive agents.

There are three basic mechanisms by which all antihypertensive drugs act: direct action on the smooth muscle of the arterioles (hydralazine, prazosin); inhibition of some part of the sympathetic nervous system (reserpine, methyldopa, propranolol, clonidine); or promotion of salt and water excretion (thiazides and related diuretics). In the geriatric patient, it may be even more difficult to match the suspected specific mechanism of the hypertension with the appropriate drug, especially if the patient has had hypertension for many years.

The joint National Committee on Detection, Evaluation and Treatment of High Blood Pressure (1977) recommends a stepped-care approach in drug therapy. These may be appropriate in the geriatric patient when diuretic therapy has not been successful and when further measures are *absolutely* indicated. Recommended in Step 1 are the thiazide diuretics. Step 2 recommends use of a sympathetic depressant. Step 3 recommends the addition of a vasodilator. Step 4 recommends the addition of a more potent sympathetic depressant.

It must be kept in mind, however, that sympathetic nervous system responsiveness may decline with aging and atherosclerotic disease. Hence, the antihypertensive drugs that are "sympathetic depressant" may be less controllable or predictive in their action and subject the elderly patient to sudden and unexpected changes in blood pressure levels, i.e., postural hypotension.

There are multiple combination tablets available of the antihypertensive drugs which may simplify drug taking after maintenance blood pressure levels are achieved. It must be kept in mind, however, that these combination tablets are difficult to modify to the individual patient's need as changes in doses affect all constituents of the combination tablet. If cost is a consideration, the combination tablets are often proportionately more expensive and may not contain sufficient diuretic component.

In summary, all of these drugs will need to be initiated in very low dosages with the aim of drug therapy at a *gradual* reduction in blood pressure. Postural hypotension is a potentially greater problem in the elderly than in the middle-aged hypertensive patient. Dose levels that may be safe and effective in the younger patient may be excessive in the elderly. Symptoms of postural hypotension may occur when a sudden and excessive reduction in pressure occurs in a patient with atheromatous inelastic arteries. Dizziness, fainting, impaired vision, and inability to walk properly may then occur and actually mimic stereotypes associated with old age. Health care workers should be aware of the side effects and precautions of commonly used antihypertensive agents indicated in Table 19-1.

Management/Assessment Guidelines

Health care providers must be conscientious and cautious in observation and approach to the elderly hypertensive patient or the therapeutic program may have diastrous consequences. Nurses with responsibility for long term management and follow-up observation of these patients will need to monitor both subjective and objective data, utilizing a management protocol appropriate to their skill level and clinical setting.

The evaluation should include a focus on:

1. Patient/family participation in the treatment program:
   a. integration of patient/health care provider plan into the lifestyle
   b. degree of impairment of quality of life and patient coping ability
2. Complications:
   a. hypertensive complications—symptoms of congestive heart failure, renal disease, stroke, hypertensive retinopathy
   b. drug complications—*hypotension*, age-related drug intolerances, side effects.

Specific information regarding the antihypertensive drugs may be carried on 3x5 note cards in the pocket for ready reference by health care providers. Similar informational cards for patient use may also be helpful and increase patient independence in the treatment program.

It is my opinion that a comprehensive follow-up program needs to include the monitoring of certain objective signs. Regular assessment should focus on:

TABLE 19-1.   Side effects of and precautions with commonly used antihypertensive drugs.

Drugs	Side Effects*	Precautions
DIURETICS		
A. Thiazide and thiazide derivative diuretics	BUN↑, uric acid↑, calcium↑, serum K+↓, glucose↑, gastrointestinal irritation, weakness, photosensitivity, blood dyscrasias, pancreatitis**	Hypokalemia, gout, renal insufficiency
B. Loop diuretics (furosemide)	Calcium↓, BUN↑, uric acid↑, serum K+↓, photosensitivity	Hypokalemia, gout
C. Potassium-sparing diuretics		
• Spironolactone	Hyperkalemia, gynecomastia, drowsiness, hirsutism, irregular menses	Renal failure, hyperkalemia
• Triamterene	Hyperkalemia, diarrhea, nausea	Renal failure, hyperkalemia
NON-DIURETICS		
A. Rauwolfia alkaloids	Drowsiness, sedation, lassitude, nasal congestion, bradycardia, depression, gastric hyperacidity, nightmares	Mental depression
B. Methyldopa	Orthostatic hypotension, drowsiness, depression, abnormal liver function tests, positive direct Coombs test	Liver disease
C. Propranolol	Insomnia, bradycardia, bronchospasm, heart failure, sedation	Asthma, heart failure, diabetes
D. Hydralazine	Headache, tachycardia, palpitations, exacerbation of angina or congestive heart failure, mesenchymal ("lupus like") reaction***	Symptomatic coronary artery disease
E. Guanethidine	Orthostatic hypotension (especially in the AM), exertional weakness, bradycardia, diarrhea, loss of ability to ejaculate	Symptomatic cardiovascular disease

Reprinted from the Report of the Joint National Committee on Detection, Evaluation, and Treatment of High Blood Pressure. U.S. Dept. of Health, Education, and Welfare. Public Health Service. National Institutes of Health. DHEW Publication No. (NIH) 78-1088, 1978, p. 16.

  * See also manufacturer's full prescribing information. Impotency may occur with any antihypertensive drug except hydralazine.
 ** Many side effects, for example, blood dyscrasias and pancreatitis, are rare with diuretics.
*** Rare with dosage under 300 mg/day.

Comparable data on side effects from clonidine and prazosin not available.

1. Physical findings:
   a. blood pressure in lying, sitting, and standing positions—observe for symptoms of postural hypotension (refer to special precautions in taking the blood pressure)
   b. pulse in lying, sitting, and standing positions—observe for changes in heart rate that may forecast heart failure
   c. heart sounds—gallops and/or murmurs, rate, and irregularities (a fourth heart sound is commonly heard in hypertensive patients and probably reflects decreased compliance of the left ventricle wall which in turn may be due to left ventricular hypertrophy)
   d. chest sounds—rales
   e. bruits—particularly carotid vessels (may help to explain depression symptoms)
   f. fundoscopic changes—papilledema, exudates, hemorrhages or presence of nicking of vessels at arteriovenous crossings
   g. weight—pattern of changes or stability
   h. presence of peripheral edema
2. Laboratory determinations as indicated in the management protocol:
   a. complete blood count and serum electrolytes, including serum creatinine or BUN —serum creatinine is the more sensitive index to renal functioning
   b. urinalysis
3. Chest x-ray picture—note changes in cardiac size or silhouette
4. Electrocardiogram—note presence of left ventricular strain or hypertrophy indicated by voltage and/or ST-T changes (other changes in the ECG, such as heart blocks or ischemia, may indicate the presence of damage secondary to associated coronary artery disease)

These management suggestions as outlined only supplement the critical role of the health care provider in assessing the individual geriatric patient in his setting—home, clinic, hospital, or long term care facility.

Evaluation

Reduction in life expectancy from hypertension is greater in the young patient. This must be kept in mind in setting the management goals and evaluating the outcomes. As discussed in the earlier sections of this chapter, hypertension in the elderly is difficult to define. We do not know who should be treated.

There has been little emphasis on study of hypertension specifically as it applies to the aged population. And it is difficult to study because it may involve withholding treatment in a group of patients who could potentially have disastrous consequences. With the advent of screening and treatment programs, hopefully, there will be a decrease in the hypertensive population before they become 70.

While antihypertensive therapy has been shown to reduce mortality in those under age 62, no similar benefit is obvious in the older age group. Therefore it should seem reasonable that the evaluation not necessarily stress attainment of the blood pressure to or at a particular level. More important is the maintenance of the quality of life and maximizing the ability of the patient and/or family to cope with the ramifications of *indicated and safe* treatment of a chronic health problem. This is, indeed, the challenge that nurses must assume.

BIBLIOGRAPHY

American Heart Association: Recommendations for Human Blood Pressure Determination by Sphygmomanometers. New York, 1972.

American Heart Association Sub-Committee on Reduction of Risk of Heart Attack and Stroke: High Blood Pressure Control: A Guide for Community Programs. New York, 1974.

Benson, H.: Systematic hypertension and the relaxation response. New Engl. J. Med. 296:1152–1156, 1977.

Borhani, N. O., Frenti, C. E., and Kraus, J. F.: An epidemiological model for evaluating community and clinical importance of hypertension intervention programs (Abstract). Circulation 52:95, 1975, Suppl. 2.

Castelli, W. P.: CHD risk factors in the elderly. Hosp. Pract. 1976.

Draye, M. A., and Roben, N.: Management of the hypertensive patient. Nurse Practitioner 1:98–101, 1976.

Esler, M., et al.: Mild high-renin essential hypertension. New Engl. J. Med. 296:405, 1977.

Freis, E.: Salt, volume and the prevention of hypertension. Circulation 53:589–594, 1976.

Freis, E. D.: Introduction to the Nature and Management of Hypertension. Bowie, Md.: Robert J. Brady Co., 1974.

Geddes, L. A.: The Direct and Indirect Measurement of Blood Pressure. Chicago, Year Book Medical Publishers, 1970.

Gifford, R. W.: Managing hypertension. Postgrad. Med. 61: 153–163, 1977.

Kannel, W. B., et al.: Role of blood pressure in the development of congestive heart failure. New Engl. J. Med. 287: 781–787, 1972.

Kannel, W. B., et al.: Epidemiologic assessment of the role of blood pressure in stroke. J.A.M.A. 214, October 12, 1970.

Kassirer, J., and Harrington, J.: Diuretics and potassium metabolism: a reassessment of the need, effectiveness and safety of potassium therapy. Kidney International 11:505–515, 1977.

Klatsky, A., et al.: Alcohol consumption and blood pressure. New Engl. J. Med. 296:1194–1200, 1977.

Mitchell, E. S.: Protocol for teaching hypertensive patients. Amer. J. Nurs. 77:808–809, 1977.

Moser, M., et al.: Report of the Joint National Committee on Detection, Evaluation and Treatment of High Blood Pressure. J.A.M.A. 237:255–261, 1977.

National Center for Health Statistics: Hypertension and Hypertensive Heart Disease in Adults, U.S. 1960–62. U. S. Department of Health, Education, and Welfare, Washington D.C., 1966.

Proceedings—National Conference High Blood Pressure Education. U. S. Department of Health, Education, and Welfare, Washington D.C., 1973.

Report of the Joint National Committee on Detection, Evaluation, and Treatment of High Blood Pressure. J.A.M.A. 237:255–263, 1977.

Sasaki, N.: The relationship of salt intake to hypertension in the Japanese. Geriatrics 19:735–744, 1964.

Shekelle, R. B., Ostfeld, A. M., and Klawans, H. L., Jr.: Hypertension and risk of stroke in an elderly population. Stroke 5:71, 1974.

The Hypertension Handbook. Published by Merck Sharp & Dohme in cooperation with the National High Blood Pressure Education Program, 1974.

Wilkie, F., and Eisdorfer, C.: Intelligence and blood pressure in the aged. Science 172:959–962, 1971.

Zweifler, A., and Esler, M.: Factors influencing the choice of antihypertensive agents. Postgrad. Med. 60:81–85, 1976.

Advanced Reading

Arch. Intern. Med. Vol. 133, No. 6, June, 1974 (Symposium issue with review of arterial hypertension).

Page, L., and Sidd, J.: Medical management of primary hypertension. New Engl. J. Med. Part 1, November 9, 1972; Part 2, November 16, 1972; Part 3, November 23, 1972.

PATIENT EDUCATION MATERIALS

General Sources

American Heart Association
National Center
7320 Greenville Avenue
Dallas, Texas 75231

State Heart Associations

High Blood Pressure Information Center
120/80 National Institutes of Health
Bethesda, MD 20014
(Pamphlets and Audiovisuals)

Recommended Materials

High Blood Pressure and How To Control It
American Heart Association, Inc.
(1974, 12-page pamphlet for patient education. Free of charge)

Watch Your Blood Pressure!
Theodore Irwin
Public Affairs Committee, Inc., New York
(June, 1974, 28-page booklet. Free of charge. High Blood Pressure Information Center)

Controlling Your High Blood Pressure
CIBA Pharmaceutical Company
Summit, NJ 08901
(1973, 10-page pamphlet for patient education. Free of charge through physician only)

Don't Take Chances with High Blood Pressure
U.S. Government Printing Office
Washington, DC 20402
(1974, leaflet. Free of charge)

The Silent Disease: Hypertension
Lawrence Galton
Crown Publishers, Inc.
419 Park Avenue S.
New York, NY 10016
(1973, 210-page booklet for patient education. $5.95/single copy)

You and Your Blood Pressure
Channing L. Bete Company, Inc.
Greenfield, MA
(1977, 15-page illustrated booklet for patient education. $0.25 each per 100)

Hypertension
Robert J. Brady Company
Bowie, MD
(1972, Flip Chart (53-page guide with take home materials). Purchase $18.20)
Robert J. Brady Company
130 Q street, NE
Washington, DC 20002

How You Can Help Your Doctor Treat Your High Blood Pressure
Marvin Moser, M.D.
American Heart Association, Inc.
(1974, 12-page pamphlet for patient education. Free of charge)

High Blood Pressure
Citizens for the Treatment of High Blood Pressure, Inc.
Suite 1630, Chevy Chase Building
5530 Wisconsin Avenue
Chevy Chase, MD 20015
(1977, condensed 4-page pamphlet. Free of charge)

Patient Education in High Blood Pressure
U.S. Department of Health, Education, and Welfare
Public Health Service
National Institutes of Health
DHEW Publication #(NIH)75-724
(A comprehensive annotated bibliography for patients, professionals, and general public)

Report of the Joint National Committee on Detection, Evaluation, and Treatment of High Blood Pressure (1978)
U.S. Dept. of Health, Education, and Welfare
Public Health Service
National Institutes of Health
DHEW Publication (NIH) 78-1088

20

Incontinence

Janet Specht and Ann Cordes

QUICK REVIEW

INCONTINENCE

DESCRIPTION	Involuntary escape of urine from lower urinary tract.
ETIOLOGIC FACTORS	Changes in central nervous system and local reflex arcs.

Psychogenic factors: regression, dependency rebellion, insecurity, attention seeking, sensory deprivation, disturbances to conditioned reflexes, symptom selection

Genitourinary factors: loss of muscle tone, urinary infection, obstruction, failure in voluntary postponement, fecal impaction

Drugs: Lasix, hypnotics, e.g., Valium, Sparine; tricyclic antidepressants, e.g., Elavil

Clothing, locomotor defects in reaching bathroom, distance to bathroom. Attitudes of self and others that one is an incontinent person versus a person with a problem of incontinence.

HIGH RISK	14 to 24 percent of elderly have problems with urinary incontinence (figures vary with studies). Females have higher incidence; incontinence is a frequent reason for loss of independent lifestyle.
DYNAMICS	Incontinence occurs when intravesicular pressure exceeds urethral resistance. Twenty reflex mechanisms involved in micturition. Postponement depends upon stimuli from bladder reaching cerebral cortex, being given significance, and on the ability then to provide additional voluntary inhibition from the central nervous system.
SIGNS AND SYMPTOMS	Dribbling or puddling. Reluctance to leave home. Telltale urine type odors about person/living quarters.
DIFFERENTIAL DIAGNOSIS	Incontinence specification: time, frequency, amount, status of voluntary control. Fecal impaction—fecal incontinence, bowel patterns. Environmental factors—clothing, location of bathroom, privacy, assistance when needed, and so forth. Reality orientation. Emotional reaction to incontinence. Medical: urinalysis (for infection), cystometry, reflex arc testing, muscle status.
COMPLICATIONS	Skin breakdown, damage to self-concept, social isolation, shrinking of bladder.
PROGNOSIS	Depends on mental status of patient and interest/skills of caretakers. Fifty percent success rate with optimum treatment.

Continued on next page.

QUICK REVIEW (cont.)

NURSING MANAGEMENT	Precise specification of nature of incontinence and factors involved: Bladder retraining programs. Modification of environment, clothing. Control of genitourinary infections and fecal impactions. Perineal exercises. Adequate sensory stimulation and physical and mental activity. Appliances as a last resort.
MEDICAL MANAGEMENT	Drug therapy, surgery, electronic devices.
EVALUATION	Episodes of incontinence decrease. Physical/social activities return to desired patterns as confidence returns. Family/staff understand nature of the person's incontinence problem and implications and participate in care or relate more effectively. Where incontinence cannot be controlled: (1) skin integrity is maintained, (2) person receives input that fosters a positive self-concept, and (3) social life and sensory environment are maintained in a way that are acceptable to the person despite continued incontinence.

Control of urine is required for social survival, and it has been described as one of the essentials for survival in old age (Fine, 1972, p. 323). The healthy older person tends to pass urine more frequently and will have a degree of urgency of micturition.

Urinary incontinence is a condition characterized by involuntary escape of urine from the lower urinary tract in a degree that imposes a social or hygienically unacceptable situation upon the individual (Caldwell, 1975, p. 12). It is a symptom of a number of underlying conditions that affect the anatomy and innervation of the lower urinary tract. There are innumerable causes that produce a single result—incontinence. It is important, when planning a successful program to reestablish continence or decrease the frequency of uncontrolled urinating, that the exact cause be established.

Etiologic Factors

Despite the high incidence of incontinence in the aged, the health professions (medicine and nursing) have shown comparatively little interest in investigating its cause. One system for classifying etiologic factors of incontinence (Willington, Incontinence-2, 1975) is presented in the following text and outlined in Figure 20-1.

Acknowledgement is made to Robert P. Gibbons, M.D., Urologist, The Mason Clinic, Seattle, Washington, for his contribution in reviewing this chapter.

Under the central nervous system heading are neurogenic and psychogenic causes. Genitourinary system causes constitute the largest group and connote any organic lesion affecting the bladder, genitalia, and associated musculature. The third group is spurious and includes incontinence caused from treatment (iatrogenic) or from mental incompetence or loss of manual dexterity (locomotor).

Central Nervous System Causes

NEUROGENIC CAUSES. There are four types of neurogenic causes of incontinence: uninhibited, automatic, autonomous, and hyperaesthetic.

Uninhibited. This cause implies loss of conscious inhibition. It appears that the premotor area of the frontal lobe is related to the action that inhibits bladder contractions and, thus, delays the point of irresistible evacuation. The characteristic pattern of elderly bladder action, in this case, probably is due to impairment in cerebral control of micturition.

Characteristic Pattern of Elderly Bladder Action

Diminution of ability to inhibit micturition
↓
Precipitate Micturition
↓
Small contracted hyperactive bladder
+
Poor neuromuscular action
↓
Incomplete Evacuation

URINARY INCONTINENCE

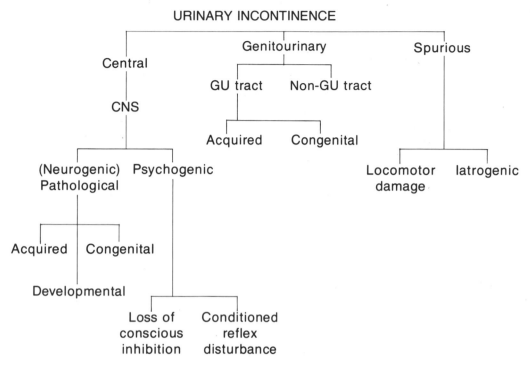

FIGURE 20-1. Classification of urinary incontinence. (From Willington, F. L.: Problems in the aetiology of urinary incontinence [Incontinence—2]. Nursing Times 71:379, 1975, with permission)

Automatic. Automatic cause denotes uncontrolled voiding that is due to reflex action of the spinal cord. It occurs with incomplete development of lesions of the spinal cord above the level of L-2.

Autonomous. The autonomous type refers to a breakdown of the primary reflex arc with damage to the nervous connections to or from the cauda equina.

Hypoesthetic. In the hypoesthetic type, damage occurs to the sensory nerves from the bladder. The primary part of the reflex arc is damaged, and a large hypotonic bladder results. The motor fibers remain intact but sensations of fullness are impaired; this results in overflow incontinence. Conditions in which this damage is present are tabes dorsalis, multiple sclerosis, and diabetes mellitus.

PSYCHOGENIC CAUSES. The psychogenic classification includes mental barriers that might result in incontinence (see box).

Willington (Incontinence-2, 1975) has shown the high incidence of incontinence with stroke may be attributed to the effects of dyspraxia, dysgnosia and body image disturbance. In a 1958 study it was found that 80 percent of incontinent patients had no physiologic reason for their condition (Lowenthal, et al., 1958).

PSYCHOLOGIC MECHANISMS IN ETIOLOGY OF INCONTINENCE*	
Regression	Response to stressful situations by return to earlier stage of development
Dependency	Control, even of body functions, turned over to caretaker, who takes over
Rebellion	Expression of anger over loss of control
Insecurity	High risk with change in environment
Attention Seeking	Means of assuring regular attention
Disturbance of Conditioned Reflexes	Usual conditions and props not present for the conditioned reflex of toileting
Sensory Deprivation	Integrity of perceptual framework lost because of inadequate environmental stimulation
Symptom Selection	Because of its vulnerability in old age, bladder frequently is the expression of emotional complications

* Adapted from Willington, F. L.: Incontinence in the Elderly. New York: Academic Press, 1976, p. 61.

Genitourinary Causes

Genitourinary causes of incontinence are probably the most familiar to nurses. A helpful way to classify these causes is to relate the cycle of micturition (filling, voluntary postponement, and emptying) with two broad types of incontinence (passive and active). Figure 20-2 shows a model for relating the stages of the cycle and the types of incontinence.

The following are causes of active incontinence:

- bladder outflow obstruction caused by enlarged prostate, fibrous bladder neck obstruction, cystocele, or trigonitis associated with atrophic vaginitis
- decline in muscle tone
- urinary infection
- fecal impaction

Spurious Incontinence

Spurious incontinence has a great bearing in the elderly. It includes iatrogenic incontinence, incontinence caused by locomotor defects, and that caused by factors in the environment.

Iatrogenic incontinence means that a "treatment" results in incontinence. Drug therapy is a frequent culprit. Brocklehurst (1972) describes these as precipitating factors and physical problems are predisposing. Most common is furosemide (Lasix) where the diuretic action is so fast that the patient becomes incontinent. Hypnotics cause such a depth of sleep that bladder sensation does not arouse. Valium and Sparine are especially troublesome. Tricyclic antidepressants (Elavil) may also cause incontinence.

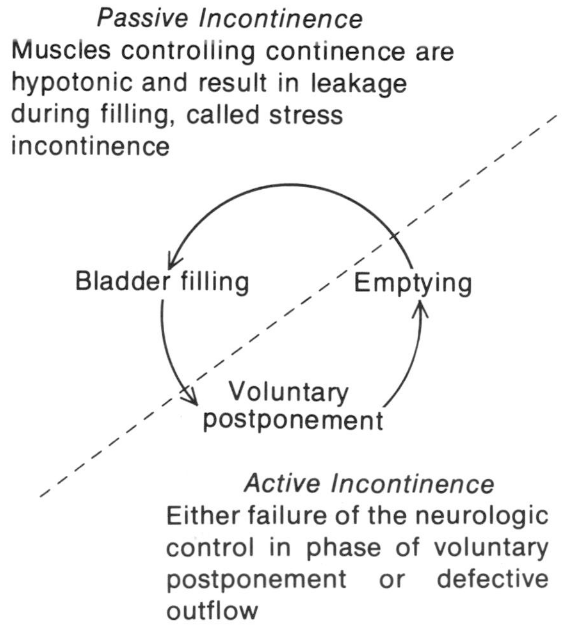

Other associated factors that lead to incontinence include locomotor defects, manual dexterity in manipulating clothing, distance to the bathroom, and other environmental factors.

The environment and attitudes of persons in the environment are causative factors in incontinence, particularly in institutional settings. The patient frequently sees himself not as a person who has a problem with incontinence but as an incontinent patient. Staff attitudes are conveyed to the patient by their mannerisms and actions. The staff accepts and expects that old people are incontinent, and it becomes a self-fulfilling prophecy as patients and families resign themselves to incontinence. Incontinence is viewed as automatic with old age. Some authorities believe that whenever a ward staff includes a doctor or nurse who believes that incontinent patients wet themselves deliberately that the ward is likely to have many incontinent patients.

A classic example of the effects of environment on incontinence occurred at the Iowa Veterans Home 10 years ago when the decision was made to have residents have personal pajamas, which they selected and bought themselves, instead of state-furnished pajamas. The rate of incontinence was reduced by one third. Persons apparently were not willing to wet their own pajamas, but the state's pajamas did not matter. The dignity of ownership prevailed. This is certainly a strong statement for personal and attractive clothing in hospitals and institutions.

Ergonomics is a concept of fitting equipment and building areas to the needs of all human beings; it has a role in incontinence. Much urinary incontinence in the elderly results from the loss of the race between the bladder and the legs.

Passive Incontinence
Muscles controlling continence are hypotonic and result in leakage during filling, called stress incontinence

Bladder filling   Emptying

Voluntary postponement

Active Incontinence
Either failure of the neurologic control in phase of voluntary postponement or defective outflow

FIGURE 20-2. Micturition cycle and two types of incontinence. (From Willington, F. L.: Problems in the aetiology of urinary incontinence [Incontinence—2]. Nursing Times 71:380, 1975, with permission)

T_1 = Time interval between the onset of desire for micturition and arrival of uncontrollable micturition

T_2 = Rate of walking in feet per minute

D = The distance to the bathroom

$\dfrac{D}{T_2}$ = Time taken by patient to the bathroom

If $\dfrac{D}{T_2}$ is greater than T_1 incontinence will result.

An example with Mrs. S will illustrate the use of the formula. Suppose Mrs. S's bedroom is 100 ft from the bathroom. She has arthritis and it takes her a while to get out of her bedroom to the bathroom (usually 5 min). She usually has about 2 min between the urge and the flow in micturition.

$$T_1 = 2 \text{ min}$$
$$T_2 = 20 \text{ ft/min}$$
$$D = 100 \text{ ft}$$
$$\frac{100}{20} = 5 \text{ min}$$

Incontinence will result approximately 3 min before she arrives at the bathroom. In this situation the environment causes incontinence. Therefore, the environment needs alteration to assist in maintenance of continence.

High Risk Populations

The elderly are high risk for incontinence and, frequently, it is the symptom that makes the difference between people staying in their own homes or going to nursing homes. Incontinence of urine is the prime cause of need for long-stay hospital care (Caird and Judge, 1974, p. 44).

Two percent of the total population have some problem with incontinence. But in the elderly, 14 to 40 percent are affected by urinary incontinence. In an Edinburgh survey of 27,000 people between the ages of 62 and 90 years, the incidence of incontinence for men was 25 percent and for women 42 percent (Milne, et al., 1972).

Persons with genitourinary infections are also high risk for incontinence. In one study, 33 percent of 166 incontinent patients had urinary infections (Brocklehurst, 1964).

Gynecologic causes of incontinence has an incidence of 600 per 100,000 persons. This includes urinary infections, vaginitis, cystocele, and so forth. Male incontinence resulting from prostatic problems is 20 per 100,000 persons.

Dynamics

Normal voiding is a reflex act under voluntary cortical control. The complexity of incontinence is demonstrated by the fact that there are about 20 reflex mechanisms in the act concerned with micturition (Willington, 1973, p. 378).

The physical basis of urinary incontinence is the existence of a higher intravesical pressure than urethral resistance can withstand. The urethral pressure profile is close to low normal when the patient assumes a sitting-resting position and drops appreciably when standing in an erect position, explaining incontinence that occurs when people get up to move about. The pelvic support is an indirect helper of the sphincteric mechanism.

The bladder neck and proximal urethra are primarily responsible for maintenance of urinary continence. It is commonly referred to as the internal sphincter. In normal patients the intraurethral pressure is higher than the resting bladder pressure because the radius of the bladder continually increases as the bladder fills, while the radius of the urethra remains zero. At maximal intravesical capacity, the collagenous fibers in the bladder wall resist further stretching, the radius no longer increases, and the intravesical pressure begins to rise rapidly. At this point, the small pressure difference between the bladder and the urethra which favors continence is lost and urine enters the proximal urethra. Continence, then, must be maintained by voluntary control of the pelvic floor skeletal muscles and external sphincter.

The desire to void is a sensation perceived in the parietal lobe of the cerebral cortex. The sensation comes from impulses that are caused by a rapid rise of tension in the bladder. These impulses pass along the pelvic splanchnic nerves (S2, S3, S4) and ascend in the spinal cord and brainstem to reach the hypothalamus.

Inhibition appears to be suppressed initially from the region of the basal ganglia unconsciously and then the cerebral cortex. Postponement of micturition depends on the following:

- condition of the relevant stimulatory impulses from S2, S3, and segments
- transmission of the stimulus to the cerebral cortex
- appreciation in the cortex of the significance
- ability to provide the necessary additional voluntary inhibition from the cerebral cortex

Signs and Symptoms

Escape of urine at unplanned times and reluctance to leave home or participate in activities may be the only signs of incontinence. Or, there may be the telltale odor in the living quarters. Incontinence is viewed as infantile behavior; it is a sure sign of regression. Great effort is often made to hide the problem.

Differential Diagnosis

History

Proper diagnosis of type and cause of incontinence requires a medical-nursing diagnostic partnership. A detailed history of the incontinence is essential with particular references to the type and duration of the incontinence and the patient's sensation and attitude to it. Bowel problems have major impact on urinary function and, as such, are an important part of the assessment.

There are areas of information needed to make an accurate diagnosis of incontinence. The nurse is in a strategic position to obtain this information in all settings. This is essential preliminary information that must be collected by the nurse and shared with the physician.

Nature of Feces and Urine. Is there constipation, diarrhea, offensive loose stool, blood, fecal staining of clothes? How does the urine smell and look? Is there visible blood or pus or gas bubbles?

Incontinence Specification. (See sample chart form.) How frequently is there incontinence and what quantity each time? Numbers of fecal incontinence and consistency of stool? Has a rectal been done to check for impaction? Is there vaginal discharge? What is it like—quantity, color, odor, and duration?

INCONTINENCE SPECIFICATION CHART*

	TIME OF DAY	6 AM	8 AM	10 AM	12 AM	2 PM	4 PM	6 PM	8 PM	10 PM	12 PM	2 AM	4 AM
Day & Date	Wet												
	Dry												
Bedtime	Used Urinal, Commode, or Bathroom												
	Amount												
Day & Date	Wet												
	Dry												
Bedtime	Used Urinal, Commode, or Bathroom												
	Amount												
Day & Date	Wet												
	Dry												
Bedtime	Used Urinal, Commode, or Bathroom												
	Amount												
Day & Date	Wet												
	Dry												
Bedtime	Used Urinal, Commode, or Bathroom												
	Amount												

* This chart usually needs to be kept three days before initiating the program.

Behavior Analysis. What were the circumstances of the episode? Can the person hold his urine and for how long (conscious inhibition)? Was the receptacle used when applied? Was the receptacle or help requested? Was there incontinence after not using the receptacle? Was the wrong receptacle used?

Emotional Reactions to the Episode. Is the person passive and dependent, aggressive, ashamed, self-deprecatory, deprived, infantile?

Associated Factors. What is the degree of mobility? Can he manage clothing, i.e., unzip zipper, pull down panties? Is he oriented? Does he understand and know his surroundings? Is he able to express needs, if not through speech, in some other way?

Medical Differential Diagnosis

The medical component of the differential diagnosis includes both laboratory examination of the urine and neurologic tests. Urinalysis is done to rule out infections as a cause of incontinence. Neurologic tests (bulbocavernous reflex and/or superficial and reflex and ice water treatment) are done to determine the type of bladder sensation. Other tests include an intravenous pyelogram to assess kidney function, cystometrogram, and cystogram. The cystometrogram reveals patterns of the emptying mechanism of the bladder. It can reflect heightened and reduced sensitivity by measuring intravesicle pressure. The motor and sensory power of the bladder is tested by cystometry, the equivalent of a neurologic examination of the bladder.

The cystometric examination is made by having the patient first empty his bladder as completely as possible. A Foley or Robinson catheter is then inserted. Residual urine is collected and measured; the catheter is then connected to an irrigating and manometric system from which the air has been expelled. Fluid is instilled in the bladder and manometric readings are taken and recorded on a graph after regular increments (usually 50 ml). The patient is asked to indicate the feeling of fullness, the first desire to void, feelings of discomfort and urgency. These sensations are noted on the graph. This test is the urologic comparison to the cardiovascular evaluations needs for an ECG.

The anal sphincter test is performed by inserting a gloved finger in the rectum and giving the Foley catheter a sudden tug. Contraction of the anal sphincter indicates that the neural arc L2 to L4 is intact; therefore, the neurogenic bladder most likely is upper motor neuron in nature. Pure lower motor neuron bladder dysfunction will be accompanied by an absent bulbocavernous reflex.

The bladder sensory arc may be tested by instilling ice water into the bladder. The catheter bulb is deflated. In the upper motor neuron bladder, the catheter and water will quickly be expelled.

A mental status test is an important part of the differential diagnosis. It is argued that incontinence that accompanies stroke is not caused by a neurogenic bladder but rather, is the consequence of impaired mental processes resulting from the stroke. Table 20-1 indicates signs to be observed in assessment of incontinence post-hemiplegic.

TABLE 20-1.   Assessment for post-hemiplegic incontinence.

Sign	Generic Disability	Special Disability	Test
Dyspraxia	Inability to perform familiar action	Inability to remember totality of voluntary muscular action for evacuation	1. Push down on bowel producing bulging of perineum and anus 2. Contraction of external sphincter on request to show a visible result
Dysgnosia	Inability to recognize or use familiar articles	Inability to recognize blood pressure equipment, commode, or urinal or position them	Test recognition of sanitary articles and demonstrate use
Body image	Loss of cortical concept of body	Inability to clean genitalia	Touch contralateral (affected) buttock with unaffected hand

From Willington, F. L.: The nursing component in diagnosis and treatment (Incontinence-4). Nursing Times, 71:464, 1975, with permission.

Complications

Skin hygiene suffers with incontinence. In a survey of 1700 elderly men, 172 were incontinent of urine. Of the 172, 5 percent had skin eruptions, 20 percent small erosions, and 2.5 percent decubital ulcers (Caldwell, 1975). Exton-Smith's (1962) assessment for risk of decubiti lists incontinence as a key factor in predisposition to decubiti.

Psychologic problems resulting from incontinence include feelings of inferiority and inadequacy, self-imposed isolation, and obsession with changing clothes and finding the bathroom.

Long-standing urinary incontinence may lead to organic shrinking of the bladder. Older people are especially prone to this. This makes it more difficult if not impossible to restore normal function.

Prognosis

Success in treating incontinence depends on an accurate physical and mental assessment of the patient and the use of a combination of available therapies. An overall success rate of 50 percent can be expected with the best management (Anderson, 1976, p. 249). The major factor governing success is the mental state of the patient and the caretakers, whether the latter be family or employed health providers.

Prevention and Management

The objective of management of incontinence is the prevention of its interfering with the person's life—to assist in maintaining current lifestyle and to allow for new growth-promoting experiences. Adequate bladder emptying with low residual urine to eliminate infections and a socially acceptable predictable voiding pattern are the goals of treatment.

Management by whom is a prime consideration. In order to decrease dependency, the patient must have an active role in and, if at all possible, direct the program. Information is essential for the patient to do this. This means nurses have to be well-informed and have positive attitudes regarding incontinence. "Old" is not synonymous with "incontinent."

Bladder Retraining

Management depends on cause; thus precise diagnosis is essential. The most important aspect of the treatment of incontinence is the patient's reeducation in bladder control. This is useful for neurogenic bladders where there is no sensation of fullness and also where mentation is impaired. It is the major nursing intervention for incontinence. The theory of conditioned reflex is the basis of this intervention. The conditioned reflex stimulus related to voiding is shown in Figure 20-3.

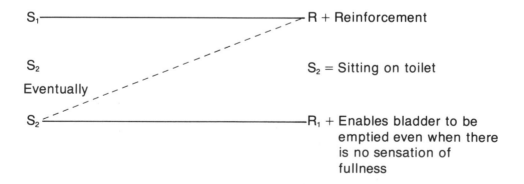

$$S = \text{Sensation of full bladder}$$
$$R = \text{Micturition}$$
$$\text{Reinforcement} = \text{Satisfaction of empty bladder}$$

FIGURE 20-3. Conditioned reflex stimulus as related to voiding. (From Willington, F. L.: Training and retraining for incontinence [Incontinence—5]. Nursing Times 71:500, 1975, with permission)

The conditioned reflex becomes a habit and demands on memory are reduced. Fluid intake and regular toileting need to be individualized. The pattern should allow for bladder fullness but prevent accidents. Prior to any training program, an incontinence record is needed. The maintenance of an incontinence chart has a therapeutic value because it focuses attention, which provides in itself a stimulus to recovery. The best guide to the bladder's capabilities is the time of evacuation with physical and mental rest, that is, the time of the first incontinent episode at night during sleep. This gives the longest possible time before the bladder will empty (Willington, 1975, p. 502). The schedule for toileting can be developed after this time interval has been established. There are five things that happen every day at approximately the same time: getting up, eating three meals, and going to bed. These regular daily activities give the patient a time reference. Used in conjunction with the time established as the longest possible time interval for the bladder to empty, a daily schedule can be established. On the scheduled times, it is essential that the patient be assisted to void in the natural manner; that is, men stand and women sit on the toilet with privacy provided.

When the bladder training program is initiated, the patient should be gotten up to the commode or toilet at the interval established, starting with a larger interval like 4 hours to ensure a full bladder, beginning with when they awaken in the morning and the last thing before retiring. He should be allowed 5 to 6 minutes to void. If the patient is unable to void, the patient or staff may try measures to encourage voiding such as stroking the inner thigh, deep breathing to promote relaxation, bearing down, and leaning acutely forward, drinking water, manual expression, or Credé's method, which is exertion of manual pressure over the lower abdomen. It is important not to keep the patient on the commode longer than 5 to 6 minutes because it then becomes viewed as punishment by the patient and acts as an inhibiting factor. If

incontinence occurs prior to 4 hours, the time interval for toileting could be adjusted to 3 or 2 hours, depending on needs. It should never be less than 30-minute intervals.

FLUIDS SCHEDULE. Fluid intake is another important component of the habit retraining program. Most adults require 2500 cc a day to maintain homeostasis.* During the training period, it is suggested that fluid intake be given from time of arising to 8:00 p.m. (Diuretics should be taken early in the day.) Serve small amounts (100 to 150 cc) frequently; establish a schedule for serving fluids. The frequent entry on care plans "force fluids" is *not* sufficient. A specific schedule establishing time, varying fluids, and prescribing amounts is important. If the patient has not been taking this amount, a *gradual* increase should be planned; it will be more acceptable to the patient.

Some authors claim that if fluid intake totals 2500 cc per day, 75 percent of patients with incontinence will be relieved of their problem. This is possible considering increased fluids reduce urinary infections, fluids reduce constipation and impactions, and fluids will fill bladder to trigger emptying if nerves are intact. There is also evidence that filling the bladder very full promotes emptying.

REINFORCEMENT MEASURES. Use of additional reinforcement has been experimented with in training programs for the incontinent. In a study by Carpenter and Simeon (1960) it was found that habit training plus reward yields the best results. In an institutional setting, socialization is an ideal reward. In a case study conducted at the Iowa Veterans Home, one patient was visited for 3 to 5 minutes whenever she was continent (used the toilet appropriately). The staff person discussed the patient's interests with her. She was praised for voiding. This served as a strong reinforcer and aided in the success of the program. When she was not continent, the patient was changed with no comment, but warm feelings were transmitted by gentle touch, unhurried manner, and smiles. In one week's time, the number of incontinences per day were reduced from six to two. This is encouraging and merits further testing.

Other Management Procedures

CONTROL OF INFECTIONS. The elimination of urinary infections frequently resolves incontinence. The

---

BLADDER RETRAINING RULES

Sequence of stimuli must always be maintained.

Inhibitory stimuli should be avoided. (Inhibitory stimuli may include lack of privacy, too long on bedpan or commode, incorrect position, sitting on bedpan or commode after evacuation has occurred.)

Put on commode whenever bladder is full.

---

* Many elderly persons have other conditions that influence fluid intake, i.e., congestive failure.

prime cause of incontinency with infections is urgency. During times of infections, an appliance, i.e., external catheter or pads, may be used.

CONTROL OF FECAL IMPACTIONS. Elimination of fecal impactions also clears incontinence. A bowel program that provides for regular evacuation frequently improves incontinence. (Refer to Chapter 16 on bowel programs.)

EXERCISES. Exercises to strengthen the pelvic muscles and sphincter will assist in maintenance of continence. Contraction of the perineum is an important part of voluntary reinforcement of bladder inhibition.

Perineal exercises consist of contracting the abdominal gluteal and perineal muscles while breathing normally. The exercises can be explained by asking the patient to hold himself as if he needed to void very badly and had no facility. Strengthening of the gluteal and levator muscles helps. This can be done by having the patient hold a paper or cloth in the fold between the buttocks. Stopping and starting the urinary stream voiding will give additional exercise.

Tanner (1966) has reported good results following electrical stimulation of the pelvic musculature. This may be done by the physiotherapist. Perineal exercises are especially helpful in stress incontinence. Perineal exercises are useless if the patient has no sensation of the need to void or ability to control the urinary stream.

MENTAL AND PHYSICAL ACTIVITY. Measures that promote the general level of physical and mental activity of the individual will contribute to the restoration of continence. Alerting consciousness by providing for environmental stimuli and active interest programs and enhanced dignity provided by humanistic care with emphasis on individuals and adaptation of the environment are all actions that nurses can take or assist families to take to enhance continence.

DRUG THERAPY. Sometimes drug treatment is useful. It is directed primarily towards a reduction of activity of the bladder reflex arc. The anticholinergic drugs are of greatest value in nocturnal incontinence. Emepronium bromide (Cetiprin) is the usual drug given. Probanthine 15 mg four times daily has also been tried (Willington, 1975, p. 160). Side effects of anticholinergic drugs include glaucoma, retention of urine, hepatic insufficiency, blurring of vision, and dry mouth.

In a Michigan study (Diakno, 1975), administration of 25 mg capsule of ephedrine sulfate was shown to be effective in improving urinary continence of varying types provided the wetting is minimal to moderate and related to decreased urethral resistance. It is of little benefit in uninhibited neurogenic bladder and severe stress incontinence.

SURGERY. Surgical intervention is most successfully used for stress incontinence. The two most common types of surgery are urethral suspension and urethral lengthening.

ELECTRONIC DEVICES. Electronic control as a treatment for incontinence is receiving increased attention but is still considered experimental. Caldwell reported his first case in 1965 and readers are referred to his book, *Urinary Incontinence*, for detailed discussion of electronic devices used for incontinence (Caldwell, 1975, pp. 89–115).

APPLIANCES. A variety of appliances are available for the management of urinary incontinence. There are two indications for use of hygienic aids for the prevention of soiling: when all other modes of treatment have failed or when treatment by other means is in progress and continence has not been regained.

The use of appliances and aids is greatly abused and frequently interferes with treatment. The expectation of incontinence is set as an incontinence pad is placed in the patient's bed on admission or in the chair before the patient is gotten out of bed. No pads should be allowed to be used with institutional admissions until a thorough evaluation has been completed. Again, once control is established, pads should not be used. It is subtly saying, "You are continent now, but at any time you could lose control." This is an area that needs careful prescription by the registered nurse because it easily becomes the routine for ancillary staff to put pads on all beds. Use of incontinent pads is costly and can cause further skin problems. With all of these disadvantages, they frequently do not serve the intended purpose of saving the necessity to change linen either. Their use must be evaluated critically.

The use of urinals by male patients is helpful in reducing incontinence, especially when locomotion is a problem. Again, they are frequently misused. Leaving the urinal in position all night is commonly done with male patients and encourages them to relax their sphincters and make no conscious effort towards continence. The expectation is also communicated that incontinence will occur. Loss of control is a factor in such practices. It is communicated, "We will take complete care of you—no need to ever worry about urinating."

The external catheter is a very helpful appliance when continence is not a possibility. Condoms can be used, attached to tubing and a leg bag, allowing the person to be dressed and participate in activities with no problems. The condom is soft and pliable and causes minimal problems as long as it is removed daily with thorough cleansing and drying of the penis. Sometimes penile clamps are used, particularly with dribbling. They are found to be unsatisfactory because of discomfort and penal swelling. Women have fewer options available to them in the area of appliances.

Pessaries have found to have too many contraindications to be useful and often cannot be managed by the disabled.

Willington (1975) describes the marsupial pants which enables the patient to be incontinent yet dry.

BIBLIOGRAPHY

Anderson, H. C.: Newton's Geriatric Nursing, ed. 5. St. Louis: C. V. Mosby Co., 1971.

Anderson, W. F.: Practical Management of the Elderly, ed. 3. Oxford England, Blackwell Scientific Publications, 1976.

Basso, A.: Genitourinary tract problems of the aged male. J. Amer. Geriatric Soc. 21:352–354, 1974.

Bates, B.: A Guide to Physical Exam, ed. 2. Philadelphia: J. B. Lippincott Co., 1979.

Brocklehurst, J. C.: Aging of the human bladder. Geriatrics 27:154–166, 1972.

Brocklehurst, J. C.: The etiology of urinary incontinence in the elderly. In Anderson, W. F., and Isaacs, B. (eds.): Current Achievements in Geriatrics. London: Cassell, 1964.

Caird, F. I., and Judge, T. G.: Assessment of the Elderly Patient. Great Britain: Alden Press, Pitman Medical, 1974.

Caldwell, K. P. S. (ed.): Urinary Incontinence. New York: Grune and Stratton, 1975.

Carpenter, H. A., and Simeon R.: The effect of several methods of training on long-term incontinent, behaviorally regressed, hospitalized psychiatric patients. Nurs. Res. 9:17–22, 1960.

Cowdry, E. V., and Steinberg, F. U.: The Care of the Geriatric Patient, ed. 4. St. Louis: C. V. Mosby Co., 1971.

Culp, D. A.: Benign prostatic hyperplasia: early recognition and management. Urologic Clin. N. Amer. 2:29–48, 1975.

Dale, G.: Iatrogenic urinary infections. Urologic Clin. N. Amer. 2:471–481, 1975.

Diakno, A. C., and Faub, M.: Ephedrine in treatment of urinary incontinence. Urology 5:624–625, 1975.

Drach, G. W.: Prostatic: Man's hidden infection. Urologic Clin. N. Amer. 2:499–520, 1975.

Exton-Smith, A. N., Norton, D., McLaren, R.: An Investigation of Geriatric Nursing Problems in Hospital. London: National Corporation for Care of Old People, 1962.

Feustel, D.: Voiding with an autonomous neurogenic bladder: the role of the rehabilitation nurse specialist. Assoc. Rehabil. Nurses J.: 1:5–8, 1976.

Fine, W.: Geriatric ergonomics. Gerontological Clinics. 14: 322–332, 1972.

Gleason, D., et al.: Active and passive incontinence: Differential diagnosis. Urology 4:693–694, 1974.

Hazards of immobility. Am. J. Nurs. 67:779–797, 1967.

Hodkinson, H. M.: An Outline of Geriatrics. New York: Academic Press, 1975.

Jaffe, J.: The genitourinary system: common lower urinary tract problems in older persons, Part VII. In Working with Older People. U.S. Department of Health, Education and Welfare, Washington D.C., 1971.

Jawetz, E.: Infections of the urinary tract. In Krupp, M., and Cratton, M. (eds.): Medical Diagnosis and Treatment. Los Altos, Calif.: Lange Medical Publications, 1975.

Kahn, A., and Snapper, I.: The genitourinary system: medical renal diseases in the aged, Part VII. In Working with Older People. U.S. Department of Health, Education, and Welfare, Washington D.C., 1971.

Krauss, D., Schoenrock, G., and Lilien, O.: Reeducation of urethral sphincter mechanism in post-prostatectomy incontinence. Urology 5:533–535, 1975.

Kropp, K.: Bacterial infections of the urinary tract (male). In Conn, H. (ed.): Current Therapy. Philadelphia: W. B. Saunders Co., 1976.

Krupp, M. A.: Genitourinary tract. In Krupp, M., and Cratton, M. (eds.): Medical Diagnosis and Treatment. Los Altos, Calif.: Lange Medical Publication, 1975.

Kunin, C.: New methods in detecting urinary tract infections. Urologic Clin. N. Amer. 2:423–424, 1975.

Lowenthal, M., Metz, D., and Patton, A.: Nobody wants the incontinent. RN 82–101, January, 1958.

Lowthian, P. T.: Portable urinals for women. Nursing Times, 1739–1741, October, 1975.

Maney, J. Y.: A behavioral therapy approach to bladder retraining. Nurs. Clin. N. Amer. 179–188, March, 1976.

McIver, V.: The extended care philosophy: a must for the long-term patient. Canadian Hospital, 34–36, November, 1973.

Metheny, N., and Snively, W. D., Jr.: Nurses' Handbook of Fluid Balance. ed. 3. Philadelphia: J. B. Lippincott Co., 1979.

Milne, J. S. et al.: Urinary symptoms in older people. Modern Geriatrics 2:198, 1972.

Moore-Smith, B.: Medicine in old age: urinary tract disease. Brit. Med. J. 29:686–688, 1973.

Pollock, D. D., and Liberman, R. P.: Behavior therapy of incontinence in demented inpatients. Gerontologist 14:488–491, 1974.

Shuttleworth, K. E. D.: Incontinence. Brit. Med. J. 4:727–727, 1970.

Sotiropoulos, A.: Urinary incontinence. Urology 6:312–317, 1975.

Specht, J.: research critique of Effect of operant conditioning on modification of incontinence in neuropsychiatric
geriatric patients, by Jeanette Grosicki, 1972.

Sturdy, D. E.: Essentials of Urology. Great Britain: John
Wright & Sons, 1974.

Tanner, E. R.: Pelvic muscle dysfunction in urinary incontinence. Physiotherapy 55:372, 1969.

Willington, F. L.: Problems in the aetiology of urinary incontinence (Incontinence-2). Nursing Times 71:378–
381, 1975.

Willington, F. L.: Psychological and psychogenic aspects
(Incontinence-3). Nursing Times 71:422–423, 1975.

Willington, F. L.: The nursing component in diagnosis and
treatment (Incontinence-4). Nurs. Times 71:464, 1975.

Willington, F. L.: Training and retraining for continence
(Incontinence-5). Nursing Times 71:500–503, 1975.

Willington, F. L.: The prevention of soiling (Incontinence-
6). Nursing Times 71:545–549, 1975.

Willington, F. L.: Incontinence in the Elderly. New York:
Academic Press, 1976.

21

Musculoskeletal Problems

Helen Wolff

QUICK REVIEW

OSTEOPOROSIS

DESCRIPTION	Progressive loss of bone mass greater than expected for age, race, and sex.
ETIOLOGIC FACTORS	Unclear but factors cited include aging (postmenopausal females); small constitutional size; genetic factors (e.g., white ancestry); low calcium, phosphorous, protein, vitamin C and D intake; lowered sex hormones; inactive lifestyle. Certain diseases involved—alcoholism, hyperthyroidism, hyperparathyroidism, chronic uremia, chronic hepatitis, malabsorption syndromes (e.g., postgastrectomy). Drugs—corticosteroids.
HIGH RISK	Postmenopausal females, sedentary/inactive persons, small-boned persons, whites, history of diet low in calcium.
DYNAMICS	From mid-30s on, bone loss begins to exceed formation. Beginning with vertebrae and moving to pelvis and long bones later.
SIGNS AND SYMPTOMS	Usually asymptomatic early. May be found on x-ray pictures after 30 percent of bone is lost. First symptom may be pain with collapse of weakened vertebrae. Signs—kyphosis, loss of height, decreased spinal mobility.
DIFFERENTIAL DIAGNOSIS	Metastatic disease, multiple myeloma, osteomalacia. Serum calcium and alkaline phosphatase remain normal in osteoporosis.
COMPLICATIONS	Fractures, falls, immobility.
PROGNOSIS	Progressive but rate varies.
MANAGEMENT	Bone loss is well established by 70, so goal is maintenance. Nonspecific—estrogens, dietary calcium, fluoride, calcitonin all are being tried and tested. Pain management: Non-narcotic analgesics. Diet: to include adequate protein, calcium, and vitamin D daily. Physical activity to place weight bearing and torsion types of stress on bones. Supportive devices, warm packs, deep heat medications for pain relief. Avoid extended periods of bedrest as much as possible.
EVALUATION	Adequacy of diet. Maintaining comfort and mobility. Daily routine incorporating weight bearing and torsion.

QUICK REVIEW

DEGENERATIVE JOINT DISEASE (DJD)

DESCRIPTION	Noninflammatory degeneration of articular cartilages in joints with formation of new bone at joint edges, a universal phenomenon of aging.
ETIOLOGIC FACTORS	Aging, wear and tear, obesity, heredity, and prior inflammatory disease.
HIGH RISK	Elderly, male and female risk about equal. Overweight.
DYNAMICS	Unclear. Possible that degeneration of cartilage triggers bone changes or that bone changes increase stress on cartilage.
SIGNS AND SYMPTOMS	Relatively asymptomatic. Principle symptom is localized *pain and stiffness,* crepitation, mild to severe nagging aches. Symptoms increase with use or on first movement after a period of inactivity with relief after "limbering up." Tends to occur in knee, hip, hands, and neck. Heberden's nodules.
COMPLICATIONS	Immobilization, leading to further disability.
MANAGEMENT	Symptomatic relief—aspirin is cheapest and most effective. Watch for side effects. Heat, isometric exercises (quadriceps) useful when knees involved. Weight control. Canes/walkers may reduce stress on knees and hips. Total hip/other joint replacement surgeries are being used.
EVALUATION	Maintaining mobility and preferred lifestyle.

QUICK REVIEW

RHEUMATOID ARTHRITIS

DESCRIPTION	A chronic, systemic disease characterized by bilaterally symmetric joint inflammation and resultant joint damage.
ETIOLOGIC FACTORS	Unclear. Current findings support immunologic reactions. Viruses may initiate condition.
HIGH RISK	Onset can occur after age 70, although younger persons are at greater risk. Equal sex distribution in older persons. Living in temperate climates increases risks. First symptoms usually occur in spring.
DYNAMICS	Decreased immunocompetence is thought to contribute to the progressive course of disease without the remissions that occur in younger persons.
SIGNS AND SYMPTOMS	Pain, swelling, and limitation of motion in small joints of hands, wrists, and feet, usually symmetric. Stiffness in early a.m., lasting one to two hours. Symptoms worse prior to changes in weather. In advanced disease, classic deformities with subcutaneous nodules around elbows/fingers, partial dislocation of cervical vertebrae, flexion contractures with ankylosis. Systemic effects: Fatigue, anemia, weight loss. Signs: x-ray findings, positive latex fixation test, poor mucin clot from synovial fluid, characteristic histologic changes—nodules and synovial fluid.
DIFFERENTIAL DIAGNOSIS	Degenerative joint disease, ankylosing spondylitis, systemic lupus. Eleven Diagnostic Criteria from American Rheumatism Association (1973).
PROGNOSIS	Tends to be steadily progressive in elderly. Changes in ADL and lifestyle exacerbate status. Poorer prognosis associated with vascular inflammation. Immobility and loss of independence.
NURSING MANAGEMENT	Determine person's perception of functional losses and impact on ADL/lifestyle. Balance rest and activities but minimize extended bedrest. Active or assisted ROM, only to point of pain, strengthening and endurance exercises several times/day. Splints/braces during acute phases. Provide assistive devices for managing ADL. Heat/cold for comfort. Aspirin (not enteric-coated)—4 to 6 gm/day (note toxic effects).
EVALUATION	Satisfying balance of activities/rest. Pain controlled so therapeutic program is possible, mobility maintenance. Living effectively with disability, prevent contractures.

The effects of normal aging on the musculo-skeletal system are pervasive. Some of the most common health problems of the elderly are associated with changes that occur in muscles, bones, and joints. The impact of these changes on the lifestyle of the older person covers a range from annoying aches and decreased ability to perform physical activity to severe nagging pain and complete immobility. Strength, speed, posture, body image, independence, and safety are all affected.

While some signs and symptoms that occur herald normal changes of aging, others are forerunners of treatable pathology where disability can be modified, delayed, or prevented by competent differential diagnosis and appropriate medical treatment. Whether normal or pathologic, these alterations are surprisingly common. By retirement, 80 percent of the population has some type of rheumatic complaint (Kolodny, 1976, p. 91). The commonality of symptoms as well as their insidious onset may contribute to the willingness of the elderly to accept or minimize their aches and pains as "normal" and delay diagnosis and management of potentially severe and treatable problems.

The high risk conditions of the elderly involving the musculoskeletal system include falls and fractures, osteoporosis, arthritis, degenerative joint disease, and gout. The normal changes of aging, in combination with the disorders that occur, have serious implications for the elderly.

GAIT AND MOBILITY

The ability of the older adult to maintain independence in a familiar environment hinges to a large extent on the efficiency of locomotion. Compromise in this critical function can seriously diminish essential coping resources, personal confidence, and initiative.

Although posture and movement in healthy aged persons covers a wide range of normal, a fairly typical pattern tends to emerge. In old age, posture tends to take on an attitude of general flexion. This hunchbacked appearance results from wedging of the vertebrae (Fig. 21-1), particularly in the thoracic area, and degenerative changes causing thinning of the intervertebral disks.

The nurse will see kyphosis of the thoracic spine (Fig. 21-2), varying in severity; forward flexion of

head and neck; and gentle bending of elbows, wrists, hips, and knees. Despite the normality of some bending, the older person *should be* encouraged to stand straight.

Secondary to the foregoing, the center of gravity shifts. This shift *leads to an increase in the amount of energy expenditure required to maintain balance and normal gait.* At the same time there is a normal loss of muscle bulk accompanied by decreased tissue regeneration, contributing not only to a changed appearance (thinning and flaccidity of muscles) but also to less strength for dealing with the increased demands created by a shift in the center of gravity. The changes imposed by this degeneration are far from insignificant.

To compensate for the anatomic changes, stance becomes wider, height of each step is lessened, movement becomes more cautious and deliberate, and hurrying tends to be avoided. In addition, an increase in reaction time, owing in part to concurrent changes in the central nervous system and loss of visual

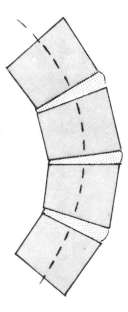

FIGURE 21-1. Wedging of the vertebrae. With thinning of the intervertebral disks, this causes a hunchbacked appearance.

acuity, accentuates locomotion difficulties. An 82-year-old lady described her ambulation ability simply, "I'm careful. I don't hurry and eventually I get there."

Studies have shown that when older persons cannot move about as freely as they once did, can't maintain their usual pace, and lose confidence in movement, they begin to see themselves as old and ill. Therefore, mobility is important not only in performance and independence but also in the person's definition of self (Shanas, 1968).

Nursing Assessment of Capacity for Activities of Daily Living

Data gathering on gait and mobility often begins with subjective data in which the nurse talks with the older person about the status of his mobility in relationship to the activities of daily living, his preferred lifestyle, and his home-neighborhood environment.

Information is obtained on what activity can and cannot be accomplished, as well as on what has had to be given up. The Shanas' Index of Incapacity may be a useful means of gathering data on basic self-care capability.

Objective data can be obtained from casual observation as well as during structured activities. In the home, clinic waiting room, senior citizen center, or nursing home corridor information can be collected about:

1. General posture—kyphosis, compensatory position of head and neck, flexion of extremities, contractures
2. Stance—distance between the feet when standing, toeing in or out
3. Gait—length of stride, height foot is lifted from the floor, shuffling
4. Normal speed in walking. Does pace decrease progressively with distance?

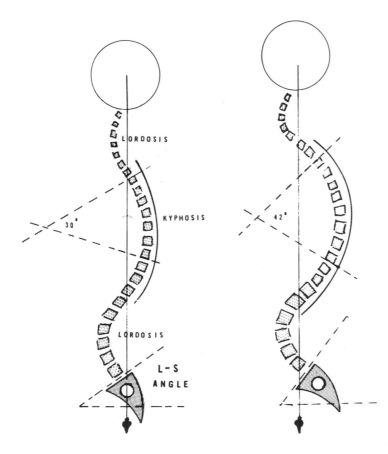

FIGURE 21-2. *Left,* Normal physiologic curve with the head directly above the pelvis. The dorsal kyphosis is approximately 30 degrees, and there is a slight lumbar lordosis. *Right,* "Round back," caused by increased dorsal kyphosis. The head is held forward of the center of gravity. Lumbar lordosis is exaggerated because of an increased lumbosacral (L-S) angle. (Reprinted from Cailliet, R.: Scoliosis. Philadelphia, F. A. Davis Co., 1975, p. 7, with permission)

5. Difficulty or ease in sitting down or standing? Note type of furniture selected to sit on
6. Support and balance provided by touching furniture, door jams, railings
7. Use of assistive devices including canes, crutches, walkers, skill in using devices, fit of the aid in relationship to size of the person
8. Ability to climb and descend stairs.

Additionally, the nurse may direct the patient to engage in certain activities to observe other capabilities:

1. Standing independently—with eyes open and eyes closed, note balance and sway
2. Range of motion—head and neck, shoulders, elbows, wrists, hands, hips, knees, ankles, back. (The height the foot can be raised in hip-knee flexion is important in assessing ability to use public transportation.) Agility and reaction time.
3. Strength in lifting objects.

Since the feet may be barriers to mobility, careful observation for corns, calluses, leg or foot ulcers, flat arches, and bunions needs to be made. The type of footwear selected for use can be a clue to foot difficulties. Are soft-soled, nonsupportive slippers worn all day?

While disturbances in gait are easily noted, the need exists to distinguish the reason for the disability and the risk areas in daily living. Only then can the nurse be useful in initiating referral for appropriate medical care, engage in nursing management, or assist the individual to develop better strategies for self-management.

FALLS

The disruption in lifestyle caused by accidents among the elderly is tremendous. In individuals over 70 the incidence of nonfatal accidents increases markedly. Falls constitute the greatest number of accidents in the older population. Often seemingly minor falls cause the older person to be confined to bed for a few days. Although immobilization would mean little to younger individuals, for older persons, bedrest increases the risk of complications and is as dangerous as the original fall. Thus the prevention and management of falls are important.

Etiologic Factors

NORMAL CHANGES OF AGING. Normal changes that occur in aging contribute substantially to falls. Altered posture with changed center of gravity, decreased muscle strength caused by atrophy, slowed reaction time, and loss of visual acuity are contributors to a large number of falls. Impaired balance, usually having its origin in central nervous system changes, further enhances the likelihood of falls. One older person summarized her propensity to fall with, "Once you start going, you've got to go" (Sheldon, 1960, p. 1687).

CHRONIC DISEASES. Chronic diseases also place the elderly at higher risk for falls. Changes in vision resulting from cataracts, glaucoma, corneal opacities, macular degeneration, and retinopathy limit visual accuracy and lead to misplaced footing or failure to recognize impending disaster in the form of barriers, slippery floors, and uneven surfaces. Cerebral hypoxia, cardiac arrhythmias, and postural hypotension

---

INDEX OF INCAPACITY*

Can you go out of doors?

Can you walk up and downstairs?

Can you get out of the house?   *Scoring*

Can you wash and bathe yourself?   0   no incapacity

                                                   1   Does the task with difficulty

Can you dress yourself and put on your shoes?   2   Unable to perform the task

Can you cut your toenails?

---

* Adapted from Shanas, E., et al.: Old People in Three Industrial Societies. New York: Atherton Press, 1968, p. 26.

cause vertigo and fainting which precipitate falls. Diabetes with concurrent peripheral neuropathy leads to diminished sensation and circulatory change, creating additional risk factors. Hemiplegia with associated loss of balance, proprioception, musculature, and sensation and often faulty awareness of the environment makes falls a high risk.

MEDICATIONS. Many drugs can be precipitating factors in falls. Antihypertensive drugs result in postural hypotension and sudden falls as the individual stands up or stands in one position for a period of time. Sedatives and tranquilizers dull perceptions in a way that decreases stability. Drugs that change fluid and electrolyte balance can contribute to the risk of falling by causing hypovolemia and arrhythmias.

DROP ATTACKS. Increasing evidence supports a fairly high incidence of falls unrelated to specific causes. Falls in this category have been labeled "drop attacks." In these situations, the individual describes a sudden loss of tone in the legs with an immediate fall. There is no corresponding loss of consciousness, identifiable neurologic deficit, or other symptoms. Some time may elapse before the individual can regain sufficient muscle tone to stand, and considerable assistance may be required.

ENVIRONMENTAL FACTORS. Many factors in the immediate environment contribute to falls. They include:

- inadequate lighting, particularly in stairwells and landings
- absence of railings on stairs and in bathrooms
- slippery surfaces in tubs and showers, on smooth surfaces with spills, or throw rugs, failure to use nonskid wax
- obstructions such as long extension or telephone cords, furniture in pathways, objects that are not picked up. Even pets and children can get underfoot

BEYOND THE HOME. Outside the home lurk the same hazards as in the immediate environment. The risk is magnified by decreased familiarity. Steps, curbs, and uneven surfaces pose the greatest danger. Buses, escalators, and building accesses are areas of high risk. Places with dim lighting or sudden changes in lighting can increase danger of falls.

CLOTHING. Clothing and shoes can contribute to falls. Loose-fitting and long robes may "catch" on furniture, doorknobs, or cooking utensils, causing a loss of balance or pulling an object into the path. Use of slippers without substantial soles, such as heelless scuffs or thongs, provide little stability, often fit poorly, and, thereby, increase the risk of falls.

Complications

Falls can cause both physical and psychologic trauma. Bruises, lacerations, and fractures are the more obvious results of falls. The complications of immobilization that may result if the person chooses or is required to recover in bed from the effects of the fall can be much more dangerous than the fall itself. Less overt, but still significant, is the loss of confidence, courage, and independence that results from fear of recurrence of falls. Older persons may experience a "sudden aging" in their approach to life as a result of the loss in pride and mobility following a fall.

The attitude of the family toward their older relative after a fall can produce guilt and fear. To convey the idea that the person should not have fallen because they were cautioned to be careful can destroy confidence and independence. If the person is unable to return to his home following hospitalization from a fall he could feel rejected by his family.

Prevention

Obviously falls are better prevented than treated. One way to minimize the hazard of falling is to restrict the area of movement to a small safe environment. However, since quality of life is as important as longevity, this is the least acceptable method of prevention. A more realistic approach is to modify the environment. Although cost may be a limiting factor, many alterations can be implemented that are both acceptable to the older person and minimal in expense.

BATHROOM. Many falls occur in the bathroom. Nonslip bathmats can be purchased at low cost and adhesive-backed nonskid strips are easily applied in tub or shower. Grab-bars may be placed at critical locations by tub and toilet to lend support. Night lights or lighted switches enable the person who gets up at night to orient himself more easily to the environment and its hazards.

STAIRWELLS. Walls and stairs should be of contrasting colors. Railings should be installed on all stairs for support and guidance in indicating position on steps. A piece of fabric or a knob can easily be attached to the rail to indicate the level of the top and bottom steps.

LIGHTING. The need for light increases with age.

Either the number of lights or the intensity of bulbs should be increased in order to keep the environment lighted at a safe level. Adequate illumination is extremely important in high hazard areas such as stairs and stairlandings.

OBSTRUCTIONS. Obviously, obstacles should be removed wherever possible. Extension and long phone cords should be avoided, taped down, or covered to minimize the possibility of tripping. Throw rugs should be avoided. Placement of furniture should be out of traffic pathways and adjusted to the best side of vision the older person has. Edges of carpeting should be blended into the adjoining floor surface as smoothly as possible. However, these changes are more easily discussed than accomplished since most older persons have adjusted to their environment without recognizing hazards and barriers.

There probably is very little that can be done effectively to control pets. However, the nurse may try to raise the consciousness of the individual about deliberately using his eyes more actively in scanning the environment. Teaching the technique of turning the head to survey the often-missed fringes of the visual field can help avoid many otherwise overlooked hazards.

ACCEPTABILITY OF PREVENTIVE MEASURES. Since most, if not all, preventive measures for falls will be undertaken in the older person's own living area, it is essential that he participate in understanding the risks and options. Time is well spent in discussing methods used to make the environment more fallproof, rather than the nurse taking the primary role in decision making. The nurse's role is to question and give positive feedback to ideas. The nurse can also play an active role in identifying community resources when labor or materials are involved and the person's resources are limited. The local office on aging is a good starting point.

Management

Where falls cannot be prevented, there are certain nursing obligations in terms of management. Nurses need to teach patients at high risk (1) the best way to fall and (2), if injuries occur, how to move across the floor to reach the telephone or furniture. When falls occur it is crucial that no blame or guilt be placed upon the patient by the nurse or family. Such criticism will only add insult to injury. Many falls among the elderly are not preventable—they just happen. After a fall the person feels badly enough; therefore, support and understanding are essential.

When risks of falls are great and the person has a preference for continuing to live independently, the nurse can help the individual to set up a "back-up situation." Many communities have a Friendly Phone Visitor program in which volunteers call the older person at a specified time each day. If the person does not answer, someone who lives nearby is notified and checks on the patient. This volunteer has a key or some form of access to the home. Thus the patient has the security of knowing he will never be left longer than a 24-hour period. With this type of system, the fear of falling and being unable to get help is less of an overwhelming concern.

The reporting of falls is extremely important. With the elderly, fractures may be difficult to see on an x-ray picture. If pain persists it should be checked out and resolved. Similarly, headaches may indicate skull fractures or head injury. When the patient relates symptoms, the nurse should determine whether a fall has occurred. If other health care providers discount the patient's reports, the nurse may need to serve as a liaison to insure that serious attention is given the complaint and that adequate x-ray studies, diagnostic tests, and medical management are undertaken.

Evaluation

The effectiveness of nursing management can be evaluated by noting such criteria as:

1. Participation of the patient in modifying the home environment for prevention of falls.
2. Behavior that assists in the prevention of falls such as increased visual awareness or changes in shoes or clothing.
3. Establishment of a daily phone call and back-up systems when indicated.
4. Continued activity and mobility in the preferred lifestyle.
5. Verbalization of what to do if a fall occurs, symptoms to observe and report, availability of emergency phone numbers.
6. Adjustment to changes that have been made.

FRACTURES

Fractures are viewed as a major catastrophe to most elderly people. Suddenly, without warning, lifestyle is disrupted and independence is dealt a severe blow. Little opportunity exists for anticipating outcomes or planning beyond the immediate situation. The more-or-less casual pace of the day-to-day events become crises waiting to happen. Coping resources are compromised by the loss of function—mobility, self-care, or both. Pain insults the ability to plan and concentrate. Reliable support systems must be available immediately to assist in short and long range planning. At best, the short term result of fracture is to be housebound for a few days; at worse, institutionalization for an indeterminate period in an unfamiliar surrounding with restricted sensory input and total dependence. Either situation leaves time to ponder the happening as well as the final outcome.

Description

Fracture refers to a break in the continuity of a bone. Fractures in the elderly occur in areas of greatest stress such as the head and neck of the femur, the weight-bearing vertebral column, or the wrist. Bones already weakened by osteoporosis are more prone to fracture. Minimal trauma such as moving or turning can result in a fracture in severely-diseased bones.

Etiologic Factors

The major factors contributing to fractures in the elderly are loss of bone mass and falls. Chronic pathologic conditions such as alcoholism, osteoporosis, and metastatic disease affect bone density, again increasing the likelihood of fracture. Drugs such as steroids used in the treatment of musculoskeletal disorders contribute to accelerated loss of bone mass. One etiologic factor that is frequently overlooked is undue cautiousness that leads to halting gait and subsequent falls.

High Risk

Old women are at greater risk of fractures than men by a ratio of 3:1. Low-income white people tend to have a higher incidence of fractures. The largest number of fractures occur in the home.

Dynamics

The bones lose strength and become more brittle with aging. Muscles, tendons, and cartilage decrease in elasticity and, consequently, are weakened. The combination of a weakened skeleton and supporting structure increases the risk that fractures will occur. Although the rate of fracture healing in the elderly is similar to that of other ages, differences in bone density and concurrent chronic conditions can alter the rate at which an aggressive rehabilitation program is introduced.

Signs and Symptoms

Undiagnosed or "silent" fractures occur more commonly among the elderly. Vertebral compression fractures often are not noticed unless an x-ray picture is taken. Impacted fractures where displacement of the bone fragments does not occur may also be ignored.

Eventually discomfort and stiffness with loss of mobility will bring the person in for attention. The nurse should be alert for signs of deformity, bruising, and abrasions when a patient complains of bone or joint pain, even when no fall has been reported. Loss of function, including refusal to bear weight, is an important sign. A high suspicion of fracture is wise.

Pain is a less reliable indicator of fracture in the elderly. Some individuals may minimize symptoms of bone and muscle discomforts as expected consequences of aging. Persons may deny pain or try to tolerate it rather than seek help because the possibility of a fracture has occurred to them and they fear hospitalization and having to leave their home should the fracture diagnosis be confirmed.

Differential Diagnosis

Differential diagnosis is to be made between soft tissue damage (sprain or strain) and actual fracture. In any injury where fracture is a possibility, x-ray studies are indicated. Sometimes roentgenography will not reveal a fracture. The patient may continue to complain of pain and on a second film a fracture is identified. Listen to the patient.

Nursing Management

MOBILITY. Following alignment and fixation, the critical component of nursing management of patients with fractures is early mobilization—ambulation and return to activities of daily living in terms of the prefracture lifestyle. Participation of the patient in planning for the return to prefracture mobility is important. The challenge is in finding activities that will help the patient retain and regain strength, flexibility, and endurance that are within present capabilities and are of sufficient interest to keep him working regularly.

Repetitive exercises, done only to please the nurse, have little value to the patient and soon will be discarded. The patient should be involved in selecting activities and planning the schedule. Participation should be more likely with patient involvement, and also helps establish a schedule that achieves an appropriate balance between exercise and rest for this person.

PAIN. Pain can be preoccupying. It makes any task more difficult, often impossible to achieve.

Response to pain varies with individuals. Discomfort is not always manifested in complaints but sometimes in withdrawal and refusal to participate. One must also consider cultural influences in assessing the patient's response to pain. (See also Chapter 27, Pain.) Control of pain and muscle spasm contributes to the person's willingness and ability to move and participate in activities. On the other hand, too much medication may make the patient too drowsy to ambulate and exercise. The response to analgesia, including the duration of relief, is important to consider when planning the administration of drugs in relationship to activities. Analgesia and muscle relaxants should be given long enough ahead of the proposed activity to be effective during the activity.

ANTICOAGULANTS. Anticoagulants frequently are used as part of therapy to prevent thromboembolic complications, particularly with hip fractures. During the acute phase of illness, prophylactic administration of short term, low dosage heparin is used. Heparin is standardized in terms of *units* rather than milligrams or milliliters. A typical dosage of "mini-heparin" is 5000 units given subcutaneously every 12 hours. The suggested site of the subcutaneous administration is the abdomen. The usual laboratory tests to determine clotting and bleeding time generally are not done in the use of mini-dose heparin, since dosages of this size alter clotting time only minimally. Use of heparin continues until the amount of time spent out of bed is greater than that spent in bed.

Acetylsalicylic acid grains 10 is given twice daily prophylactically to prevent thrombus in the actue phase following hip fracture. This regimen may be continued following discharge.

If anticoagulant therapy is required following hospital discharge, Coumadin or Dicumarol are used. Careful monitoring of bleeding and clotting times must be done. Prothrombin time is the test of choice used to determine the effectiveness of therapy. The patient needs to understand the importance of keeping appointments to have laboratory tests done. Written instructions including the date, time, and location of the appointment should be provided. Patients receiving Coumadin and Dicumarol should be advised not to take aspirin. Interaction of the drugs increases the likelihood of bleeding. Tylenol, Motrin, and other new nonsteroid anti-inflammatory agents also interact with anticoagulants and prolong prothrombin time. The patient on anticoagulants should be cautioned to avoid other nonprescription medications because of possible adverse interaction.

Both the patient and family need to know the implications anticoagulant therapy has for daily living. They should observe and report bleeding gums, bruising, or dark-colored stools.

ANTIEMBOLIC STOCKINGS. Antiembolic stockings should be used for patients who are immobilized for long periods of time. This includes patients with fractures of the hip and vertebra. The decision to use these stockings can be a nursing judgment.

Antiembolic stockings must fit properly to be useful. Those that do not fit are worthless. Stockings may constrict circulation if they are too tight or too long, or they will slip down around the ankles if they are too large. The entire foot should be encased in the stocking. They should extend over the knee to midthigh.

To insure a proper fit, patients should be individually measured. These stockings are expensive and, once used, cannot be returned.

The stockings come in knee length, thigh length with gusset top, and full leg with stabilizer belt top. For knee length stockings, measure, as in Figure 21-3: (1) the circumference of the calf at the widest point and (2) the length from heel to the bend in the

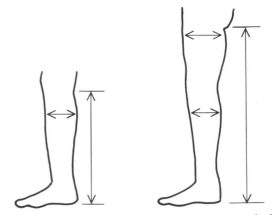

FIGURE 21-3. Measurement guide for antiembolic stockings. *Left,* Knee length; *Right,* Full length. (See text.)

back of the knee. For full length stockings, measure, as in Figure 21-3: (1) the circumference of the calf at the widest point, (2) the circumference of the thigh, just below the gluteal fold, and (3) the length from heel to gluteal furrow. Do not apply stockings if the measurement of the circumference of the thigh is more than 32 inches (81.3 cm).

While the patient is in a health care facility, the stockings should be removed for 30 minutes every shift. The person at home should be instructed to remove the stockings once daily. When the stockings are off, the skin should be observed for breakdown, particularly in the area of the heel, ankle, and knee. Keep the stockings off for 30 minutes so that air can reach the skin.

The care of the elderly person with a cast, splint, or brace is the same as that for any other age group. Refer to a standard orthopedic textbook for a review of these principles of care.

Complications

Loss of independence and mobility are the general high risk complications of fractures in the elderly. Mobility is decreased by loss of joint function, contractures, decreased strength, and decreased endurance. Fear of recurrence and the associated undue caution also complicate the individual's subsequent lifestyle. Sensory deprivation may be a secondary complication to the loss of mobility and independence.

Locally the complications are related to interruption of the nerve and circulatory supply either in the surrounding soft tissue or to the bone itself. These can result in nonunion or malunion and need for further treatment.

The associated bedrest or physical immobilization contribute to all the known hazards of immobility for each system. For the older person they occur earlier and last longer.

Thrombophlebitis and pulmonary emboli are life-threatening complications of fractures caused by immobilization. They are less likely to occur presently than in the past because of improved surgical techniques, prophylactic medications, and early mobilization. Because of increased risks during the period of immobility, legs should be checked daily for evidence of phlebitis. Measurement of the calf provides a baseline for comparison if signs of phlebitis develop. Daily assessment of the legs includes comparison of affected and unaffected leg and observation of edema and redness. Any complaint of tenderness should be treated immediately. Homan's sign (discomfort behind the knee or in the calf on forced dorsiflexion of foot) can be used as a reliable indicator of thrombophlebitis. (For a full discussion of thrombophlebitis, its diagnosis, management, and complications, see Chapter 13.) The purpose of this assessment is early identification so medical treatment can be implemented.

Pulmonary emboli can occur post-fracture. This is a serious and often fatal complication. Shortness of breath, chest pain, hemoptysis, and fever are presenting complaints. Even sophisticated tests such as lung scans and pulmonary angiography can fail to confirm the diagnosis. Medical treatment is instituted when symptoms suggest pulmonary emboli.

Prognosis

Following fracture, a good prognosis for return to previous lifestyle is associated with *having been previously active and involved* so that there is a reason for getting better. Recovery from illness and trauma is so much slower in the over-70 group that frustration and hopelessness can occur. It becomes important to recognize small gains and point them out to the patient and family so that there is continued motivation to work to improve, rather than give up.

Another factor influencing prognosis is the promptness with which rehabilitation exercises are instituted—whether the person is in bed, confined to a chair, or ambulatory. Some form of activity can always be undertaken. Conversely, it is rarely too late to begin a rehabilitative program that can influence prognosis in some manner.

High Risk Fracture Sites

Hip

The most common site of fracture in older people is the hip. Hip fractures occur in two main locations —those involving the neck of the femur, referred to as the subcapital or intracapsular, and the intertrochanteric region or extracapsular. The shaft of the femur is a relatively uncommon site of fracture. Owing to marginal circulation to the neck of the femur, fractures in this area carry greater risk of nonunion.

Characteristically, hip fractures result from falls. Frequently a fracture seems unlikely in view of the minimal trauma incurred. A rapid assessment of the classic signs and symptoms that correspond to hip fracture leave little alternative to the diagnosis of fracture. Typically, the individual complains of pain in the hip or thigh, adduction, external rotation, shortening, and reluctance to move or bear weight on affected extremity. If the fracture is impacted or undisplaced, the person may experience little discomfort, still be able to walk, and *shortening of the leg may be the only evidence of injury.*

For a variety of reasons, from denial of injury to lack of a support system, the individual with a hip fracture frequently is not seen for treatment for one to four days. This undesirable delay in initiation of therapy can represent time during which complications get an unyielding foothold. Relatively minor problems with poor nutrition, fluid imbalances, skin breakdown, and joint stiffness can be magnified in a few days to cause arrhythmias, decubuti, and contractures.

Choice of treatment depends on (1) the location and severity of the fracture, (2) time elapsed since the initial injury, and (3) general health of the individual. Major surgery using either a nail or prosthesis to stabilize the fracture is the treatment of choice. Recent use of a prosthetic femoral component has nearly eliminated the incidence of avascular necrosis of the head of the femur and has made early ambulation a reality. Pinning or nailing of femoral neck fractures, while extremely satisfactory, can carry the risk of a second surgical procedure if problems caused by circulatory inadequacy develop. Pins also may require removal at a later date because of the ongoing discomfort they cause. Mobilization normally progresses to nonweight-bearing ambulation with a walker and eventual independence in a period of four to six weeks.

Occasionally a fracture of the femoral head is stable without surgical intervention either because it is impacted into the acetabulum or shows only a hairline break. Bedrest ranging from a few days to a week is recommended to decrease muscle spasm and reduce pain. At the conclusion of the time, ambulation with weight bearing to tolerance can be resumed.

The period of bedrest inherent in all of the above treatments carries the threat of complications that astute nursing care often can prevent. Fractures of the hip are the most devastating to the elderly in terms of time required for healing, extent of treatment required, limitation of mobility, and the wide range of associated complications that occur. In recent years health care providers and patients have seen evidence that hip fractures do not necessarily mean an end to independence. Attitudes and expectations are gradually changing with more positive outcomes being anticipated and experienced. With this should come a more assertive approach by both nurses and patients to initiating and maintaining the rehabilitative activities that will make return to normal a reality for as many patients as possible.

Wrist

Fracture of the wrist, i.e., Colles' fracture, is an unfortunate result in many falls. Typically, the distal radius is broken as the older person attempts to avert disaster by falling on an outstretched hand. The fracture that results is described as a "dinner fork" deformity with displacement of the wrist backward and toward the radius.

The goal of therapy is to restore joint function. This is accomplished by manipulation of bone fragments into alignment and immobilization, using a rigid plaster dressing or splint. Stability is difficult to achieve because of the many small bones in the wrist.

Following a wrist fracture, the patient must be alert to any change in circulation or nervous function in the lower arm and hand. The person should be taught to check for warmth, color, capillary refilling in the nailbeds and any abnormal sensation including tingling, burning, and numbness and report these changes immediately. The weight of the cast can be a deterrent to movement of the shoulder in older people. To prevent this complication the person should be encouraged to resume activities that promote this movement, such as combing the hair. Raising the arm above the head several times each day will also prevent development of a stiff shoulder. To prevent dependent edema both before and after removal of the cast/splint the arm and hand can be supported in a sling.

While in place, the cast or splint provides a secure feeling that the fracture is healing and that additional damage cannot occur. When the device is removed the joint feels weak and painful and swelling may occur. Many patients have concern that they will damage the fracture site if they participate in activities. They may need reassurance that it is safe to resume activity. Light housework, folding laundry, setting the table, doing dishes, knitting, and trimming grass with garden shears are all activities that assist in regaining lost function.

Older persons who have had fractured wrists also need to know that it is common for some pain and stiffness to persist. This is particularly true with changes in the weather.

Vertebrae

Crush or compression fractures of the spine are relatively common in the elderly. Fractures of this type are sustained with minimal trauma, such as a jolt, sitting down abruptly, or even turning over in bed, in people with osteoporosis, metastatic disease, or those who have been on long term steroids.

When seen for treatment the patient's main complaint is localized pain in the back. The amount of pain is a poor indicator of the extent or severity of damage, so roentgenography is necessary to confirm the diagnosis. If multiple fractures have occurred, deformities of the back will be apparent, accompanied by loss of total body height. A more critical indicator of compression is the measurement of trunk height in relationship to total body height. The latter seems a justification for measurement of height and trunk height on routine examination as part of a patient's baseline data. If there has been a delay in seeking treatment, symptoms of abdominal distention with nausea, vomiting, and constipation may indicate a paralytic ileus.

Since compression fractures seldom cause neurologic deficit, the treatment is directed at reduction of symptoms. Muscle spasms that cause back pain are alleviated by bedrest of 5 to 10 days. Mild analgesics are ordered for comfort. Rib belts and corsets provide support in the low thoracic and lumbar spine where the majority of these fractures occur. Braces, while helpful in providing support, are usually too encumbering for the old person and are soon discarded. The effect of these devices on restricting lung expansion is also a consideration in their use.

Following the initial period of immobilization, gradual resumption of activity is encouraged. The individual should be cautioned against extremes of flexion or extension of the back.

OSTEOPOROSIS

Osteoporosis refers to progressive loss of bone mass greater than normally expected for age, race, and sex. The remaining bone is normal in mineral composition although decreased in volume (Avioli, 1976). The skeleton is less dense, weaker, and takes on the appearance of being spongy or moth-eaten. So common is this condition among elderly women, it is often called "senile" or "postmenopausal" osteoporosis. The skeletal areas having the greatest impact on the lifestyle of the older person include the vertebrae with risk of compression fractures and the long bones with increased risk of fractured hip.

Etiologic Factors

The cause of age-associated bone mass decrease is unclear. A variety of factors have been implicated in producing bone loss. Those commonly cited include:

- female sex
- small constitutional size
- genetic factors, including white ancestry
- deficiency in calcium and protein
- lowered level of sex hormones
- inactive lifestyle
- aging

Some diseases and conditions in which osteoporosis is commonly seen are hyperthyroidism, hyperparathyroidism, Cushing's syndrome, chronic uremia, chronic hepatitis, alcoholism, malabsorption syndromes, and postgastrectomy state. Long term administration of corticosteroids is also associated with bone loss causing osteoporosis.

NORMAL AGING. Normal aging is in itself an etiologic factor in bone loss. A fairly typical pattern of bone changes occurs with advancing age. Between age 30 and 40 there is an 8 percent bone loss in women and 3 percent in men. The reduction in bone begins earlier in women and is accelerated following menopause.

RACE. The atrophy of bone is similar among races. However, black people and males have a greater initial skeletal mass and, therefore, show symptoms of loss at an older age.

INACTIVITY. Inactivity, which frequently accompanies advancing age, is also recognized as a factor in osteoporosis. Stresses on long bones, such as normal weight bearing, stimulates bone formation. Immobility imposed by disease or limited physical activity reduces the necessary stress and accentuates bone resorption.

NUTRITION. Nutritional status has been investigated as a factor potentially contributing to bone loss. In order to maintain skeletal integrity, calcium, phosphorus, vitamins C and D, and protein must be available in sufficient amounts. Ninety-nine percent of the body's calcium is stored in bone. When intake is inadequate, bone is resorbed. The addition of 1 gram of calcium daily to the diet of postmenopausal women will reduce bone loss (Nordin, 1975). To maintain serum calcium in equilibrium, vitamin D is needed either in the form of a supplemental source or synthesis from sunlight. The latter frequently is lacking in the elderly who are institutionalized or spend most of their time indoors. Recently sodium fluoride is being studied regarding its role in providing "hardness" to bones. Individuals who were raised in areas with high levels of fluoride in the water have tended to have less pronounced osteoporosis.

HORMONES. By far the largest number of individuals with osteoporosis are postmenopausal women. A direct relationship between estrogen deficiency and bone loss has been identified. Replacement therapy with cyclic natural estrogen has been moderately successful in providing symptomatic relief. Latest evidence would tend to support that menopause accelerates bone loss and this can be retarded or prevented by estrogen replacement therapy (Lindsay, 1976). Calcium absorption is increased in postmenopausal women by estrogen therapy. These observations suggest that part of the mechanism by which estrogen deficiency increases bone loss is to raise the level of dietary calcium required to maintain positive calcium balance (Gallagher, 1978).

High Risk Populations

From the foregoing discussion, osteoporosis looms as a fairly certain event of aging. The mere circumstance of growing old makes one vulnerable. None of the various suggested treatments for osteoporosis have been fully satisfactory either in arresting the progression of bone loss or in producing increase in bone mass.

A composite of high risk factors would suggest that the person at highest risk of osteoporosis is the small, slender, white, relatively inactive, postmenopausal female who has avoided dairy products in her diet through a lifetime.

Dynamics

Until some point between the third and fourth decade, the skeleton maintains an equilibrium between bone formation and resorption. Bone loss affects the entire skeleton, but the rate at which it proceeds in the various parts of the body is not uniform. The vertebrae begin to be affected by 25 to 30 years,

while changes in cortical bone become obvious much later.

Many explanations have been offered on the dynamics of excessive loss. These include proposals that:

1. Osteoblasts fail to deposit osteoid tissue because of lack of estrogen.
2. Calcium deficiency occurs as a result of dietary intake.
3. An imbalance exists between either adrenal or parathyroid and gonadal hormones.
4. There is depression of calcium absorption in the intestine or there is a disturbance in renal processing of calcium.
5. There is an abnormal adrenal response to corticotrophin and defective growth hormone secretion.

The single explanation for accelerated bone loss and/or reduced bone formation is still undetermined.

Signs and Symptoms

Typically, osteoporosis is asymptomatic. Recognition of the condition generally follows a fracture or medical examination for a different reason. For some individuals the first symptom is severe pain resulting from fractures of a vertebra or femur. Lumbar and thoracic pain is due primarily to the collapse of vertebral bodies.

Physical signs include kyphosis and reduced lumbar lordosis (see Fig. 21-2), decreasing body height (particularly in the trunk), and decreased mobility of the spine. Roentgenography will show the demineralization only after 30 to 60 percent of the bone mass is lost.

Differential Diagnosis

Many disorders mimic osteoporosis and make precise diagnosis difficult. Metastatic disease, multiple myeloma, and osteomalacia present with x-ray appearances similar to osteoporosis. Laboratory tests such as serum calcium and alkaline phosphatase frequently are of value in ruling out other conditions. These tests remain normal in osteoporosis. Bone biopsy is the most reliable way of establishing the diagnosis; however, this is not usually done in old people since, even if accurately diagnosed, treatment is symptomatic.

Complications

Osteoporosis in its advanced stages contributes to fractures, falls, and nerve compression. The associated kyphosis can contribute to breathing and cardiac difficulties as a result of compression of the lungs and heart and the decreased mobility of the thorax.

Management

The ideal treatment of osteoporosis would be to find some means to slow down bone resorption and increase bone formation. Since the mechanisms are not well understood, the treatment remains nonspecific at this time, with the goals of therapy being to maintain a sense of well-being, decrease discomfort, and maintain a realistic level of activity.

Drug and mineral therapy for the treatment of osteoporosis is an area of ongoing study. Estrogen replacement, once thought to be a means of halting or slowing postmenopausal osteoporosis, has been found in some studies to have an initial short term favorable effect in decreasing the rate of bone resorption but, after longer treatment intervals (9 to 15 months), resulted in a secondary decrease in bone formation (Jowsey, 1977). While estrogen can retard osteoporosis, remineralization of bone does not occur. Because of the increased risk of breast and uterine cancer, women receiving estrogen should be taught breast self-examination and should have yearly mammography and pelvic examination. Estrogens improve feelings of well-being and are reasonable choices of therapy. Androgens are also being tested.

Dietary calcium intake of 1 gm per day is required to maintain physiologic function of muscle and nerves. Without an intake of milk or milk products, deficiency will develop and the skeletal reservoir of calcium will be utilized. Nordin reported that the greatest amount of calcium loss occurs at night in the elderly. A dish of ice cream or a glass of milk at bedtime could be suggested. Sardines are a good source of calcium that is seldom considered (Nordin, 1971).

Fluoride has been suggested as a therapy in osteoporosis because of a decreased incidence of osteoporosis noted where the level of natural fluoride in drinking water is high. Some reserach has shown improvement in osteoporosis with supplementation of fluoride. New bone formation is stimulated but mineralization is poor and, consequently, not structurally sound. However, the decreased incidence of fractures and pain relief using fluoride has been promising.

Calcitonin, a peptide hormone secreted by cells in the thyroid gland, is known to suppress bone resorption. Some good results have been reported in slowing bone resorption with use of this substance; however, it does present some complications. The use of this substance, as with others, is still being evaluated as effective therapy.

Because of the chronicity of osteoporosis, nonnarcotic analgesics are prescribed for relief of back and leg pain. Skeletal muscle relaxants are of some use in relieving discomfort of spasms of the paravertebral muscles.

Because bone loss tends to be well established in the over-70 age group, goals of providing support and promoting adjustment are more realistic than prevention. Nursing management is concerned with helping the individual to include sufficient calcium, vitamin D, and protein in the diet, given the established eating patterns, financial situation, and other existing medical problems. Helping the person to include daily physical activity involving weight bearing and torsion on bones that are not at high risk of pathologic fracture is also important. Data gathered through discussion with the patient on usual activities of daily living will assist in identifying the best or most acceptable alternatives for incorporating additional exercise.

It is important to relieve pain/discomfort. Analgesics should be given judiciously. Drug dependency, however, is not a major concern in treating people over 70 even though osteoporosis is a chronic condition. The goal is to keep them comfortable.

Supportive devices such as back braces, corsets, and belts are useful in providing pain relief. Because the device is often cumbersome to handle, difficult to get on and off, and further restricts mobility, it may be discarded by the older person. Warm packs, "deep-heat" ointments and gentle massage are selectively useful for relief of annoying discomforts.

The immobilization of bedrest hastens the process of bone demineralization. Avoiding prescriptions of bedrest or limiting inactivity to the shortest time compatible with healing or recovery from illness is advisable. When bedrest is needed, muscle setting exercise may be instituted to continue torsion-type bone stress even where weight bearing is not possible. Because these people are often fearful of turning or moving, it is helpful to teach methods of turning and getting up from a bed or chair. Nurses need be aware that fractures can result both from proper and improper turning of a person with *severe* bone loss.

Evaluation

Evaluation areas should include (1) the absence of new fractures, (2) freedom from symptoms, and (3) ability to participate in activities of daily living. It is useful to gather data in the following areas:

1. The patient is ambulatory and there is daily physical activity that involves muscle torsion on bones and weight bearing.
2. The individual knows how to protect the bones at high risk of fracture.
3. Discomfort is controlled to the extent that an acceptable level of participation in usual activities of daily living is possible.
4. Dietary intake of calcium, protein, and vitamin D within recommended limits is maintained.
5. Devices to aid posture or mobility are available and used (braces, corset, walker).

DEGENERATIVE JOINT DISEASE

Degenerative joint disease (DJD), sometimes called osteoarthritis, is a universal phenomenon of aging characterized by noninflammatory changes in the articular cartilage of joints and formation of new bone at the joint edges. The condition is asymmetric in distribution and is progressive.

Etiologic Factors

Aging, trauma, obesity, heredity, or prior inflammatory disease are contributing factors.

High Risk Population

All older people are subject to degenerative joint disease. Obesity contributes to its severity. Under-age-60 females report symptoms of DJD twice as often as males. In older ages the sex distribution is equal. Wear and tear of joints increases the severity of DJD.

Dynamics

The mechanism for cartilage destruction has not been clearly defined. One explanation is that degeneration of cartilage triggers secondary bone changes.

Another theory is that bone changes increase stress on weight bearing surfaces of joints, leading to breakdown of cartilage.

Signs and Symptoms

Although degenerative joint disease is common in older people, few are bothered by symptoms.

Pain is the main symptom. It occurs in motion and weight bearing, and it can increase before changes in weather. While most people experience only mild aching confined to the joint area, a few have constant nagging pain that persists even at rest and is referred to nearby muscles. Joints are usually more painful after overuse. Conversely, joints may be particularly painful when first moved after a long period of inactivity. In contrast to the pain of rheumatoid arthritis, which persists for hours, relief in DJD occurs in a short time with "limbering up."

Typically, the symptoms will be those of pain in knee, hip, hand, neck, or lower back. Initially, the pain occurs with movement or weight bearing. As the degeneration progresses, pain may occur even during rest and may interrupt sleep. People affected also complain of stiffness and "crunching" sounds with movement.

Loss of joint mobility is another common symptom. Initially this is recognized by the patient as stiffness and inability to do simple movement without pain. Muscle weakness may occur as stiffness increases, leading to abnormalities of posture and gait.

Crepitation, a grating sound heard when the joint is moved through its range, can often be noted. Knees, hips, interphalangeal joints, and the spine are most often involved.

Heberden's nodes are bony enlargements that occur at the end joints of the fingers. The potentially-deforming nodes occur most often in females and tend to run in families.

Subjective complaints tend to be affected by the lifestyle and expectations of the person rather than the extensiveness of the degenerative joint disease. Some people expect the "aches and pains of growing old" and continue to be active and ignore discomfort. Lonely, unhappy persons with time on their hands may find the joint pains intolerable.

Complications

The most serious complication associated with degenerative joint disease is that the discomfort and stiffness may cause increasing immobilization and unwillingness to retain the desired lifestlye. Deformity owing to nodules is minimal but may be a threat to women who have had pride in their hands. In turn, the immobilization creates further disability.

Management

Treatment is aimed at symptomatic relief. More than many other conditions, the "rheumatism" of old age is affected by folkways or personal ideas of treatment. Many old people view particular elements in the diet, such as "acids," as a cause of disease and, therefore, avoid these substances. Others single out a particular food touted as a cure and ingest this to the exclusion of other nutrients. Lamps, vibrators, exercise, and salves—all have their proponents. The nurse needs to be astute in determining the belief system of the individual about joint disease and attempt to develop an articulation with these beliefs and the professionally prescribed regimen.

Several kinds of drugs are used for DJD. At present aspirin (ASA), Darvon, and Tylenol are used for mild pain. Because of excellent pain relief and low cost, aspirin should always be tried first. The side effects of aspirin should be a constant concern of patients on long term therapy. Medication should be taken regularly so severe pain does not occur. Analgesics should be given before undertaking activities that could be painful.

Occasionally, stronger drugs such as indomethacin and phenylbutazone will be used. These drugs tend to cause severe gastrointestinal upsets and blood dyscrasias and are poorly tolerated by some patients. If phenylbutazone is prescribed, it should be given for a limited time and the patient should be monitored while taking it. Injections of hydrocortisone into intra-articular surfaces provide temporary relief. Systemic corticosteroids are seldom prescribed.

Sometimes heat, ultrasound, and massage are helpful in relieving the discomfort caused by cervical or lumbosacral degenerative joint disease. Isometric exercises can strengthen the quadriceps when knees are involved.

Where weight-bearing joints are involved and obesity is present, weight reduction may be helpful. However, weight reduction in the over-70 group is difficult because of lowered BMR and calorie requirement, reduced activity, set eating habits, time on their hands, and low food budget with deficits in protein, low calorie fresh fruits, and vegetables. Walking with two canes helps reduce stress on knees and hips and increases mobility.

When possible, the nurse should try to keep the person mobile. Where periods of bedrest for acute illness and trauma occur, older persons will need encouragement to face the discouragement of the slower road back to full activity and sometimes the "push" to work at coming back even when it would seem easier not to try.

Surgery

When symptoms of hip and knee pain are not relieved by other measures, surgery can be performed. Hip and knee replacements are done with good success in elderly people. Any surgery carries a risk that must be weighed against the complication of long term immobility and its consequences.

Total joint replacement is a recent technique devised to treat pain and loss of joint mobility caused by disease and injury. All are important factors in maintaining mobility, especially in older persons. While virtually all major body joints are replaceable, the most common surgery involves the hip, knee, elbow, and finger joints. Through use of artificial joints, many people with degenerative joint disease, rheumatoid arthritis, and fractures have obtained relief of symptoms and regained independence.

TOTAL HIP REPLACEMENT. This procedure involves surgical reconstruction of the hip joint using a metal ball and stem and a plastic socket. The artificial parts are stabilized in place with a bone "cement," and the new joint is realigned so that it moves freely through a normal range of motion.

The individual who understands total hip surgery and knows what to expect before and after the operation will be able to participate actively throughout all phases of the surgery and rehabilitation process. Ideally, preparation of the patient for total hip replacement begins several months prior to the scheduled surgery. During the early phase of preoperative care, emphasis is placed on teaching muscle strengthening exercises and providing opportunity to practice crutch walking. Because of rising high costs of hospitalization the preoperative preparation is done on an outpatient basis with hospital admission usually a day or two before surgery.

All of the following areas should be reviewed before preoperative preparation is considered completed:

- history and physical examination
- laboratory tests (complete blood count, electrolytes, sedimentation rate)

- roentgenography of chest and both hips
- exercises for muscle strengthening, including quadricep and gluteal setting (see the end of this chapter)
- learning crutch walking
- measurement for abduction splint and anti-embolic stockings

It is helpful for the patient, family, and friends to know that the surgical procedure requires several hours.

Rehabilitation progresses in a predictable fashion following total hip replacement. The older person should be informed of the expected progression of activity. Although some variation in the rehabilitation schedule exists based on the operative approach and physician preference, a usual pattern of postoperative recovery included:

- bedrest for one to four days
- head of bed elevated up to 60 degrees for comfort
- turning to unaffected side or back
- overhead trapeze to help lift and turn self
- ambulation using a walker or crutches following period of bedrest
- abduction splint, triangular bolster or pillows between knees while on bedrest and at night
- discharge in one to three weeks

Infection and dislocation are serious complications of total hip replacement. When infection occurs, removal of the prosthesis is necessary and the person is left with a less functional hip than before undergoing surgery. Prophylactic antibiotics are routinely administered for 72 hours postoperatively to avoid this complication. Dislocation is a complication preventable by careful positioning of the affected hip. The patient is taught to *avoid* hip flexion greater than 90 degrees, adduction beyond the midline of the body, and internal rotation.

Discharge instructions stress the importance of proper hip positioning and increased activity. Instructions for the person going home following a total hip replacement include:

1. Continue exercises as instructed in the hospital.
2. Do not cross one leg over the other in any position. Do not even cross ankles until the physician permits (up to 3 months).
3. Do not sit for longer than 1 hr at a time without standing, stretching, and walking a few steps.
4. Avoid sitting in low or overstuffed chairs that require bending forward to stand up. Do not stoop down to pick things up or bend over to tie shoes (slip-on shoes are best).
5. When lying on your side, lie on unoperated hip.
6. Use abduction splint or pillows between legs when in bed or 6 to 8 weeks following discharge.
7. Use crutches when ambulating until the physician indicates (usually 4 to 6 weeks). When permission is given to use one crutch or a cane, use it on the unoperated side.
8. Use a raised toilet seat for 4 wk after discharge.
9. Continue to wear support hose for 6 wk postoperatively.
10. May start driving in 6 wk.
11. May resume sexual activity in 6 wk.
12. Put away scattered rugs.

Total hip replacement has given many elderly people a new outlook on life. Although the replacement cannot be considered a normal joint, this procedure has contributed immensely to improvement in qualify of life through pain relief and increased mobility.

Evaluation

The problems of people with DJD are related to stiffness, difficulty moving, and pain. An effective plan of care addresses these issues. The person should carry out activities relatively free from pain if medications are taken regularly and devices that assist with walking and moving are used. If weight cannot be reduced, at least it should not increase. The person who has had total hip replacement surgery should have a new lease on life.

GOUT

Gout is an acute disease in which crystals of monosodium urate are deposited in the joint space. Although any joint can be involved, the single joint most commonly affected is the great toe. Gout is not a single disease but a syndrome resulting from different biochemical abnormalities that lead to hyperuricemia (Harrison, 1977).

Etiologic Factors

Gout results from either overproduction or under-excretion of uric acid. The mechanism of overproduction is unknown. Thiazide diuretics have been found to inhibit excretion of uric acid; therefore, people on this type drug have a higher incidence of gout. Heredity is also a contributing factor.

High Risk Population

Gout increases with age. Primarily it affects males over 50 but, after age 50, incidence in females increases.

Dynamics

High serum uric acid levels result in deposition of monosodium urate crystals in the joint and trigger an acute inflammatory reaction.

Signs and Symptoms

Classically, the patient will be male, complaining of severe pain in the great toe developing in the middle of the night. The joint and the surrounding tissue appear red and swollen and are extremely painful. The person may seem ill and feverish. Bed clothing touching the joint or someone walking in the room produces pain. Any joint can be involved. In individuals where gout is poorly controlled, nodules called tophi, formed by crystals, may be found on ears, elbows, and hands.

The past history of symptoms is important. Usually there will have been previous acute brief attacks with complete relief between. There will also be a family history that "gout runs in the family."

Blood tests show elevated serum uric acid, sedimentation rate, and white blood count. Attacks may recur after several years of being asymptomatic.

Differential Diagnosis

Cellulitis, tendonitis, and infectious arthritis must be ruled out. The presence of the crystals in the synovial fluid confirms the diagnosis (Harrison, 1977, p. 615).

Complications

Renal damage may occur where blood levels of uric acid run higher than 11 mgm percent (normal 2 to 7 mg percent). Destructive joint changes occur if the patient does not respond to treatment.

Management

Gout is a disease in which complete remission is possible. Gout can be managed effectively with medication, preventing recurrence of attacks. Phenylbutazone, indomethacin, and colchicine are used to treat acute attacks. Steroids are used selectively, taken for 2 to 6 days. They should result in complete elimination of symptoms. Narcotics are indicated for relief of severe pain during acute attacks.

Recurrent attacks are treated by drugs that act to lower the serum uric acid (allopurinol probenecid, sulfinpyrazone). Low doses of aspirin (under 1 gm) tend to inhibit excretion of uric acid while high doses (greater than 4 gm) increase excretion.

Treatment is aimed at eliminating attacks, preventing complications caused by deposits of sodium urates in joints, and preventing formation of uric acid kidney stones. While special dietary restrictions are not indicated, reduction in alcohol intake and purine-containing foods such as organ meats may be useful. Weight reduction for the overweight patient has helped some.

Evaluation

Understanding of signs and symptoms enables the person with an acute attack to seek immediate assistance. Compliance with prescribed drug therapy can prevent recurrent attacks.

RHEUMATOID ARTHRITIS

Older persons can be afflicted by a variety of over 100 disorders grouped under the heading of rheumatic disease. Over 20 million people in the United States experience symptoms of "rheumatism" or "arthritis" severe enough to cause them to seek treatment. Many elderly people are debilitated by symptoms of joint pain and stiffness referable to one of these conditions. Unfortunately, living with mild discomfort that has developed insidiously over the years tends to cause older persons to disregard additional symptoms as being just more evidence of "old age." The end result is that they fail to seek medical evaluation because they feel, often incorrectly, that "nothing can be done anyway."

Description

Rheumatoid arthritis is a chronic, systemic disease characterized by bilaterally-symmetric joint inflammation. The synovium lining the joint space becomes inflamed and edematous, eventually resulting in irreversible joint damage.

Etiologic Factors

Although several theories have been suggested, the cause of rheumatoid arthritis has not been identified. Current findings support the belief that immunologic reactions occur to trigger destructive changes in the synovium. Rheumatoid factor, an antibody found in the serum of many patients with this disease, is thought to play an important role in perpetuating inflammation through reactions with the body's immunoglobulins. Synovial aspiration has failed to yield a microorganism responsible for inflammation. The incidence of transient rheumatoid arthritis associated with various viral infections gives support to the idea that a virus may be responsible for initiating the condition.

High Risk

While rheumatoid arthritis is often considered a disease of younger persons, the elderly can experience initial acute attacks. Although females are more frequently affected by rheumatoid arthritis in younger age groups, the sex distribution becomes about equal after age 70. Persons who live in temperate climates are also at higher risk.

Dynamics

The onset of rheumatoid arthritis, while variable, is usually insidious, with the first symptoms occurring more commonly in the spring (Grob, 1978). Periods of nearly complete relief of symptoms alternating with acute inflammatory flare-ups are characteristic. In elderly people, however, the course of the disease often progresses in a "malignant" fashion without episodes of remission, although generally symptoms are less severe than in their younger counterparts (Kolodny, 1976, p. 93; Ditunno, 1970, p. 165). This is thought to be related to the diminished immunocompetence that accompanies aging.

Signs and Symptoms

The appearance of signs and symptoms, whether subtle or explosive, is characterized by early morning stiffness that lasts one to two hours, pain, swelling and limitation of motion in hands, wrists, or feet. Joint involvement is symmetric.

In contrast to the joints affected in degenerative joint disease and gout, the small joints of the hands, feet, and wrist are most vulnerable. Pronounced swelling, pain, and stiffness are the symptoms most aggravating to the patient. In advanced disease, classic deformities such as subcutaneous nodules around the elbows and fingers (25 percent of patients), partial dislocations of cervical vertebra and wrist, and flexion contractures with ankylosis involving the fingers and hands help to expose the diagnosis (Kolodny, 1976). In addition there are systemic manifestations of fatigue, anemia, and weight loss. Many people with arthritis express an innate ability to predict the weather based on subjective changes in joint discomfort.

Because of the many diseases that masquerade as rheumatoid arthritis and the diversity of symptoms of persons seeking treatment, the American Rheumatism Association (1973) has identified eleven Diagnostic Criteria for Rheumatoid Arthritis:

1. Morning stiffness
2. Pain on motion or tenderness in at least one joint
3. Swelling (soft tissue thickening or fluid, not bony overgrowth alone) in at least one joint continuously for not less than six weeks)
4. Swelling of at least one other joint
5. Symmetric joint swelling
6. Subcutaneous nodules
7. X-ray changes typical of rheumatoid arthritis
8. Positive latex fixation test
9. Poor mucin clot from synovial fluid
10. Characteristic histologic changes in synovial membrane
11. Characteristic histologic changes in nodules.

These criteria must have been present for at least six weeks in order to establish a diagnosis. The diagnosis of "probable" disease is given a person with three of the symptoms, "definite" disease with five, and "classic" with seven symptoms.

Laboratory tests are inconclusive for establishing a diagnosis. Latex fixation test, rheumatoid factor, detects the presence of the specific antibody in the blood. While eventually present in about 85 percent of persons with rheumatoid arthritis, the substance occurs in numerous other collagen diseases as well as in some persons without the disease. Synovial fluid aspiration usually reveals an elevated white count but no specific organism has been identified.

Erythrocyte sedimentation rate (ESR Sed rate), a nonspecific indicator of inflammation, is used to determine the course of rheumatoid arthritis. During an acute inflammatory episode values elevate markedly. The test is used to determine when an episode has subsided to the extent that activity can be resumed.

Differential Diagnosis

Rheumatic symptoms are common to many systemic diseases and frustrate efforts to confirm a diagnosis. Other conditions, principally those affecting joints, must first be excluded from consideration. Degenerative joint disease, ankylosing spondylitis, and systemic lupus erythematosus may, in some instances, be indistinguishable from rheumatoid arthritis.

Prognosis

Poor prognosis is associated with the presence of systemic complications such as pericarditis and vasculitis. High titers of rheumatoid factor are indicators of poor prognosis (Anderson, 1975). Hydralazine and procainamide, drugs seen in common use in the elderly, may produce arthritis-like symptoms as a side effect.

Changes in daily routine, emotional upsets, and alterations in dietary patterns are frequently identified as factors that can provoke exacerbation of symptoms.

Nursing Management

A thorough review of the presenting signs and symptoms is needed. Discussion with the patient to obtain a complete history and *indication of the person's perception of functional losses is crucial.* Information can be obtained by asking such questions as: "What activities are most difficult for you to perform?" "In what way has your ability to move about been affected?" and "When did you last feel well?" Unless asked specific direct questions, the basis for some problems will not be identified. Either through deliberate denial or failure to recall an event such as a fall, data can remain undiscovered. Bruises, lacerations, and other physical findings can provide a starting point for discussion.

Rheumatoid arthritis is a chronic and progressive disease. Although a cure has not been identified, there is much that can be done to promote comfort and maintain or increase functional ability. All therapy is directed toward assisting the person to meet these goals.

A balance between rest and exercise is of primary concern. Just as too little assistance can be disastrous, in rheumatoid arthritis too much help can be damaging.

The use of bedrest is restricted to periods of acute joint swelling when activity would cause further damage. The ill effects of prolonged inactivity can lead to rapid development of weakness, muscle atrophy, contractures, and osteoporosis.

Exercises

Range of motion, strengthening, and endurance exercises are used. Active, assistive, or passive ROM of all involved joints is indicated several times each day. This activity should be continued only to the point of pain. Isometrics are used in all phases of the disease. They are well tolerated and are more likely to be continued than strenuous exercises. Strengthening exercises should be repeated frequently. They are best suited to upper extremity functioning (Ditunno, 1970).

Splints and Braces

Splints and braces can decrease pain and prevent deformity. Splints are effective in acute episodes of joint inflammation and at night to prevent development of contractures. Braces are used under the same circumstances. However, braces provide greater support and are more costly. They must be custom made and the individual must be trained in the use of such devices. If problems arise, the bracemaker should be notified so the problem can be resolved before damage results and a helpful piece of equipment discarded. Splints and braces are not substitutes for exercise.

Assistive Devices

Devices or gadgets made by the patient or a family member to aid in maintaining function are more likely to be used than expensive equipment produced commercially. Devices are not just gadgets but are valuable tools to help the person maintain independence. The nurse's attitude should support this value.

Modifications that can be made in the home include use of straight back chairs and raised toilet seat. Stacking sofa pillows provides a higher and

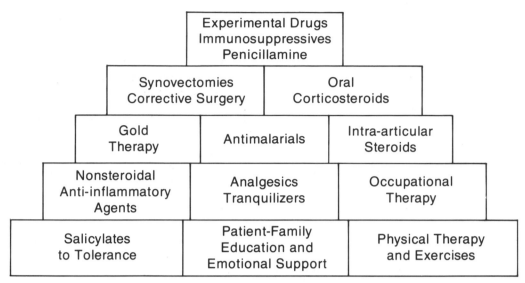

FIGURE 21-4. Drug pyramid for treatment of rheumatoid arthritis has aspirin at the base. If base modalities are inadequate, the next level is tried, and so on to the top, where extreme caution in drug use is essential. (From Kolodny, A. L., and Klipper, A.: Bone and joint diseases in the elderly. Hosp. Pract. 11:94, 1976, with permission)

more firm place to sit. Additional suggestions are available in a pamphlet from the Arthritis Foundation. (See end of chapter for address.)

Consultation with a registered physical therapist is useful to identify areas of retraining and plan a program to meet this goal. The physical therapist can also provide assistance in periodic evaluation of the ongoing program and retraining in activities of daily living so stress on joints is reduced to a minimum. Any program developed for people with rheumatoid arthritis must be practical. Patients must have input into the plan since they are to carry it out. Ongoing evaluation of the program is needed or the goals may be forgotten and the program soon discarded.

Application of heat and cold are useful in relieving pain and joint stiffness. With this relief a more effective exercise program can be undertaken. Heat is applied through packs, paraffin bath, whirlpool, and Hubbard tank. Ice packs and tubs of ice are also used. The amount of relief achieved by the patient determines which therapy will be selected.

People with rheumatoid arthritis should be encouraged to maintain as much of their normal lifestyle and activity as possible. Swimming is one activity that provides diversion and exercise. Since there is less resistance to movement in water than in air, increased amounts of exercise can be accomplished with less energy expenditure. For those with limitations of neck motion a snorkel can be used in swimming.

Drugs

The aim of drug therapy is relief of pain, inflammation, and arrest of the progress of the disease. This is important because a person in pain will be unable to carry out any program of exercise.

Aspirin is the drug of choice in rheumatoid arthritis. Four to six grams a day may be required to relieve discomfort and control inflammation. The anti-inflammatory properties of aspirin should be explained to the patient. Enteric-coated aspirin is not recommended, since in this form salicylate absorption may be erratic. It has been found that enteric-coated aspirin has passed through the gastrointestinal tract in the same form in which it was ingested.

The therapeutic dose of ASA is found by producing ototoxicity in the form of ringing in the ears and reducing the dosage until tinnitus stops. Serum levels of salicylates should be monitored. Hemorrhage, ulcer, and other gastrointestinal problems are side effects of aspirin.

Anti-inflammatory medications such as indomethacin, tolmetin, naproxen, and fenoprofen are used when aspirin cannot be tolerated. These drugs also cause gastrointestinal irritation. Many nonsteroid anti-inflammatory agents are being tested currently. Hopefully a drug will be found which will be effective, well-tolerated, and have few side effects.

Gold salts have been found to be effective in the treatment of elderly people with rheumatoid arthritis. Several months of use are required before the benefit from gold can be determined. Serious side effects associated with gold therapy include bone marrow depression, skin rash, and kidney damage. Evidence of any of these side effects necessitates discontinued use.

Corticosteroids are anti-inflammatory drugs. Their major action in rheumatoid arthritis is to relieve inflammation, which will lead to remission of acute symptoms. In acute stages of the disease they can be most useful. These drugs given for short term may be useful until other drugs take effect. Small doses of Prednisone (2.5 to 7.5 mgm daily) may enable the person to tolerate pain and, thus, maintain activities of daily living.

Summary of management is described in the pyramid in Figure 21-4.

Evaluation

Rheumatoid arthritis is a chronic, progressive disease. The aims of treatment are:

- balance between rest and activity
- control of pain so that a therapeutic program can be followed
- maintaining interests and mobility in so far as possible
- adjustment/acceptance of deformity
- prevention of contractures

Plans of care are designed to achieve these goals. Modifications are made as the condition changes.

FADS AND QUACKERY

Musculoskeletal problems, because of their chronicity and failure to respond to therapy lead to frustration with usual forms of treatment. As patients seek relief, they are vulnerable to fad remedies that are generally worthless, almost always expensive, and may be harmful. A neighbor may have read that a diet of grapefruit or beets is a sure cure for arthritis. There are books about the efficacy of copper bracelets. Vibrators have their advocates. Persons seeking

relief through quackery are often reluctant to discuss their "remedy" with a member of the health team for fear of being ridiculed or reprimanded. It is important for the nurse to be a sensitive listener and a nonjudgmental resource in helping the persons to make wise choices from the options available.

EXERCISE

Exercise takes many forms, from encouragement of activities of daily living to formal classes. Classes in techniques of exercise for older people are now being offered in many areas. Exercises can be planned to maintain mobility of joints in normal aging, in diseases like arthritis, and preoperatively and postoperatively in total joint replacements. Sharing the philosophy of organized group activity is essential. Some attitudes about group exercise include:

Exercise is fun.
A social situation is created and interaction is encouraged.
Exercise can be done sitting, standing, lying, or in bed.
Each person competes only with himself.
Props such as rubber bands, balls, and sticks can be used as "adult" toys.
Do only what you feel you can.
Practice at least three times a week.
Repeat each exercise only four times.
Anyone can "invent" an exercise.

The goals of exercise are both psychologic and physiologic: to strengthen and increase tone of muscles, to improve range of motion or flexibility, to relieve boredom, and to reduce social isolation. Some examples of movements that can be taught:

1. Lifts—movements against gravity. Ex: While in a sitting position, extend the knee, raise the leg straight and return to the floor.

2. Swings—back and forth movements originating in a large joint. Ex: Starting with arm at the side, swing the arm forward to shoulder height and backward as far as possible.

3. Twists—turning or rotating movements. Ex: Sitting in a chair with feet on the floor, reach across the body with right hand and attempt to grasp left back of chair.

4. Stretches—movements that produce a pull. Ex: Spread fingers as far apart as possible and return to resting position.

5. Circles—full rotation motion. Ex: With arm straight out from shoulder, draw a circle with the hand, or with the neck.

Kamentz (1971) suggests some ground rules for exercises for the elderly. The purpose of exercise is to get rid of muscle pain, to create relaxation, to improve circulation, and not to cause pain, produce anxiety, or tax the heart. Exercise daily (preferably twice a day). Do not rush but, rather, pace and feel comfortable doing the exercises.

Some patients are immobile. For them, many of the same exercises can be done in bed as well as sitting in a chair. If patients can be put on a stretcher, they can be moved to the area where exercises are being done by those who are ambulatory. This gives the bed patient a feeling of being part of the group.

Exercises for Persons with Rheumatoid Arthritis*

Exercises for patients with rheumatoid arthritis suggested by Watkins are listed:

1. After learning the motions to be performed, begin with only one or two repetitions of each exercise and repeat two to four times daily as ordered. Every few days, when possible, gradually increase the number of repetitions of each exercise to a maximum of ten repetitions.

2. Rest should follow each series of exercises. As improvement occurs, the rest periods will be shorter and exercise periods longer.

3. All exercise movements should be done slowly, carefully, and forcefully. Each active movement should be done through as great a range of motion as is possible.

4. An increase in pain or excessive fatigue that lasts for more than two hours following exercise indicates that the exercise has been too strenuous and fewer repetitions should be performed at the next exercise session.

5. Other physical therapeutic procedures such

---

* This section is reprinted with permission from Watkins, A. L.: Therapeutic exercise in rheumatoid arthritis. Courtesy Arthritis Rheum. 2:21, 1959. Reprinted in Marmor, L.: Arthritis Surgery. Philadelphia: Lea and Febiger, 1976.

as local use of heat, hydrotherapy, and massage are often prescribed to facilitate exercise.

Shoulders

1. Supine position with elbows comfortably bent, abduct the arms to shoulder level. (Do not allow scapular or clavicular motion.)

2. Now from position of abduction externally rotate as far as possible. (Point hands to head of bed.)

3. Then internally rotate as far as possible (point hands to foot of bed) and return to starting position.

4. Place each palm or forearm on top of head, then bring elbows together in front and back to sides.

5. With elbows straight at sides lift arms forward and up over head to extreme elevation.

6. Use pulleys as instructed.

Elbows

1. Fully and forcefully flex and extend.

2. Repeat above exercise with hand alternately in pronation and supination.

3. Add resistance of weights to exercise 1 as instructed.

Wrists

1. With elbow flexed and fingers relaxed completely extend wrist.

2. Now fully flex wrist.

3. With elbows flexed fully supinate.

4. Now fully pronate.

5. Do radial deviation (lateral movement towards thumb).

Fingers

1. Make a tight fist.

2. Fully extend fingers and spread apart.

3. With distal joints of fingers relaxed, fully extend at proximal joints (metacarpophalangeal).

4. Full radial deviation of thumb, then move finger in the same direction individually.

5. Oppose thumb to each fingertip, opening hand as wide as possible between each movement.

6. Gentle assisted stretching of contractures as specified.

Neck

1. Recumbent: flatten cervical spine, chin down and in.

2. Rotate head to left and right.

3. Flex neck laterally, chin straight ahead.

4. Head traction as instructed: ____ minutes, ____ pounds

Jaw

1. Open jaw fully.

2. Full lateral motion to both sides.

3. Protrude jaw forcefully.

Upper Back

1. Lying with small towel under midspine, extend back against bed with knees flexed.

2. Breathe deeply with prolonged inspiration.

3. Breathe deeply against sandbag on chest.

4. Breathe deeply while stretching ribs with hands.

Low Back

1. Gluteal setting. Forcefully tighten buttocks and pinch together.

2. Contract lower abdominal wall, bringing pelvis up slightly.

3. Alternate straight leg raising with feet in dorsiflexion.

4. With hands behind head, lift head and shoulders off bed.

5. Lying face down, raise head and shoulders off bed with back muscles.

Hips

1. Abduction in internal rotation:
   a. With knees straight and toes pointing slightly together, spread legs laterally.
   b. Standing, raise one leg, then the other, as far laterally as possible.

2. Internal rotation:
   a. Rotate entire extremity toward (toes pointing together).
   b. Standing, feet 12 inches apart, turn foot and leg inward and outward.

3. Fully flex the hips and knees, alternating each leg.

4. Extension:
   a. Lying face down, lift thigh off bed.
   b. Standing with trunk stationary, move thigh backwards.

5. Stationary bicycle riding.

Knees

1. Extension:
   a. With pillow under knees lift heels till knees are straight without hip motion.
   b. Quadriceps setting.
   c. Sitting on edge of support, straighten leg.
   d. Repeat with weights on feet as instructed.

2. Lying face down, fully bend knee.

3. Lying face up with hips flexed, flex and extend knees as though riding bicycle.

4. Standing: mark time with full hip and knee flexion.

5. Bicycle riding as instructed.

Ankles and Feet

1. Full dorsiflexion and slight inversion.

2. Repeat with toes curled downward.

3. Circling motions of ankle through dorsiflexion, inversion, planter flexion, and eversion.

Exercises for Persons with Prosthetic Hip Joints

As indicated earlier in this chapter, an exercise program is instituted with persons who are about to have hip joints replaced. The following exercise regimen is typical of those prescribed. Patients are taught the exercises preoperatively then the regimen is instituted while they are still in the hospital and continued as they convalesce at home.

1. A. Active Ankle Movement:
     (1) lie flat on back
     (2) slowly move ankles up and down
     (3) slowly move ankles in circles (both direction)
   B. Quad Sets
     (1) slowly tighten thigh muscles by straightening the knee
     (2) hold ____ seconds
     (3) relax
   C. Gluteal Sets
     (1) tightly pinch buttocks together
     (2) hold ____ seconds
     (3) relax
   D. Hamstring Sets
     (1) pull heel into bed
     (2) hold ____ seconds
     (3) relax

2. A. Pull Ups
   (1) lie flat on back
   (2) grasp trapeze bar above head with both hands
   (3) pull head and upper body towards bar as far as possible
   (4) hold ____ seconds
   (5) relax
   B. Arm Pushing
   (1) lie on back and grasp bottom rung of each side rail with hands
   (2) push down against rails
   (3) hold ____ seconds
   (4) relax
3. Active Hip and Knee Flexion, Quad Setting
   (1) lie flat on back
   (2) bend hip and knee by sliding heel up toward buttock
   (3) straighten leg all the way down and tighten thigh muscle as hard as possible
   (4) hold ____ seconds
   (5) relax
4. Bridging
   (1) lie flat on back with both knees bent and arms crossed over chest
   (2) raise hips and buttocks off bed
   (3) hold ____ seconds
   (4) slowly lower the hips to the bed
   (5) relax
5. Terminal Knee Extension
   (1) lie flat on back with small pillow under back of knee to be exercised
   (2) bend opposite knee
   (3) straighten the knee to be exercised all the way
   (4) hold ____ seconds
   (5) slowly let the knee bend so that the foot is again touching the bed
   (6) relax
6. Partial Sit-Ups
   (1) lie flat on back with both knees bent and arms crossed over chest
   (2) raise head and shoulders off the bed just so the shoulder blades no longer touch the bed
   (3) slowly lower the head and shoulders back to the bed
   (4) relax
7. Full Arc Knee Extension
   (1) sit on the edge of the bed or in a chair
   (2) lean backward slightly
   (3) straighten the knee all the way
   (4) hold ____ seconds
   (5) slowly bend the knee
   (6) relax

8. Hip Abduction
   (1) lie flat on back with your knees straight and your unoperated leg out to the side
   (2) take the operated leg out to the side as far as possible, keeping the knee and toes pointing straight up toward the ceiling
   (3) return the leg so that it is again straight down from your body
   (4) relax

BIBLIOGRAPHY

Anderson, R. J.: The diagnosis and management of rheumatoid synovitis. Orthopedic Clin. N. Am. 6:629–639, 1975.

Asher, M. A.: Management of adult hip disease. Postgrad. Med. 54: 73–79, 1973

Avioli, L. V.: Senile and postmenopausal osteoporosis. Advances Intern. Med. 21:391–415, 1976.

Avioli, L. V., and Krane, S. M.: Metabolic Bone Disease. New York: Academic Press, 1977.

Barzel, U.: Common metabolic disorder of the skeleton. In Reichel, W. (ed.): Clinical Aspects of Aging. Baltimore: Williams & Wilkins, 1978, pp. 277–288.

Berghan, F. R., Kupperman, A. S., Parfitt, M.: Thwarting the erosion of osteoporosis. Patient Care 7:50–70, 1973.

Bienenstock, H., and Fernando, K. R.: Arthritis in the elderly. Med. Clin. N. Am. 60:1173–1189, 1976.

Bollet, Al. J.: An essay on the biology of osteoarthritis. Arthritis Rheumatism 12:152–161, 1969.

Brocklehurst, J. C. (ed.): Textbook of Geriatric Medicine and Gerontology. Edinburgh: Churchill Livingstone, 1973.

Castelden, C. M.: Who is responsible for elderly patients on orthopedic wards? Geriatrics 32:65–68, 1977.

Chiroff, R. T.: An overview of osteoarthritis. Geriatrics 32:57–59, 1977.

Cobey, J. C., et al.: Indicators of recovery from fractures of the hip. Clin. Orthopaed. June 1976, pp. 258–262.

Cohn, S. H., et al.: Effect of aging on bone mass in adult women. Am. J. Physiol. 230:143–148, 1976.

DeCarlo, T. J., Castiglione, L. V., and Cavusoglee, M.: A program of balanced physical fitness in the preventative care of elderly ambulatory patients. J. Am. Geriatric Soc. 25:331–334, 1977.

Ditunno, J. and Erhlich, G. E.: Care and training of elderly patients with rheumatoid arthritis. Geriatrics 25:164–172, 1970.

Ehrlich, G., Katz, W. A., and Cohen, C. H.: Rheumatoid arthritis in the aged. Geriatrics 25:103–113, 1970.

Frankel, L. J., and Richard, B. B.: Exercises to help the elderly—to live longer, stay healthier, and be happy. Nursing 77. 7:58–63, 1977.

Freehaver, A. A.: Injuries to the skeletal system of older persons. In Reichel, W. (ed.): Clinical Aspects of Aging. Baltimore: Williams & Wilkins, 1978, pp. 289–302.

Gallagher, J. C., and Riggs, B. L.: Nutrition and bone disease. New Engl. J. Med. 298:193–195, 1978.

Gordon, G. and Vaughan, C.: The role of estrogen in osteoporosis. Geriatrics 32:42–48, 1977.

Grob, D.: Common disorders of muscles in the aged. In Reichel, W. (ed.): Clinical Aspects of Aging. Baltimore: Williams & Wilkins, 1978, pp. 245–260.

Grob, D.: Prevalent joint diseases in older persons. In Reichel, W. (ed.): Clinical Aspects of Aging. Baltimore: Williams & Wilkins, 1978, pp. 261–276.

Harris, R., Rodstein, M., and Still, C. N.: Look beyond hurt when an oldster falls. Patient Care 11:80–94, 1977.

Harrison, T. R.: Principles of Internal Medicine, ed. 8. New York: McGraw Hill Book Co., 1977.

;Heaney, R. P., Recker, R. R., and Saville, P. D.: Calcium balance and calcium requirements in middle-aged women. Am. J. Clin. Nutrition 30:1603–1611, 1977.

Hollander, J. L., and McCarty, D. J. (eds.): Arthritis and Allied Conditions, ed. 8. Philadelphia: Lea and Febiger, 1972.

Hunt, J. E.: Rehabilitation of the elderly. Hosp. Pract. 12:89–97, 1977.

Jowsey, J.: Osteoporosis: Dealing with a crippling bone disease of the elderly. Geriatrics 32:41–50, 1977.

Kamentz, H. L.: Exercises for the Elderly, American Pharmaceutical Company, P. O. Box 1022, Chicago, Ill., 1971 (Seicom Inc.); also in Am. J. Nurs. Vol. 72, August, 1972.

Kolodny, A. L., and Klipper, A.: Bone and joint disease in the elderly. Hosp. Pract. 11:91–101, 1976.

Lindsay, R., et al.: Long-term prevention of postmenopausal osteoporosis by oestrogen. Lancet 1:1038–1041, 1976.

Marmor, L.: Arthritis Surgery. Philadelphia: Lea and Febiger, 1976.

Mayne, J. G.: Planning a treatment program for rheumatoid arthritis. Geriatrics 28:92–102, 1973.

McBeath, A. A.: The aging skeleton—osteoporosis and degenerative arthritis. Postgrad. Med. 57:171–175, 1975.

Montgomery, R. M.: Relieving painful feet. Geriatrics 29:137–142, 1974.

Moskowitz, E.: Rehabilitation in extremity fracture. Am. Family Physician 11:107–112, 1975.

Moskowitz, R. W.: Osteoarthritis: A new look at an old disease. Geriatrics 28:121–128, 1973.

Newton-John, H. F., and Morgan, D. B.: The loss of bone with age, osteoporosis, and fractures. Clin. Orthopaed. July–August, 1970, pp. 229–252.

Nordin, B. E. C., Horsman, A., and Gallagher, J. C.: Effect of various therapies on bone loss in women. In Kulencordt, F., and Krause, H. P. (eds.): Calcium Metabolism, Bone and Metabolic Bone Diseases. New York: Springer Verlag, 1975, pp. 233–242.

Nordin, B. E. C.: Clinical significance and pathogenesis of osteoporosis. Brit. Med. J. 1:571–576, 1971.

Olsen, E. V.: The hazards of immobility. Am. J. Nurs. 67:779–797, 1967.

Peck, W., Recker, R. R., and Saville, P. D.: Osteoporosis: Exploring options and odds. Patient Care 11:71–79, 1977.

Rodnan, G. P., McEwen, C., and Wallace, S. L. (Eds.): Primer on the Rheumatic Diseases, ed. 7. New York: The Arthritis Foundation, 1973. Reprinted from J.A.M.A. 224 (Supplement), April 30, 1973.

Rogoff, B., and Sergent, J., Rheumatoid arthritis. Hos. Med. 11:54–69, 1975.

Rossman, Isadore (ed.): Clinical Geriatrics, ed. 2. Philadelphia: J. B. Lippincott Co., 1979.

Rowe, C. R.: The management of fractures in elderly patients is different. J. Bone Joint Surg. 47[Am]:1043–1059, 1965.

Shanas, E., et al.: Old People in Three Industrial Societies. New York, Atherton Press, 1968.

Sheldon, J. H.: On the natural history of falls in old age. Brit. Med. J. 1:1685–1690, 1960.

Smith, C.: Accidents and the elderly. Nursing Times 72:1872–1874, 1976.

Smith, D. M., and Edmondson, J. W.: Common adult osteopenic states: Osteoporosis and osteomalacia. Am. Fam. Physician 14:160–166, 1976.

Steinberg, F. U.: Gait disorders in the aged. J. Am. Geriatr. Soc. 20:537–540, 1972.

Watkins, A. L.: Therapeutic exercise in rheumatoid arthritis. Arthritis Rheumatism 2:21, 1959.

Wheeler, M.: Osteoporosis. Med. Clin. N. Am. 60:1213–1224, 1976.

Zvaifler, N. J.: Further speculation on the pathogenesis of joint inflammation in rheumatoid arthritis. Arthritis Rheumatism 13:895–901, 1970.

Additional information can be obtained by writing to:

The Arthritis Foundation
475 Riverside Drive
New York, NY 10027

22

Respiratory Problems

Suzanne Bither

QUICK REVIEW

CHRONIC OBSTRUCTIVE PULMONARY DISEASE

DESCRIPTION	Group of diseases with persistent obstruction to bronchial air flow leading to ventilation-perfusion abnormalities in the lung.
ETIOLOGIC FACTORS	Smoking, air pollution and occupation, infection, heredity, aging, allergy.
HIGH RISK	Smokers, occupations with high air pollution, males, family history, elderly.
DYNAMICS	*Chronic Bronchitis:* Airway obstruction resulting from excessive mucosal swelling and hypertrophy, inflammation, and excessive sputum production.
	Asthma: Reversible airway obstruction caused by smooth muscle hypertrophy, spasm, mucosal edema, and increased mucus production.
	Emphysema: Airway obstruction owing to loss of supporting structure of the lung and impairment of elastic recoil, resulting in collapse of distal airways on expiration, destruction of alveolar walls causing uneven ventilation, and mismatching of blood flow and ventilation.
	COPD: A combination of chronic bronchitis, asthma, and emphysema. Breathing becomes more difficult as secretions increase and more energy is needed to maintain ADL. Lifestyles change to adapt to life of chronic illness.
COMPLICATIONS	Bronchopulmonary infections, cor pulmonale, congestive heart failure, respiratory failure, peptic ulcer, and spontaneous pneumothorax.
SIGNS AND SYMPTOMS	Cough, sputum, breathlessness, wheeze, changes in pulmonary function studies and ABG.
MANAGEMENT	Drugs (bronchodilators, antibiotics, oxygen), adequate hydration and nutrition, maintain activities within physical limitations, airway management (breathing treatments, chest drainage, and percussion). Patient education about details and specifics of total management. Recognition and reporting of complications. Modification of life because of increased work of breathing.
EVALUATION	Symptom relief, improvement of quality of life, development of a life that is satisfying within limitations of breathing and the schedule of prescribed therapies.

QUICK REVIEW

PNEUMOCOCCAL PNEUMONIA

DESCRIPTION	Inflammation of the lungs, an acute infectious disease.
ETIOLOGIC FACTORS	Pneumococcus normal inhabitant of nose and throat. Upper respiratory infection (URI) often precedes disease. Imbalance between virulence of bacteria and defense of host determines occurrence.
HIGH RISK	Elderly, persons with COPD, URI. Seasons of higher risk are winter and spring.
SIGNS AND SYMPTOMS	Sudden chills and fever peaking in P.M.; increased pulse, respiratory rate, and pulse pressure; pleuritic pain. Leukocytosis, abnormal x-ray picture; cough productive of pinkish-rusty sputum. Crackles (rales).
DIFFERENTIAL DIAGNOSIS	Gram stain, culture, and sensitivity of sputum. Roentgenography.
COMPLICATIONS	Atelectasis, pleural effusion, pericardial effusion, herpes simplex.
PROGNOSIS	Most individuals will recover. Recovery is slower in elderly, particularly with COPD or cardiac disease. Recurrence must be guarded against. Fourth highest cause of death in 75+ age group.
MANAGEMENT	Hospitalization and bedrest. Antibiotic therapy, O_2, hydration, vital signs. Observe for symptoms of complications.
EVALUATION	Monitor vital signs and acute signs and symptoms; roentgenography. Monitor ADL, fatigue, and frustration during convalescence.

CHRONIC OBSTRUCTIVE PULMONARY DISEASE

Chronic obstructive respiratory problems present a real challenge to the patients and their families and to the health care providers as they work together to maintain optimal health and activity in the face of diminishing oxygenation and increased discomfort and disability. These people are aware of every breath they take.

Persons who suffer from chronic obstructive pulmonary problems have a progressive, chronic disease. Therefore, they are required to continually modify their activities of daily living and cope with new symptoms, equipment, medications, and complications. They must conserve their resources and utilize their support systems in different ways. This strongly suggests an area for nursing involvement in health care management.

Description

Chronic airway obstruction (CAO), chronic obstructive lung disease (COLD), and chronic obstructive pulmonary disease (COPD) are terms that are used to describe a group of overlapping disorders— chronic bronchitis, reactive airway disease, or asthma and emphysema. More commonly than not there is a mixture of all components, and so we are treating the patient who lies where the circles overlap, as depicted in Figure 22-1.

CHRONIC BRONCHITIS. Chronic bronchitis is a disease characterized by a chronic or recurrent productive cough. If this cough is present for at least three months of the year for two successive years and other diseases that cause cough such as tuberculosis, abscess and tumors, bronchiectasis, or cardiac disorders have been ruled out, the diagnosis of chronic bronchitis can be made. The condition is characterized by excessive mucus secretion in the bronchial tree. Smoking is the primary cause but more and more air pollutants are being implicated as contributory factors (Oregon Thoracic Society, 1977).

ASTHMA. Asthma or reactive airway disease is characterized by reversibility of airway obstruction. The trachea and bronchi are hyperreactive to various stimuli, resulting in generalized narrowing of the airways secondary to bronchospasm, mucosal edema, and hypersecretion of mucus (Oregon Thoracic Society, 1977). A term used to describe reactive airway disease is "twitchy lung."

EMPHYSEMA. Emphysema is an anatomic alteration of the lung characterized by an increase in size of the air spaces distal to the terminal, nonrespiratory bronchioles, accompanied by destructive changes of the alveolar walls (Oregon Thoracic Society, 1977).

Etiologic Factors

Recently it has been recognized that chronic bronchitis and emphysema are two distinct diseases. They may each occur alone and their etiologic factors and pathogenesis may be unrelated. However, they so frequently occur together that it is suggestive that some etiologic factors may be common to both and that in some circumstances chronic bronchitis may actually cause emphysema (Rodman, 1969). The emphysematous lesion that complicates chronic bronchitis usually is morphologically different from that which occurs as a separate disease entity. Centrilobular emphysema causes dilation of the respiratory bronchioles, affects the upper lungs more commonly but is unevenly distributed, and is associated with chronic bronchitis. Centrilobular emphysema is sel-

Acknowledgment is made to Dr. James F. Morris, Section Chief of Pulmonary Disease, Veterans Administration Hospital, Portland, Oregon, for his contribution in reviewing this chapter.

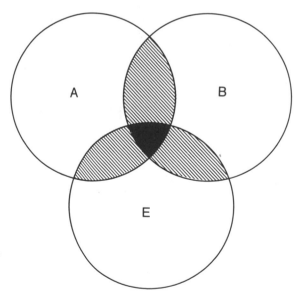

FIGURE 22-1.   In chronic obstructive pulmonary disease, there is overlapping of various disorders: *A,* asthma; *B,* bronchitis; and *E,* emphysema.

dom seen in nonsmokers. Panlobular emphysema causes enlargement and destruction of the alveoli. It is usually diffuse but is more severe in the lower lung areas.

Genetic Factors

Panlobular emphysema is a characteristic finding in those with "pure emphysema," specifically those with an alpha-1-antitrypsin deficiency (Oregon Thoracic Society, 1977). This is an inherited form of emphysema. It occurs in people who have an inherited deficiency in a protein, alpha-1-antitrypsin (A_1AT). A_1AT inhibits trypsin, which is an enzyme that is released from white blood cells and is useful in fighting infection. If there is a deficiency in A_1AT, trypsin is uninhibited and can destroy lung tissue. The deficiency may be severe if it is a homozygous abnormality, that is, an abnormal gene is inherited from both mother and father. This usually means that symptoms of emphysema occur at an early age even without a smoking history. If only one parent donates an affected gene it is a heterozygous abnormality. There is moderate A_1AT deficiency in this case and the person is apt to develop emphysema by 45 years of age (Lieberman, 1975).

Smoking

Cigarette smoking is by far the most damaging etiologic agent and the relationship of the substances inhaled in tobacco smoke and chronic bronchitis is fairly well substantiated. The normal cleansing mechanism of the airway consists of a thin layer of mucus and the movement of this mucus upward through the action of the cilia. Any foreign substance that reaches distal to the terminal bronchioles is removed by phagocytosis or by direct absorption into the lymphatics or bloodstream. Smoking has been shown to inhibit this mucociliary clearance by paralyzing the cilia (Wynder, 1967). The paralysis is followed by mucus stasis which impairs clearance of bacteria and particulate matter from the airways. Chronic inflammatory changes and infection result. Prolonged exposure to tobacco smoke is followed by permanent loss of cilia, goblet cell hypertrophy, submucous gland hyperplasia and lymphocytic infiltration; all the changes of chronic bronchitis (Fletcher, 1968). Population mortality studies have shown that men who smoke 25 or more cigarettes per day are about 20 times more likely to die from bronchitis than nonsmokers and the risk increases regularly with the amount smoked (Lowe, 1969). Postmortem studies have shown close relationships between severity of bronchitis and emphysematous changes and the amount of cigarette smoking before death (U.S. Public Health Service, 1967).

Dynamics

Normal Ventilation

The ventilatory volume of a normal resting adult is about 6 L per minute. Of this 6 L, approximately 2L is ventilation that does not participate in respiratory gas exchange or *dead space ventilation*. The cardiac output of a normal resting adult is about 5 L per minute. Nearly 100 percent of this blood flow passes through the pulmonary capillary bed so that the ratio of alveolar ventilation to pulmonary perfusion is normally 4/5 or 0.8. This *relationship of ventilation to perfusion is called the* $\dot{V}/\dot{Q}$ *ratio*. There are enormous variations in the $\dot{V}/\dot{Q}$ ratios in normal subjects in different portions of the lung. For example, in the upright position, the base of the lung has both increased ventilation and increased blood flow because of the effects of gravity, but the blood flow increase is much greater than the airflow so that perfusion is proportionately greater than ventilation and the $\dot{V}/\dot{Q}$ ratio is reduced to about 0.65. A respiratory unit at the lung apex has both diminished ventilation and low perfusion but the perfusion is proportionately more decreased than the ventilation. The result is a $\dot{V}/\dot{Q}$ ratio of about 3.0.

Although airflow and blood flow relationships are far from ideal even in normal subjects, the lungs have a regulatory mechanism for matching airflow and blood flow at the regional level. A reduction in local blood flow such as from a pulmonary embolus is quickly followed by a drop in the carbon dioxide concentration in the corresponding airway because the source of carbon dioxide in the airway is the pulmonary capillary blood. Respiratory bronchiole and alveolar duct constriction follows, so that ventilation is not wasted. If ventilation is reduced to a small area of lung tissue such as by atelectasis, the resultant decrease oxygen concentration is sensed by the adjacent pulmonary arteriole. Arteriolar spasm occurs with shunting of blood away from the poorly ventilated lung tissue. In this way lungs function with a minimum of wasted ventilation and blood flow. As long as there is matching of ventilation and perfusion, arterial blood gases will be normal (Rodman, 1969).

Ventilation/Perfusion Changes

Chronic obstructive lung disease results in many areas of lung which have grossly abnormal $\dot{V}/\dot{Q}$ ratios. The "pink puffer" has alveolar septal disruption, which tends to destroy both alveoli and capillaries. Although there might be a great deal of lung destruction, the alveoli and blood vessels are destroyed evenly so there is still matching of ventilation and perfusion in the remaining lung. Therefore the blood gases will be reasonably good. In contrast, the patient with chronic bronchitis, or "blue bloater," has a relatively well-preserved pulmonary capillary bed and continues to perfuse an area of lung that he is unable to ventilate adequately. As a result he suffers from a much more severe ventilation imbalance than does the pink puffer, and his blood gases will reflect the mismatching by a low partial pressure of oxygen in the arterial blood (P_aO_2).

Increased Resistance to Flow

The resistance to airflow is increased in all patients with obstructive lung disease. Depending upon the severity, it may be increased in both the inspiratory and expiratory phases of respiration, but the expiratory resistance is by far the most prominent. Overcoming the resistance to airflow in the normal tracheobronchial tree requires about 30 percent of the total mechanical work of respiration (Rodman, 1969). Resistance to airflow is increased in COPD as a result of (1) increased sputum production and plugging of airways; (2) mucosal hypertrophy due to chronic irritation; and (3) destruction of the lung parenchyma with resultant loss of support and hyperreactivity of the airways to various stimuli.

Increased Work of Breathing

Dyspnea is an uncomfortable subjective symptom perceived by the sufferer as a conscious awareness of inappropriately heavy or labored breathing. It seems to be related to the work of breathing. Emphysema causes loss of elastic recoil in the alveoli with resulting retention of air in the lungs. The hyperinflated lungs press on the diaphragm, causing it to lose its effectiveness and other muscles must be brought into play to carry on the function of breathing. Whenever you start bringing into play accessory muscles there is a cost and the cost in this case is in the work of breathing. People with COPD must work very hard to breathe owing to increased resistance to airflow and increased muscle work. They become very tired during the day just because they are working so hard at something others can take for granted —breathing.

Changes in Lifestyle

Besides the physiologic effects of COPD, there is a large psychologic component. The disabling effects of COPD usually strike between the ages of 45 and 55. It is the over-40 age group that is normally the most stable and economically productive in our society, but this is the group commonly affected. The gradual respiratory impairment and the subsequent decrease in activity capacity may precipitate work cessation and a loss of self-esteem in any role (Schwaid, 1970; Scott, 1969).

Barstow (1974) presented the progression of emphysema in the following sequence:

Pulmonary emphysema . Problem in body oxygenation

Decreased oxygenation .. Decreased energy source for activity

Alteration in activity ... Changes in roles

Role change .... Changes in style of living

Changes occur in ...... Self
Work life
Intrafamily relationships
Social relationships

Kimbel (1971) gave the Minnesota Multiphasic Personality Inventory (MMPI) to all patients with COPD in an inhospital program for rehabilitation. He found abnormalities in the first three scales: somatic concern, depression, and conversion tendencies (the neurotic triad). There was a progressive increase in the mean scores for each of the groups as severity of symptoms and restriction increased.

Adaptation to Chronic Illness

The model of adaptation to chronic illness follows the grieving process as described by Engel (1964). He states that the process involves five events:
- shock and disbelief
- developing awareness
- restitution
- resolution of the loss
- idealization

Adaptation to chronic illness follows a similar pattern:

- disbelief
- developing awareness
- reorganization of relationships with others
- resolution of the loss
- identity change

The person does not necessarily go through each stage in order. He may skip a stage or may be in several stages at one time. With each loss of function he goes through part or all of the stages again.

The stage of disbelief begins when the person learns either by diagnosis or change in function that he has a particular condition. This represents a threat to self. He resorts to denial to protect himself against the impact of it. Behaviors may include a refusal of the diagnosis or statements to the fact that something else is causing his symptoms. For example, he may attribute his shortness of breath to old age or lack of exercise. He may avoid medication by refusal or forgetfulness. This is particularly damaging to people with early to moderate lung disease, since many continue smoking.

As symptoms progressively worsen, even with decreased activity, he becomes less able to deny. He begins to become aware of what has happened and the implications of it. Some patients react to their need for dependence on others with anger. They may blame those on whom they depend for care, family, friends, a supernatural power, or themselves. When they turn their anger inward, they become depressed. Their fear of the unknown may lead to anxiety. They may exhibit overdependence. Emotional lability and/or withdrawal may be observed.

In his reorganization of relationships with others he remakes contact with his support system, generally his family. The family may go through the same stages of adjustment as the patient when they are learning to accommodate him as a person with a disability. They may react with fear, resentment, disgust, and anxiety, especially in the initial contacts. As the disability increases, a significant other assumes more and more responsibility, including the role of breadwinner. Loss of self-respect occurs because of role change and the need to be more dependent.

In the stage of resolution, he begins to acknowledge changes in how he sees himself and he begins to identify with others who have the same problem. He acknowledges himself as a person with a loss. Behavior may include making derogatory statements about himself. He may overemphasize his pain or disability. He may seek out others with the same condition and foster similarities.

Finally, in the stage of identity change, he feels he is a person worthy of respect. He begins to be able to recognize himself as an individual with a specific disability. He is able to utilize his strengths and recognize his liabilities. Behaviors might include his acceptance and participation in the treatment plan and his willingness to be dependent when necessary. His emotional state will have attained a greater degree of stability. He will be making some plans for the future in various aspects of his life. This does not mean that he does not mind being ill, but he is better able to live with his illness.

Signs and Symptoms

The cardinal symptoms of COPD are shortness of breath and cough. Shortness of breath is caused by the increased work of breathing and the cough is due to the accompanying bronchitis. There is a marked decrease in breath sounds owing to decreased movement of air. Wheezing and prolonged expiration occur because of obstruction to airflow from collapsed airways, excessive mucus, or bronchospasm. The presence of a "barrel chest" with an increased anteroposterior diameter suggests the presence of advanced COPD with resultant hyperinflation. However, a barrel chest is a common finding as a result of the aging process so the finding by itself can be quite misleading. In the advanced state of disease, there may be evidence of weight loss, depression of the liver, hyperpnea and tachycardia with mild exertion, and a low, flat, and relatively immobile diaphragm. Heart sounds may be distant and cyanosis may be present.

Diagnosis

The single most important diagnostic tool in verifying the presence of obstructive lung disease is the pulmonary function test. By a simple vital capacity and forced vital capacity maneuver, restrictive and obstructive lung disease can be determined.

Vital Capacity (VC)

The vital capacity is the maximal amount of air expelled after a maximal inspiration. The patient is allowed all the time he needs to complete the maneuver. The vital capacity measures the amount of restrictive disease present. Restriction is defined as an interference with easy or adequate lung expansion. Several factors affect expansion of the lung and, thus, cause a decrease in vital capacity*:

Insufficient effort on the part of the person.

Reduction in functioning lung tissue as with surgical excision, atelectasis, and lung tumors.

Limitation of chest expansion due to obesity, decreased diaphragmatic excursion caused by ascites or pregnancy or absent diaphragmatic movement in phrenic nerve paralysis.

Reduction in lung expansion due to pneumothorax, diaphragmatic hernia, pleural effusion and fibrosis. Engorgement of blood vessels secondary to left ventricular failure where the increased space they occupy limits expansion of alveoli

Airway obstruction or loss of lung elasticity as in asthma, emphysema, and bronchitis.

Depression of the respiratory center in brain or cervical spinal cord injuries that interfere with neural conduction or neuromuscular transmission to the respiratory muscles.

Forced Vital Capacity (FVC)

The forced vital capacity is the maximum volume of air expired rapidly and forcefully after a maximal inhalation. The difference between the vital capacity and the forced vital capacity is *time*. The patient is told to blow out as rapidly and forcefully as possible. Patients with emphysema show marked airway collapse on expiration because of loss of surrounding supportive tissue. Rapid forceful breathing increases the collapse, resulting in a decreased forced vital capacity. Therefore, the forced vital capacity may better reflect obstructive disease than the vital capacity.

The forced expiratory volume in one second (FEV_1) is the volume of gas exhaled over a given time interval (one second) during the performance of the forced vital capacity. Ordinarily 75 to 80 percent of the forced vital capacity should be exhaled during the first one second. If airway obstruction occurs, less air is exhaled during this interval. The FEV_1 is also reduced in restrictive disease because the amount of

air the patient is able to take into his lungs is decreased; therefore the amount of air he can exhale in the first second will also be reduced.

The ratio of FEV_1 to FVC (FEV_1/FVC percent) offers a rough distinction between restrictive and obstructive disease. The FEV_1/VC percent is preferable to the FEV_1/FVC percent for distinguishing between restrictive and obstructive impairment because the VC is less affected by air trapping due to obstruction to airflow than the FVC (Morris, 1976). A ventilatory defect with a low FVC and a normal flow (FEV_1) is restrictive in nature. If the defect causes a decrease in flow (FEV_1) and a normal volume (VC or FVC) it would be categorized as obstructive disease (Gordon, 1960). Because the FEV_1 is also reduced in restrictive disease, you must look at the ratio to determine which impairment is causing the reduction. If the ratio between the FVC and FEV_1 is normal (80 to 100 percent of predicted), the lowering of the FEV_1 is due to restriction.

The following components of the test are called flow rates. Flow rates are measured at specific intervals of the FVC curve and are useful in specifying the area of obstructive disease (Fig. 22-2).

MAXIMUM EXPIRATORY FLOW RATE (MEFR OR FEF). The maximum expiratory flow rate (MEFR or FEF 200-1200) is the average rate of flow for a specified portion of the forced expiratory volume between 200 and 1200 ml. This test measures resistance to airflow in the large airways or larynx and varies with patient effort.

FORCED MID-EXPIRATORY FLOW RATE (FEF). The forced mid-expiratory flow (FEF 25–75 percent) is the rate of flow during the middle half of the forced expiratory volume. This test indicates damage to the small airways and is considered to be effort-independent in that the subject cannot voluntarily increase the result by trying harder.

FORCED END-EXPIRATORY FLOW (FEF). The forced end-expiratory flow (FEF 75–85 percent) is an even more sensitive measure of obstruction in the small airways.

Maximum Voluntary Ventilation (MVV)

The maximum voluntary ventilation (MVV) is the volume of air that a subject can breathe with voluntary maximum effort for a given time, usually 12 to 15 seconds. If the percentage of volume predicted for the FEV_1 and the MVV are nearly the same, it is fairly good evidence that the patient has used maximum effort during the test. With COPD, the volume

---

* Gordon, B. L. (ed.): Clinical Cardiopulmonary Physiology, ed. 3. New York: Grune and Stratton, 1969.

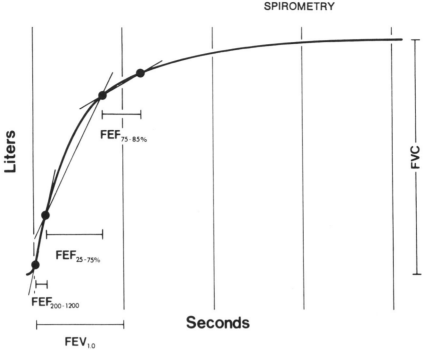

FIGURE 22-2.   Components of the forced expiratory vital capacity curve. (From Morris, J. F.: Spirometry in the evaluation of pulmonary function [Medical Progress]. Western J. Med. 125:113, 1976, with permission)

of air that can be moved in one minute is less as a result of loss of elastic recoil, airway obstruction, and fatigue of respiratory muscles. Generalized weakness and pain can also affect this test.

Sometimes pulmonary function tests are ordered before and after the administration of an aerosolized bronchodilator. This test gives an indication of the reversibility of the disease. It would always be used to rule out asthma.

INTERPRETATION OF PULMONARY FUNCTION TEST. Table 22-1 may be used to determine the severity of ventilatory impairment. The numbers indicate the percent of predicted normal that the patient has achieved, that is, the actual figures observed in testing compared to those predicted for a nonsmoker of similar age and height. The predicted normals for men and women (Figs. 22-3 and 22-4) were obtained by Morris and coworkers (Morris, 1976).

Based on spirometric testing, patients are grouped into categories of ventilatory impairment (Table 22-2). These categories are normal, mild, moderate, severe, and very severe. Reduction of vital capacity indicates restrictive disease. Reduction of the FEV_1/FVC distinguishes between restrictive and obstructive disease. Reduction in the flow rates indicates precisely where the obstruction is occurring.

Advanced COPD is relatively easy to diagnose. There is a simple method for measuring FEV_1 to determine if airway obstruction is present. The person is asked to take a deep breath and blow the air out as hard and fast as possible. At the same time the nurse

TABLE 22-1.   Categories of ventilatory impairment.

	VC, FVC, FEV₁, MVV	FEF200–1200, FEF 25–75% FEF75–85%
Normal	>80*	>75
Mild	65–80	60–75
Moderate	50–64	45–59
Severe	35–49	30–44
Very severe	<35	<30

From Morris, J. F.: Spirometry in the evaluation of pulmonary function (Medical Progress). Western J. Med. 125:116, 1976, with permission.
* Percent of predicted normal
VC = vital capacity
FVC = forced vital capacity
FEV_1 = one-second forced expiratory volume
MVV = maximum voluntary ventilation
FEF200–1200 = maximum forced expiratory flow
FEF25–75% = forced midexpiratory flow
FEF75–85% = forced end-expiratory flow

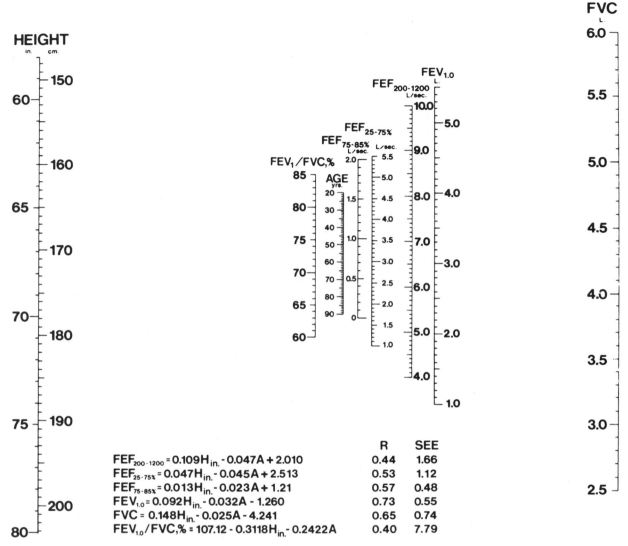

FIGURE 22-3. Prediction nomogram for normal men (BTPS).

BTPS = body temperature, ambient pressure, saturated with water

FEF200–1200 = maximum forced expiratory flow

FEF25–75% = forced midexpiratory flow

FEF75–85% = forced end-expiratory flow

FEV$_1$ = one-second forced expiratory volume

FVC = forced vital capacity

(From Morris, J. F.: Spirometry in the evaluation of pulmonary function[Medical Progress]. Western J. Med. 125:114, 1976, with permission)

places a stethoscope over the trachea and times how long it takes for the air to be expelled. Someone without disease can empty the lungs in 3.5 seconds or less. If the maneuver takes 4 seconds or longer, airway obstruction is present (Judge, 1974).

Hodgkin and associates published the guidelines in Table 22-3 for differentiation of stable obstructive airway disease (Hodgkin, 1975).

Complications

Patients with COPD are most vulnerable to bronchopulmonary infections that predispose to cor pulmonale which can lead to respiratory failure and eventual death. Congestive heart failure with cor pulmonale can be treated and does not mean a rapid

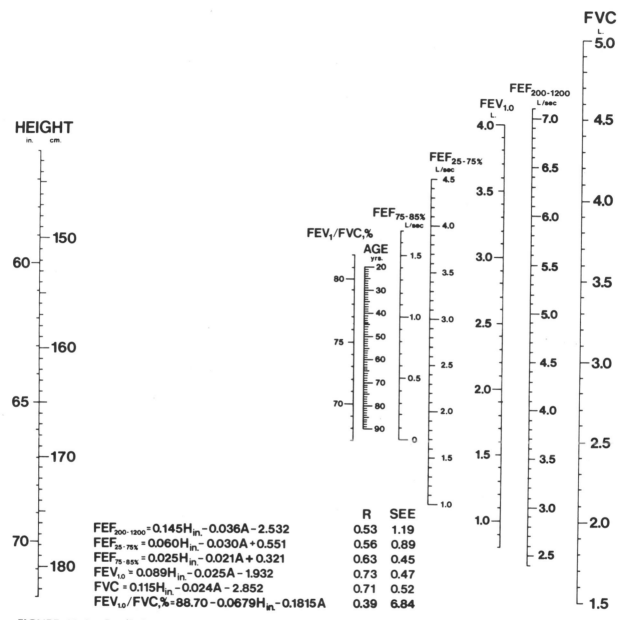

FIGURE 22-4. Prediction nomogram for normal women (BTPS). See Figure 22-3 for abbreviations. (From Morris, J. F.: Spirometry in the evaluation of pulmonary function [Medical Progress]. Western J. Med. 125: 115 1976, with permission)

death. Management of underlying factors, hypoxemia, and acidosis aims to prevent heart failure. The stress of chronic illness, long time steroid therapy, increased gastric acidity, decreased arterial saturation, and carbon dioxide retention predispose to peptic ulcers. Approximately 25 percent of patients with COPD will have an ulcer at one time (Oregon Thoracic Society, 1977, p. 93). Other complications are spontaneous pneumothorax and pulmonary emboli.

Prognosis

COPD is a progressive disease, though the rate of progression varies with individuals. In the following study designed to document the course and prognosis of patients under conservative and individual management, data were gathered from a group of 200 patients with chronic obstructive pulmonary disease. "At the end of one year follow-up, 186 patients were

TABLE 22-2. Categories of ventilatory impairment.

FEV₁/FVC	Category	Manifestations
80%	Normal	Clinical impairment absent. Breathlessness appropriate to activity.
65–80%	Mild impairment	Chest x-ray picture may be normal. Cough with or without sputum during upper respiratory infection. No dyspnea with usual activities but person may be able to perform ADL by pacing self. Drives rather than walks and takes energy-saving short cuts in all activities.
50–64%	Moderate impairment	May have persistent cough; intermittent wheezing made worse with chest colds and sputum production. With upper respiratory infection, ordinary activities may cause unusual shortness of breath.
35–49%	Severe	Seeks medical care because of inability to control shortness of breath. Often shortness of breath at rest. Major changes in lifestyle—unable to work, hunt, fish, garden.
35%	Very severe (end stage)	Cannot function even in basic ADL without help. Dressing, shaving, toothbrushing, and so forth are exhausting. Shower causes a suffocating feeling. Tight-fitting clothing increases SOB—males may wear suspenders instead of belt. May require slip-on shoes. Requires smaller, frequent feedings to avoid distending stomach and compromising breathing. Rushing is avoided because of anxiety and dyspnea.

TABLE 22-3. Guidelines in differentiation of stable obstructive airway diseases.

Test	Emphysema	Chronic Bronchitis	Asthma
Spirometry	Obstructive pattern with no bronchodilator improvement	Obstructive pattern may shows some bronchodilator improvement	Obstructive pattern usually shows definite bronchodilator improvement
Sputum	Not helpful	Predominantly neutrophils	Predominantly eosinophils
Chest roentgenogram	Helpful, if evidence of bullous lesions or loss of peripheral vascular markings; suggestive if presence of flattened diaphragms (hyperinflation)	Often normal; may have increased lung markings; may have hyperinflation	May be normal; no loss of vascular markings; may be hyperinflated during an acute attack
Allergy testing	Not helpful	Not helpful	May be helpful
Diffusing capacity	Less than 50% of predicted; higher values do not exclude the presence of emphysema	Diffusing capacity normal to moderately reduced	Diffusing capacity normal in stable patient
Lung compliance, static	Increased	Normal	Normal; may be increased during sustained hyperinflation

From Hodgkin, J. E., et al.: Chronic obstructive airway diseases, current concepts in diagnosis and comprehensive care. J.A.M.A. Vol. 232, June 23, 1975, p. 1245. Copyright 1975, American Medical Association. Reprinted with permission.

alive. At the end of seven years, 35 were alive, 104 were known dead and four were lost to follow-up. The overall mortality was 50% before six years." (Burrows, 1969). The study concluded that emphysema is a progressively deteriorating disease.

An investigation was undertaken cooperatively with 15 Veterans Administration Hospitals to relate the life expectancy of COPD patients to the pulmonary function of the patient at the beginning of the observation period. At four years of follow-up, the mortality rate for 98 patients with FEV_1 >1.49 liters was 26 percent. For 320 patients with FEV_1 0.5–1.49 liters the mortality rate was 44 percent and for 64 patients with FEV_1 <0.5 liters the mortality rate was 89 percent.

When the arterial oxygen saturation (SaO_2) was >92 percent and the partial pressure of carbon dioxide (PCO_2) was lower than 48 mm Hg, the 4-year mortality was 33 percent. When the SaO_2 was less than 92 percent the death rate was 44 percent; when both oxygen and carbon dioxide deviated abnormally from these quantities, the mortality rate was 72 percent (Renzetti, 1966).

Death often results from an acute bronchopulmonary infection, with or without right heart failure. There is often organized pneumonia or scarring of the lung parenchyma from previous infections. Other causes of death include pulmonary thromboembolism, bleeding or perforating peptic ulcer, spontaneous pneumothorax, or cardiac arrhythmias associated with disturbances of blood gases or electrolytes (Oregon Thoracic Society, 1977).

Management

Chronic obstructive pulmonary disease, contrary to the opinions of many professionals and patients, does lend itself to treatment. There are many treatments that can be employed to improve the quality of life for people with these diseases. Because there are so many new developments, consultation with a specialist who keeps abreast of trends of treatments can be an excellent investment of time and money for the patient. Patients are best managed when physicians and nurses work closely, integrating their diagnoses and management activities.

Drug Management

Most persons with COPD will be on a large number of drugs, probably for the rest of their lives. These drugs include bronchodilators, antibiotics, steroids,

and oxygen. To participate in the drug regimen effectively, each patient needs to know:

1. The names of the medications he is taking.
2. The purpose of each medicine—what it does for the patient.
3. The side effects of each drug.
4. An appropriate schedule for self-administration of medications that is compatible with his lifestyle.
5. How to evaluate over-the-counter drugs used for respiratory problems.
6. The proper method for using an inhaler.
7. The symptoms to report to nurse and physician.

Bronchodilators

Bronchodilators cause a response by their action on the alpha and beta receptors of the sympathetic nervous system (Fig. 22-5). Stimulation of the alpha (or excitatory adrenergic receptors) causes bronchial vasoconstriction and, thus, are useful as bronchial mucosal decongestants.

Stimulation of beta$_1$ receptors primarily affects the heart. It increases the force of contraction (inotropic effect) and the heart rate (chronotropic effect). Stimulation of beta$_2$ receptors primarily affects the smooth muscles of the tracheobronchial tree by relaxing them.

Bronchoconstriction occurs in reactive airway disease, causing decreased airflow in and out of the lungs. The bronchoconstriction stage is set when cholinergic receptors are stimulated by local irritating factors either inhaled or ingested. IgE, an immune globulin antibody is formed and mediates the reaction by attaching to the antigen (Ag), setting into motion a chain of events which causes it to react and narrow the airway (Burton, 1977). Normally this action is opposed by release of beta stimulator catecholamines which stimulate adenylcyclase and promotes the conversion of ATP (adenosine triphosphatase) to cyclic AMP (adenosine monophosphate).

$$ATP \xrightarrow[\text{Adenylcyclase (enzyme)}]{} cyclic\ AMP \xrightarrow[\text{Phosphodiesterase (enzyme)}]{} AMP$$

From cyclic AMP comes all good things as far as treatment of reactive airway disease. Cyclic AMP promotes relaxation of smooth muscle. An increase in cyclic AMP results in bronchodilation while a decrease in cyclic AMP results in bronchospasm. One limitation of cyclic AMP is that it is short lived. It is

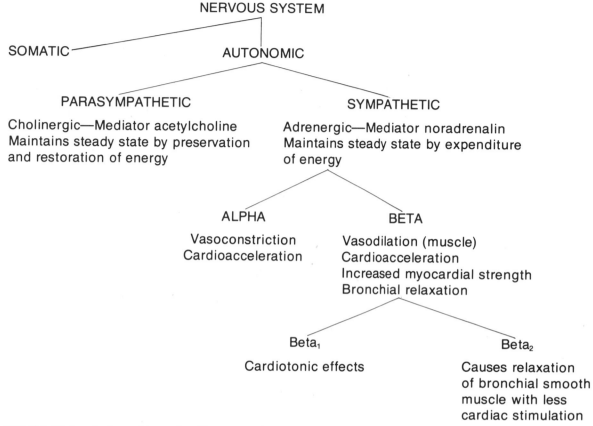

NERVOUS SYSTEM

SOMATIC — AUTONOMIC

PARASYMPATHETIC

Cholinergic—Mediator acetylcholine
Maintains steady state by preservation
and restoration of energy

SYMPATHETIC

Adrenergic—Mediator noradrenalin
Maintains steady state by expenditure
of energy

ALPHA

Vasoconstriction
Cardioacceleration

BETA

Vasodilation (muscle)
Cardioacceleration
Increased myocardial strength
Bronchial relaxation

Beta$_1$

Cardiotonic effects

Beta$_2$

Causes relaxation
of bronchial smooth
muscle with less
cardiac stimulation

FIGURE 22-5. Action of bronchodilators on the sympathetic nervous system.

constantly being hydrolyzed by a catalyst called phosphodiesterase to AMP. Drugs that stop rapid hydrolysis are those in the xanthine family. In general, catecholamines increase production of cyclic AMP by stimulating the formation of adenylcyclase and the xanthines decrease the breakdown of cyclic AMP (Mathewson, 1977, p. 16).

Bronchodilators have many side effects, most commonly heart palpitation, upset stomach, jittery, insomnia, and urinary retention. The medication that is effective for one person may aggravate another. So frequent changing of medication and dose is common. It is important that symptoms probably related to medication be promptly reported. Another medication most likely can be prescribed.

CATECHOLAMINES. Ephedrine stimulates both alpha and beta adrenergic receptors directly as well as through release of noradrenalin from storage sites. The longer it is used, the less effect it has and the more side effects it produces, such as nervousness and bladder neck obstruction. Recent controlled studies have suggested that the bronchodilator effect of ephedrine 25 mg is not significantly different from that of a placebo (Geumei, 1977, p. 267).

Noradrenalin acts mainly on alpha receptors and has little effect on the beta receptors, except in the heart. It has a marked constrictor action on blood vessels and positive inotropic (force of contractions) and chronotropic (rate) effects on the heart. Because of its alpha action of constriction of blood vessels it is good for mucosal swelling but has little effect on the airways (AMA Drug Evaluation, 1973, p. 34).

Adrenalin affects both alpha and beta receptors. It shrinks mucosa and dilates smooth muscle of the tracheobronchial tree. It stimulates the heart a great deal. *Adrenalin is not indicated in the hypoxic patient* because it can cause arrhythmias owing to increased demand for oxygen in the myocardium.

Isoproterenol stimulates beta receptors more than alpha but beta$_1$ and beta$_2$ are equally affected; therefore, there is as much cardiac effect as lung effect.

Isoetherine possesses a preferential action on beta$_2$ receptors while exerting a minimal action on the beta$_1$ receptors. This drug starts to achieve the action desired. Bronkosol 2 contains 1 percent iso-etherine HCl.

Several synthetic beta adrenergic agonists are now in use clinically. They are more potent broncho-dilators in that they have greater beta$_2$ and less beta$_1$ effects. The new drugs are longer acting and are ad-ministered orally.

Four drugs—metaproterenol, terbutaline, feno-terol, and albuterol (salbutamol)—currently are being used clinically, but only two (metaproterenol and terbutaline) are presently available in the United States. Metaproterenol (10 to 20 mg) is a more potent bronchodilator and has fewer side effects than ephedrine 25 mg with effects lasting 4 hours (Geu-mei, 1977, p. 267).

Terbutaline and fenoterol are more selective beta adrenergic stimulants than metaproterenol. Terbuta-line 5 mg given by mouth has been shown to have a greater bronchodilating effect and lasts longer than 20 mg of metaproterenol or ephedrine 25 mg (Geu-mei, 1977, p. 267). An increase in heart rate and a slight decrease in diastolic blood pressure may be noted with terbutaline therapy. Headaches, sweating, nausea and vomiting, and muscle tremor are frequent side effects which usually decrease with continued therapy. Albuterol 5 mg has been shown to be com-parable to terbutaline in every way.

Feneterol 5 to 10 mg has a more potent broncho-dilating effect than 20 mg of metaproterenol or 4 mg of albuterol and has minimal side effects. The medi-cation peaks at 2 to 3 hours and lasts up to 8 hours.

XANTHINES. The use of an adrenergic drug with theophylline or one of its derivatives often provides bronchodilator action superior to that produced by either used alone. Oral aminophylline can be given in a plain tablet or in an alcoholic solution. Examples of oral aminophylline are Elixophyllin, Theolair, Cho-ledyl, Quibron, and Lufyllin. Long-acting prepara-tions are now on the market with effects lasting to 8 hours. Slo-Phyllin, Aminodur, and Theo-Dur are ex-amples of long-acting preparations. Combination drugs containing aminophylline, ephedrine, and a barbiturate are also available. Examples include Tedral, Marax, and Amesec. Combination drugs are not as desirable as single drugs, since increasing the dose of one of the drugs in the combination might cause an overdose of another.

There is a very narrow therapeutic range for theophylline, 10 to 20 ug/ml of serum. Below 10, the dose is usually ineffective. Above 20, side effects are extremely common. The most serious side effects are seizures and supraventricular tachycardia. Minor symptoms include nausea, vomiting, anorexia, head-ache, nervousness, and sleeplessness (Jenne, 1975, p. 407). The gastrointestinal symptoms are now be-lieved to originate in the central nervous system and are not relieved by taking the drug with food. Serum theophylline levels add an element of excellence to patient care and are important in providing comfort to the patient who will depend upon the drug for a lifetime.

Steroids

Steroids are anti-inflammatory drugs that are sometimes used in severe reactive airway disease. Their action includes preventing antigen-antibody reactions by inhibiting antibody formation, inhibi-tion of some cellular mechanisms involving broncho-constriction and by directly increasing the intra-cellular concentration of cyclic AMP, thereby caus-ing bronchial muscle relaxation (Burton, 1977, p. 485).

Some patients have heard many things about steroids—fact or fantasies—and they refuse to take them. The nurse or physician may be able to share the realities of effects and side effects in such a way that the patient will be willing to try them rather than base a decision on hearsay evidence.

The role of steroids in the relief of symptoms is important. All patients seem to get some relief from shortness of breath and have a greater sense of well-being. Although many side effects have been at-tributed to long term steroid therapy, one must weigh these for the elderly against the well-being achieved by taking the drugs for their remaining years. It is also true that the elderly are more vulner-able to the side effects, particularly skin fragility and bleeding. If a decision is made to discontinue ste-roids, it should not be done abruptly—a psychotic break is a real possibility, as well as adrenal dysfunc-tion. In ambulatory care settings where receptionists or nurses take incoming calls from pharmacists re-garding drug renewals, the decision to refuse a re-newal on the basis of the patient's failure to have been seen by the physician recently should be tem-pered by the judgment regarding the potential com-plications if the drug is stopped. It is a decision that should be made by a physician or nurse who under-stands the risks.

The lesser side effects include moon face and

trunk obesity, acne, and purplish striae on the skin. More serious side effects include systolic and diastolic hypertension, hyperglycemia, osteoporosis, particularly of the vertebrae, gastric or duodenal ulcers, sodium and water retention, potassium loss, cataracts, glaucoma, and decreased resistance to infections. The person on steroids has a sense of well-being.

Patients on long term steroids will have some of these side effects. In those instances the nurse will have to accept this as a reality and help the patient and the family to deal with the particular problem rather than necessarily stopping the drug.

The administration of steroids varies. Prednisone may be given in a large dose (40 to 60 mgm) once a day or once every other day. The rationale for this approach is that there is less adrenal suppression this way than when given in smaller divided doses. At other times they are administered on a q.i.d. basis, though not interrupting the sleeping hours. They are usually given orally, but may also be given intravenously or intramuscularly for faster effect. Steroids are also given by inhalation. The steroids that are usually ordered are prednisone, prednisolone, Decadron, hydrocortisone, Aristocort, and Solu-Medrol.

A recent advance in medicine has been the introduction of a new steroid, Vanceril (beclomethasone). It is a medication that is inhaled directly into the lungs and has minimal side effects. Only patients who are already receiving systemic steroids and whose disease is stabilized should be considered for Vanceril therapy. Initially Vanceril is administered concurrently with the patient's usual dose of systemic steroid. After a week, gradual withdrawal of the systemic steroid is begun at 1-to-2-week intervals. This must be done slowly as there is a risk of adrenal insufficiency with withdrawal of systemic steroids. Recovery from impaired adrenal function may take up to 12 months. Localized infection with Candida albicans or Aspergillus niger have occurred in the mouth, pharynx, and, occasionally, the larynx secondary to Vanceril therapy. Gargling with mouthwash after each dose may decrease the incidence. Use of an inhaled bronchodilator before Vanceril enhances penetration into the bronchial tree. Several minutes should elapse between the inhalation of the bronchodilator to reduce toxicity of propellants in the two aerosols (Schering Corporation).

Symptoms of steroid withdrawal may include joint or muscular pain, lassitude, depression, hypotension, and weight loss. Psychiatric manifestations can occur if the patient is taken off high dose long term therapy too rapidly. These include euphoria, depression, and hallucinations.

People on steroids should be given Med-Alert bracelets and carry a card stating the dose and purpose of the medication in order to prevent disaster if an accident occurs.

Antibiotics

Early recognition and treatment of upper respiratory infection is essential because such infections may progress to pneumonia, bronchitis, or bronchiolitis. Appropriate therapy should be begun at the first sign of bronchopulmonary infection. Patients must be taught to be alert for any signs of lung infection (see box).

Some physicians keep patients supplied with antibiotics with instructions to begin treatment whenever they note a change in sputum color— feeling that immediate treatment is essential. However, it is still important for the patient to communicate with the physician's office to share the information as to what is occurring and how it is being managed.

Tetracycline or ampicillin are the drugs of choice. If the patient has not improved in two days or has recently been on antibiotics, a Gram stain should be done before antibiotics are given or changed (Lertzman, 1976). A common misconception among patients is that they can take a few doses of antibiotics until they are feeling better and then stop.

SIGNS AND SYMPTOMS OF LUNG INFECTION IN PERSONS WITH COPD

Increased cough

Increased sputum production

Change in color of sputum from clear or white to yellow, green, or grey

Change in consistency of sputum from thin and watery to thick, sticky, and stringy

Increased shortness of breath and decreased exercise tolerance

Fever and/or chills (temperature >100 should call doctor)

Sudden decrease in the amount of sputum coughed up

Feeling of tightness in the chest

Once antibiotics are begun, a course of 7 to 10 days must be completed.

Some COPD patients are on continuous antibiotic therapy prophylactically. The medications can be given one week, off one week, and on one week. Another way is to take antibiotics three weeks of a month and off one week. Nurses should not be concerned that the patient is on antibiotics for long periods of time for this is the best way to keep infections under control in some patients.

Sputum cultures are expensive and chancy diagnostic tools. They must be collected in a special way and in special containers and then must be analyzed promptly in the laboratory or they are of questionable value. If it is determined that a culture is important in either diagnosis of the type of infection or to determine response to treatment, the laboratory should be called prior to collecting the specimen to assure that proper collection and handling will occur. It is usually not appropriate to wait until the results of a sputum culture are returned before starting antibiotic therapy in the elderly and/or with the patients with COPD.

COUGH MEDICINE. If a cough is due to an acute infection, the antibiotic given for the infection will usually be effective. Mild cough mixtures to soothe the throat are used in place of strong sedatives which depress the cough. Medicines with codeine are not usually ordered. Robitussin is useful especially when it is added to a glass of warm water. When taken several (three to four) times a day, it increases hydration as well as relieves the cough.

If the cough is due to dryness, humidity should be checked and increased by setting out a pan of water or boiling water. Smoking or smoke from others can produce a cough; the treatment of this is obvious. Antihistamines are drying and may cause discomfort. For the person with COPD, use of over-the-counter drugs for respiratory problems should be discouraged.

Oxygen and Oxygen Equipment

OXYGEN AS A DRUG. Oxygen is a drug, and this is the way it should be presented to the person who is to use it. It is a drug that many people resist, even though it would give them greater freedom to participate in activities which they have forfeited as a result of shortness of breath.

OXYGEN RATES AND BLOOD GASES. Administration of oxygen in COPD is not based upon appearance of the patient but by drawing arterial blood and measuring oxygen, carbon dioxide, and pH. Based on these factors, the physician will prescribe the liter flow of oxygen. Fairly rigid criteria should be adhered to when prescribing home oxygen. Those patients who are severely hypoxic (PO_2 on room air less than 55) demonstrating cor pulmonale, secondary polycythemia, or oxygen desaturation during exercise are candidates. The on-again-off-again prescription for oxygen does little more than addict the patient to an expensive form of therapy with little physiologic benefit. Oxygen is expensive and, once on it as a treatment for chronic shortness of breath, the individual rarely comes off it.

Adjustments in dosage should not be made either by the patient or others without consultation with the physician. It is a general rule never to give someone with COPD more than 2 liters without checking arterial blood gases. This would not apply to other conditions. The risk in giving too much oxygen to patients with long standing hypoxemia with high levels of PCO_2 is that there will be further depression of the respiratory center. *Oxygen then, instead of being helpful, can be fatal.*

OXYGEN SYSTEMS AND LIFESTYLE. Oxygen therapy used to mean a life of seclusion, tied to a tank in the house. With the present oxygen systems, mobility not only in the home and about the community but also in longer travel is quite possible.

Mobility can be achieved about the home, apartment, or garden by attaching a long hose to the reservoir. Up to 90 ft of oxygen tubing has been tested and will deliver the same liter flow, but a maximum of 50 ft is recommended and will allow a fair amount of freedom. Liquid oxygen systems are ideal for movement in and out of the home because the reservoirs are compact and not extremely heavy. The Linde reservoir weighs 68.4 pounds when full and the Liberator weighs 83.8 pounds when full. Tanks are also available. M tanks are set up for travel; these weigh 70 pounds and contain approximately 4000 L of oxygen. They are placed on a carrier and *pulled* by the patient.

There are several portable systems available. The Linde System (Union Carbide) is perhaps the most well-known as it has been on the market for a longer period of time. This is a liquid oxygen system and its containers can be compared to giant thermos bottles. When they are not in use, the liquid oxygen forms a gas as it warms and will be discharged into the atmosphere through a pop-off valve on the container. It is a low pressure system with approximately 50 PSI in the reservoir compared to 2400 PSI in the J Tank.

The Linde reservoir is 13½ inches high and $9^{11}/_{32}$ inches in diameter and contains 13,700 L of oxygen. The Linde Walker is a compact container that can be carried over the shoulder and contains enough oxygen to last 8 hr at 2 L. It weighs 10.2 pounds when full. A carrier can be obtained to pull the walker if the weight is a problem. The Linde system cannot be purchased and must be rented.

Another liquid system has been introduced recently. This is the Liberator/Stroller (Cryogenic Associates). The Liberator reservoir is 27 inches in height and 12 inches in diameter. It contains 17,000 gaseous liters of oxygen. The Stroller can be carried over the shoulder and weighs 10.4 pounds when full. It will last approximately 9.6 hr at 2 L. It can be purchased for under $3000. It also has a pop-off valve to release oxygen as it heats and becomes a gas, so some must be used each day if there is to be no waste.

The Traveler (Erie Manufacturing Company) is a portable tank of oxygen that can be refilled from any large tank as long as it contains 2000 pounds of pressure. It contains 360 L of gas. It will last approximately 3 hr at 2 L, 5½ hr at 1 L. The system can be purchased for under $200.

The newest system on the market is the Oxygen Concentrator (DeVilbiss DeVO$_2$) which is only portable within the home. This is an electrically operated machine which extracts nitrogen, carbon monoxide, and hydrocarbons from room air and delivers an enriched oxygen supply. It looks like a piece of furniture and has a gentle hum as it works. It has a built in analyzer which monitors the concentration of oxygen. It requires minimal maintenance and can be purchased for under $3000. The cost of electricity may be anywhere from $8 to $25 per month, depending on the cost of electricity for the area. This system must have a back-up tank in case of power failure and must also have a portable system for mobility.

Individuals needing continuous low-flow oxygen are not restricted from traveling on commercial forms of transportation. They cannot be discriminated against because of this, but it is wise to check with the local carrier early in planning a trip to alert them to the plans. Private oxygen supplies in any form are not allowed aboard the aircraft. In flight, the airline supplies the oxygen. Arrangements must be made for oxygen to be available upon arrival at the destination. The patient should have a written statement from the doctor concerning need for oxygen and flow rate during the flight.

SAFEGUARDS/DANGERS. Tank oxygen has its peculiar dangers because of its being a high pressure system. If for any reason the valve should break, the tank would become a missile as all the pressure is released through a small opening no larger than a quarter. It has been known to smash through brick walls and fly through the air. Because of this it is important that the tank be firmly fastened to a carrier rack or chained to a structure that will prevent it from falling over. It should be placed away from small children.

Certain safeguards apply to all oxygen systems. Oxygen containers should be kept away from heat sources because the Linde system will vent oxygen as it warms; tank oxygen obeys Charles Law which states "A given volume of gas at a constant pressure will expand proportionately to the absolute rise in temperature." Oil, grease, and other combustible material should never come in contact with any part of the oxygen set-up. Hand lotions, mentholatum, and Vicks Vaporub are common substances that might be on the hands of those coming in contact with gauges, valves, hoses, and so forth. A good rule to follow is *always wash hands before touching the equipment.* Valves should always be closed on tanks when the oxygen is not in use. Smoking should never be allowed around oxygen.

Drugs for Other Symptoms

ANTIALLERGY AGENTS. Cromolyn sodium (Intal) is a relatively new drug on the market. It acts through inhibiting release of histamine and other mediators from MAST cells (Farzan, 1978). It has no intrinsic bronchodilator, antihistamine, or anti-inflammatory activity. It has no direct effect on smooth muscles. It is an effective prophylactic agent in allergic asthma. It will not inhibit allergic response if given after an antigen challenge (Brogden, 1974); therefore, it has no role in treatment of acute attacks of asthma.

Cromolyn is given by inhalation by a specially developed turbo-inhaler (Spinhaler). The Spinhaler punctures the capsule containing 20 mg of cromolyn and 20 mg lactose, and the patient's inhalation causes the micronized powder to be distributed in the lungs. It must be used regularly, four times a day. Cromolyn should be introduced during a period of relative freedom from symptoms. Lungs should be relatively free from mucus plugging so that the patient is able to inhale a sufficient quantity of air necessary to disperse the powder effectively from the inhaler (Fisons Company). Improvement will occur within 2 to 4 weeks if the drug is effective.

Local irritation of the throat and trachea frequently is reported. Occasionally cough or broncho-spasm will occur following inhalation. Some advocate the use of an inhaled bronchodilator prior to cromolyn dose to improve distribution in the lungs.

DIGOXIN. Pulmonary disease predisposes to atrial arrhythmias when there is concurrent atrial dilatation and hypoxia. Digitalis may be used to control premature atrial contractions and rapid ventricular response in atrial fibrillation and flutter and may convert or control paroxysmal atrial tachycardia not caused by digitalis excess. Sinus tachycardia and multifocal atrial tachycardia are poorly controlled by digitalis (Green, 1977, p. 459). Although the role of digitalis in controlling right heart failure is controversial it is sometimes used for its contractile force effect on the right ventricle.

Pulmonary disease enhances the susceptibility of patients to digitalis toxicity. Several factors are associated with these increased risks: acute hypoxemia increases sensitivity to digitalis preparations; hypokalemia that tends to occur in chronic stable patients, particularly those on diuretics; and over-ventilation leads to acute alkalosis (Green, 1977). Early signs of toxicity may include anorexia, nausea, vomiting, and diarrhea. Visual disturbances include a halo effect around dark objects and a tendency for objects to appear yellow or green. Cardiac arrhythmias may be the first evidence of digitalis intoxication. The most frequent arrhythmias are premature ventricular contractions and any degree of atrioventricular block. Bigeminy or ventricular tachycardia also can occur (AMA Drug Evaluation, 1973). (For side effects peculiar to the elderly, see also Chapter 10, p. 173.)

Persons living independently who are taking digoxin should be taught to take their pulse. This is done by teaching them to place their index and middle finger of one hand on the wrist artery on the other arm, count the pulse for 30 seconds and multiply by two. If it is below 60 beats per minute, above 100, or as directed by the physician, they should be told to hold the dose and notify their doctor. They should also report any changes in rhythm from regular to irregular or the reverse that begin after receiving the drug.

DIURETICS. Diuretics decrease the volume of extracellular fluid by causing a loss of salt and water through the kidneys, thus preventing or eliminating edema. Their mechanism of action differs depending on the type of drug.

The thiazides accomplish their action through inhibition of sodium reabsorption in the distal convoluted tubule. The thiazides also reduce arterial pressure by reduction of blood volume and reduction of peripheral vascular resistance owing to their direct action on the smooth muscles of the arteriolar walls.

Side effects include hypokalemia and metabolic alkalosis because there is increased exchange of sodium for potassium and hydrogen ions at the distal convoluted tubule; hyperglycemia because of their direct effect on insulin release and because hypokalemia also reduces release of insulin; and hyperuricemia because thiazides interfere with excretion of uric acid by the distal convoluted tubule (Chrysant, 1976).

Furosemide (Lasix) is a loop diuretic and acts by interfering with sodium reabsorption by the ascending portion of Henle's loop. The side effects are the same as other thiazides but the hypoglycemia may be milder and the hypokalemia, metabolic alkalosis, and hyperuricemia may be more severe.

Certain diuretics are potassium-sparing in that they interfere with the exchange of sodium for potassium and hydrogen ions in the distal convoluted tubule. Spironolactone is the drug of choice in hypertension resulting from steroids.

Patients taking diuretics should be instructed to weigh daily and report any sudden changes to the doctor. They should also be told of possible problems caused by potassium loss. Symptoms to watch for are fatigue and weakness, "a washed out" feeling. Eating foods high in potassium may be sufficient to prevent deficiency. Some examples are canned salmon, baked potato, frozen lima beans, dried prunes, raisins, bananas, and oranges.

Occasionally potassium supplements such as potassium chloride may be ordered. They should be diluted before ingestion, usually with fruit juice or water. Giving them after meals may minimize gastric irritation. They taste bad and it is difficult to disguise the taste. Potassium that is enteric-coated is not effective. If diuretics are ordered b.i.d., patients should be encouraged to take them early in the day or they may have nocturia.

NARCOTICS, SEDATIVES, TRANQUILIZERS, AND MOOD ELEVATORS. Respiratory depression is the action of most narcotics and *can be lethal.* This does not mean that tranquilizers cannot be used or that people must suffer pain. The wearing effect of a chronic disease may necessitate regular use of low dose tranquilizers or mood elevators. Remember, too, that CO_2 retention is manifest in sleepiness.

Management of Lifestyle

Hydration

Maintaining adequate hydration is one key to keeping secretions thin enough to be coughed up. A desired fluid intake for these patients is about 3000 cc per day. The nursing role includes the following:

1. Assess the usual pattern of fluid intake, types of fluids, amounts, and timing.
2. Assure that the patient accepts the importance of fluid intake and understands the relationship between fluids and thinner, less viscous sputum, decreased work of coughing and raising sputum, greater availability of oxygen in cleared air spaces, and decreased risk of infection where the stasis of sputum is less.
3. Work with him to develop a workable schedule of fluid intake. (With those who take multiple medications, a full glass of water with each medication will often enable them to meet the goal.)
4. Set expectations of maintenance of a diary of fluid intake until the pattern is set and the patient is satisfied with the schedule.

For the patient with uncompromised cardiac status and adequate renal function the maintenance of this type of a fluid schedule is one of taking fluid. However, with patients who have some congestive failure, or who must have fluids restricted for other reasons, the maintenance of hydration to the point where secretions are reasonably thin becomes a real problem. The requirements of management of one disease must be balanced with the complications posed for the other. Often this means lower fluid levels, thicker secretions, and higher risk of infection with more reliance on machines than on physiologic coping mechanisms.

Another complication of high fluid intake is concerned with its effect on appetite and food intake. The person who increases fluid intake may feel too full to eat. This can be harmful because patients with COPD need to maintain adequate food intake or they become weak, lose weight, and are less able to maintain their schedule of activities.

The scheduling of fluid intake is no routine matter to be handled with a "be sure to take 3000 cc per day." It takes perceptive assessment and careful work with the patient to accommodate as much as possible to the variables that are interwoven with increased fluid intake. One example which might be helpful to some patients is to fill a 2-quart plastic container with water each morning and drink from it throughout the day along with other fluids such as coffee and juice. Liquids should be taken throughout the day and not pushed only in the day time. It is an area of professional nursing accountability, whether the nurse does it, checks the patient in his management, or works with another health care provider in achieving an acceptable outcome.

The greatest challenge is trying to maintain liquid secretions in the face of fluid restriction. Hot liquids may help. Periods of increased humidity can be achieved by running hot water first in the tub or shower to create steam and then adding the cold, or standing at the sink while hot water is running, or standing near the dishwasher during the drying stage. All these may create some additional moisture and usually stimulate a cough reaction. On the other hand, some persons find that humidity increases their problems in breathing. It is obvious that the nurse and the patient need to balance the effects of fluid restrictions necessary for cardiac status with the increased oxygen deficit created by thickened unraised secretions.

Urine color is a good indicator of hydration. Too little fluids are being ingested if urine is dark. Fluid intake probably is adequate if urine is pale.

Coughing and Spitting

Our society considers coughing and spitting as nonacceptable behavior. It is not only acceptable for COPD patients; it is essential. Their motto must be "Sputum is Beautiful." Repressing the urge to cough is something they cannot afford to do.

Given this, the nurse may wish to explore with patients and families their reservations (or lack of them) about coughing and spitting. Then they can attempt to discover ways that are acceptable for engaging in coughing and spitting in varying situations they encounter in their lifestyle. Planning ahead may enable them to cope more effectively and comfortably.

Sleep

Many individuals with chronic illness experience difficulty in sleeping. Many older persons without illness complain of being unable to sleep enough to suit themselves. The older person with COPD has a high risk of being dissatisfied with his sleep patterns.

Secretions tend to accumulate at night because of the horizontal position, and some people awaken with a choking situation and the need to expectorate the retained secretions. Fear keeps them awake even after they have cleared their airways. Some spend nights sitting up or frequently using their machines. However, reports of orthopnea, actually having to sit up to breathe, should alert the nurse to cardiac complications beyond the pulmonary pathology.

As with other areas of nursing management, one begins with an accurate assessment of the situation:

1. Are fluids or diuretics being taken late in the day so that sleep is interrupted to go to the bathroom?
2. Are they consuming any stimulants (coke, coffee, etc.) in the evening hours?
3. Are they involved in stimulating or distressing discussions, seeing disturbing TV programs, becoming excited to the point where sleep is difficult?
4. Are they sleeping in a room with another person who is keeping them awake or whom they fear to awaken?
5. Do they sleep at all during the day time hours?
6. How many hours a night do they sleep? from what hours?
7. When they are not sleeping, what do they do to occupy the time?

It is very important that persons with COPD avoid fatigue, and so they should rest at intervals throughout the day.

Many people choose to spend their entire day in a chair in front of the TV, dozing on and off. More often than not the dozing is due to boredom rather than to real fatigue. They then find it difficult to sleep at night. They should be encouraged to participate in activity during the day in increasing amounts to build up exercise tolerance. Leaving the house for rides or short excursions to an enclosed shopping mall can be accomplished even during inclement weather and will stimulate more interest in the waking world. If they are dozing on and off, perhaps the total is enough through 24 hours. They might be encouraged to keep a record of the hours they sleep so that they can see the total and worry less. That, in itself, might solve part of the problem.

Those who are awake a great deal in the night are concerned that the noise they are making coughing and breathing will keep others in their home awake. They worry about their partner's being kept awake. Some people move into separate rooms to avoid the worry of keeping the partner awake and find this a satisfactory solution. Usually, in this case, some sort of call system must be arranged should trouble arise. If this is not worked out both partners will lie awake worrying about the one in the other room.

Diuretics taken late in the afternoon can cause many trips to the bathroom during the night. Diuretics should be taken no later than 3:00 p.m. and a b.i.d. schedule must take this into consideration. Beverages containing caffeine, such as coffee, coke, and chocolate, taken before bed could cause sleeplessness because of their stimulating as well as diuretic effects. Patients should be warned to avoid stimulating substances in the evening. Instead, a light snack may be the key to at least a few hours sleep. Stirring television shows, arguments, or other distressing situations can cause difficulty in sleeping and should be avoided.

Sedatives may be used with caution. Some over-the-counter preparations that are promoted as safe agents to ease tension or overcome insomnia contain an antihistamine, usually methapyrilene, as their principle ingredient. Antihistamines are contraindicated in chronic pulmonary disease because of their drying effect on secretions. Barbiturates cause respiratory depression and, therefore, are contraindicated in patients at home. Chloral hydrate provides a rapid short term effect with minimal respiratory depression and is sometimes used. The benzodiazepines (Librium, Valium, and Dalmane) are long-acting sedatives and usually are free from significant side effects in therapeutic doses.

Persons with chronic lung disease must be observed for fatigue. If they are not getting sleep and rest, they may become so tired they will have to be hospitalized and possibly placed on a ventilator to get rest.

Environment

People with chronic lung disease are very sensitive to conditions in the environment, particularly temperature extremes, humidity, and air pollution. Many who can manage in earlier stages of the disease in the northern areas with the cold and humidity can find comfort only in drier, warmer climate as the disease progresses. Certainly all need to have real respect for air pollution and smog alerts, staying indoors and keeping windows closed to minimize contamination of their environment. Aerosol cans, cigarette smoke, greasy smells from frying, and freshly painted rooms are a few examples of respiratory irritants that should be avoided. Extremely hot climates cause a sense of smothering to some people. Extremely cold air may cause bronchospasm. If it is necessary to go out in cold weather, the protection of a scarf over the face to warm the air may be helpful. Geographic relocation is a choice some make from areas of cold, high humidity, and pollution to dry, clear, warm climates, but this should not be done without a 2-to-3-month trial. Sometimes a change in surroundings itself will have a positive effect for a short time but the effects are not lasting.

The barometric pressure, which is the total pressure of all the gases in the air, decreases progressively at higher altitudes. The barometric pressure at sea level is 760 mm Hg; at 10,000 ft, 523 mm Hg; and at 60,000 ft, 64 mm Hg (Guyton, 1976). Naturally, when the barometric pressure falls the PO_2 also drops, and this is the cause of hypoxia at higher altitudes. For this reason, a person with lung disease may get along well at sea level in Portland, Oregon, but develop respiratory distress when disembarking from a plane in Denver, Colorado, at 5000 ft (Silver).

If mild to moderate disease exists, travel at 6000 ft is possible but 8000 ft would seriously limit activities. It is recommended that persons with severe disease stay below 6000 ft or, if they must go to higher altitudes, they sharply curtail activities or investigate the possibility of using supplementary oxygen (Silver).

Mates

COPD is an invisible illness; thus it presents risks of being difficult to understand and make accommodations for. In at least one practice it seemed that there were fewer problems in marital relations when it was the husband who was ill with the disease than when the wife was ill.

The patient and the mate need to be involved in decisions about the aggressiveness of treatment as the disease becomes more severe or terminal. This includes decisions regarding hospitalization, use of intensive care facilities, tracheostomies, and other life-saving maneuvers. Both the patient and the mate need support during terminal stages of the illness, even down to such pragmatics as the symptoms or situations that should be reason to call the doctor. The nurse can be a supportive person in opening these discussions and helping couples or families relate effectively to each other in the midst of these ongoing stresses.

Another area for counseling by the nurse, doctor, or some other health provider, perhaps even another patient, is in the area of sexual activity. Both partners may need to have an opportunity to discuss this separately and together. It may be less of a problem for older persons than it is for young COPD patients, but it should not be overlooked solely on the basis of age. What is important is that the person have someone to talk this over with as needed, one who has expertise but who is also comfortable talking about it. Reading material may be provided for those who are too reticent to discuss sexual needs, or the reading may suggest the questions they need to ask.

Airway Management

The impairment of the normal mucociliary clearance mechanism and the excessive production of mucus and bronchial inflammation in chronic bronchitis causes a decrease in airway diameter. In emphysema, loss of effective elastic support for the bronchi causes the airways to collapse and readily obstruct when cough is forceful, which reduces the effectiveness of clearing the lungs. This ineffective cough is exhausting to the already compromised patient and retention of secretions further adds to the problem and can lead to respiratory failure.

POSTURAL DRAINAGE. Postural drainage is a simple method of helping clear the chest of excessive secretions. Few studies have evaluated this technique and those that have are conflicting in their results (March, 1971; Lorin, 1971; Clarke, 1973; and Anthonisen, 1964). From the evidence it would seem that if a patient has excessive secretions that are difficult to raise, postural drainage may aid in the removal but not without some potential dangers.

Because secretions are thick, postural drainage should be done following the use of bronchodilator therapy, if prescribed. It should be performed before meals or at least two hours after a heavy meal.

A realistic approach to postural drainage as an effective means of removing secretions must take into consideration other factors that would make breathing more difficult because of the shift in gravity and external pressure. Patients with congestive failure, or any other cardiac complications, air swallowers, obese individuals, and persons on long term steroids may have difficulties with positioning where the chest and head are in a dependent position. The head-down position is also contraindicated in patients with increased intracranial pressure and the procedure should not be performed on those patients who have had a recent myocardial infarction. Extreme caution must be used in those who have bleeding tendencies; the results of stroke or bruising will be far worse than the benefits. Hyperemias and arrhythmias have been found in patients during postural drainage (Tyler, 1977).

People have thought of some ingenious ways of positioning for postural drainage at home. They include:

- An ironing board with one end supported by a chair or stool and the other end on the floor.
- A lawn chair can be used by leveling the head section and lowering the foot portion to the ground.
- The foot of the bed can be elevated on 20-inch blocks if the head of the bed is safely stabilized against the wall.
- Tightly rolled blankets and pillows can be used on the bed to reach the desired angle.
- An inverted four-legged kitchen chair padded with pillows will also provide a good drainage position.

Four drainage positions are recommended:

- lying face down with hips elevated 18 to 20 inches
- lying on the right side with hips elevated 18 to 20 inches
- lying on the left side with hips elevated 18 to 20 inches
- semireclining or sitting upright

Each position should be held for 5 min or until secretions diminish. Coughing should be attempted after each position.

PERCUSSION. Percussion may be done by cupping a hand and striking the chest over the area to be drained. The motion should come from the wrists, shoulders, and elbows in a relaxed manner. This is thought to change the pressures in the airways, allowing air to get around the secretions so that cough is more effective in dislodging the plugs. Percussion should never be done over the spine, kidneys, or breasts and should not be done on the bare skin. A thin sheet or hand towel will protect the skin during the procedure while still allowing effective percus-

sion. Percussion should be carried out for 2 min over each area. Coughing should be encouraged after each drainage position is carried out. Nurses should consult with a chest physiotherapist before beginning percussion and if they have problems later. Ribs and vertebrae can be fractured, especially in older patients, if percussion is done improperly. There are commercial devices which really are vibrators that can be used to help loosen secretions. They are useful for older people with arthritis who cannot cup their hands or who have decreased strength. The effectiveness of these devices, however, is questionable. Nurses and family members should know what they are doing since, because of the force they exert when using a vibrator, they can be harmful.

Graded Exercise

GOALS. It is very important to get the patients involved in goal setting. Without their involvement, motivation will not be as great and performance will not be at a maximum. Questions to be answered are "What would you like to be doing in one month? Three months? Six months?" It is important that patients are assisted to set realistic goals so they can experience some needed successes in their activities.

BREATHING TECHNIQUES. Breathing techniques are taught to control the rate, depth, and speed of respiration. Probably the simplest and most helpful technique is pursed lip breathing. Breathing out through pursed lips forces the patient to slow his breathing down, to relax the air out rather than forcing it out. The beauty of this is that the patient has a simple method to use to control his dyspnea. There is less of the panic that accompanies lack of control. This can easily be taught by having the patient blow through a straw.

Another helpful technique which is easily taught is controlled breathing during various activities. The patient is taught to exhale on any motion which tends to force air out of the lungs. For example bending over to pick up something, sitting up from a supine position, pushing an object, would all be performed during exhalation. All of these motions tend to decrease the angle that the legs make with the upper body so the patient can also be told to exhale on any activity that decreases this angle, and inhale on any activity that tends to increase this angle. Inhaling is also proper during activities that tend to bring air into the body such as pulling and reaching. An example of breathing control during an activity such as vacuuming would be to inhale when pulling and exhale when pushing.

Abdominal breathing may be taught also, but this takes much longer to learn. It is believed that relaxing the abdominal muscles on inspiration aids in pulling the diaphragm down, thus aiding the inspiratory process. Contracting the abdominal muscles on expiration is thought to push the diaphragm upward, decreasing the size of the thoracic cavity aiding in expiration. Voluminous literature on the anatomy and physiology of breathing lends support to this traditional method of treatment, but extensive clinical testing is limited and nonconclusive.

STAIR CLIMBING. Stair climbing is an activity that may seem overwhelming to a patient with chronic lung disease, but it can be accomplished by learning how to perform it using energy conserving techniques. The pattern would be to climb one or two stairs on inhalation then exhale on two or three steps, repeating the process as tolerated. Another method is to climb three to five steps on exhalation and to rest until recovered for a few breaths, then climb again on exhalation. The key is not to hold the breath at any time. Such simple breathing techniques open up a new world to patients who have been limited from going anywhere that has stairs.

Living with Breathing Equipment

EQUIPMENT. Occasionally bronchodilators are ordered to be given by aerosolization. There are a number of devices available to deliver aerosolized medications. All of the equipment breaks up the drug into droplets small enough to reach the lungs when inhaled. The simplest device and the least expensive to the patient is the handbulb nebulizer. The cost is under $10.00. With each squeeze of the bulb a fine aerosol of medication is delivered. In order to use this device the patient must be able to take a deep breath and coordinate the squeeze of the handbulb with the inhalation of the medication. Some muscle strength is also required to squeeze the bulb. Although this sounds simple it is not easy for an older person who has difficulty with hands or coordination to learn.

A compressor-driven device might be more suitable to the needs of those patients who cannot coordinate their movements or have poor muscular strength. These machines such as Pulmo-Aide or Maximyst run by electricity and cost under $100.00. They provide the power for a fine mist to be generated. The patient must be able to take a deep breath and coordinate this with occlusion of the port on the nebulizer.

The most complicated as well as the most expensive form of nebulization is the Intermittent Positive Pressure Breathing (IPPB) machine. Cherniack (1974) stated that there is no added benefit to obstructed patients when bronchodilators are delivered by IPPB. However, if patients cannot take a deep breath or are unable to hold it long enough to let the aerosol deposit, then IPPB may be of benefit. IPPB will not insure this effect, however, unless an adequate tidal volume is delivered. The patient must be taught how to relax and let the machine do the work of delivering the aerosol under positive pressure. Without adequate instruction in slow, relaxed, deep breathing, the added benefits of IPPB therapy will not be achieved (Berkow, 1977, p. 602).

Another use for IPPB may be to loosen sputum and to encourage patients to cough. Areas of lung that are obstructed by secretions are poorly ventilated. These poorly ventilated areas tend to cause inspissation of mucus. One reason for this is that negative pressure occurs behind the plug as air is gradually absorbed in the occluded area. This holds the mucus in the airway. IPPB opens up some of these areas increasing the pressure distal to the plugs. It may also force air, which enters well-ventilated areas through the pores of Kohn and canals of Lambert, into the poorly ventilated areas with the same effect (Berkow, 1977). All breathing equipment is used with a solution: know the medication, the strength, and the dose.

Coughing is absolutely essential after any form of inhalation treatment. The medications, water, or saline that are used also stimulate mucus production with or without loosening inspissated secretions. If the patient cannot cough there may be increased plugging of the airways with the additional fluid, actually worsening the condition.

EVALUATION. Patients who have equipment at home should be able to (1) explain the purpose of the equipment, (2) demonstrate self-reliance in its use, (3) clean the equipment properly, and (4) explain concepts of infection control.

EXAMPLES OF WRITTEN INSTRUCTIONS. Whatever device is used to deliver the aerosol, proper instruction and cleanliness are essential. Written instructions should be provided so that the patient can refer to them when at home with no professional help available. An example of an instruction sheet is given on the next page.

INSTRUCTIONS FOR PULMO-AIDE
Model 645

1. Measure the prescribed amount of bronchodilator* and place into nebulizer outlet. Dosage_____
2. Place measured amount of prescribed sterile water* or normal saline* into outlet of nebulizer. Dosage_____
3. Make sure nebulizer is held in upright position at all times or solution will be lost.
4. Attach tubing to nebulizer.
5. Remove white plug from slot on side of nebulizer.
6. Turn on compressor. Place finger over control until mist is seen, then release.
7. Exhale as much as is comfortably possible.
8. Position mouthpiece of nebulizer just inside teeth. Close lips around mouthpiece.
9. Put finger over the fingertip control to release mist and inhale slowly and deeply with an abdominal breath.
10. Hold breath at the end of full inspiration for a few seconds to allow the medication to settle in the airways. Otherwise you may exhale some of the droplets.
11. Remove mouthpiece from mouth. Exhale through pursed lips. This allows better distribution of the medication in the airway.
12. Repeat the deep breaths until the medication is gone. Rest at intervals to prevent overbreathing and dizziness.
13. Clean nebulizer after each use by rinsing with warm water and mild detergent (Ivory Liquid, Joy, etc.) after each use. Rinse and then soak in a solution of ⅛ cup *white* vinegar and 2 cups of water overnight. This kills bacteria. Actually, 20 to 30 minutes is sufficient to kill the bacteria but it may be easier for you to leave it soaking all night. Before the next treatment, remove the nebulizer from the solution, shake off excess vinegar, and rinse well with warm water.
14. The vinegar solution can be reused twice more if kept refrigerated and covered.
15. Always wash nebulizer in a bowl away from the sink as small parts are easily lost down the drain.

* Once opened store in refrigerator

INSTRUCTIONS FOR MAKING NORMAL SALINE. If normal saline is used with the bronchodilator, an inexpensive solution can be made at home in the following manner:

Place an uncovered, clean, quart jar and its lid in a clean saucepan and completely cover with water. (A smaller jar, such as a baby food jar, can be used if smaller amounts are required.) Cover the saucepan and boil for 10 min. In another clean saucepan, place 1 tsp *uniodized* table salt in 1 qt water from the tap. If smaller amounts are required place ½ tsp uniodized salt in 1 pt of tap water. Cover the pan and boil for 10 min. Do not tamper with this concentration or boil much longer or the concentration of the solution will change. Turn off heat and allow both pans to cool with covers on. Carefully pour the water from the pan containing the jar and its lid into the sink. Do not touch the insides of the jar or the lid. Pour the salt solution into the jar and screw the lid on tightly. If the jar is tightly sealed and the inside not touched, the solution will remain sterile for a week if stored in the refrigerator.

INHALERS. The Bronkometer, DuoMedihaler, and Alupent Spray are examples of metered dose medications that are dispensed in a pocket-sized cartridge. The medication is inhaled into the lungs. It is very important that the cartridge be shaken several times before inhaling. In addition to the medication, the cartridge contains a propellent gas. The medication is heavier than the propellent and tends to settle in the bottom. If not shaken, the dose might be the propellent alone. When the propellent is gone there is no way of getting the medication out, money is wasted and the patient does not get the benefit of the medication.

After shaking the cartridge, the patient should exhale completely, beginning as deep an inspiration as possible while vaporizing the medication, hold his breath for 3 to 4 seconds at the end of inspiration, and then exhale slowly through pursed lips. This will better insure deposition of the medication into the lungs. This handy device can be carried around in a pocket to be used as ordered. The problem with these devices is that they are too handy and some patients tend to abuse them. Another disadvantage is that the drug is not diluted and the higher concentrations can be somewhat irritating.

In gaining information about patients with respiratory problems, find out how often they are using these devices. Someone who is using them frequently (every 2 to 3 hr) needs to be evaluated and placed on appropriate therapy. Complications can ensue unless this is done.

Morale

Living with chronic oxygen deficit, shortness of breath, cough, and high risk of infectious complications is difficult. Some patients tend to be casual in maintaining their treatment regimen and monitoring their activities. When these folks encounter complications, they may be unhappy or disgusted, but they may also feel they paid the price. There are other patients who are truly conscientious about following the prescribed regimen. At times these people get infections and complications too. For them there is real discouragement, when all their diligence does not have a better payoff. The nurse needs to be willing to listen without trying to cut off their reported low morale with platitudes or "shoulds." The same may hold true for families whose morale may vary directly with that of the patient's.

Activities

Life becomes a paced schedule for the patient with oxygen deprivation associated with COPD. Each activity requires increasingly longer amounts of time as the pace is slowed to accommodate to less oxygen and longer recovery times. Between activities there are the treatments involving breathing equipment and medications. For the patient with severe COPD there are few moments during the day when they are not involved in ADL or compliance with treatment regimens.

A problem the nurse faces is in the degree of emphasis to place on the treatment schedule. On the one hand, if regular treatments with breathing equipment and medications are not carried out, secretions thicken and clog the airways. If, on the other hand, too much emphasis is placed on the treatments, some patients do nothing else. With each patient this need for balance becomes a matter for rational planning. The nurse can help by gathering data on the usual patterns of daily living the person is maintaining and what he would like to do. A plan can be developed with the patient and family on how both can be accommodated.

It takes time in the morning for patients to "get going." They may take a medication and treatment upon awakening. Rest. Then they may do respiratory toilets. Rest. Followed by breakfast. Rest. Go to the bathroom. Rest. All this is an example of why activities such as doctor's appointments are best scheduled late in the morning or early afternoon. If the person must be somewhere at 9:00 a.m. he must move his schedule back, causing him to get up as early as 4:00 or 5:00 a.m.

Evaluation

Although respiratory therapy measures, IPPB, chest percussion, and drainage have been used in the treatment of COPD, these therapies have not been evaluated. They have been helpful to some patients. Whether improvement was due to changed physiology or provided psychologic benefit is not known in many instances. All aspects of the therapies are under study now. Until the outcomes are known their use will continue (Cherniak, 1974).

The nurse's evaluation of patient response is based upon the quality of life that can be maintained by those with COPD. Adherence to the therapeutic regimen does not guarantee freedom from hospitalization, infection, and gradual respiratory decline. The patient is a full partner in plans and decisions which must be made relative to his care. This requires that he know/understand fully about the disease process, the purpose of drugs, the meaning of pulmonary function tests and ABG, the signs and symptoms of complications, especially pulmonary infections, and what to do for each. Care of patients with respiratory problems is truly a team effort— patient, family, nurse, therapist, physician.

The prognosis is one of deterioration. This can be better accepted by the patient/family when they have been involved and know that their opinions are respected and expected.

The Nurse's Relationship

COPD is a progressive disease. While the rate of change may vary with individuals, it is ultimately a terminal disease. Given its chronicity and the declining patient resources, the relationship with the nurse can be an important one for the patient. One characteristic in this relationship that is significant in helping the patient to manage his daily living and lifestyle is honesty and openness on the part of the nurse(s). If this behavior is initiated early, maintained consistently, and done with sensitivity, it encourages similar reciprocal openness on the part of the patient. For example, the disease process, medications, and other associated therapies and issues should be explained to the patient and those who are involved— family, others. Implications for daily living need to be explored so that they can make informed decisions and engage in realistic planning. The result of such ongoing encounters between providers and patients is a mutual engagement in dealing with the often difficult problems of living with this disease and its complications—day in, day out, over the years.

PNEUMONIA

Pneumonia is a bacterial or viral lung infection for which the elderly, particularly those with COPD, are at high risk. Bacterial pneumonias comprise the largest number found in the elderly. Ninety percent of all bacterial pneumonias are caused by streptococcus (streptococcus pneumoniae). The other pneumonias are caused by four classes of organisms: virus, mycoplasma, chlamydia (parrot fever) and rickettsia (Q fever). There is no effective treatment for viral pneumonia and, considering that mycoplasma, chlamydia, and rickettsia are fairly uncommon in the elderly, attention will be given to pneumococcal pneumonia.

Etiologic Factors

The pneumococcus is a normal inhabitant of the nose and throat. Whether or not pneumonia results depends on the virulence of the bacteria versus the defenses of the host. The pneumococcus is a gram-positive encapsulated coccus. The capsular substance is a complex polysaccharide and there are 84 types of pneumococci with differing capsules. All cause disease in humans, but types 1, 3, 4, 7, 8, and 12 are the most frequently found types in clinical practice. Types 6, 14, 19, and 23 are most often found in children (Thorn, 1977). The capsule is what protects the pneumococci from being phagocytized, so the greater the capsule the more virulent the organism (Lerner, 1975).

High Risk

All old people are at high risk for pneumonia; however, persons with COPD have greater susceptibility. They have *increased* bronchial secretions which provide a warm moist breeding ground for bacteria and *decreased* capability for clearing the bacteria out.

Upper respiratory infections increase the risk of pneumonia. Seventy-five percent of those who acquire pneumococcal pneumonia have had a preceding upper respiratory infection. Aspiration of this infected material into the lower respiratory tract probably begins the infectious process.

Winter and spring seasons are the time periods of greatest risk. These are the months when pneumococcal pneumonia most frequently occurs.

Dynamics and Signs and Symptoms

The person usually experiences a sudden, shaking chill. The cause of this is not clear, but it may be due to a specific pyrogenic component of the pneumococcus. Bacteremia is present in a third of the cases and may be detected after the chill has occurred (Sodeman, 1974).

FEVER. Fever can rise to 102 to 106°F. (39 to 41.5°C.), usually peaking in late afternoon or evening. (Whenever an elderly person is febrile, a pulmonary infection should be considered as this is the most common cause after urinary tract infections.) Increases in temperature are accompanied by tachycardia, increased respiratory rate, and widened pulse pressure (Lerner, 1975).

LEUKOCYTOSIS. The white blood count (WBC) may reach 30,000, usually reaching its peak on the third day. Polymorphonuclear leukocytes make up 70 to 90 percent of the leukocytes (Hoeprich, 1977). A normal or low WBC is indicative of a fulminating infection with bacteremia.

X-RAY FINDINGS. The x-ray picture shows consolidation. This is due to the outpouring of edema fluid in response to the bacteria. This fluid carries the organisms through the pores of Kohn to adjacent alveoli with each breath. Polymorphonuclear leukocytes enter the infected area, fill the alveoli, and produce consolidation. The consolidation remains in one lobe unless there is aspiration of the infected fluid into the bronchial tree with infection of several lobes (Sodeman, 1974).

PHYSICAL SIGNS. Physical signs over areas of consolidation include dullness to percussion, increased tactile fremitus (vibration felt with hand on chest during talking), bronchial breath sounds, whispered pectoriloquy (distinct transmission of whispered sounds), and egophony (long e; sound transmits as ay). Crackles (rales) are also present (Forgacs, 1978). There is decreased motion on the affected side. The trachea is midline unless pleural effusion or empyema are present (Thorn, 1977).

COUGH. The accumulation of purulent material and irritation of the lower respiratory tract results in cough, producing pinkish or rusty mucopurulent sputum (Sodeman, 1974). Inflammation and bleeding into the alveoli account for the color.

CYANOSIS. Cyanosis of the lips and nailbeds may be evident in severe cases owing to the ventilation-perfusion abnormalities caused by blood's traveling through unventilated alveoli, as exudate replaces air in the lung. Arterial hypoxemia results.

ANXIETY. The person with pneumococcal pneumonia is alert but apprehensive because of his inability to get enough air.

Differential Diagnosis

It is very important that diagnosis be made as early as possible, because the organisms double rapidly and can become overwhelming within a few hours. Specific therapy must be instituted, and harm can come to the patient who is started on the wrong antibiotic.

Before starting antibiotics, sputum for culture and sensitivity and Gram stain must be collected. Sputum must come from the lower respiratory tract for accurate diagnosis. This material is usually thick and yellow, green, or pink-tinged (mucopurulent) compared to the thin, clear, frothy material from the mouth. If an aerobic infection is suspected the patient can cough and expectorate the specimen. If the patient is unable to produce a specimen, sputum induction may be necessary. To do this the patient is given an ultrasonic mist treatment with sterile distilled water or normal saline. This is irritating to the respiratory tract and will cause the patient to cough. A nasotracheally suctioned specimen using a mucus trap may be necessary if the patient cannot expectorate sputum.

Because anaerobes are normal flora in the mouth, other methods must be used to obtain a specimen if an anaerobic infection is suspected. Suctioning with a mucus trap is one method and percutaneous transtracheal aspiration is another. A small plastic catheter is passed by a physician through the anterior neck into the trachea. A small amount of sterile water is injected and immediately aspirated, bringing with it organisms from the lower respiratory tract. This specimen can be used for both aerobic and anaerobic cultures. The specimen should be processed as soon as possible after collection. The longer the time elapsed, the more possibility of overgrowth from contamination by other organisms. At least two blood cultures should be obtained before antibiotics are started because the possibility of bacteremia is so high.

Complications

Complications in the lung include atelectasis, manifested by sudden recurrence of pleuritic pain and rapid respirations; delayed resolution beyond the normal two to three weeks, and abscess which causes persistent fever and expectoration of large amounts of purulent sputum.

Pleural effusion occurs in 5 percent of patients with pneumococcal pneumonia. Rarely does it require aspiration but absorbs spontaneously. Empyema is a very rare complication and also causes pleuritic pain and fever. Spread of the infection to the pericardial sac causes pericarditis. Precordial pain, accompanied by a friction rub on auscultation, is a sign of this complication. Arthritis resulting from growth of pneumococci in the joints may occur as well as pneumococcal meningitis, both caused by bacteremic spread. Liver damage occurs occasionally, resulting in mild jaundice (Thorn, 1977).

Good observation of the patient includes inspection and auscultation and awareness of the possible complications that might occur.

HERPES SIMPLEX. Herpetic blisters about the mouth are common.

PLEURISY. Inflammation of the pleura result in pleurisy. There is sharp stabbing pain, accentuated by inspiratory movement, referred directly to the overlying chest wall. This results in splinting of the affected side and rapid shallow respirations. If the diaphragmatic pleura is involved, pain is referred to the shoulder (Thorn, 1977).

GASTROINTESTINAL SYMPTOMS. Ileus may occur. It is thought to be the result of low oxygen saturation of the blood supplying the bowel. This causes abdominal distention and further complicates the work of breathing.

Prognosis

With prompt and adequate therapy, most patients recover uneventfully. Older persons, however, need to anticipate a longer period of convalescence and a slower return of energy, often a major frustration to them. COPD and cardiac disease may slow recovery rate even more and can increase risks of complications. Pneumonia and influenza are the fifth leading causes of death for all ages and both sexes. At age 75+ these diseases are the fourth cause of death (Vital Statistics, 1975).

Medical and Nursing Management

BEDREST. The older person with pneumococcal pneumonia should be hospitalized. Bedrest is instituted to decrease the body's demand for oxygen. This can be an added danger to someone who is already experiencing airway obstruction. The patient must be reminded constantly to deep breathe and cough. An incentive spirometer is helpful in assuring deep breathing and can prevent further complications if used faithfully every 1 to 2 hours. The patient must be encouraged to change position frequently, and a footboard should be provided so that leg exercises can be practiced at regular intervals.

ANTIMICROBIAL THERAPY. Aqueous crystalline penicillin 100,000 units IM should be given immediately after collection of the sputum and Gram stain has indicated pneumococcal pneumonia. This is followed immediately by procaine penicillin G, 300,000 units daily for a week. Other effective antibiotics include erythromycin 0.5 gm q 8 hr IV or P.O. or cefazolin 0.5 gm q 8 hr IM or IV (Oregon Thoracic Society, 1977).

Before giving the medication the patient should be asked if he is allergic to penicillin and should be inspected for skin rash or other unusual symptoms after antibiotics have been started.

HYDRATION AND AIRWAY MANAGEMENT. As mucus increases and fills the airways, water is absorbed from it, making it difficult to raise sputum and causing airway obstruction. If this occurs in enough airways, the patient is unable to meet his oxygen needs. The patient must be kept well-hydrated to keep the mucus thin and easily expectorated. This is best done by forcing fluids to 2000 to 3000 ml daily, orally or intravenously. Intake and output must be monitored closely to insure adequate intake as well as providing clues to another complication of hypoxia, namely, renal shutdown.

Coughing should be encouraged if it is productive. If the patient becomes fatigued by unproductive coughing, a cough suppressant such as codeine might provide relief.

Postural drainage may aid in the removal of secretions. Auscultation should be done before drainage to assure proper positioning and afterward to assess the results.

OXYGEN. An increased concentration of oxygen is needed if the arterial blood gases indicate hypoxemia. Hypoxemia results from the ventilation/perfusion mismatch caused by fluid-filled alveoli and the increased metabolic needs for oxygen caused by fever. The patient may appear restless, confused, or aggressive—symptoms similar to acute alcoholic intoxication. These are signs of cerebral hypoxia. Decreased urinary output progresses to renal shutdown

if hypoxia is prolonged. The heart rate increases in response to hypoxia. A slight increase in blood pressure and epistaxis are additional signs of decreased oxygen (Beland, 1975). In some patients the blood pressure falls as the disease progresses. This is due to a lowered cardiac output caused by depressed myocardial function and fluid loss secondary to fever (Sodeman, 1974).

The arterial blood gases must be monitored closely because giving oxygen to patients who retain CO_2 is potentially dangerous. The patient's stimulus to breathe is low oxygen and, if oxygen is given in flow rates above 2 L per minute, the patient may cease breathing.

VITAL SIGNS. Because tachycardia and hypotension are signs of cardiac stress, pulse and blood pressure should be monitored frequently. Elevated temperature causes an increase in the basal metabolic rate. This increases the need for calories and protein. Weight loss will occur if these are not provided. An increased metabolic rate also causes water and sodium loss by means of diaphoresis. An adequate fluid intake must be maintained and is measured by an output of at least 1000 ml per day (Beland, 1975). Because the patient's skin must be kept dry, frequent gown and linen changes may be necessary. The headache that may accompany fever is better treated with codeine than by aspirin since the diaphoresis that follows administration of aspirin may be more uncomfortable than the headache. Temperature, pulse, and respiration should fall within 12 to 36 hours after initiation of penicillin, but may not reach normal for four or more days. Roentgenography will show evidence of clearing also.

PLEURITIC PAIN. Codeine may be given for pleuritic pain unless cough suppression is contraindicated. An intercostal nerve block may offer temporary relief (Harrison, 1977).

PREVENTING SPREAD. Bacterial pneumonia is spread by airborne droplets. The patient should be taught to cover coughs and sneezes. If no tissues are handy, the hand can catch most of the escaping droplets and can be easily washed. Tissues should be placed in a paper bag which is then burned.

PREVENTING RECURRENCE. Patients with secretions should be taught methods of bronchial hygiene. They must be encouraged to be faithful in carrying out the routine at home.

A new vaccine (Pneumovax) has recently been introduced on the market and is effective against certain strains of pneumococci. Fourteen pneumococcal capsular types are included in the vaccine. These types—1, 2, 3, 4, 6, 8, 9, 12, 14, 19, 23, 25, 51, and 56 —account for at least 80 percent of all pneumococcal pneumonias. The antibody levels may remain for up to 5 years and revaccination is recommended at no more than 3-year intervals to minimize local reactions in those whose antibody levels remain high. The vaccine is recommended in all persons having chronic debilitating diseases, including chronic pulmonary disease. Those persons receiving immunosuppressive therapy may not respond as well to the vaccine (Merck and Company, 1977).

FLU SHOTS. All persons over 65 are advised to be immunized yearly against influenza. Those with COPD are particularly vulnerable to the flu. There are basically two major types of influenza—Type A which tends to drift and shift in terms of different strains and Type B which is fairly stable. Older persons should check with their local health departments or their private physicians to determine their need for initial injections or boosters. These injections should never be given to those who are allergic to eggs because eggs are the media used to produce the vaccine.

Many older persons are reluctant to have these injections because they do not believe in them. Some report developing side effects of a cold after the injections and find it difficult to understand that the injections will protect against more severe illness.

It is important for the injections to be taken early in the fall so that they can be of maximum benefit. They do no good if given when the infection is in progress. The injections take from 2 to 3 weeks to become effective after they have been given.

Evaluation

Fortunately, pneumonias usually respond to the prescribed therapy. The older patient usually begins to feel better in 2 to 3 days after treatment begins, especially if the organism is identified and is sensitive to the antibiotics. An x-ray picture is taken frequently during therapy to check the resolution of the infection.

Since it will take longer to be fully recovered than the older person may like, it becomes important for the nurse to be aware of the patient's response to activities and demands of daily living and see how he is pacing himself. With time he should return to his pre-illness state.

BIBLIOGRAPHY

Chronic Obstructive Pulmonary Disease

AMA Department of Drugs, AMA Drug Evaluations, ed. 2. Acton, Mass.: Publishing Sciences Group, 1973.

Anthonisen, P., Rus, P., and Sgaard-Andersen, T.: The value of lung physical therapy in the treatment of acute exacerbations of chronic bronchitis. Acta Med. Scand. 175:715, 1964.

Barstow, R. E.: Coping with emphysema. Nursing Clin. N. Amer. 9:140, 1974.

Berkow, R. (ed.): The Merck Manual of Diagnosis and Therapy, ed. 13. Rahway, N. J.: Merck Sharp and Dohme Research Laboratories, 1977.

Breon Laboratories: Product Information (Bronkosol-2).

Brogden, R. N., Speight, T. M., and Avery, G. S.: Sodium cromoglycate (cromolyn sodium): A review of its mode of action, pharmacology, therapeutic efficacy and use. Drugs, 7:164–282, 1974.

Burrows, B., and Earle, R. H.: Course and prognosis of chronic obstructive lung disease. New Engl. J. Med. 280: 397, 1969.

Burton, G. G., Gee, G. N., and Hodgkin, J. E.: Respiratory Care: A Guide to Clinical Practice. Philadelphia: J. B. Lippincott Co., 1977.

Cherniack, R. M.: Intermittent positive pressure breathing in management of chronic obstructive disease: current state of the art. Amer. Rev. Respir. Dis. 110:188, 1974.

Cherniak, R. M., and Svanhill, E.: Long term use of IPPB in COPD. Amer. Rev. Respir. Dis. 113:721–727, 1976.

Chrysant, S. G.: Effects of antihypertensive agents. Drug Therapy 12:22–31, 1976.

Clarke, S. W., Cochrane, G. M., and Webber, B.: The effects of sputum on pulmonary function. Thorax, 28:262, 1973.

Conference on the Scientific Basis of Respiratory Therapies. Amer. Rev. Respir. Dis. 110:July–December, 1975.

Diener, C. F., and Burrows, B.: Further observations on the course and prognosis of COLD. Amer. Rev. Respir. Dis. 111:719–724, 1975.

Engel, G. L.: Grief and grieving. Amer. J. Nurs. 64:93–98, 1964.

Farzan, S.: A Concise Handbook of Respiratory Disease. Reston, Virginia: Reston Publishing Co., 1978.

Fisons Company Package Information (Cromolyn Sodium), 1978.

Fletcher, C. M.: Cigarettes and respiratory disease. In Goodman, H. A. (ed.): World Conference on Smoking and Health: A Summary of the Proceedings. New York: American Cancer Society, 1968.

Geumei, A. M., and Miller, W. F.: New oral bronchodilator drug with relatively selective stimulation of beta-2 adrenergic receptors. Chest 72:267–268, 1977.

Gordon, B. L. (ed.): Clinical Cardiopulmonary Physiology, ed. 3. New York: Grune and Stratton, 1969.

Green, L. H., and Smith, T. W.: The use of digitalis in patients with pulmonary disease. Ann. Intern. Med. 87:459–465, 1977.

Guyton, A. C.: Textbook of Medical Physiology, ed. 5. Philadelphia: W. B. Saunders Co., 1976.

Hodgkin, J. E., et al.: Chronic obstructive airway diseases, current concepts in diagnosis and comprehensive care. J.A.M.A. Vol. 232, June 23, 1975.

Jenne, J. W.: Rationale for methylxanthines in asthma. In Stein, M. (ed.): New Directions in Asthma. American College of Chest Physicians, Park Ridge, Ill., 1975, pp. 391–413.

Judge, R. D., and Zuidema, G. D.: Methods of Clinical Examination: A Physiologic Approach, ed. 3. Boston: Little Brown & Co., 1974.

Kimbel, P.: An in-hospital program for rehabilitation of patients with chronic obstructive pulmonary disease. Chest (Supplement) 60, 1971.

Lertzman, M. M., and Cherniak, R.: Rehabilitation of patients with chronic obstructive pulmonary disease. Amer. Rev. Respir. Dis. 114:1145–1165, 1976.

Lieberman, J.: This inherited deficiency can lead to a devastating form of emphysema. Amer. Lung Assoc. Bull. 61:10–13, 1975.

Lowe, C. R.: Industrial bronchitis. Brit. Med. J. 1:463–486, 1969.

Lorin, M. I., and Denning, C. R.: Evaluation of postural drainage by measurement of sputum volume and consistency. Amer. J. Phys. Med. 50:215–219, 1971.

March, H.: Appraisal of postural drainage for chronic obstructive pulmonary disease. Arch. Phys. Med. Rehabil. 52:528–530, 1971.

Mathewson, H. S.: Pharmacology for Respiratory Therapists. St. Louis: C. V. Mosby Co., 1977.

Morris, J. F.: Spirometry in the evaluation of pulmonary function. Western J. Med. 125:110–118, 1976.

Oregon Thoracic Society (COPD Manual Committee): Chronic Obstructive Pulmonary Disease. New York: American Lung Association, 1977. (Excellent resource available without charge from local Lung Association, 118 pages.)

Renzetti, A. D., Jr., McClement, J. H., and Litt, B. D.: Mortality in relation to respiratory function in COPD. The Amer. J. Med. 39:115, 1966.

Rodman, T., and Sterling, F. H.: Pulmonary Emphysema and Related Lung Diseases. St. Louis: C. V. Mosby Co., 1969.

Schering Corporation, Product Information (Vanceril).

Schwaid, M. C.: The impact of emphysema. Amer. J. Nurs. 70:1247–1250, 1970.

Scott, B. H.: Tensions linked with emphysema. Amer. J. Nurs. 69:538–540, 1969.

Silver, H. M.: Travel for the patient with COPD. The Rehabilitation Research and Training Center, The George Washington University Medical Center, Washington D.C. (No date given on the pamphlet.)

Tyler, M. L.: Arterial Blood Gases, Arterial Oxygen Saturation, Blood Rate and Blood Pressure During Chest Physiotherapy. Unpublished Master's Thesis, University of Washington School of Nursing, Seattle, Wash., 1977.

U.S. Department of Health, Education and Welfare: The Health Consequences of Smoking: A Public Health Service Review (PHS Publication No. 1696), Washington D.C., 1967.

U.S. Public Health Service: Smoking and Health: Report of the Advisory Committee to the Surgeon General of the Public Health Service. (PHS Publication No. 1103), Washington D.C., 1964.

Wynder, E. L., and Hoffman, D.: Tobacco and Tobacco Smoke, Studies in Experimental Carcinogenesis. New York: Academic Press, 1967.

Pneumonia

Beland, I. L., and Passos, J.: Clinical Nursing: Pathophysiological and Psychosocial Approaches, ed. 3. New York: London: Macmillan Co., 1975.

Capell, P., and Case, D.: Ambulatory Care Manual for Nurse Practitioner. Philadelphia: J. B. Lippincott Co., 1976.

Forgacs, P.: The functional bases of pulmonary sounds. Chest 73:399–405, 1978.

Hoeprich, P. D.: Infectious Diseases, ed. 2. Hagerstown, Md.: Harper & Row, 1977.

Lerner, A. M., and Jankauskas, K.: The classical bacterial pneumonias. DM (Disease a Month), February 1975.

Merck & Co., Product Information, Pneumovax (Pneumococcal Vaccine Polyvalent, MSD), November 1977.

Oregon Thoracic Society, COPD Manual Committee: Chronic Obstructive Pulmonary Disease. American Lung Association, N.Y. 1977.

Sodeman, W. A., and Sodeman, W. A., Jr.: Pathologic Physiology, Mechanisms of Disease, ed. 5. Philadelphia: W. B. Saunders Co., 1974.

Thorn, G. W., et al. (eds.): Harrison's Principles of Internal Medicines, ed. 8. New York: McGraw-Hill Book Co., 1977.

Vital Statistics of United States, U.S. Bureau of Census, Washington D.C., 1975.

23

Skin Problems

Pauline Bruno

QUICK REVIEW

DRY SKIN (OSTEOTOSIS)

DESCRIPTION	Age-related loss of moisture in tissues and loss of effectiveness of skin as a barrier to moisture loss lead to increased dryness of skin.
ETIOLOGIC FACTORS	Dry skin in the elderly results from decreased endocrine secretion, sebaceous gland activity and sweating; degeneration of papillary capillaries; washing away of protective lipids with soap and water.
HIGH RISK	Elderly with previous history of dry skin and chapping, dry climate, frequent exposure of skin to water and soap or detergents.
DYNAMICS	Moisture in dermis determines suppleness and elasticity of skin. Dryness excites cutaneous nerves leading to itching.

SIGNS AND
SYMPTOMS

Back: Pale, rough texture, small scales.
Lower legs: smooth and shiny; possible fine fissures on red moist cracks.
Dorsum of hands: wrinkled fissures.
Itching: reported as intense. Most severe at retiring and on arising. It is exacerbated by rough-textured cloth or wool next to skin, change in temperature, increased air movement (wind, fans), chemicals, e.g., detergents.

COMPLICATIONS	Skin breaks and infection.

MANAGEMENT

Dry Skin: Restrict use of soap to axillary and genital areas. Rinse thoroughly. Use tepid rather than hot water. Bathe less frequently. Apply nonperfumed emolient containing lanolin immediately following washing to prevent loss of moisture absorbed. Increase humidity of environment. Wear cotton undergarments. Add oil to rinse water in laundering undergarments, hose, bedlinen.
Itching: Minimize static electricity by using antistatic rinses or dryer additives. Use topical antipruritic preparations, oral antihistamines. Finger pressure over areas to override stimulus to nerve endings. Diversion or social activities to distract and lower itch-awareness.

EVALUATION	Signs and symptoms of dryness and itching reduced. Incorporates prevention and management of skin dryness into lifestyle.

The skin is the outermost tissue layer of the body. It provides a protective covering for the inner tissues and organs and is the part of self that is visible to others. The content of this chapter addresses (1) functional changes with age and actions to offset the detrimental effects of these changes; (2) assessment of the skin of the elderly; and (3) commonly occurring skin disorders. The latter section outlines the dominant etiologic factors, the underlying pathophysiologic changes, the manifestations, prevention measures, and management of the condition.

The skin is an essential organ for life. Anatomically, it is a boundary and a shield between the body and its environment. It assists in perception of the environment and performs or initiates many of the adaptations resulting from this perception. It enables identification of the individual by providing shape to the facial and body contours and distinctive markings such as fingerprints. The skin reveals emotions such as anxiety (sweating), embarrassment (blush-ing), fear (paleness), and anger (redness). The appearance of this dynamic, reactive organ is markedly changed with age and by a variety of external forces.

Structurally, the skin consists of three distinct layers: the epidermis, corium (dermis), and subcutaneous tissue (Fig. 23-1). Contained in these layers are glands, nerves, blood vessels, lymphatics, and muscles.

FUNCTION CHANGES AND ADAPTIVE ACTIONS

The skin has four significant functions which are modified as a result of normal changes that occur with aging. These changes affect a persons comfort and interaction with the environment and are important considerations in the management of health care for the elderly. The principal functions of the skin include protection, heat regulation, sensation, and body image.

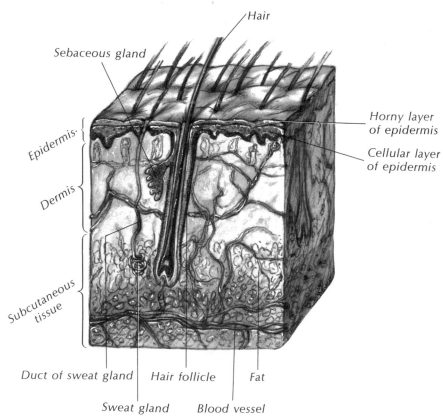

FIGURE 23-1. Cross section of the three layers of the skin. (From Bates, 1979)

Body Image

Skin is the part of oneself visible to others. The readily observable changes in appearance with aging are in the epidermal layer; these changes often reflect alterations in the dermis and subcutaneous layers. The variables influencing the timing and extent of skin changes include environmental traumas, genetic inheritance, and disorders of other body systems. A youthful, attractive appearance of the skin and appendages, the hair and nails, is highly valued in American society, resulting in considerable expenditure of time, energy, and money to promote this effect. A skin problem perceived as being unattractive may for a person of any age result in a change in body image, lowering of self-esteem, and avoidance of contact with other people.

There is considerable individual variability in the quality of skin changes that occur with aging and in the time of onset in the life cycle. The extent of skin pigmentation, heredity, and environmental influences contribute to this individual variability; however, even with similar exposure to sunlight, some persons have marked skin changes and others very little. In general, nonexposed skin or skin protected by pigment undergoes slight epidermal atrophy and dermal connective tissue changes. Characteristics of aging skin and its appendages that tend to impinge on one's appearance include the following (Verbov, 1975):

1. *Furrowing,* which may be marked, is thought to be associated with degeneration of elastic fibers in the dermal connective tissue and with loss of subcutaneous fat. The facial lines reveal not only exposure to sunlight but also something of the person's dominant disposition, i.e., "happy" lines, "sad" lines.

2. *Mottling and roughness of exposed areas* occurs especially in persons with little pigment in the skin such as blond or red-haired individuals. Racial groups with more permanent pigment such as blacks, American Indians, and Asians, are protected against the damaging effects of solar rays and demonstrate less mottling and roughness.

3. *Pigment accumulations* occur on the back of the hands, the face, and in the genitoanal region. Patches of pigment accumulation may reflect a spotty increase in pigmentation but, in general, there is a decrease in the number of functioning melanocytes (Carlsen, 1975). The patches are cosmetically unattractive but have no pathologic significance.

4. *Losses and excesses of hair and changes in color and structure* are cosmetic factors that concern people. Greying and loss of hair is attributed respectively to a reduction of melanocytes and melanin pigment and to a decrease in the density of hair follicles. Blacks tend to become grey about ten years later than whites. Males are prone to more extensive alopecia than females. Females lose axillary and pubic hair but often have an increase in facial hairs secondary to decreased estrogen production to oppose androgens. Males often have hair growth occurring in the ears and nares.

5. *Areas of purpura* occur especially on the back of the hands and on the forearms because dermal blood vessels become fragile and tear easily.

6. *Nails grow more slowly and the nail plate becomes thicker.* The nails are brittle and lack luster. The skin around the nails of the fingers may have yellow stains from years of smoking cigarettes.

7. *Decrease in rosy appearance* of the skin and mucous membrane probably is associated with changes in blood vessels and diminished blood supply.

8. *Telangiectatic areas* consist of a group of dilated dermal capillaries appearing as red, raised areas. The most common site is the trunk.

9. *Decreasing tissue resiliency* is present when lifting the skin and releasing it results in a slow rate of return to normal position and contour in contrast to the immediate return noted in young people. This characteristic is probably related to collagen changes in the dermal layer.

Nursing Implications. The nurse should promote pride in appearance and safety in actions used to minimize aging changes. The latter includes counselling in use of face lifting, hair dying, and cosmetics to cover blemishes.

Protection

The effectiveness of the skin in withstanding mechanical traumas and serving as a barrier to chemical and bacterial substances diminishes with age. However, the regenerative capacity is retained, thereby permitting repair of wounds.

DECREASED PROTECTION FROM TRAUMA. The conforming, soft, elastic-skin characteristics that protect against trauma and invasion diminish with age because of changes in the epidermal and dermal skin layers. The life span of epidermal cells (keratinocytes and melanocytes) decreases with age, the dermoepidermal interface becomes flattened, and cell shapes change. The epidermis becomes thinner in areas of exposed skin (face, arms) and skin with little pigment protection. This atrophy of the epidermis is associated with atrophy of the papillary vessels in the dermis; the epidermis depends on this vascular supply for nutrition. Skin protected by pigment and nonexposed skin undergoes only slight tissue atrophy.

The outermost horny keratinized cells retard the inward and outward movement of substances in the skin. Atrophy of keratinized cells may account for an increase in aged-skin permeability to some chemical substances. Keratin holds water; a decrease in this water-holding capacity contributes to a loss of the soft, supple skin characteristics. The collagen fibers in the dermal layer provide tensile strength and have a structural protective effect, but this effect decreases with aging as the fibers tend to become thicker. Elastic fibers become fragmented, thus losing elasticity and pliable support. There is a gradual decline in the amount of subcutaneous fatty tissue that furnishes shock absorption. These structural and functional changes result in a thin, fragile skin which is susceptible to mechanical trauma and chemical and bacterial permeability.

Nursing Implications. Teach actions to prevent trauma and raise the person's level of awareness of potential problems. The following are some suggestions:

1. Wear hat, gloves, and long-sleeved garments when out-of-doors to protect from actinic exposure.
2. Wear gloves for dishwashing and other household chores where detergents are used.
3. Rinse hands well with plain water following use of household chemicals if gloves are not worn.
4. Wear gloves and take extra safety precautions when working with sharp equipment such as gardening and hobby tools.
5. Laundering precautions: wash new undergarments before wearing; rinse all clothes well to remove detergents.
6. Pad body surfaces being subjected to mechanical trauma, i.e., the knees when gardening, thimbles when sewing.
7. Avoid contact with extremes of hot and cold water, electric blankets, radiators, and so forth.
8. Avoid tight and constricting clothing such as elastic waistbands and stockings to prevent friction trauma as well as restriction of circulation.

9. Keep areas of skin abrasions clean; expose to the air for drying.

DECREASED EFFECTIVENESS IN WATER RETENTION. Not only does the skin become a less effective barrier to external elements but it also becomes less efficient in retaining water. The keratinized cells of the outermost section of the epidermis have the capacity to hold and absorb water. The amount of water is governed by the water supply of the body as a whole as well as by environmental factors such as temperature and humidity. When the water content of the air is low, the skin surface may lose water faster than it can be replaced internally, and symptoms of chapping may result. With aging there is an absolute decrease in intracellular water.

Insufficient water is the primary reason for dry skin; however this is influenced by the decreased secretion of skin lipids as they help to retain water. With aging there is a decrease in both sebaceous gland (sebum or skin oil secretion) and sweat gland activity. Loss of this barrier permits water evaporation from the skin. Washing with soap further removes the protective oils and increases skin dryness.

Nursing Implications. Measures to minimize skin dryness:

1. Restrict use of soap in bathing to the axillary and genital areas. Be sure all soap is removed.
2. Use tepid water rather than hot water for bathing.
3. Bathing twice a week is usually sufficient.
4. Apply a nonperfumed emollient containing lanolin to the skin immediately following washing or bathing to prevent loss of the moisture absorbed during these activities. The water necessary for oil absorption is present. Increase the moisture in the environment, i.e., room humidifiers, placement of containers of water over heating elements.
5. Wear cotton undergarments.
6. Rinse undergarments and bed linens in water to which oil has been added.

DECREASED EFFECTIVENESS OF TEMPERATURE REGULATION. The vascular system of the skin has both nutritional and protective roles. It is essential for body heat regulation, provides defenses against microbial and physical damage, provides nutrient supply to the avascular epidermis, and promotes wound healing. The body must maintain a balance between heat production and heat loss to sustain critical enzyme reactions. The skin mechanisms for regulation of heat conservation and dissipation are control of blood flow and blood content in the skin vessels, evaporation of sweat which cools the blood circulating in the skin, and subcutaneous fat which provides heat insulation. The epidermis depends on the vascular supply of the dermal layer for its nutrition. Any variation in this supply could adversely affect the activity of the cells located in the epidermal layer. The dermal layer of the skin has extensive papillary capillaries close to the body surface; these permit a large flow of blood for rapid heat dissipation. Deeper horizontal arteriovenous plexuses are responsible for shunting the blood to the papillary capillaries (Ryan, 1966).

The control of blood flow through the skin during temperature regulation is influenced primarily by hypothalamic changes transmitted through the sympathetic nervous system. Local changes in skin blood flow are effected by local neurogenic activity; direct stimulation of the skin results in afferent impulses that are converted into efferent vasomotor impulses near the site of stimulation. The efferent impulses pass down a branch of the nerve axon associated with regional vessels. The skin blood vessels are also sensitive to humoral factors of a vasoconstrictor and vasodilator nature. The most effective vasodilator factors are histamine and acetylcholine; the vasoconstrictors are epinephrine and norepinephrine.

The papillary capillaries, which are responsible for epidermal nourishment and heat dissipation, degenerate, with aging, leaving only the horizontal arteriovenous plexuses lying beneath the skin surface. This progressive impairment of vascular circulation and tissue nutrition and loss of subcutaneous tissue predisposes to a feeling of being cold, especially in cool environments. It also depresses the response to trauma and increases susceptibility to infection. When the environmental temperature is low, the protective response is peripheral vasoconstriction to conserve body heat, but this response in the elderly diminishes blood flow in the skin because of the fewer papillary capillaries. Some vascular disturbances that occur in older persons, such as Raynaud's disease and arteriosclerosis, may further inhibit epidermal blood supply, contribute to atrophy of epidermal cells, and promote the feeling of being cold.

The horizontal vessels are visible on the skin surface of the elderly because of the decreased papillary capillaries and the separation of the horizontal vessels from the epidermis because of a decrease in tissue fluid. The vessels, now lying on a crinkly or indenting skin surface, cause dispersal of superficial fluid and result in red marks on the skin. These marks are, for the most part, due to exposure of the horizontal vessels, an event that occurs with prolonged positional pressure on bony prominences.

The central control area for eccrine sweating is the hypothalamus. The hypothalamic area responds to an increase in skin temperature and in blood temperature; glandular work is governed by secretory nerves of the sympathetic nervous system. The sweat center also responds to other types of stimuli such as emotions, nausea, and hypoxia. Sweat contains 99 percent water, some sodium chloride, and a trace of urea. The sweat glands are one source for loss of body water. The other source of loss is caused by osmosis—insensible perspiration. The decrease in size, number, and function of sweat glands with aging impairs adaptation to elevated internal and environmental temperatures.

Nursing Implications. Promote actions to maintain adequate blood flow to the skin and maintain body temperature:

1. Maintain room temperature constant around 72° F. (22.5°C.) in cold weather.
2. Wear close knit (not tight) undergarments in the winter to prevent heat loss.
3. Wear hat and gloves in cold weather because heat is lost from head and hands.
4. Wear wool in preference to synthetic fibers; wool provides better insulation.
5. Stocking or bedsocks prevent cold feet during the night.
6. Sheet blankets are warmer than regular sheets as bedclothing.
7. Stay indoors on windy days to avoid the windchill factor, which stresses adaptive mechanisms.
8. Frequent, small meals and warm liquids help to provide heat to the body.
9. Early morning is the period of lowest body metabolic activity; add extra clothes until food and physical movement stimulates the circulation.
10. Body movement stimulates circulation; therefore, alternate physical and sedentary activites.
11. Sedatives and some tranquilizers depress cerebral function and circulation, requiring extra effort to prevent chilling.

12. Wear light, loose but protective, clothing in hot weather.

13. Wear a hat to protect against the intense heat on the head.

14. Do outdoor work in the early morning and when the area is in the shade. Work for limited periods of time.

Sensation

The skin serves as a protective sense organ. The epidermis and dermis contain specific receptors for each of the various sensory modalities: touch pressure, pain, and temperature. These nerve endings are of two types: free endings and those terminating in a corpuscular arrangement (pacinian corpuscles). The pacinian corpuscles decrease numerically with age but the free nerve endings remain unchanged. The sensory receptor converts the stimuli into electric energy which is the mechanism for transmission of nerve impulses to and from the central nervous system. The magnitude of the electrical response is proportional to the intensity of the stimulus, i.e., the lower the external temperature the greater the sensation of cold. The nerve impulse's perception of pain, touch, pressure, warmth, or cold takes place in the cerebral cortex and depends on the specific nerve ending stimulated.

The cutaneous touch and pressure receptors provide information that is synthesized in the brain with information received from the proprioceptive receptors in the muscles and joints to derive information about the position of the body in space. A slowing of transmission of impulses from one or more receptors may result in disharmony of impulse arrival in the brain and may interfere with data synthesis and with accuracy of information about position of the body in space. Slowing of the pulse transmission accompanies the aging process. Elderly people frequently express feelings of positional and movement instability.

Nursing Implications. The nurse must help the patient become aware of safety measures necessary because of diminished sensitivity to touch, pressure, pain, and local temperature change. This involves attention to position, movement, and touch, and includes (1) checking temperature of bath and dish washing water, water bottles, and ice packs; (2) observing pressure areas (from clothing, prostheses, position); and (3) moving cautiously on uneven walking surfaces.

EVALUATION OF INTEGUMENT

One observes the characteristics of aged skin when doing an initial health history and examination in a clinic or in an acute or long term care setting. A mental comparison of the person's stated age and skin appearance may suggest something of the person's genetic endowment and lifestyle. The prolonged skin exposure to sun of a farmer, sailor, or outdoor enthusiast will be evident in skin appearance. The aims of a skin assessment include:

- Usual patterns of skin care
- Aging changes and the person's response to these changes
- Pathologic changes and effect on the person's lifestyle
- Earlier and current lifestyle as this relates to past and present pathologic conditions and to potential problems in the future

History

The following items are of particular interest in the history portion of assessing the skin.

Past Illnesses. Inquire about any condition and its treatment that could affect the skin, e.g., liver disease with jaundice and pruritus, allergic reactions to medications, long term steroid therapy causing bruising and open lesions.

Treatments Earlier in Life. Earlier treatments may increase the risk of skin disease. Examples are depilation and x-ray treatment for acne. The latter increases the risk of malignancy.

Grooming and Attire Preferences and Patterns. Note the value placed on appearance. This pertains to usual care of both hair and skin, i.e., hairdresser, hair coloring, cosmetic use, cosmetic surgery, attire.

Occupation and Hobbies. Long exposure to sun and weather increases the risk of senile keratoses and skin malignancies, especially in persons with relatively little skin pigment. Evaluate activities that produce characteristic changes in particular areas such as fingers, palms, soles, knees, ankles, e.g., corns, calluses.

Travel and Recreational Activities. Note exposure to sun and wind and to agents of an infectious or allergic nature.

Nutritional Habits. Inquire about diet and possible relationship to present health status. Look for food allergies.

Body Image. Observe the relationship of the person's body appearance to current lifestyle. Does current skin status interfere with preferred lifestyle? Is there anxiety regarding status and/or prognosis of skin conditions? Fear of disfigurement?

Resources. The negative and positive aspects of resources must be studied. Is the patient financially able to afford desired care or prescribed treatment? Is transportation available for required visits for treatment? Does the home situation allow carrying out prescribed therapy and/or preferred hygienic practices? Does the patient have adequate motor skills and physical strength to perform self-care? Does he have control of his physical environment, such as temperature and humidity? Are there plants and animals in the environment that may contribute to allergic reactions?

Physical Assessment

Physical assessment of the patient follows a methodical study from head to toes.

General Observations

Hair and scalp assessment includes color, texture, and patterns of growth. It includes searching for pediculosis, scalp lesions, and lesions behind ears.

Observe the skin for moisture (dryness/oiliness); temperature, which includes differences between extremities; texture (rough, smooth); edema; thickness and areas of increased thickness; color and areas of discoloration; and turgor as determined by raising a section of skin over the sternum. (Normally turgid skin regains shape quickly; loss of turgor is evidenced by a slow return to previous shape.) Examine areas of opposing skin surfaces, groin, axillae, and submammary in females.

The amount of melanin present in the epidermis determines skin color—the more pigment the darker the color. The number of functioning melanocytes decreases with age, often resulting in a blotchy, irregularly-pigmented appearance, particularly of exposed skin. Other factors contributing to abnormal skin color in the elderly are degeneration of elastic tissue, which causes yellowish papules and plaques, and degeneration of supportive connective tissue surrounding the dermal vasculature, which results in senile purpura, extravasation of blood to the interstitial spaces, and slow reabsorption.

Circulation also influences color. Vasodilatation perfuses the cutaneous blood vessels and gives a red color to the skin. This occurs in warm temperatures as a means of dissipating heat, as a result of alcohol intake, and in the inflammatory response to trauma. Vasoconstriction decreases blood flow and the skin becomes pale. Pallor is apparent on exposure to cold. Anemia from malnutrition or some other causes imparts a pale color to mucous membrane, nailbeds, and ear lobes. Decreased oxygenation of hemoglobin with respiratory problems or excessive deoxygenation in the peripheral circulation, as occurs with impaired circulation, may lend a bluish tinge to the skin, whereas retained carbon dioxide, as with chronic obstructive pulmonary disease, may result in vasodilation and a reddening of the skin. Edema increases the distance of capillaries from the skin surface and decreases the intensity of color.

Skin texture and thickness reflect environmental exposure and persistent traumas throughout life. Accumulations of keratic cells and dried cornified epithelium result in rough, thick areas such as calluses and exfoliative dermatitis. Skin turgor decreases with age because of loss of subcutaneous fat. It worsens with dehydration.

Lesions

Observe lesions for anatomic location, description of structural characteristics (use standard nomenclature), size (use metric measurement), color and grouping patterns, e.g., in folds of tissue, along nerve pathway.

Observation of anatomic distribution is necessary because some skin diseases have characteristic distributions. These specific distributions may depend on skin features in a particular region. For instance, monilial infections occur in moist skinfolds such as under the breast and in the axillae. Bandlike distributions following a peripheral nerve pattern suggests herpes zoster, whereas keratosis occurs in areas exposed to sunlight. Patterns in the grouping of skin lesions may also have diagnostic significance. The lesions may be in a semicircle, or circular configuration or a combination of these. The absence of a discernable pattern may be significant; often this is a characteristic of urticaria. Table 23-1 consists of descriptive terminology for categorizing lesions according to structural characteristics.

SECONDARY LESIONS. Secondary lesions are modifications or changes that appear after the pri-

TABLE 23-1. Basic primary skin lesions.

Type	Lesion	Characteristics	Examples
Non-elevated	Macules	Nonpalpable localized areas of color change. Various shapes. May be associated with scaling.	Drug eruptions; petechiae
Elevated solid, and localized	Papules	Lesions of approximately 0.5 cm in diameter or less. Top and borders of various shapes. Color—lighter, darker, or same as skin.	Pedunculated—neurofibromas; round or irregular—senile angiomas; flat-topped psoriasis; pointed—insect bites
	Nodule	Lesions ranging in size from about 0.5 cm to 1.0 cm. in diameter. Extend deeper into skin than papules. Palpation—when lesion is below the dermis the skin slides over it, whereas a dermal lesion moves with the skin.	Erythema nodosum; gouty tophi
	Tumor	Lesion larger than 1.0 cm.	Basal cell carcinoma
	Wheal	Irregular. Circumscribed area of edema. Color varies from pale to red.	Insect bite; hives
Fluid-filled elevations	Vesicle	An accumulation of serous fluid within or below the epidermis depending on the site of cell damage. Diameter less than 1.0 cm.	Blister; second degree burn
	Bullae	Serous fluid accumulations greater than 1.0 cm.	Bullous pemphigoid
	Pustules	Vesicles or bullae filled with pus. The translucent skin overlying the lesion reveals the color of the contents, i.e., yellow, green, milky.	Infected pimple

mary lesion (Table 23-2). For example, burn vesicles may dry and form a crust, may ulcerate, or may heal by scar tissue formation (Bates, 1974).

PIGMENTED SKIN LESIONS. The presence of pigment in skin lesions is an important diagnostic characteristic. Pigmented lesions are either macular or papular. The macular lesions usually occur on solar exposed skin. The color of skin lesions may be changed if blood pigment is present, because it gives a brown-black discoloration. For instance, angiomas may be black nodules because of the presence of extravasated blood. Table 23-3 lists common pigmented lesions.

Nursing Diagnosis and Therapy

Analysis of the data obtained from the history and from observations of the skin results in a nursing diagnosis and planning of nursing interventions. The goals of intervention are to prevent skin problems, to maintain maximum level of skin function and structure, and to promote a return to a healthy skin status when disease is present.

This section deals with nursing problems commonly encountered in the elderly. Common problems of elderly persons with skin disorders include:

- Low self-concept—related to disfigurement
- Disruption of lifestyle—dependency on others for assistance with therapy and with activities of daily living; need for prescribed therapy
- Discomfort from manifestations—pruritus pain, oozing, or dry lesions
- Systemic disturbances—sleep loss, fatigue, fluid loss
- High potential for complications—the elderly have lower tolerance for stress, a lowering of physiologic responses, often have one or more chronic illnesses

TABLE 23-2. Basic secondary skin lesions.

Lesion	Characteristics	Examples
Crusts	Formed from materials that seep out of the skin and dry; may be pus, blood, or serum.	Impetigo
Scales	Accumulations of thin plates of dried, cornified epithelium.	Psoriasis; exfoliative dermatitis
Lichenification	Thickening of skin layers, often as a result of repeated rubbing. Normal skin furrows are accentuated.	Atopic dermatitis
Erosion	Removal of the upper epidermal layer, resulting in a moist surface that does not bleed or scar.	Syphilitic chancre
Ulcer	Removal of skin to a depth below the basal cell layer with healing by scar tissue.	Stasis ulcer; decubitus ulcer
Scar	Replacement of normal tissue with fibrous tissue.	Keloid (hypertrophied scar)
Atrophy	Decrease in size and number of cells, resulting in thinning and loss of normal skin furrows.	

Self-Concept

The appearance of the skin receives considerable attention in our society. It is an important aspect of self-image and of the image one presents to others.

TABLE 23-3. Pigmented skin lesions.

Macular	Papular
Atrophic pigmentation and depigmentation (mottling)	Malignant melanomas
Senile purpura	Melanocyte nevus
Senile lentigo	Keratosis
Lentigo maligna	Thrombosed virus wart
Freckle (ephelis)	Thrombosed angioma
Melanocyte nevus	Pigmented basal cell epithelioma; histiocytoma

By facial expressions, by color changes with emotions, through grooming, and through touch, the skin is a means of communication. It is sensitive to touch, and it is a means of conveying love, concern, and empathy. Unfortunately, cutaneous disorders are aesthetically unappealing and carry the stigma of physical and moral uncleanliness. The afflicted person receives messages of rejection from others and inwardly may feel guilty or unworthy, believing the condition to be a punishment for past actions and, thus, self-inflicted. Self-esteem becomes low when it is apparent that other people avoid social contact, looking, and touching. The whole aspect of guilt may date back to Biblical times when people with leprosy were considered to be sinners and the disease was punishment for their sins.

Feelings of shame and fear increase the stress level of the afflicted person and contribute to exacerbations of the disorder or prevent a positive response to therapy. The elderly have difficulty coping with stress, and stress remains high because of the constant irritation of the disease, the reactions of others, and the persons own beliefs about the disorder. The person is prone to sleeplessness, anxiety, and depression.

Nursing actions to promote self-esteem include:

1. Convey acceptance by touching. Use a handshake or touch on the arm. In the presence of infection, explain the purpose of avoiding hand-lesion contact and deliberately establish physical contact on the nonaffected site.

2. Look at the person and the lesion with control of facial expression. Words cannot erase a message conveyed by a look of distaste or disgust. Establish eye contact—this communicates interest and provides an opportunity to assess the person's response.

3. Talk to the person, using techniques to promote expression of feelings.

4. Listen to what the person says about his feelings and those of the family concerning the illness and its manifestations.

5. Explain the disorder, clarify misconceptions, and promote assistance with care.

Disruption of Life Style

Factors inherent in a cutaneous disorder and its treatment that bring about a change in lifestyle are the disease manifestations (pruritus, oozing), therapy (dressing, lotions) and systemic responses. The afflicted person may be unable to carry out the therapy because of other disabilities or fatigue. For instance, a person with a disabling arthritis of the hands may be unable to apply lotion or dressings, or the lesion site may not be accessible (the back). The need for assistance can be costly, it may necessitate hospitalization or assistance of a health team member in the home or it may mean a role reversal for family/ friend with whom the patient lives. Dependence on others in itself may provoke feelings of inadequacy.

Interventions to assist the person to cope with the disorder include assessment of the home situation to be certain the environment permits adequate therapy (i.e., hot water, tub for bathing, clean area for preparation of dressings) and that the necessary supplies are available or can be purchased. Teaching the methods of therapy and providing for assistance are nursing responsibilities. Helping the person to adapt to receiving assistance from others is another nursing responsibility.

Assessment of the socioeconomic implications of the illness for the afflicted person and interventions to obtain assistance with the cost of supplies and medical attention are often necessary. Sugges-

tions to promote maintenance of contact with friends and to prevent sensory deprivation are important. The basis for suggestions should be an understanding of the persons previous lifestyle. Socioeconomic aspects likewise are important to consider in the long term or acute care facility.

Pruritus

Itching is a manifestation of dry skin; therefore it occurs frequently in the elderly. It also accompanies some skin diseases and can be an indication of an internal disorder. The sensation arises from stimulation of free nerve endings in the papillary dermis and lower epidermis. The nerve impulse travels via C nerve fibers through the spinothalamic tract to the thalamus and then to the cortical area for interpretation. The pruritic sensations vary from those of urticaria which induce a desire to rub gently to those of eczema which provokes vigorous rubbing or scratching. This action traumatizes the skin and perpetuates both the eczema and the pruritus.

Common causes of generalized pruritus in the elderly are:

- Dry skin (osteotosis)
- Systemic disorders—liver and kidney disturbance, anemia, polycythemia neoplasms, drug withdrawal (barbiturates)
- Oozing, weeping lesions—pemphigus, eczema, localized excoriations (intertrigo, pruritis ani and vulvae)

Dry Skin (Osteotosis)

Dry skin is the most common cause of generalized pruritus in the elderly.

ETIOLOGIC FACTORS. Factors contributing to osteotosis include decreased endocrine secretions, degeneration of papillary capillaries, decreased sebaceous gland activity and secretion, decreased sweating, and washing away of protective lipids with soap and water.

HIGH RISK. Persons with history of dry skin and chapping.

DYNAMICS. The amount of moisture in the dermis determines the degree of suppleness and elasticity of the skin. Dryness excites the cutaneous nerves and results in the sensation of itching.

MANIFESTATIONS. The appearance of dry skin varies on different areas of the body. On the back the skin looks pale and has small, rough-feeling scales. On the lower legs, where circulation may also be impaired, the skin appears smooth and shiny and may have fine fissures on red, moist cracks. The dorsum of the hands appears wrinkled and fissured with dry skin.

The itching associated with dry skin will be reported as intense. It tends to be most severe upon preparation for retiring at night and on arising in the morning. This may be related to the air exposure and the irritation of undressing and dressing. Certain factors tend to exacerbate the itching: rough textured clothing next to the skin, wool clothing next to the skin, change in temperature, increased air movement (wind and fans), or chemicals such as detergents.

PREVENTION. The best way to avoid pruritus associated with dry skin is to manage the dry skin problem. Basically this consists of modifying washing and bathing practices to preserve the lipid barrier (sebaceous secretions) and minimize water loss from the skin.

MANAGEMENT. (See management of dry skin given earlier in this chapter.) Treatment of pruritus that accompanies pathologic states depends upon identification and treatment of the cause.

Temperature and humidity control are important. Pruritis present with hypersensitive reactions decreases with low, cool temperatures and low humidity. Lesions dry out. Avoid hot liquids and warmth which produce vasodilatation. Use cool, wet dressings to decrease blood flow and promote evaporation.

Sodium bicarbonate and oatmeal baths are overrated. Oatmeal gives a slippery feeling to water. After the bath, both solutions leave a dry covering on the skin. One useful home remedy, which minimizes static electricity that stimulates itching, is the changing of only one bedsheet at a time. Also, use antistatic rinses or dryer additives.

There are topical antipruritic preparations. Oral antihistaminic agents include trimeprazine tartrate (Temaril) and cyproheptadine hydrochloride (Atorax). Tranquilizers may be necessary temporarily while awaiting results of therapies to control cause.

Finger pressure over the site may present an overriding stimulus to nerve endings. Diversional therapy is helpful, as is socialization. Lower the level of itch awareness by direction of interest to issues and activities of a nonemotional nature. This promotes relaxation and directs concentration on events rather than self.

Skin Eruptions

Purposes of treatment in skin eruptions are:

1. Protect lesions from further trauma.
2. Protect from complications associated with loss of skin barrier: infection, fluid loss.
3. Alter blood flow and cell metabolic rates.
4. Deliver medications.
5. Provide comfort.

Methods of therapy are:
1. Dressings: closed wet, open wet, dry.
2. Soaks, baths.
3. Topical medications: antihistaminics to control hypersensitive reactions, corticosteroids for anti-inflammatory reaction, antibiotics to control infection, and antipruritic agents.

Dressings accomplish the following:
1. Protect from trauma, i.e., scratching, irritation of bedclothes, dust and other environmental irritants, extremes of temperature and humidity.
2. Provide a barrier to microorganism entry and fluid loss.
3. Cover lesions during socialization periods, and time applications of intermittent dressings to mealtime and visiting periods. (Laundered and ironed rags are inexpensive dressings for use in the home.)

The aims of baths, soaks, and wet dressings are:

1. Remove skin debris such as scales and crusts. Discomfort is decreased if debris is softened prior to debridement.
2. Protect bed linen from moisture of wet dressings.
3. Wet dressings—evaporation of moisture results in cooling and vasoconstriction. This decreases blood flow, heat, and itching; it slows metabolic rate and decreases extent of inflammation.
4. Warm soaks and heat lamps increase blood flow and, thus, oxygen and nutrient supply to promote healing and comfort.

Topical medications are available in different bases— the base influences the mode of action. Powders increase effective area for evaporation; absorb moisture, thereby producing a drying effect; and reduce maceration and friction in intertriginous areas. Lotions are suspensions of insoluble powders in water. They must be shaken before application to resuspend particles. Creams and ointments are emulsions of water and oil. The water evaporates and a thin, nonapparent film of oil remains on the skin. This oil film retards further water loss through the skin. Topical medications promote absorption of medications. They retain heat, and, therefore, are contraindicated in infected areas where heat may promote bacterial growth. Pastes are powder and ointment mixtures that produce dryness in conjunction with lubrication.

Application with clean hands prevents waste, provides even spread and conveys acceptance of the condition. Gloves are used when the lesion is infected. Wet dressings may be open or closed. Open consists of saturated gauze applied directly to skin. In this case, evaporation of moisture occurs and microorganism attachment is a danger. Closed dressings consist of a moistened layer with dry coverings to prevent water evaporation, heat loss, and trauma. The danger of this dressing is skin maceration and infection from organism growth in a warm, dark environment.

Antibacterial agents have minimal absorption through the skin, low potential for contact dermatitis, and local action against common bacteria. They include Polymyxin B, Gentamicin, and Bacitracin.

The advantages of topical corticosteroids are:

1. They are safe and effective anti-inflammants in low doses (1 percent hydrocortisone).
2. They probably cause vasoconstriction which decreases edema and itching. They have a slow rate of cell mitosis and enzyme activity.
3. High strengths are not used, or a reservoir of the drug accumulates under occlusive dressings.

Side effects may occur if topical corticosteroid therapy is prolonged. Side effects are transient and localized and may include atrophy and telangiectasis.

Isolation precautions include:

1. Explanations to person afflicted to promote understanding and emotional comfort. Isolation emphasizes the stigma attached to skin lesions and lowers the persons level of sensory stimulation.
2. Protective isolation to prevent infection.
3. Prevention of organism spread when infection is present.

ALTERATIONS IN THE SKIN OF THE ELDERLY

Skin disorders are relatively common in the elderly. Some disorders are the same as those found in younger persons; others are, for the most part, confined to the elderly. Likewise, some alterations are within the realm of normal changes and others are not. The incidence of skin disorders in adult age groups varies with race, climate, occupations, and extent of melanin present in the skin.

Factors that influence the development and course of skin diseases in the elderly are:

1. Decrease in peripheral vascular circulation influencing the response to physical trauma and cold.
2. Atrophy of the reticular endothelial system leading to depression of the immune response.
3. Malnutrition.
4. Life-long history of exposure to sunlight.
5. Exposure during life to radiation therapy and drugs.
6. Genetic predisposition to aging changes.
7. Emotional responses to stresses of life.
8. Changes in responsiveness of nerve endings to sensory stimuli.

Classification of lesions according to type of pathologic disturbance separates them into infectious and noninfectious. Noninfectious skin disorders arise from degenerative changes, changes in growth patterns, hypersensitive reactions, and vascular disturbances or are skin indicants of systemic disorders. A subdivision of this classification is based on whether or not the lesion is pigmented.

Common skin alterations that often involve the nurse in health care management are listed in Table 23-4.

Alterations in Cell Growth

The nature of alterations in cell growth determines the classification as benign, premalignant, or malignant. Benign cell growths may expand and compress adjacent tissues but their growth is self-limiting—they do not undergo malignant changes nor do they metastasize to distant sites. Premalignant lesions may undergo changes of a malignant nature and, therefore, are a threat to the well-being of the person. Characteristics of malignant lesions are un-

TABLE 23-4. Common skin alterations in the elderly.

Infectious	Noninfectious
Infestations (scabies, body lice, ringworm) Infections (bacterial, viral, fungal)	Alterations in cell growth Benign epidermal (skin tags, seborrheic keratosis, keratoacanthoma)
	Benign vascular (senile angiomas, venous lakes, angiokeratomas)
	Premalignant (solar and radiation keratoses, leukoplakia)
	Malignant (basal cell carcinoma, squamous cell carcinoma, malignant melanoma)
	Degenerative changes (Pemphigus, lichen simplex chronicus, seborrheic dermatitis)
	Hypersensitive reactions (contact dermatitis, bullous pemphigoid, pemphigus)
	Alterations in vascular patterns (stasis dermatitis, positional tissue trauma)
	Foot problems (corns, calluses, ingrown toenails)

COMMON TYPES OF ALTERATIONS IN SKIN CELL GROWTH IN ELDERLY

Benign epidermal tumors—skin tags, seborrheic keratoses, keratoacanthoma

Benign vascular tumors—senile angiomas, venous lakes, angiokeratomas

Premalignant tumors—solar and radiation keratoses, leukoplakia

Malignant tumors—basal and squamous cell carcinomas, malignant melanoma

---

controlled growth and sometimes metastasis to distant sites. Skin tumors are readily visible and easily observed for changes such as nonhealing and increase in size. A major nursing function is assessment of skin changes, early detection of possible malignancies, and referral to a physician. Malignant skin lesions usually grow slowly in the elderly and usually are amenable to curative therapy. They are recognizable and treatable at an early stage, thereby preventing the discomfort, disfigurement, and death that follows from nontreatment.

Benign Epidermal Tumors

Benign epidermal tumors include skin tags, seborrheic keratosis, and keratoacanthoma. These are common, unsightly, hyperkeratotic lesions which should be treated for cosmetic reasons.

ETIOLOGIC FACTORS. Unknown.

DYNAMICS. The stalk of a skin tag has a connective tissue core and the epidermis may be thickened.

MANIFESTATIONS. *Skin tags* are small (pinhead to pea size), soft, pedunculated protrusions of normal-colored skin. Usually they are located over the front and sides of the neck, the upper trunk, and eyelids. *Seborrheic keratoses* (seborrheic wart, basal cell papilloma) are slightly raised, yellowish or tan plaques which are sharply circumscribed and covered with a greasy scale. The size is about 1 cm in diameter. They often are multiple and appear to be "stuck on" the skin. As the lesion ages, it thickens and becomes more brown or brownish black and may have a granular appearance as a result of follicular plugging. *Keratoacanthoma* is a crater formed by a rolled elevated epidermis. The crater has a keratinous plug. It grows rapidly to a size of 1 to 3 cm; then it slowly regresses and leaves a scar. It usually is located on exposed, hairy skin in whites but is rare in blacks.

TREATMENT. Skin tags and seborrheic keratosis may be removed for cosmetic reasons in an office or outpatient clinic. The technique for removal is cautery or surgical excision. Because keratoacanthoma has a histology similar to that of squamous carcinoma, biopsy is indicated. If the biopsy confirms the diagnosis, then the natural course of regression may be permitted. Sometimes therapy consists of surgical excision or curettage with cautery.

Benign Vascular Tumors

Senile angiomas (cherry spots), venous lakes, and angiokeratomas are benign vascular tumors.

ETIOLOGIC FACTORS. Unknown.

MANIFESTATIONS. *Senile angiomas* are cherry or ruby-red vascular papules that increase in size and number with age. The usual site is the trunk. The papules consist of tufts of dilated capillaries which may bleed when traumatized but do not empty on pressure. *Venous lakes* are blue or bluish-black papules composed of dilated thick-walled vessels. They usually occur on lips and ears of the elderly. *Angiokeratomas* are superficial, distended, thin-walled blood vessels covered with a hyperkerotic epidermis. These occur as multiple or discrete lesions on the scrotum or vulva.

TREATMENT. Venous lakes are removed for cosmetic reasons. No treatment is indicated for senile angiomas or angiokeratomas.

Premalignant Conditions

Actinic (solar) and *radiation keratoses* are important keratolytic lesions since they may be the origin of basal or squamous cell carcinoma. *Leukoplakia* occurs as spots or patches on the mucosal or mucocutaneous tissues such as lips, buccal mucosa, and vulva.

ETIOLOGIC FACTORS. Cell damage or possible genetic mutation are possible causes. Excessive exposure to radiation of either solar or radiotherapy origin is a factor. On the lips it is associated with chronic irritation of tobacco smoking. In the oral cavity the irritant is mechanical, such as that caused by dentures or jagged teeth, or from such agents as snuff, betel nut chewing, and hot, highly-spiced foods. Some of these agents relate to cultural practices which a complete history would reveal.

HIGH RISK. At high risk are persons in occupations requiring work with radiation therapy (radiologist, technicians, dentists) or outdoors (sailors, farmers, persons living in tropical sunny climates); persons treated with radiation earlier in life for eczema or acne; and persons with habits predisposing to leukoplakia.

DYNAMICS. Uncontrolled cell growth.

MANIFESTATIONS. *Keratoses* are slightly-elevated, scaly papules of light brown-black color on exposed body surfaces. The surface may be flat, round, or verrucous (wartlike). The scale is adherent and returns each time it is removed. Sometimes excessive cornification occurs and the lesion presents as a cutaneous horn. The chronicity of the lesion and its enlargement, induration, and ulceration are significant factors in consideration of the need for dermatologist referral. *Leukoplakia* are discrete, persistent, white plaques that may be either smooth or warty and may fissure or ulcerate. Usually they are free of induration or inflammation unless they transform to squamous cell carcinoma.

PREVENTION. Prevention of keratoses involves wearing protective clothing and keeping exposure minimal. Sunscreen containing para-aminobenzoic acid should be used before sun exposure (persons with history of actinic keratoses as well as young persons). Blacks seldom develop solar keratoses because of the pigment and horny protective layer of their skin. To prevent *leukoplakia*, avoid tissue-irritating habits mentioned previously.

TREATMENT. Refer to a dermatologist. A variety of methods are used to remove lesions: surgical excision, cauterization, cryosurgery with liquid nitrogen, and topical application of a 1 to 5 percent concentration of 5-fluorouracil in propylene glycol. Diagnostic confirmation. Results usually are curative, especially if the source of irritation is eliminated.

Malignant Conditions

Malignant conditions include basal cell carcinoma, squamous cell carcinoma, and malignant melanoma.

BASAL CELL CARCINOMA. This carcinoma has the highest incidence of skin cancers.

Etiologic Factors. Unknown.

High Risk. Fair-skinned persons exposed chronically to sunlight are at risk.

Dynamics. Arising in the basal cell layer of the epidermis, the malignant cell retains the property of cell replication but does not have the ability to mature and keratinize normally. The tumor grows slowly but invades surrounding tissue by direct extension. It rarely metastasizes. Usually develops in persons over 45 years of age.

Manifestation. Begins as a small, slowly enlarging papule, growing over months or years. The borders develop a semitranslucent pearly appearance; the center erodes, ulcerates, and becomes depressed. Pigment in varying amounts may be dispersed throughout the lesion. Telangiectatic blood vessels may be visible over the border. Crusting often occurs about 6 months to a year after the lesion is first observed. The untreated lesion may extend inward even to the bone.

Prevention. Avoid chronic exposure to sun.

Treatment. Refer to a dermatologist. Many modes of therapy effect a cure: surgical excision, cautery, freezing, and radiation therapy. Selection depends on the general health of the affected person, the location, size, malignant characteristics of the biopsied tissue, and the cosmetic implications.

SQUAMOUS CELL CARCINOMA. *Etiologic Factors.* Unknown.

High Risk. Elderly whites are at risk but squamous cell carcinoma rarely occurs in blacks. Often the site is where another skin lesion occurred earlier, e.g., actinic keratosis, radiation scars, chronic irritation, leukoplakia, and varicose ulcers.

Dynamics. The cell of origin is the squamous (prickle cell) of the epidermis. It grows more quickly than a basal cell carcinoma and may metastasize early, especially tumors on the lip, tongue, and external genitalia.

Manifestations. It usually appears as a single, hard, conical nodule which grows by invasion and destruction of the surrounding skin. This results in an area of induration, and the border of the ulcer is often indistinct and elevated. As the lesion enlarges, it attaches to the underlying tissues and becomes fixed and firm to touch.

Treatment. Refer to a dermatologist. Early recognition is necessary for a cure. Treatment of choice is removal.

MALIGNANT MELANOMA. *Etiologic Factors.* Unknown.

High Risk. Malignant melanoma occurs most frequently in exposed areas of skin.

Dynamics. It invades and metastasizes. Malignant melanoma is apt to occur in moles because of the predominance of melanocytes in this area, not because moles are premalignant (Parrish, 1975).

Manifestations. Malignancy is suggested by its irregular border, varied colors of a blue or red shade within the lesion, and an irregular surface such as uneven elevation and loss of skin markings.

Treatment. Refer to a dermatologist. Usually surgical excision is made with wide and deep tissue removal and coverage with a skin graft.

Infectious Conditions

Some infectious conditions are relatively prevalent in the elderly; they are uncomfortable and disfiguring. Such infectious conditions prevalent in the elderly are herpes zoster (viral), erysipelas (bacterial), furunculosis (bacterial), chronic paronychia, candidiasis (fungal), and scabies (infestation). Skin infections in the elderly may indicate underlying systemic disorders such as diabetes, lymphoma, or anemia.

The systemic manifestations associated with infectious processes (elevated temperature, increased perspiration, and elevated neutrophilic count) are not as pronounced in the elderly as in younger persons; therefore detection of these processes requires close scrutiny of all indicants.

Pain, unsightly lesions, and the need for techniques to prevent disease transmission often accompany infections of the skin. All three factors influence nursing interventions aimed at promoting comfort and patient self-care, administration of prescribed medical therapies, and education for prevention of future recurrences.

Herpes Zoster

ETIOLOGIC FACTORS. The causative agent is the herpesvirus.

HIGH RISK. Herpes zoster is common in the elderly, and is the infection that causes the highest morbidity. Persons with Hodgkin's disease and lymphomas and persons receiving immunosuppressive therapy or irradiation are at high risk.

DYNAMICS. Pathogenesis is thought to be a reactivation of a latent viral infection of the dorsal root ganglia with retrograde spread to the skin. Cause of reactivation is unknown; it may occur in situations listed under high risk.

MANIFESTATIONS. It appears as groups of papulovesicular lesions following a unilateral dermatomal pattern down an arm or more frequently around one side of the lower chest from posterior to anterior midline. The lesions become cloudy about a week later and a crust develops. Pain of a burning nature with varying duration and often of extreme severity occurs in most persons. The disorder clears in about 3 to 4 weeks but the pain may persist longer if a postherpetic neuralgia is present, in which case the pain may persist for months. Sometimes the eye may become involved.

PREVENTION. One specialist recommends zoster immune globulin (Judelsohn, 1972).

TREATMENT. Treatment aims at relieving discomfort since no therapy is known to shorten the course. Sedatives allow for sleep, and high doses of analgesics may be necessary to relieve pain. Calamine lotion and menthol camphor are beneficial. Isolation precautions are not necessary since transmission of the disorder is not by contact.

COMPLICATIONS. Post-herpetic neuralgia is a common complication. Eaglstein and coworkers indicate that cortisone therapy will prevent post-herpetic neuralgia in the elderly (Eaglstein, et al., 1970). Eye complications are referred to an ophthalmologist. Cervical sympathetic nerve blocks have been found to relieve herpetic pain and speed up resolution of the eruption in eye lesions (De Backer, 1978).

Erysipelas

ETIOLOGIC FACTORS. Streptococcus is causative. Organism entry is through skin abrasion.

HIGH RISK. There is danger of break in skin continuity, especially in elderly people with leg edema who sit for many hours.

DYNAMICS. Cellulitis spreads rapidly and involves the dermis and superficial lymphatics.

MANIFESTATION. It manifests itself as a raised, reddened area with a sharp edge. Signs of toxicity may not be marked.

TREATMENT. Report to the physician. Penicillin usually is ordered. Isolation isn't necessary unless an open lesion is present.

Furunculosis

ETIOLOGIC FACTORS. A staphylcoccal organism is causative.

HIGH RISK. Persons with chronic debilitating diseases are at high risk.

DYNAMICS. Acute, localized infection of hair follicle may develop.

MANIFESTATIONS. A raised, soft lesion with yellow or white center occurs. Intense throbbing pain may be present. Rupture of the abscess releases a thick, creamy yellow pus.

TREATMENT. Refer to physician. Warm compresses are used to relieve pain, and incision and drainage when the center becomes soft. Drainage is contagious; use dressing isolation procedures. Antibiotics.

Chronic Paronychia

Chronic paronychia is a frequent problem in the elderly.

ETIOLOGIC FACTORS. Bacteria or fungus are causative.

HIGH RISK. Persons with debilitating illnesses are at high risk. Also those who have been exposed for years to wet work with frequent traumas, e.g., cleaning, canning, dishwashing, fishing.

DYNAMICS. Separation of cuticle from the nailbed allows organism or fungus to enter.

MANIFESTATIONS. There is swelling and tenderness of posterior nailfold, accompanied by pus under nailfold.

TREATMENT. Use topical applications of thymol in chloroform, the thymol being an effective bactericidal and fungicidal agent and the chloroform a drying agent. Nystatin cream is also effective. Avoidance of moisture is necessary.

Candidiasis (Moniliasis)

ETIOLOGIC FACTORS. Candidiasis is a fungus infection.

HIGH RISK. Persons with a debilitating disease are at high risk, and those taking broad spectrum antibiotics.

DYNAMICS. Candidiasis needs moisture to grow. It establishes colonies in intertriginous areas, especially at the angle of the mouth, under dentures, and around the anus and perineum.

MANIFESTATIONS. It occurs as excoriated, inflamed areas with sections of white plaques (yeast colonies).

TREATMENT. Dry with a heat lamp and/or topical dehydrating medications. Nystatin is specific for both skin and mucous membrane lesions.

Scabies

ETIOLOGIC FACTORS. Sarcoptes scabiei, the itch mite, is the causative factor.

HIGH RISK. At risk are persons in unhygienic conditions or who bath infrequently.

DYNAMICS. The organism burrows and moves along under the skin.

MANIFESTATIONS. It appears as a dark line under the skin and itches over the site. Usually it occurs on inner surfaces of thighs and forearms, under breasts, between the fingers, and around the perineum.

PREVENTION. Personal and environmental hygienic practices will aid in preventing scabies.

TREATMENT. Give a prolonged hot bath, using a brush on the skin. Apply benzyl benzoate emulsion (25%) or gamma benzene hexachloride cream or lotion. Calamine lotion is applied for itch. Antibiotics are used for secondary infections.

Hypersensitive Responses

Dermatoses of an immune (hypersensitive) nature occur at any age. The disorders seen in the elderly may be exacerbations of previous conditions, may be newly acquired, or may result from therapy for other pathology. Two disorders of an immune nature are specific to the older person. They are bullous pemphigoid and pemphigus. As noted earlier in this chapter, the decrease in the protective oily secretions permits increased epidermal permeability and the decreased blood flow in the dermis slows percutaneous absorption (rate of clearance of substances following entry). These changes enhance the possibility of occurrence of contact dermatitis. The incidence of systemic allergic reactions are lower in the elderly than in young persons, perhaps because of a decrease responsiveness of the humoral immune system; however, ability to cope with an intense allergic response is lowered. Careful questioning for a history of allergic responses is an essential preventive measure. Individuals with a personal or family history of hay fever, asthma, or other allergies are at risk to hypersensitive responses to drugs.

Bullous Pemphigoid

ETIOLOGIC FACTORS. This is possibly an autoimmune response (Jordan, 1967).

DYNAMICS. Bullous pemphigoid runs a chronic course of exacerbations and remissions. It usually occurs in persons over 70 who are generally in good health. Lesions are subepidermal; the entire thickness of the epidermis forms the roof of the vesicle, thereby providing resistance to rupture. Autoantibodies probably are present at the site of vesicle formation (Jordan, 1967). When lesions are extensive, the tendency is toward general debilitation and danger of a superimposed infection.

MANIFESTATIONS. Multiple tense vesicles and bullae present most frequently on the lower abdomen and thighs, but may be generalized, including the oral cavity. Usually pruritus accompanies the eruption. Regardless of location, lesions do not rupture easily.

TREATMENT. Anti-inflammants (corticosteroids) and immunosuppressive agent (Methotrexate) are employed. Use of both agents seems to produce a remission with less danger of untoward side effects than with steroid therapy alone. However, both agents produce iatrogenic effects; therefore persons on these medications must be followed closely. Afflicted persons often need nursing assistance to cope with the puritus and general discomfort.

Pemphigus

ETIOLOGIC FACTORS. Possibly it is autoimmune.

DYNAMICS. Epidermal cells lose the desmosomes that attach them to each other; the cells separate and fluid collects within the spaces. The vesicular lesions tend to be soft and rupture easily because of the intra-epidermal nature of fluid accumulation. Experimental work by Beutner (1965) on serum antibody titers raises the possibility of the etiologic basis being an immune response. Most common form is pemphigus vulgaris. Onset is usually in the 50 to 60 age group. The denuded weeping areas permit loss of body fluid and an avenue for microorganism invasion; therefore fluid and electrolyte problems and infections are potential complications.

TREATMENT. Initial high doses of corticosteroids will improve the situation and permit tapering of the dosage level. Titers of serum antibodies serve to monitor therapy. Methotrexate may enhance effectiveness of steroids to allow use of lower doses. Compresses and emollient creams control weeping and crusting.

Bullous conditions in the elderly have potentially serious primary complications. Because of this, nurses should obtain immediate attention for elderly persons afflicted with this type of disorder.

Degenerative Conditions

Degenerative conditions result from changes in the skin that are associated with aging. Repeated pressure or friction over time may result in a thickening of the stratum corneum (hyperkeratosis) known as corns and calluses. Usually the number of active melanocytes decrease with aging, but in some localized areas the number of melanocytes increase and remain in the basal layer. This change is apparent as lentigines. The decrease in number of capillaries and in the supporting connective tissue elements influence the development of vascular changes such as purpura, vasculitis, stasis dermatitis/ulcerations, and positional pressure lesions.

Purpura is relatively common in the elderly. It presents as ecchymoses on the arms and legs. An apparent initiating factor is disruption of blood vessels by minor trauma. Another factor is the cutaneous atrophy associated with long term corticosteroid therapy for a chronic disorder such as rheumatoid arthritis. Purpuric lesions are often present along with atrophic changes. Investigations of newly acquired purpuric lesions should include a consideration of hematologic disorders as evidenced by changes in platelet count, bleeding, and prothrombin time. Purpura usually is not palpable; it is a macule. Vasculitis, by contrast, includes changes in vessel walls and loss of fluid and cells into the dermis. The changes result in edema and cell infiltration and are palpable as tissue elevations.

Corns and Calluses

These benign hyperkeratotic lesions, corns and calluses, are often disabling because of interference with mobility. The stratum corneum (outer surface of skin) is made up predominantly of a tough hard protein (keratin) synthesized by the prickle cells. Keratin is hard and brittle when dry, pliable and strong when hydrated. Maintenance of a balance between production of new keratinocytes in the basal cell layer and sloughing off from the outermost layer is essential for barrier function. Formation of new cells at a faster rate than cells are sloughed off results in a thickened or scaly outer surface.

ETIOLOGIC FACTORS. Chronic pressure and friction from poor-fitting shoes or chronic excessive stresses from occupational/recreational activity, i.e., postman, lumberman, are causes. Corns result from friction to tissue overlying bone.

DYNAMICS. Corns and calluses are a protective response, since thicker skin can absorb more pressure and withstand more friction. Excessive growth over bone leads to a core which causes inward pressure and pain (corn). Calluses often are on plantar surface, especially when the metatarsal arch lowers in later years, thus increasing pressure on the sole.

MANIFESTATIONS. Callus is a slightly elevated area of hyperkeratosis; retains normal skin markings after trimming with scalpel. A corn is also a thickening of the stratum corneum, but the area is more localized and sharply demarcated, skin markings are lost, and it has a center core of keratin. When trimmed, the core of soft, avascular tissue is apparent.

PREVENTION. Pads, adequate fitting shoes, weekly inspection of feet are helpful.

TREATMENT. Soak in water to soften. Rub with emory board after soaking or very fine sandpaper afixed to a tongue depressor (Brown, 1978). Calluses and corns usually respond to the use of keratolytic agents which aid in softening and removal of the material. A 20 percent salicylic acid ointment on a pad cut to size and held in place for a few days re-

moves outer layer of tissue. The central core may be removed with liquid nitrogen by the physician. Devices such as metatarsal pads will help to avoid direct pressure and prevent recurrence. Place small pad with center cut-out over corns to relieve pressure. If core is not removed, a new layer of skin forms unless pressure is relieved. Attention to the fit of shoes will also assist in preventing further trauma. Visual disturbances and diminished joint mobility may prohibit self foot care. Family members may need to be instructed.

Ingrown Toenails

ETIOLOGIC FACTORS. With lack of proper care, the nails curve inward.

HIGH RISK. At high risk are persons with mobility problems, i.e., unable to reach their feet. Persons not practicing hygienic care are at risk also.

DYNAMICS. Nails become thickened, adherent to skin, and turn inward.

MANIFESTATIONS. Thick, deformed nails pressing into skin tissue.

PREVENTION. Soak feet in water to soften nails. Slide orange stick around under nail to loosen skin adherence. Cut nails regularly—use clippers, keep nail corners above skin line, cut straight across. Teach family member if person unable to do self-care.

TREATMENT. Following above treatment, place wisp of cotton/lambs wool gently under edge of nail if it can be changed daily.

Lentigines

ETIOLOGIC FACTORS. Long term exposure to active radiation is a cause of lentigines.

HIGH RISK. Fair-skinned persons with chronic sun exposure are at risk.

DYNAMICS. Increased number of melanocytes in basal layer.

MANIFESTATIONS. Hyperpigmentation of dorsa of hands and face. Small, tan-to-dark-brown macules that do not disappear. In contrast, freckles are brown-pigmented macules that increase in size with sun exposure (increased pigment production in response to ultraviolet radiation) and fade when no longer exposed.

TREATMENT. Lentigines are benign and no treatment is necessary except for cosmetic reasons.

Stasis Dermatitis/Ulcerations

ETIOLOGIC FACTORS. Ischemia of lower extremities is the cause.

DYNAMICS. Single or multiple variables are present: chronic venous insufficiency, venous stasis, atherosclerosis, and age changes in cutaneous vascular supply. There is interference with oxygenation of tissue and removal of waste products of metabolism. Healing is slow because of circulatory inadequacy, and secondary infection is a potential complication. The underlying pathology often is not curable; therefore condition becomes chronic.

MANIFESTATIONS. This condition is manifested in erythema, vesicular lesions, edema, and thin, dry skin. With chronicity there is thickened epidermis, indurated scaly papules or plaques, and accentuated skin markings (lichenification). A brownish discoloration produced by hemosiderin is secondary to petechial hemorrhages. Ulcerations may follow from trauma to the area.

TREATMENT. Goals are to prevent/cure infection, promote healing, relieve pruritus, promote circulation, and relieve edema. Preferred position/mobility is bedrest or limited mobility. Elevation of foot of bed and sitting with the legs elevated as much as possible will help drain the veins and minimze edema. This is contraindicated if the ulcer accompanies arterial insufficiency.

Agents used in the care of an ulcer include wet dressings of normal saline or bacteriocidal solutions such as ¼ to ½ percent silver nitrate and aluminum acetate or topical antibiotic ointments. Topical steroid creams decrease inflammation. Sometimes oral antibiotics are necessary depending on the results of laboratory studies for organisms and sensitivity or for prophylaxis. Measure ulcers to evaluate healing. Keep them covered. When an ulcer is clean, a zinc paste boot (Unnas boot) provides an occlusive medicated bandage for 7 to 10 days. This allows for reepithelialization and healing without the trauma of frequent dressings. Mobility is possible with a boot. Cleanliness is necessary to prevent infection.

With arterial insufficiency, Buerger's exercises may promote circulation. Vascular surgery may be necessary to attain adequate blood flow. Persons with these problems must not use constricting clothing such as round garters or knotting of stockings, actions that occlude blood flow. Avoidance of these practices is a sound preventive measure for anyone.

Duration of treatment is prolonged, sometimes months. Hospitalization is not necessary if adequate support is available at home. Public health nurse can evaluate adequacy of care and response to therapy and assist person and family to cope with the situation.

Positional Trauma

Positional trauma is a descriptive phrase for excoriations and ulcerations of tissue overlying weight-bearing bony prominences. The danger of this condition is high in elderly people with mobility restrictions. These people may be living in a long term care facility or in their home. Pressure of sufficient extent and duration to interfere with adequate tissue nutrition and oxygen will result in necrosis. The extent and duration of pressure necessary to result in tissue damage are not consistent from one person to another.

Many variables apparently influence whether or not an individual will develop positional trauma. Determination of individual susceptibility depends on knowledge of the following principles of developmental dynamics.

Etiologic Factors, Risk, and Dynamics

1. Duration of pressure on weight-bearing bony prominences—the longer the sustained pressure the greater the danger of interference with circulation and, hence, with nutrition and oxygenation of tissue. Mean capillary pressure is 25 mm Hg; therefore positional pressure readily occludes the microcirculation. High pressure for a short time is safer to skin than low pressure for long periods (Husain, 1953).

2. Extent of pressure varies with position. The extent of pressure on ischial tuberosities is greater when sitting in a chair with the feet supported than when the feet hang free. The latter situation distributes the weight along the posterior thighs and, thus, does not focus pressure on one site. The pressure on the sacral area varies directly with the extent of the elevation of the head of the bed (Lindan, 1965). Persons in semi- or high Fowler's position for cardiovascular respiratory problems are at increased risk to postural pressure lesions.

3. Shearing forces on sacral tissues vary directly with increasing elevation of the head of the bed (Goth, 1942). With head elevation, the outer skin

tissues adhere to the bed linen but gravity pull displaces the underlying subcutaneous tissue downward. This uneven tissue shift distorts the anatomy of blood vessels within the tissues, causing angulation and interference with circulation. As noted under principle 2 above, maintenance of a semi-sitting position increases susceptibility to sacral tissue trauma.

4. Extent of pressure varies with body build (Lindan, 1965). Weight-bearing pressure is concentrated over the bony prominences of thin persons, whereas the tissues of an obese person disburse the weight over a larger surface. However, the blood supply to the subcutaneous tissue of an obese person is impaired because blood vessels are not proportionately increased and overall tissue nutrition and oxygenation may be marginal. Additionally, the interstitial area for transport of nutrients is greater in an obese person than one of normal height-weight relationships.

5. Tissue compressibility contributes to pressure effects (Lindan, 1965). The tissues of the elderly are relatively inelastic and compress readily under postural pressure. Lindan (1965) demonstrated that in young, healthy subjects the regain of tissue depth following release of pressure required twice the duration of compression, that is, two hours of pressure required four hours to regain normal tissue depth. The tissues of elderly people compress readily and may be slower to regain normal depth. A reoccurrence of postural pressure prior to regaining normal tissue depth may increase susceptibility to tissue damage. Tissue compressibility is a factor to consider when establishing scheduled for positional change.

6. Perception of and response to painful stimuli are decreased in depressed persons and absent in paralyzed areas of the body. The apathetic, withdrawn person may not change position even when capable of self-mobility. The stimuli may not be perceived or, if perceived, may not generate a response. To protect tissues a person capable of self-movement must change position in response to painful stimuli. The person who becomes depressed or who is incapable of self-movement is prone to postural trauma. Persons who are incapable of self-movement include the comatose, the very weak and debilitated, those in severe pain, and some persons who are partially paralyzed.

7. Oxygen and nutrients are essential for tissue viability. Normal changes in dermal capillaries de-crease skin blood supply in the elderly and contribute to postural pressure hazards. The person who in addition has vascular pathology is highly susceptible to this trauma.

8. Nutrient supply to tissues is dependent upon nutritional intake. Less than adequate nutritional intake, a relatively common practice with the elderly, predisposes to postural tissue trauma.

9. Susceptibility to postural tissue trauma seems to vary inversely with the extent of melanin in the skin. (Bruno, 1971). Persons with a light complexion are probably at greater risk to postural pressure than persons of darker skin tones.

10. The presence of systemic disorders, particularly infections with an accompanying temperature rise, increases the metabolic rate and needs of cells and heat and body fluid losses. Tissues in this situation are less resistant to trauma, particularly if circulation and nutritional intake are compromised and dehydration occurs. Systemic disorders predispose to tissue trauma from postural pressure.

11. Rough, wrinkled, damp bed linen may contribute to skin maceration and irritation, especially in the elderly who have thin, atrophic skin. The greater the number of layers of bed linen, the greater the risk of wrinkling and pressure. Dampness may result from the heat of plastic draw sheets or from incontinence. Prompt changing of damp or wet linen or clothing is necessary to prevent skin maceration and irritation.

Manifestations

An initial assessment must be made of skin color, height-weight relationships, cardiovascular status, thickness of the skin, positional patterns, appearance of tissues overlying weight-bearing bony prominences, general health including emotional and nutritional status, and mobility. This assessment provides baseline data for determining susceptibility to postural trauma.

Manifestations of tissue trauma are:
1. Redness that persists for longer than 20 minutes after pressure release.
2. Positive blanching test—slow capillary filling following digital pressure.
3. Persistent redness or dusky redness.
4. Softened (mushy) and/or hardened area under site.
5. Blister or break in continuity of skin.

Detection of a change toward increased susceptibility to positional tissue trauma is a nursing responsibility. Assessment on a daily basis for changes in mobility status, emotional outlook, nutritional intake, general health status, and condition of bed linen should provide the data necessary for making judgments about susceptibility.

Prevention

Preventive measures should be initiated promptly. The type of measures selected will vary with the extent of danger. Sheepskin may be effective for some persons, while others may need an alternating pressure mattress, or perhaps a gel pad under the buttocks area and an hourly turn schedule. The turn schedule should use all positions possible before returning to the initial position, thus avoiding the cumulative effects from compressed tissue that did not regain normal depth.

Treatment

The incidence of trauma to tissues overlying weight-bearing bony prominences remains high (Bruno, 1971), The literature is replete with suggestions for therapy, but controlled studies of the efficacy of therapies are few. At the present time, no one method appears to promote healing of superficial lesions to an extent greater than other methods. Cleanliness of the area, exposure to the drying effects of air or a heat lamp, and avoidance of further trauma usually results in healing if nutrition is maintained and the general physical status of the person does not worsen. Superficial lesions do not penetrate the full thickness of the skin. They tend to be painful but usually heal quickly if kept clean and free of pressure interference with circulation.

Large positional ulcerations include full skin thickness and deeper muscle layers. The trauma may originate with necrosis of the deeper areas and lie beneath a slightly reddened external surface until it breaks through, exposing a large crater. The rim is often undermined extensively. This ulcer is dangerous and the physician should know of its existence. The area may need surgical debridement and skin grafting, although cleansing with hydrogen peroxide, irrigating the undermined area, exposure to air, and elimination of weight bearing on the site may permit healing by granulation and scar tissue.

SUMMARY

Functions of the skin include protection from the inward transmission of noxious physical and chemical agents and the outward loss of critical substances such as water; regulation of body temperature through the sweat glands and blood vessels; and transmission of sensory stimuli. Gradual changes occur in the skin with aging, especially on surfaces exposed to solar and other environmental traumas. These changes include thinning of the epidermis, decrease in water content and elasticity, and development of wrinkles, keratoses, and lentigines. Skin disorders present in the elderly may result from structural and functional changes in this tissue with age, exposure to solar radiation and other environmental noxious agents, and abnormalities in other body systems. A dermatologic health history includes data about habits of hygienic skin care, sociopsychologic factors possibly related to skin problems, normal aging changes, and apparent pathologic changes including the person's reaction to these changes. Observations of eruptions consist of anatomic distribution, structural characteristics, color, and grouping patterns. Necessary information to communicate about eruptions is developmental changes, response to therapy, and accompanying systemic manifestations.

Classification of skin disorders are infectious and noninfectious. The noninfectious are pathologically classified as degenerative, hypersensitive, and neoplastic. Nursing goals are planned to assist the afflicted person and family/friends to cope with dermatologic problems. Coping includes maintaining or regaining a positive self-concept, understanding the problem and expected results from therapy, participating in care to the extent possible, and preventing complications. Collaborative aspects of nursing goals requires ongoing assessment and evaluation of therapy and consultation with or referral to a physician when necessary and consultation with social workers when indicated to obtain assistance with socioeconomic aspects of care. Nursing interventions include assistance with environmental factors (temperature, humidity, cleanliness, sensory stimulation) family care, and prescribe therapy (dressings, baths, and lotion applications). The elderly person with a skin disorder may have special needs in regard to self-concept and socialization. The obvious disfigurement compounds the frequent feeling of unattractiveness that accompanies aging skin changes.

BIBLIOGRAPHY

Alliston, J. R., and Rist, T.: Skin infections may be outward signs of inner disorders. Geriatrics 30:87–95, February, 1975.

Bates, B.: A Guide to Physical Examination, ed. 2. Philadelphia: J. B. Lippincott Co., 1979.

Beutner, E. H., et al.: Autoantibodies in pemphigus vulgaris: response to an intercellular substance of epidermis. J.A.M.A. 192:682–688, 1965.

Brouner, G. J.: Cutaneous diseases in the black races. In Moschella, S. L., et al. (eds.): Dermatology. Philadelphia: W. B. Saunders, 1975, vol. 2, pp. 1704–1737.

Brown, B.: Verbal suggestion, Seattle, 1978.

Bruno, P.: Variables Associated with the Development of Postural Tissue Trauma. Unpublished Doctoral Dissertation, University of California, San Francisco, 1971.

Carlsen, R.: Aging skin: understanding the inevitable. Geriatrics 30:51–54, February, 1975.

DeBacker, L. J.: Sympathetic block for herpes zoster. N. Engl. J. Med. 299:664, 1978.

DeGowin, E., and DeGowin, R.: Diagnostic Examination. New York: Macmillan Co., 1969.

Eaglstein, W. H., et al.: The effects of early corticosteroid therapy on the skin eruption and pain of herpes zoster. J.A.M.A., 211:1681–1683, 1970.

Epstein, W.: Melanoma: value of early detection and treatment. Postgrad. Med. 61:82–89, 1977.

Fitzpatrick, T., et al. (eds.): Dermatology in General Medicine. New York: McGraw-Hill Book Co., 1971.

Fleischmajer, R., et al.: Aging of human dermis. In Frontiers of Matrix Biology, Volume 1, 90–106, Basel, Switzerland: Karger, 1973.

Goldman, R., and Rockstein, M. (eds.): Proceedings of a Symposium: The Physiology and Pathology of Human Aging. New York: Academic Press, 1975.

Goth, K. E.: Clinical observations and experimental studies of pathogenesis of decubitus ulcers. Acta Chira Scandia, 87:Supplement 76:198–200, 1942.

Hanna, M., and MacMillan, A. L.: Aging and the skin. In Brocklehurst, J. C. (ed.): Textbook of Geriatric Medicine and Gerontology. London: Churchill Livingston, 1973, pp. 593–618.

Hurwitz, N.: Predisposing factors in adverse reactions to drugs. Brit. Med. J. 1:536, 1969.

Husain, T.: An experimental study of some pressure effects on tissues with reference to the bedsore problem. J. Pathol. Bacteria 66:347–358, 1953.

Johnson, S.: (ed.): Coping with common skin conditions. Geriatrics 30: Part I: 50–131, February, 1975; Part II: 44–92, March, 1975.

Johnson, S.: Problems of aging: relieving itching in the geriatric patient. Postgrad. Med. 58:105–109.

Jordan, R. E., et al.: Basement zone antibodies in bullous pemphigoid. J.A.M.A. 200:751–756, 1967.

Judelsohn, R. G.: Prevention and control of varicella-zoster infections. J. Infect. Dis. 125:82–84, 1972.

Kennedy, J. A.: Skin problems of blacks. J.A.M.A. 236:301, 1976.

Korting, G. W.: The skin in old age and its clinical aspects. In Vogel, H. G. (ed.): Connective Tissue and Aging. Amsterdam, Excerpta Medica, 1973.

Kosiak, M.: Etiology and pathology of ischemic ulcers. Arch. phys. Med. Rehabil. 40:62–69, 1959.

Lantis, L., and Lantis, S.: Allergic dermatoses in the older patient. Geriatrics 30: 75–84, February, 1975.

Lee, J. A., and Merrill, J. M.: Sunlight and the etiology of malignant melanoma: a synthesis. Med. J. Australia. ii:846–851, 1970.

Levene, G. M., and Calnan, C. D.: Color Atlas of Dermatology. Chicago: Year Book Medical Publishers, 1974.

Lindan, O., et al.: Pressure distribution in the surface of the human body. Arch. Phys. Med. Rehabil. 46:378–385, 1965.

Moschella, S., et al.: Dermatology. Philadelphia: W. B. Saunders Co., 1975.

Montagna, W.: The skin. Scientif. Amer. 212:56–66, 1975.

Parrish, J. A.: Dermatology and Skin Care. New York: McGraw-Hill Book Co., 1975.

Pearce, R. H., and Grimmer, D. J.: Age and the chemical constitution of normal human dermis. J. Invest. Dermatol., 58:347–61, 1972.

Prunievas, M.: Aging of the epidermis. In Robert and Robert, (eds.): Frontiers of Matrix Biology. Basel, Switzerland: Karger, 1973.

Robert, L. (ed.): Aging of connective tissue. Frontiers of Matrix Biology. Basel, Switzerland: Karger, 1973.

Rook, Arthur, et al. (eds.): Textbook of Dermatology. Oxford: Blackwell Scientific Publishers, Vol. 1, 1972.

Rossman, I.: Clinical Geriatrics, ed. 2. Philadelphia: J. B. Lippincott Co., 1979.

Ryan, T. J.: The microcirculation of the skin in old age. Gerontology Clinician 8:327–337, 1966.

Ryan, T. J.: The direction of growth of epithelium. Brit. J. Dermatol. 78:403–415, 1966.

Selmanowitz, V., et al.: Aging of the skin and its appendages. In Finch and Hayflick (eds.): Handbook of the Biology of Aging. New York: Van Nostrand Reinhold Company, 1977.

Soloman, L. M., et al.: The adult skin and its potential for allergic reactions. Med. Clin. N. Amer. 58:165–183, 1974.

Spencer, S. K., and Kierland, R. R.: The aging skin: problems and their causes. Geriatrics 24:81–89, 1970.

Verbov, J.: Skin Diseases in the Elderly. Philadelphia: J. B. Lippincott Co., 1974.

Verbov, J.: Skin problems in the older patient. Practitioner 215:612–622, 1975.

Verzár, F.: The aging of collagen. Scientif. Amer. 208:104–117, 1963.

Watson, W., and Farber, E.: Controlling psoriasis. Postgrad. Med. 61:103–112, 1977.

Young, A. W., Jr., and Miller, L.: Skin problems in the geriatric and general hospital. J. Amer. Geriat. Assoc. 16: 1140, 1968.

24

Vision Problems

Gretchen G. Boyer

QUICK REVIEW

CATARACTS

DESCRIPTION	Clouding or opacity of the lens.
ETIOLOGIC FACTORS AND HIGH RISK	Aging, chronic disease (diabetes, hypoparathyroidism), radiation, trauma. Medications: cortisone, phospholine iodide.
SIGNS AND SYMPTOMS	Temporary improvement of vision (second sight). Poor vision, eye fatigue, headaches, increased light sensitivity. Irritability as patient works harder to see. Visualization of clouded lens.
DYNAMICS	Opacities vary in density and location—central, scattered, peripheral. Signs, symptoms, and coping difficulties depend on location.
PROGNOSIS	Few cataracts mature to the point where surgery is warranted.
NURSING MANAGEMENT	Help patient define visual needs and expectations for self as a basis for decision regarding surgery. Assist in planning time of surgery in relation to lifestyle—realistic time schedule. Assist in preoperative planning for least stressful postoperative ADL—food supplies, placement of utensils and materials, counter height, activities to avoid, need for cleaning and maintenance, safety proof home against falls. Teach management of lifestyle and ADL with cataract glasses or contacts.
EVALUATION	Satisfaction with means of making decision to have or not to have surgery. Reality of expectations—experience and outcomes of surgery and appliances. Adequacy of preoperative preparations at home for effective postoperative ADL. Effectiveness of managing lifestyle before/after cataract lenses.

QUICK REVIEW

GLAUCOMA

DESCRIPTION	Increased intraocular pressure secondary to chronic or acute obstruction of normal flow of aqueous humor resulting in loss of peripheral vision or blindness.
ETIOLOGIC FACTORS	Age-related changes in area of canal of Schlemm, infection, injury, swollen cataracts, tumors.
HIGH RISK	Risk increases with age and family history.

SIGNS AND
SYMPTOMS

Chronic: Symptoms: Morning headache that disappears after arising, sense of eyestrain. Late: tunnel vision. Signs: Elevated pressure, field defect, change in optic nerve.

Acute: Intense eye pain, injected watery eye, blurred vision, red and green halos around lights, dilated pupil.

COMPLICATIONS   Blindness

PROGNOSIS

Acute: Depends on promptness of treatment. Blindness can occur in 24 to 36 hours.
Chronic: Depends somewhat on compliance with medical regimen.

NURSING
MANAGEMENT

Acute: Refer for emergency immediate medical treatment.
Chronic: Support the person in adjusting to glaucoma as a lifelong disease requiring careful compliance even without signs and symptoms. Assist patient in adjusting lifestyle to minimize situations and conditions that cause (1) dilation of pupils and (2) physical emotional stress. Help patient develop reliable system for instilling eye drops or taking related medications. Serve as liaison/advocate for retaining patient's medication routine if admitted to different care setting.

EVALUATION

Intraocular pressure values in normal range. Lifestyle has accommodated to minimal pupil dilation in a satisfying way. Transition to health care settings insures continuity of eyedrop routine.

Changes in vision are age related, becoming more pronounced as an individual grows older. In addition to the normal vision changes that everyone experiences, there are some pathologic conditions that become an increased risk as people age—cataracts, glaucoma, and macular degeneration. When visual changes occur simultaneous to the experience of other age-related problems, the balance between the demands of daily living and coping abilities may become increasingly precarious.

The ability to see is closely linked with the way in which people manage their daily lives. Any loss of vision makes a significant impact upon lifestyle:

- Use of medication becomes hazardous when labels are difficult to read and all the bottles are shaped and colored alike.
- Nutrition becomes poorer as difficulties with cooking and shopping are compounded. Labels on cans cannot be read or amount of seasoning determined. Burns while cooking become an increased risk.
- Falls and bruises increase with failure to observe objects in the environment or notice surface changes.

There is also reason to be concerned about the emotional health of the person whose vision is failing:

- Boredom can ensue when usual forms of diversion—reading, watching television, writing letters, doing crafts, gardening—are lost.
- Isolation results from the failing ability to get out caused by either the difficulty of reading street and bus signs or the embarrassment (or fear) of looking clumsy or awkward to others.

These only begin to sample the areas of difficulty an older person may experience with failing vision. It suggests that nursing expertise can be a useful support system to help these people modify their lifestyle and learn new coping skills.

ASSESSMENT OF LIFESTYLE AND VISION PROBLEMS

A realistic understanding of an older individual's lifestyle is the key to assessment of the impact of failing vision on a person's ability to cope with daily living. As in any other condition, it is crucial that the nurse assess this lifestyle from the perspective of visual influences prior to formulating and instigating any plan of care. This assessment is as important for nursing care as the physician's examination of the eye is for medical care.

Questions found useful for determining the areas of high risk problems in failing vision include the following:

How do you spend your day?

What kind of work do you do? (Even if retired, older people use the word work to describe their daily activities.)

What do you do for pleasure? (Check reading, television, crafts, handiwork, gardening, and so forth.)

Do you live alone? in a house? apartment? retirement complex? If alone, are there people/relatives nearby?

Do you do your own cooking? How do you get your groceries?

What kind of transportation do you use? drive? get rides from others? take a bus?

Do you get out much? Does your eyesight interfere with your getting about?

What kinds of problems are you having because of your poor vision? (Social life, taking medications, concerns, fears).

In practice, one question leads to another and, depending on the responses, the nurse will follow where the patient leads.

Objective data are equally important. In a clinic setting the nurse can observe the patient in the waiting room and as he walks to the examining room. Things to notice are:

Does he touch door jambs and chair edges?

Are there spots on his clothing?

Are there burns on hands or forearms?

Does he wear sunglasses and broad-brimmed hats? (to cut down on the glare caused by cataracts)

Does he look at you when he talks or just past your ear? (seeing you with peripheral rather than central vision)

Does he test floor surfaces with his feet when he comes to the edge of the rug? (loss of depth perception)

Acknowledgment is made to Dr. Roger Johnson, Clinical Associate Professor of Ophthalmology, University of Washington School of Medicine, Seattle, for his assistance in reviewing the manuscript.

In home visits the nurse can note:

Does he use his hands in place of his eyes to orient himself (e.g., touching edges of tables or stoves as a basis for placing objects)

Does he appear to be listening more intently?

In grooming—do stockings match? color combinations appropriate? other aspects? (These observations should be made in terms of the individual's preferred lifestyle and not that of the nurse)

Are there burns on the individual or the furniture?

How are lights and glare controlled?

All these observations provide objective data on vision problems and coping behavior.

In addition to obtaining data on daily living and coping skills, a highly significant area to assess is the individual's perception of the handicap and what is seen as *usable* support systems. For example:

> Mrs. Parsons came to the office complaining of poor vision. "It is just terrible. I can't see. You've got to do something for me! I can't read menus. I don't recognize people's faces. My eyes feel like they are coming out of my head when I sew. It's terrible—I used to be able to sew all day." A vision check showed no change in the small cataract that had been found six months earlier, distance vision was unchanged, and there was only a one line change in near reading.

On the other hand:

> Mrs. Albright, who is temporarily unable to wear her contact lenses, refuses to wear her cataract glasses because they make her "look funny" and she feels sick and dizzy with them on. Without correction she sees only shapes and shadows, yet she walks surely and unhesitantly. Without knowing, one could not tell that she is virtually blind. For her, the loss of vision is acceptable while loss of appearance and discomfort is not.

Some people seem to have trouble accepting small changes in their vision while others tolerate major loss and still function at a high level.

NORMAL CHANGES IN THE AGING EYE

The aging eye and the pathology that affects it require understanding of the formation and structure of the eye. Significant components include those shown in Figure 24-1.

Like all other body systems the eye is subject to the effects of time. Throughout life, structural and functional changes occur gradually in the eye. Since the pathologic conditions that affect vision in the elderly are closely related to these changes, normal aging of the eye is reviewed here before considering specific pathology.

CORNEA. The cornea tends to cloud with age, losing its luster and transparency. The epithelium develops minor irregularities and corneal fibers thicken as a part of the general decrease in tissue water content that occurs with aging (Friendenwald, 1942, p. 541). A white or yellowish ring may develop around the cornea. This arcus senilis may be related to high blood cholesterol levels.

IRIS—PUPIL. Changes in the iris result in an increased need for light, and loss of speed in accommodating to light and dark. These changes, caused by sclerosis, cause a narrowed pupillary diameter and a slowed pupillary response. Therefore, the pupils of older people normally are small and somewhat fixed.

The narrowed pupil affects the amount of light the older person needs for effective vision. It may become necessary to increase the size of light bulbs to promote good vision and to carry purse or pocket-size flashlights for greater ease in seeing steps and keyholes in the dark.

The slowed response to light changes presents several coping difficulties. As the pupillary sphincter response slows, more time is needed to adjust to light changes. Entering a darkened room or building results in a period of time when it is difficult to distinguish objects or people. Alternatively, moving out of doors into bright day or having a light suddenly turned on in a darkened room causes a glare that is equally blinding. In each case, hazards are posed for the older person if he tries to adjust to the environment quickly. Night lights, canes, and a helpful arm promote safety and aid adjustment at these times.

Night driving becomes an increasing problem. The inability to accommodate quickly to oncoming headlights, particularly with the glare of wet streets and raindrops, plus the subsequent blackness after a car has passed, causes many older individuals to give up night driving completely. This has the effect of changing social lifestyles for many. Unless alternative transportation can be arranged, evenings must be spent at home.

LENS CHANGES. The changes in the lens have the greatest impact on vision and are associated with major coping problems. The lens is formed like

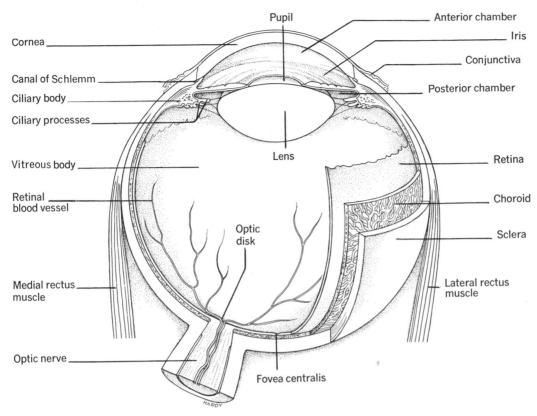

FIGURE 24-1. Transverse section of the eyeball. (From Chaffee, E. E., and Greisheimer, E. M.: Basic Physiology and Anatomy, ed. 3. Philadelphia: J. B. Lippincott Co., 1974, p. 239, with permission)

an onion. The oldest tissue is in the middle and the youngest at the periphery. As cellular growth slows with age, the lens comes to have a larger proportion of old tissue. Its center gradually becomes yellowish and rigid. This results in a lack of flexibility that makes it difficult for the ciliary muscle to change the shape of the lens; a slowed and less complete accommodation for near and far vision results. This loss of accommodation begins to be noticeable in the forties.

CILIARY MUSCLE. Over a period of time, the ciliary muscle also becomes stiff and less functional. This, along with the decreased compliance of the lens, contributes to the problems of accommodating to distances. Because the eye brings visual images to focus on the retina by changing the shape and thus the refractive power of the lens, near vision requires the greatest amount of work by the ciliary muscle. Therefore, as the muscle loses its ability to contract, near vision is compromised. People who

have never worn corrective lenses before will need to wear reading glasses and others may add bifocals or trifocals to existing corrections.

VITREOUS. Gradually the gelatinous vitreous shrinks and the collagen material of which it is composed tends to clump (Duke-Elder, 1969, p. 335). This causes shadows to be projected on the retina and results in vitreous opacities or floaters in the field of vision. To some degree these opacities are normal, but they may also be diagnostic of such eye problems as uveitis, retinal hemorrhage, or retinal detachment. Therefore, any sudden change in the kind or amount of floaters warrants a complete fundoscopy.

The extent to which normal floaters bother people is highly variable. A recreational sharpshooter or seamstress will complain of them much more than someone who plays bridge or cooks as a hobby.

RETINA AND MACULA. Except for the macula, the retina shows the fewest changes associated with age alone. Only when vascular changes interrupt its blood supply or changes in pigment occur is its function compromised.

In contrast, the macula is highly vulnerable to age-related sclerotic changes. Since its function is associated with detailed vision, very small changes in the macula will be readily noted by the patient as either distortion or loss of visual acuity. Such changes are referred to as macular degeneration.

CATARACTS

The term "cataract" refers to any clouding or opacity of the lens.

Etiologic Factors and High Risk Populations

It is likely that everyone will develop some degree of cataract if he lives long enough. The age of onset varies widely and is somewhat predictable by heredity. Cataracts commonly occur later in life. In a population 65 years of age, 95 percent of all people can be expected to have some clouding of the lens (Duke-Elder, 1969, p. 63). Diabetes and hypoparathyroidism increase the risk of cataracts as do some drugs such as ophthalmic drop preparations of cortisone and phospholine iodide. Other causes of cataracts include radiation, trauma, infrared light, electric shock, uveitis, and congenital anomalies.

Types of Cataracts

Cataracts vary primarily in terms of location and density. The opacity may be diffused or scattered. It may be located centrally or peripherally. The location determines the nature of coping difficulties the individual will experience and the types of compensatory behavior in which they must engage.

CENTRAL CATARACTS. If the cataract is located in the central area of the lens, individuals will see better in dim light that causes the pupil to dilate. In bright light the pupil constricts and the person may become almost totally blind. Therefore, the nurse can expect to see people with central cataracts reading in dim light and keeping room lights at a minimum level. Coping behavior to deal with sudden exposure to bright light or managing in brightly lit areas becomes more important to enhance safety and maintain activity.

SCATTERED CATARACTS. Scattered cataracts produce an effect of multiple, minimirrors in the eye.

Since light refracts differently off each opacity, people with this type of cataract complain predominately of glare. They read better with an eye shade and often wear a broad-brimmed hat outdoors. Habitually they use their hands to shield their eyes from glare or wear tinted or dark glasses.

PERIPHERAL CATARACTS. Opacities located in the periphery of the lens usually do not cause coping problems until they grow into the pupillary area. Often they are diagnosed only in the doctor's office when the pupil is widely dilated. Occasionally a spike will invade the central portion of the pupil and cause a splitting or doubling of images.

Signs and Symptoms

The earliest symptoms of cataract are caused by a swelling of the lens prior to the formation of any visible opacity. This swelling artifically increases the power of the lens and for some people causes a temporary improvement in their near vision, commonly referred to as "second sight." Some people experience a need for frequent prescription changes as the lens swelling changes their refractive error. This early stage of cataract development is highly variable; it may be either so short or so long as to go unnoticed.

Almost all cataract patients complain of poor vision, eye fatique, headaches, increased light sensitivity, and blurred or multiple vision. It is not unusual for some people to become irritable as they work harder to see through their growing cataracts.

Diagnosis

Diagnosis of cataracts is confirmed by direct visualization of the lens opacity. Being informed of this diagnosis can be very traumatic to some patients, especially if by past experience, they equate cataracts to blindness. Accurate information, appropriate to each patient's presenting situation, needs to be provided. Sometimes, however, the shock of the diagnosis makes patients unable to hear or assimilate the information provided at this time. Therefore followup explanations by the nurse become important when the patient is ready to hear and participate.

Nursing measures at the time of diagnosis include listening to the patient's concerns or, where the individual does not express them, introducing fears commonly held by others and checking them out. It is important for the nurse to have knowledge of the person's prior experience with individuals who have had cataracts and/or surgery in order to gain some sense of their expectations and ideas about coping patterns.

Many people ask what causes cataracts. The best answer to this is "age." Some blame excessive reading, sewing, or television watching as the cause of their cataracts. They need to know that such activity has neither caused nor will it worsen their condition.

Prognosis

Although cataracts are common, relatively few mature to the point where surgery is warranted. Older persons need to know that most cataracts grow very slowly over many years, and so they should not become inappropriately fearful of impending blindness or immediate surgery. Only when glasses can no longer improve vision and normal activities such as reading or driving are being compromised is surgery indicated.

Decision Regarding Cataract Surgery

Numerous factors enter into the decision as to whether or not to proceed with cataract surgery. The nurse plays an important role in helping the person understand the types of surgery available and how lifestyle may be changed as a result of surgery. It is especially important that the nurse explore with older persons their understanding of what the doctor has told them and help them acquire enough knowledge to make informed decisions. The nurse can expect to be called many times both before and after the decision about surgery is made. Often the same questions will be asked. This is the expected, usual behavior, but it requires patience and understanding.

At times a decision is made to have surgery before vision becomes severely limited. Some of the factors that contribute to this decision include:

- having surgery done prior to retirement for insurance purposes
- having met that year's deductible charge for Medicare coverage
- ensuring adequate vision to pass a driver's license renewal examination (Older persons often have a more difficult time reacquiring a driver's license once it has been lost.)
- being able to enjoy anticipated travel

Timing

The timing of surgery should be discussed and arranged so as to fit most comfortably into the person's lifestyle. Many people decide to have surgery during the winter months so as to be able to garden in the summer. Others want their surgery done in the early fall in order to see well enough by the holiday season to participate in family preparations and activities.

Information also should be given so that patients can not only schedule surgery to meet their needs but also plan their lives to accommodate any limitations they may experience.

Time considerations for an *intracapsular* cataract extraction:

1–4 weeks	scheduling time
3–4 days	hospitalization
6–8 weeks	recovery period
1–2 weeks	for lenses to be made
2–4 weeks	to adjust to glasses
2–4 months	post-surgery for contacts

Expectations

In addition to the time elements involved, other considerations include the patient's expectations about the experiences he will have in the process of having surgery and the nature of his vision postoperatively. The following areas have been found to be important:

- the types of experiences friends and acquaintances have reported to them about cataract surgery and its associated vision changes
- the desire to retain binocular vision for work or hobby
- the fear of becoming dependent or having to function without the assistance of a mate or companion
- the expectation of wearing contacts or glasses, or having an intraocular lens

Occasionally the nurse will encounter a patient who does not complain despite a large amount of visual loss. This person may be waiting for the doctor to suggest surgery or may be overly frightened of having eye surgery. Talking with this person about his fears of surgery and the types of problems he is having will provide the nurse with an accurate understanding of the factors influencing his decision making. Where appropriate, the nurse can clear up any misunderstanding about the surgery and its risks. These data can then be incorporated into the doctor's discussion with the patient.

Cataract Surgery and Nursing Management

Nursing management associated with the care of the patient who contemplates or has cataract surgery is multifaceted. It begins early in the decision-making process and continues through the preoperative period, the immediate postoperative period, and into the often long, postoperative readjustment period. Since the surgery or failure to have it affects almost all aspects of daily living, the areas for nursing diagnosis and management are wide and potentially crucial.

This section of the chapter deals with many of the day-to-day issues and problems the patient faces when cataract surgery is contemplated or undertaken. If nurses understand the nature of the problems and some of the solutions, they are in a much better position to be of assistance to patients in the small frustrating areas of trouble as well as in the major areas. Additionally, since nurses are expected to have a better data base on the individual's lifestyle, they are excellent consultants to physicians in the plans of medical management.

Much of what is discussed here will be useful not only to the nurse in the surgeon's office or in a clinic or hospital setting but also to the nurse in the home health care agency, senior citizen center, or retirement or nursing home. Whether for spotting problems or reinforcing learning at a time when the person is less stressed and more prepared to listen, the nurse is often crucial to the adjustment of the patient who undergoes cataract surgery.

Preoperative Planning

Once the decision is made to proceed with cataract surgery, the nurse plays an important role in assisting the patient prepare for the experience and organize his environment and resources to cope with daily living during the postoperative adjustment period. Because of the limited vision following surgery and restrictions placed on bending and lifting, patients should be helped preoperatively to arrange their environment accordingly:

- arrange with a friend, family, or home health aid to help with weekly grocery shopping and laundry
- lay in supplies or prepare meals that involve minimal preparation—frozen dinners, casseroles, salads
- place commonly used eating and cooking utensils and needed supplies at counter-top level
- do any crucial house or garden work, and then plan to ignore dust and weeds for six weeks
- arrange transportation for doctor's appointments
- have hair cut/washed just prior to surgery as shampooing generally is restricted for two to three weeks

A complete physical usually is required and may be done by the patient's private physician prior to hospitalization or at the time of admission.

Types of Surgery and Implications for Nursing Management

The exact method of cataract removal varies and depends on the patient, the ophthalmologist, and to some extent the area of the country. The objective in each case is the same—the removal of the opaque natural lens and restoration of vision by using glass, contact, or intraocular lens.

Hospitalization can range from two to six days and only rarely will both eyes be operated at the same time. Local anesthesia usually is preferred for the standard intracapsular extraction to eliminate the risk of postoperative vomiting with its associated rise of intraocular pressure; however, a general anesthetic may be used. Preoperative teaching is similar to that done for any surgical patient.

Operative Procedure

Intracapsular extraction is the traditional method of cataract removal. It involves making an incision halfway around the cornea and extracting the lens through a widely dilated pupil. A partial iridectomy is done to ensure that secondary glaucoma does not result, should the vitreous humor move forward and block the flow of the aqueous humor from the eye. The corneal incision is closed with silk, nylon, or vicril sutures. If silk is used, the stitches will be removed about three weeks postoperatively.

**GUIDELINES FOR MANAGEMENT OF
ADL WHILE HOSPITALIZED**

Ambulation is usually allowed the day of surgery.

Only the operated eye is patched for the first 24 hours.

Avoidance of all bending, stooping, lifting, and rapid head movements.

A stool softener such as Colace is used to avoid straining.

Pillows can be placed at the patient's back to prevent rolling to the operated side.

Pain is minimal after the first 24 hours.

Only shapes and shadows can be seen with the operated eye.

A temporary glass can be worn if the unoperated eye is blind.

Postoperative Nursing Management

Although there is some variation in the prescribed care for the cataract patient postoperatively, the goals are the same. They are to *prevent* increased intraocular pressure, stress on the suture line, and hemorrhage into the eye.

During the next six weeks at home while the corneal incision is healing, some restrictions continue and affect management of ADL. These constraints on activity for the first six weeks postoperative are the following:

1. Continue to avoid all bending, stooping, and lifting.
2. Avoid long car trips and crowds where one might be jostled.
3. Exercise caution in bathing or walking in hazardous areas where falls might occur.

Medications

Eyedrops and ointment are a routine component of postoperative therapy. Some patients are fearful that they may injure their eye when instilling these for themselves. Discharge planning should incorporate teaching patients how and when to instill any ophthalmic medications prescribed.

Steps in instillation of eyedrops are:

1. Lie down. Close the eyes.
2. Rest the eyedropper on the bridge of the nose.
3. Place a drop of the medication into the nasal corner of the eye. (Only one drop is necessary.)
4. Gradually open the eye. (The medication will roll into the appropriate area.)

For instillation of ointment, follow these steps:

1. Stand before a mirror in good light.
2. Pull down the lower eyelid.
3. Place a small amount of ointment (¼ inch) on the inner surface of the lower lid.
4. Blink the eyes several times to distribute the medicine.

Temporary Glasses

While waiting for the cornea to heal, temporary cataract glasses may be used to help the patient ambulate and begin adjustment to a new way of seeing. If the unoperated eye is blind or has been removed, these glasses provide the patient with some limited amount of vision.

Temporary glasses are inexpensive ($15 to 20) and can often be borrowed from the operating surgeon or an optometrist. They are poorly made and intended only for interim use while the cornea is healing. Wearing them helps the person prepare for the changed image size and altered way of seeing that all cataract glasses cause.

Alternative Types of Surgery

As in other areas of medical management, research continues in improving the management of cataracts.

PHACOEMULSIFICATION. Recently a new instrument and surgical procedure has been developed that uses ultrasound to break up the lens. The procedure, called phacoemulsification, is done through a 3 mm incision that can be closed with a single suture. The surgery requires a high degree of technical skill and is used only for selected patients.

Because the cornea is not disturbed, contacts can be worn almost immediately and the patient is able to return to full activity soon after surgery. Presently phacoemulsification is preferred for patients in their 40s and 50s who have a softer lens and whose lifestyles preclude the longer recovery period of the traditional surgery.

INTRAOCULAR LENS REPLACEMENT. Currently new materials and new methods of fixation have lead to the development of the intraocular lens. Although the long range effect of this surgery is not fully known presently, it increasingly is being done on carefully selected patients. The intraocular lens has the advantage of eliminating the visual distortion of cataract glasses and, unlike contact lenses, does not need to be inserted and removed daily.

Adjustments in Daily Living after Cataract Surgery

Once sutures are removed, visual distortion begins to clear and trial lenses show a gradual increase in vision. After two months corneal changes stabilize and permanent lenses can be prescribed. Because cataract glasses (costing upwards of $100 plus frames) and contact lenses ($180 to 300) are so expensive and need to be exactly ground, it is worthwhile to wait until the best possible fit can be made. The nurse who prepares her patient preoperatively for a long recovery period will have a happier, less frustrated person to care for.

Choice of Glasses or Contacts

Glasses or contact lenses serve as a replacement for the opaque lens that is removed during cataract surgery. Each has advantages and disadvantages that must be considered in conjunction with the lifestyle and abilities of the patient when making the replacement choice.

Glasses position the lens 14 to 15 mm in front of the natural lens position, which causes objects to be magnified about 33 percent. For this reason, glasses following surgery never incorporate a cataract and a regular lens together, as double vision results if each eye receives a different size visual image. In order to use both eyes, the postoperative patient must either have both eyes operated or wear a contact lens on the operated eye and a corrective glass lens on the unoperated eye.

Contact lenses approximate the position of the natural lens, reduce the magnification to 8 percent, and allow binocular vision. When contact lenses are not a feasible option, both eyes usually are operated and the patient adjusts to cataract glasses.

Currently the intraocular lens presents the best

option for binocular vision. Image size varies by about 1 percent with this lens.

Adjustment to Glasses

Learning to wear cataract glasses following surgery can be the most difficult part of having a cataract removed. After making the decision to have surgery, going through the operation, waiting two months for the glass prescription and another week for the lenses to be made, the patient puts on his new glasses to discover that they make him dizzy, nauseated, and throw him off balance when he tries to walk. It is at this time that important nursing functions are understanding what the patient is experiencing and giving concrete suggestions of help and encouragement.

The ease with which a person adjusts to cataract glasses is often predicted by whether or not bilateral surgery is done and, if not, the amount of vision in the unoperated eye. The better the vision in the unoperated eye, the more the patient will be bothered by the blur and distortion of the cataract glass. For these people, adjustment takes longer because they have a tendency to take off the glasses and use the poorer but more natural vision of the unoperated eye. When there has been surgery in both eyes, there is no longer a choice and the patient must adjust to his new glasses. In time, the brain automatically compensates for the increase in object size.

In helping patients adjust to cataract glasses, the nurse should suggest that the patient wear the glasses initially when sitting, and then only gradually start walking around the safe level areas at home. Driving should never be attempted until the patient has completely adjusted to the glasses.

The 33 percent size increase makes everything appear closer than it really is and causes poor

---

VISUAL CHANGES CAUSED BY CATARACT GLASSES

Thirty-three percent increase in object size

Distortion

Increased brightness of images

A circular scotoma or blind area around the edges of the glass that gives a "jack-in-the-box" effect when persons or objects suddenly jump into the visual field, startling the patient depth perception. Arms of chairs, counter tops and stove tops, and coffee cups and utensils are not where they appear to be. The patient must be warned particularly about pouring hot liquids, setting objects down, and going up and down stairs and curbs. Feeling for the edges of tables and counters helps determine where surfaces really are. He should be told to use both hands when handling breakable objects and to avoid machinery with moving parts.

Nausea and dizziness result from the wavy jerky appearance of objects viewed through the edges of the thick glass. This can be lessened by looking through the center of the lens and consciously turning the head to see objects to the side. The nurse needs to remind the patient that the more he wears his glasses the less discomfort he will experience.

Occasionally the nurse will encounter some patients whose temperament is such that they never seem to adjust to cataract glasses unless both eyes are operated or unless the other eye becomes blinded by its cataract. It is difficult to help older persons, who already have experienced the frustration and complications of trying to adapt to glasses after the first surgery, understand that their vision will be improved by having another operation. Yet at times (assuming they are unable to manipulate a contact lens and the intraocular lens is not an option) this is the only solution to the problems of adjustment.

Care of Cataract Glasses

Usually cataract glasses are thick and, therefore, normally made of plastic in a lenticular cut to decrease the weight—the lighter the glasses the better they will comfortably stay in place. Because these glasses are expensive and worn constantly, the choice of frame is very important. Patients should select frames that are not overly large and are durable and well made so that they fit comfortably and stay in adjustment. Because a 1 mm position shift can markedly alter visual acuity, it is crucial that these glasses fit properly. If hearing aids are incorporated into the ear pieces, these must also be considered.

Nurses should notice if cataract glasses have slid down a patient's nose or become crooked from being taken off and put on. Helping the patient locate a good convenient optometrist is worthwhile, since frequent adjustments may be necessary to maintain a good fit. Wise shopping at this time can save time, money, and exasperation in the purchase of glasses.

The expense and precious nature of cataract glasses usually ensures that they are properly cared for. Plastic lenses are much more likely to scratch than those made of glass. For this reason, when being cleaned, they should *always be rinsed before* being wiped with a *soft cloth* in order to prevent dust particles from being rubbed across the lens surface, thus causing scratches. When not in use, glasses should be stored in a safe place and never laid upon the lens surface.

Using Contact Lenses

For those patients who are able to use them, contact lenses eliminate much of the visual distortion created by cataract glasses. Because they more closely approximate the position of the natural lens, there is very little problem with magnification and, even when only one eye has been operated, binocular vision is possible. Many active persons prefer contacts since peripheral vision and depth perception approximate the natural eye. Others prefer the contacts for cosmetic reasons. Soft lenses, some which do not have to be removed, have been developed in cataract strengths and are now available for persons who previously were unable to wear hard contact lenses.

Learning to use contacts can be difficult for many patients, especially those with parkinsonian tremors or arthritis, or those who psychologically are uncomfortable placing an object in their eye. Patience and practice will help to overcome many of these problems.

It is important that the patient be instructed in the proper methods of inserting and removing the contacts. Steps for insertion of both hard and soft contact lenses follow:

1. Wash hands.
2. Place a large flat hand mirror on a towel spread over a well-lighted flat surface.
3. Remove the contact lens from its case and place it on the tip of the index finger (middle finger if a two-handed approach is used) convex side down.
4. Place a drop of wetting solution on the lens.
5. *Then* remove the cataract glasses.
6. Bending over the towel and looking into the mirror, spread the eyelids with the fingers of one hand (or with two hands: hold the upper lid with the hand that does not hold the contact lens and pull down the lower lid with the index finger of the hand holding the lens).

7. Brace the finger with the lens against the one holding the lower lid and insert the lens onto the cornea.

Steps for removal of a *hard* contact lens are:

1. Wash hands.
2. Place a large flat hand mirror on a towel spread over a well-lighted flat surface.
3. Bending over and looking into the mirror, pull the eyelids taut and blink quickly.
4. The lens should pop out.
5. If the lens becomes dislodged, manipulate it back onto the cornea and repeat the procedure.

Instructions for removal of a *soft* contact lens are:

1. Wash hands.
2. Place a large flat hand mirror on a towel spread over a well-lighted flat surface.
3. Bending over the mirror, pull the lens down off the cornea with an index finger.
4. Using thumb and index finger, pinch the contact and remove.

The patient who has had surgery on both eyes and who chooses to wear contacts must also plan to have a regular pair of cataract glasses to wear when the contacts are not in place. These enable the person to see well enough to handle his contacts and are necessary in case the contacts are lost or broken. Additionally, since contacts presently can only be ground for distance vision, reading glasses must be purchased also. This creates quite an expense for what is often a limited budget.

For more information and pictures on care and insertion of contact lenses by the patient or others, see "Handling of the Lens—Insertion, Removal, Cleaning, and Storage" (1970).

SENILE MACULAR DEGENERATION

Senile macular degeneration (SMD) is a condition in which the macula (the point in the retina where visual acuity is greatest) no longer functions well. The cause is unknown, although it is thought to be related to a decreased blood supply to the sensitive nerve endings in this region. Both eyes almost always are affected.

People who are afflicted with senile macular degeneration complain that their central vision is either so dark or so distorted that they no longer can see what they are looking at. Usually the condition worsens gradually and, in the more advanced cases, it is as though a hole had been punched in the center of the visual field. Usually the best corrected vision for these people is the large E on the charts; therefore, they are classified as *legally blind*.*

Lacking acute vision, people with SMD no longer can read, watch television, drive a car, play cards, do handwork, or recognize a face. By *scanning* to use peripheral vision, they are able to get around, cook, clean, garden, and, in general, manage much of their daily routines. A nurse can often recognize the person who has SMD, because he tends to look just past the object of his attention.

SMD responds poorly to medical treatment. It often becomes a problem for nursing management. Data on previous lifestyle will enable the nurse to determine problem areas in accommodating to the loss of central vision, as well as alternative activities that the individual can find reasonably satisfying. These people need a great deal of reassurance that they will never become totally blind from macular degeneration. By using peripheral vision they should be able to care for themselves and function with a relative degree of independence.

GLAUCOMA

There are two types of glaucoma: wide angle and narrow angle. The first is an insidious chronic condition. The second, often characterized by an acute condition, may require surgery if blindness is to be avoided. The incidence of glaucoma increases rapidly from ages 40 to 70 and is a common disease of later life. Therefore all eye exams and physicals on persons over 40 should routinely include tenometry readings to check for glaucoma. Where there is a family history of the disease, members should be checked annually. Glaucoma can also occur secondarily to infection, injury, swollen cataracts, and tumors.

---

* Legal blindness: The best corrected vision in the best eye is 20/200 or less, or visual field is limited to twenty degrees.

Wide Angle Glaucoma (Chronic, Simple)

Wide angle glaucoma results from an obstruction to the normal flow of aqueous humor from the eye caused by changes in the area of the canal of Schlemm (venous sinus of the sclera). The resultant backup of fluid causes an increase in the intraocular pressure that gradually damages the tender structures of the retina and optic nerve, which causes a progressive loss of visual field.

Signs and Symptoms

Wide angle glaucoma is most often diagnosed during a routine eye examination when the eye pressure is above normal or changes are seen in the optic nerve. Because the symptoms of wide angle glaucoma are so vague, few people are ever aware that they have anything wrong with their eyes. These unrecognized symptoms may include:

- morning headache that disappears shortly after arising
- a feeling that it is getting hard to see and/or a sense of eyestrain.

Signs are:

- elevated pressure
- a change in the angle formed by the iris and cornea
- a field defect
- a change in the optic nerve

It is only after the disease has advanced and nerve damage has occurred that the patient becomes aware of visual loss. At this stage, blind areas and tunnel vision will be noted.

Treatment and Nursing Mangement

The treatment of glaucoma is aimed at maintaining eye pressure within normal limits either by decreasing the production of fluid or aiding its outflow.

The strength, frequency, and type of medication is regulated on the basis of tenometry readings, peripheral field examinations, and changes seen in the optic nerve. To aid in fluid outflow, miotic drugs are given to constrict the pupil and widen the drain angle. Various types of preparations are available and different physicians will have their own preferences of drugs and management.

In talking with patients about their medications, there are some fundamental principles the nurse should emphasize and reinforce. The first of these is that, *once a diagnosis of glaucoma is made, treatment must be continued for the rest of one's life.* Glaucoma, like diabetes, at this time can be treated only; it cannot be cured. Patients find this difficult to comprehend or believe, particularly when they are experiencing no discomfort. Others, believing modern medicine can cure any condition, may mistrust a care provider who tells them they must take medication for the rest of their lives.

The second principle that should guide the lifestyle and disease management of glaucoma patients is *eye pressure tends to rise whenever the pupils are dilated or the system is placed under physical or emotional stress.* This has implications for the timing of medications. Drops should always be taken before retiring and the first thing in the morning since the pupils dilate during sleep. During periods of life change, emotional excitement, or anxiety pressure readings often indicate the need to increase either the strength or frequency of medication. Nurses may alert patients to be aware of these times or may notify the patient's family or physician to discern stressful events.

When drops are prescribed to be taken several times during the day, they should be spaced at *regular intervals.* Often older patients complain that they think about taking their drops and then can't remember if they have. In such instances it is best to have the patient take additional medication rather than continue with the possibility of none at all. The same is true if a patient must skip or misses a dose. In this instance patients should be told to take their drops as soon as they remember or are able to do so, and then to return to their regular schedule even though the time interval may be short. For many older people who have memory problems it is best to link their eyedrop schedule to another activity such as lunch, dinner, a television show, or before an afternoon nap.

When treatment is initiated, patients should be told that the drops may give them a slight headache or "pulling" sensation to their eyes. People with central cataracts may complain of a visual loss because the smaller pupil prohibits them from looking around their opacity. Nurses in any setting need to be aware of the specific cataract status of individuals to whom they offer nursing care so that they can be alert to predictable problems and institute assistance in management of daily living activities where indicated.

All glaucoma patients have difficulty seeing in dark places. Advanced planning strategies they can use to compensate for this may enable them to feel more secure in such situations. Night driving is particularly difficult and hazardous. This suggests implications for nursing management in acceptance of a changed mobility status not only by the patient but also by family and friends. Coping behaviors will need to be found that enable them to acceptably modify their lifestyle. The use of night lights, canes, flashlights, and larger light bulbs may become necessary.

If intraocular pressure is difficult to control or drops pose a problem either for compliance or administration, a carbonic anhydrase such as Diamox tablets may be used to decrease the production of aqueous humor.

Carbonic anhydrase is a diuretic and may deplete the body of potassium. If taken in combination with other diuretics, hypokalemia may occur. Increasing the dietary intake of potassium or taking a potassium supplement may be necessary to maintain an adequate potassium level. Patients with a history of kidney stones or infection also need to be alert when these medications are prescribed, since some physicians feel they increase stone formation.

Carbonic anhydrase is often prescribed at bedtime because of its longer lasting effect; however, this can result in increased nocturia and interfere with adequate rest and sleep. Restricting fluids in the late afternoon and evening may help. Other patients who routinely get up during the night are not particularly inconvenienced. The nurse needs data on sleep patterns to predict and manage these attendant problems.

Patients who have both kidney disease and/or hypertension and glaucoma often find themselves caught between the medical management of these problems. Frequently it is the alert nurse who, by careful questioning of her patients' general health and lifestyle, discerns potential problems and helps to keep other health care providers aware of the risks their mutual patients may be experiencing. Persons with glaucoma need to be alerted to the effects that other medications may have on their eyes. They should be advised to do the following:

- Read the labels of all over-the-counter preparations and/or check with the pharmacist about effects the drugs may have on their intraocular pressure.
- Avoid all cold medications containing antihistamines.
- Avoid all medications containing caffeine, e.g., Anacin, APC, No-Doz.
- Tell anyone who is prescribing or giving medications in an emergency that they have glaucoma.
- Wear a Medalert identification tag.
- Avoid all stomach medications that contain atropine-like substances.

Adjustment to Living with Glaucoma

Glaucoma patients vary markedly in their ability to adjust to having a chronic condition. Most become *very* faithful in adhering to their "drop schedule" and can become acutely distressed if their schedule is altered. Because these patients tend to be rather high strung and tense, they often experience a great deal of anxiety if hospitalized, particularly in adherence to their drops schedule. For this reason it is recommended that they be allowed to keep their eye medication at their bedside and retain control of their own schedule of administration. If this is not possible, nurses should attempt to adhere closely to the schedule the patient has been maintaining prior to hospitalization. The same caveat should hold true for any change in living situation where the patient risks losing control of his medication schedule, e.g., nursing homes or some retirement settings where staff control dispensing of medications. Most of these patients have been taught that if they do not comply to the prescribed schedule they risk retinal damage and blindness. Having internalized this risk, they become fearful when others do not comply to their schedules. This fear is real and nurses should give it the attention and urgency that is appropriate to its reality.

Surgical Treatment

Surgery may be proposed if field loss and pressure cannot be controlled with medication or if drops are used so frequently that the patient's lifestyle is disrupted. There are several operative procedures for glaucoma; all attempt to establish an alternative pathway for circulation of the aqueous humor. Patients need to know that surgery may or may not alleviate the need for drops. It has no effect on vision already lost, a fact that patients need to understand, not merely be told. Further, although surgery may substantially lower intraocular pressure, it does not decrease the need for medical follow-up to ensure that the pressure remains normal and the drain continues to function.

Another possibility of change following glaucoma surgery is that a glass prescription may no longer be correct. This results either from an alteration in fluid pressure or from the surgery's changing the shape of the cornea. Similarly, some people who have always been able to read without glasses because of a small pupil, now discover that they must wear reading glasses for close work. These changes not only create additional expense but also may be upsetting to the patient if he has not been forewarned.

Whether or not the patient maintains on drops or has surgery, *tenometry readings should be done at least every four to six months.* The nurse should schedule (or patient request) appointments for tenometry readings at different hours of the day to ensure that the treatment is maintaining a normal pressure throughout the day. Early morning checks are particularly important because pressure tends to elevate during sleep (when the pupils are dilated) and when coffee (with caffeine) is consumed. Field examinations to plot peripheral vision changes should also be done on a regular basis—at least every year. These are tedious examinations and should be done in the morning when the patient is well rested.

Narrow Angle Glaucoma (Acute Closure)

Narrow angle glaucoma is less common than wide angle. It is characterized by acute attacks that may be severe enough to lead to blindness unless promptly treated. With this type of glaucoma there is a sudden rise in intraocular pressure caused by the complete closure of the drain angle by the iris.

Signs and Symptoms

Symptoms of narrow angle glaucoma relate to the extreme increase in intraocular pressure. These include intense eye pain, secondary nausea and vomiting, injected watery-appearing eye, blurred smoky vision, red and green halos around lights (secondary to corneal edema), and dilated pupil. If pressure is unrelieved, blindness can occur within 24 to 36 hours.

Medical Treatment

Immediate treatment is to use miotic drops every 5 to 10 minutes to constrict the iris and pull it away from the drain angle. Usually a carbonic anhydrase such as Diamox or a hyperosmotic solution such as Mannitol is given to diurese the patient and slow the production of aqueous fluid. Narcotics are given for pain. Surgery is performed following the acute attack or if the pressure cannot be relieved. The surgical procedure consists of bilateral peripheral iridectomies since the disease almost always involves both eyes.

Because this condition poses such a severe visual risk, any patient with a history of suspect symptoms or prodromal attacks should be examined thoroughly.

DRY EYES

Just as age affects secretions of other glands so also may lacrimal secretions lessen over time. For some individuals this results in a chronic condition referred to as "dry eye." While never a cause of blindness, it is the source of a great deal of discomfort for many older people. Hormonal changes seem to play a part in these changes because the condition is more frequently seen in postmenopausal women.

Symptoms include a dry sensation in the eyes, a tendency to close the eyes, and a desire to rub them frequently. Since mild infections are usually present secondary to these symptoms, the patient may complain of itching, burning, and a scratchy sandy feeling in the eyes. When examined with a microscope the surface of the cornea appears to have been superficially stippled with a pin, a condition referred to as punctate keratitis.

Unfortunately there is no cure for dry eyes. Treatment is directed toward eliminating the secondary infections and providing some lubrication for the eye itself. During the day artificial tears purchased over the counter can be used. At night a greasy ointment such as Lacrilube provides relief. This condition is so uncomfortable that it is often difficult for patients to accept that the doctor can do little to help them. Frequently nurses provide the best help by simply listening and being sympathetic toward the problem. At present it is the best that is available.

NURSING MANAGEMENT OF THE OLDER PERSON WITH POOR VISION

When vision becomes limited, for whatever reason, individuals must learn new styles of coping with activities and demands of daily living and of adaptations in their lifestyle. Memory and the other senses—hearing and touch—become increasingly important in maintaining some degree of independence. Routine tasks become increasingly more difficult and fatiguing. Usual sources of diversion are less possible. Where age limits agility, the increased fear of falling keeps some people from venturing into unknown areas. Stairs and curbs create new hazards. Even a change in the texture of floor surface, from carpeting to smooth surface, can create uncertainty and one can observe the patient testing the edges with the sole of the shoe to determine the changes in level.

Canes

Canes serve a dual purpose for the elderly with a visual handicap. They enable the person to test for surface changes and identify objects in the path. They also provide stability in walking. In addition, canes alert others to a person's poor vision. For this latter reason some older persons refuse to use a cane because they do not want others to know they are handicapped.

Assisting the Visually Handicapped

When helping persons with limited vision get about there are some useful guidelines.

1. *Identify yourself if there is a chance.* They may not remember your voice.
2. *Give advance verbal notice of directions.* For example, "A few more steps and we will turn to the right," "The carpet edge is here," "The chair is just to your left."
3. *Approach blind individuals from the front,* not from the rear.
4. *Ask if they wish assistance; do not assume.*
5. *Choose restaurants in terms of amount of light.*
6. *Help them locate (touch) both arms of the chair before seating themselves.*
7. *Take their hand and place it on your arm.* This enables them to sense direction of movement and maintain their balance without feeling that they are being pushed or pulled. It also appears less obvious to others. Do not grab their arm to guide them.
8. *Let them know where they are if it is an unfamiliar area.*
9. *Teach them to use their hands to locate* edges of tables, shelves, stoves, and so forth. In eating, suggest using clock locations of foods (meat at 6, potatoes at 9).
10. *Help them to become effective in using the assistance of others in ways that increase not decrease their independence.* Find ways to let others know what kind of help is useful and that which is not (Bindt, 1952). This may mean exploring with others what they do and do not like. It may also mean the nurse's making a contact with the family, friend, or homemaker and making some suggestions.

Loss of acute vision may seem less traumatic than blindness, but it too can be incapacitating in subtle ways. Being unable to read print means more than missing the evening paper or a good book. It means the inability to read labels on cans and packages, making food shopping and preparation either guesswork or impossible. Taking medications becomes more hazardous as the labels blur.

CONCLUSION

For those with sight, it is difficult to realize the limitations imposed upon a person's lifestyle by poor vision. Since there is no substitute for experience, the nurse should listen to the patients and share what they have learned with other health care workers.

BIBLIOGRAPHY

Anderson, B., and Palmore, E.: Longitudinal evaluation of ocular function. In Palmore, E. (ed.): Normal Aging II. Durham, N.C.: Duke University Press, 1974.

Bindt, J.: A Handbook for the Blind. New York: Macmillan Co., 1952. (Offers ideas for the blinded person on adjustments in everyday activities of daily living as well as to those who wish to be of assitance to the visually handicapped.)

Boyd-Monk, H.: Cataract surgery. Nursing 77. 7:56, 1977.

Camp, R., et al.: Handling of the lens—insertion, removal cleaning, and storage. In Gerard, L. (ed.): Corneal Contact Lenses. St. Louis: C. V. Mosby, 1970, pp. 205–217.

Corso, J. F.: Sensory processes and age effects in normal adults. J. Gerontol. January 26:90–103, 1971.

Duke-Elder, S.: System of Ophthalmology, Vol. XI. St. Louis: C. V. Mosby, 1969.

Friedenwald, J.: The eye. In Cowdry, E. V. (ed.): Problems of Aging. Baltimore: Williams and Wilkins, 1942.

Gordon, D. M.: Eye problems of the aged. In Chinn, A. B. (ed.): Working with Older People, Vol. IV, Clinical Aspects of Aging. Washington D.C.: U. S. Department of Health, Education, and Welfare, July, 1971.

Jaffe, N.: Current concepts in ophthalmology: Cataract surgery—A modern attitude toward a technological explosion. New Engl. J. Med. 299:235, 1978.

Schwartz, B.: Current concepts in ophthalmology: The glaucomas. New Engl. J. Med. 299:182, 1978.

RESOURCES

(addresses follow list)

An In-Depth Study of Blindness and Aging, by Father Thomas Carrol.*

An Introduction to Working with the Aging Person who is Visually Handicapped, 1972.*

Caring for the Visually Impaired Older Person, by R. M. Jolicoeur, Sr. (A practical guide for long term care facilities and related agencies. This consists of an illustrated manual in print, a 16 mm film strip and a script for the film both in print and on a cassette.)†

How to Intergrate Aging Persons who are Visually Handicapped into Community Senior Programs, 1972.*

The Relocation of Blind Persons from a Residential Home for the Blind and the Development of Specialized Community Services for the Older Visually Handicapped Population, by M. Saterbak, J. Sineps, and R. Relaford. (Handling charge $1.00.)†

Mobility

Basic Components of Orientation and Movement Techniques, by L. Widerberg and R. Kaarlela, 1970.‡

How Does a Blind Person Get Around? (Pamphlet)*

Parameters of Posture and Mobility in the Blind. Prepared by Illinois Visually Handicapped Institute and Western Michigan University, 1969.‡

Eating

Techniques for Eating—A Guide for Blind Persons, by L. Widerberg and R. Kaarlela.‡

Homemaking

A Step-by-Step Guide to Personal Management for Blind Persons.*

Catalog of Blind Aids and Appliances. (Available free of charge)§

Homemaking Goes Creative, by B. M. Yank, 1970. (Rehabilitation Teaching Services, Services for the Visually Impaired, State of Nebraska, Division of Rehabilitation)

Housekeeping Skills—Self Study Court #1. (This publication comes in large print with six cassettes) ‖

Ideas for Better Living—A Special Blind Aids and Appliances Catalogue. (In print and braille—free)*

International Catalog of Aids and Appliances for Blind and Visually Impaired Persons.*

Large Type Books in Print, by R. A. Landau and J. S. Nyren (eds.), 1970.#

So What About Sewing. (several volumes)**

Various catalogues on general and tangible aids and appliances, available in print only, free of charge.††

For Persons Who Work With Visually Impaired

Directory of Agencies Serving the Visually Handicapped in the U.S.*

Outcome Measure System. (A report by the Committee on Reporting and Evaluation of the National Council of State Agencies for the Blind, Inc., 1975.)‡‡

Rehabilitation Teaching for the Blind and Visually Impaired: The State of the Art, 1975.‡‡

Social Services for Persons Who Are Blind, 1975. (A guide for staff in departments of public social services. Prepared by U.S. Dept. of Health, Education and Welfare, Social and Rehabilitation Service.)§§

When Your Patient is Blind. (short illustrated pamphlet)##

ADDRESSES

* American Foundation for the Blind, Inc.
  15 West 16th Street
  New York, NY 10011

† Minneapolis Society for the Blind, Inc.
  1936 Lyndale Avenue, S.
  Minneapolis, MN 55403

‡ Graduate College
  Western Michigan University
  Kalamazoo, MI 49001

§ Howe Press
  Perkins School for the Blind
  Watertown, MA 02172

‖ Center for Independent Living
  New York Infirmary
  310 East 15th Street
  New York, NY 10003

R. R. Bowker Company
  1180 Avenue of the Americas
  New York, NY 10036

** The Catholic Guild
  Services for the Visually Impaired
  67 West Division Street
  Chicago, IL 60610

†† American Printing House for the Blind
   1839 Frankfurt Avenue
   Louisville, KY 40206

‡‡ American Association of Workers for the Blind
   1511 K Street NW
   Washington, DC 20005

§§ SRS Publications Distribution Center
   Room G-115-b, HEW, Mary E. Switzer Bldg.
   330 C Street SW
   Washington

Industrial Home for the Blind
   57 Willoughby Street
   Brooklyn, NY 11201

Part 4

Other High Risk
Problems
of Aging

Introduction to Part 4

Some phenomena that are at high risk for the elderly cut across diseases. They may make the individual more vulnerable to disease or they may add subtle complications. Part 4 deals with four such phenomena. As in Part 3, the format is one of organizing the concepts into a diagnostic/treatment approach so that clinicians can identify high risk persons or situations, recognize signs and symptoms, and understand the dynamics as a basis for logical management and evaluation strategies.

Three of the four chapters deal with losses—interpersonal losses, intrapersonal losses, and loss of influence. The other chapter deals with pain as a nursing concept, highlighting what is known about differences in pain for the elderly.

Most persons who reach their 70s have experiences involving each of these phenomena. The majority cope with the experiences without help from providers. However, where the risks are high or the presenting situation suggests that the individual does not have the resources to cope with the situation, it is essential to have knowledgeable, sensitive, effective nursing diagnosis and management.

25

Loneliness

Doris Carnevali

QUICK REVIEW

LONELINESS

DESCRIPTION	Personal suffering associated with a deficit in needed or desired intimacy.
ETIOLOGIC FACTORS	Failure to develop intimate relationships or loss of existing relationships.
HIGH RISK	Risk of loneliness is increased by loss of a spouse, companion, sibling, child; living in an urban area and in high risk neighborhoods; being housebound; changing residence; loss of usual mode of transportation; illness/disability; time on one's hands; inadequate income.
	High risk times include evenings, weekends, anniversaries of events, holidays.
DYNAMICS	Loneliness is generated by some degree of loss quantitatively or qualitatively of a relationship characterized as intimate in that it gives a sense of belonging, familiarity, repetition, sharing, sameness. It can be triggered by memories of past loneliness or by current or anticipated loneliness. The discomfort tends to be communicated—creating anxiety in others because all are vulnerable.
SIGNS AND SYMPTOMS	Complaints of too much time or being abandoned; change in pattern to over- or under-activity—physical/verbal; increased presence or reporting of signs and symptoms of ill health; loss of ability to concentrate; indecisiveness; increased irritability. Complaints of sense of unreality or depersonalization, *denial*.
DIFFERENTIAL DIAGNOSIS	Solitude, lonesomeness, or aloneness that produces none to mild discomfort.
COMPLICATIONS	Anxiety, depression, anger, illness, suicide.
PROGNOSIS	Good prognosis associated with good health or positive view of it, being able to get out and around the community, adequate income, being single, male, having meaningful time-occupying activities, having a pet, sharing housing.
NURSING MANAGEMENT	*Prevention:* Identify risk factors and intervene early. *Management:* Take initiative in working with problem, gather data on nature of loneliness (loss, times, current coping, goals, usable support systems). Time contacts for high risk periods: evenings, meals, holidays, anniversaries. Assist as needed with activities to occupy time, transportation, or protection to get out and around. Deal with work of bereavement. Assist in repeopling their world.
EVALUATION	Abatement of signs and symptoms. Reported satisfaction with new relationships or substitutes for them.

Loneliness is a high risk personal and health problem for many older people. Mates, relatives, and friends of one's own generation die or become housebound. Members of the younger generations become preoccupied with the multiple demands of their own lives. Thus, long-standing personal relationships, sources of human intimacy, decrease and change. At the same time financial, physical, and transportation constraints may limit mobility and the ability to maintain contacts or make new friends.

Nurses and other health care providers might view loneliness as a purely personal problem were it not for its impact on the health of the lonely person (Fromm-Reichman, 1957; Guptan, 1971; James, 1963). Holmes' study (1961) of deaths among patients with lung pathology gave evidence that the significant difference between those who died of lung disease and those who did not was not the extensiveness of the loung damage. Many who died had less extensive involvement than did the survivors. Instead the significant difference was that those who died lacked close personal ties with others. Another example of symptoms related to loss or loneliness is the increase in angina associated with recent death of a mate or close companion. Nutritional status is also compromised by loneliness (Hood, 1974; Howell, 1969; Palmore, 1971), as are drinking patterns (see Chapter 11). Thus, while not a health problem in itself, loneliness has the potential for affecting health negatively. It is a "complication" that can influence existing illness and treatment and can apparently increase the risk of illness.

> A woman in her 70s living in a retirement community comments, "When there is a death here I seem to suffer a setback. I don't know whether I'm sick or lonesome." Her daughter confirms that it takes days, sometimes weeks, for her mother to regain her usual appearance and lifestyle.

As a factor influencing health, loneliness is, therefore, a nursing concern and an area to be identified for nursing diagnosis. It is a significant factor in planning for nursing management of daily living. To ignore it because it is difficult to treat would leave many unanswered questions in understanding the dynamics of patients' health and responses to illness or treatment.

Description

Loneliness is a deficit in needed or desired human intimacy. It results in personal suffering characterized by feelings of abandonment, emptiness, dissatisfaction, anxiety, and depression. It may be generated by the absence of a particular person, lack of contacts for human intimacy, or failure of interactional partners to give the kind of relationship the person desires.

In a study made on loneliness, the elderly talked about it in various ways:

I can't stop thinking about it.

It's a peculiar sensation, I don't know what to do. I can't handle it until it's over.

I get depressed enough to do something real bad.

I get fed up with things and wish it (life) were ended.

It's a depressed feeling that no one loves me—I have no friends.

It hurts from the bottom of my feet to the top of my head. It can keep you from sleeping—can even make you a maniac.

It's too personal to talk about.

I don't let myself think about it.

It's an ache for my children and an emptiness for my husband.

It's like a toothache.

It comes over you like a wave.

It happens quickly. Sometimes in the middle of a crowd I'll think, "I wish Mary were here."

Loneliness is a painful and threatening experience.

Etiologic Factors

If loneliness has its roots in separation from those who provide needed and desired interpersonal intimacy, then etiologic factors must be related either to the failure to generate these relationships or the loss of established relationships. Persons over 70 have experienced past losses, and the likelihood of future losses are high. Compensatory behavior in finding new sources of caring and contact may be limited.

Data in any of the following areas should alert the nurse to the increased risk of loneliness as a problem in the over-70 age groups.

Loss of Spouse, Sibling, Child, or Friend

One of the most potent factors in producing profound loneliness, particularly among the elderly is the death of a mate, sibling, child, housemate, or dear friend. Each loss deprives the person of a source of caring and of a support system. Being unable to turn to a person who is genuinely caring and interested in time of need has been found to be a definite factor in producing loneliness (Hood, 1974). Loss of siblings tends to produce greater loneliness than the loss of a child; however, it is difficult to generalize because it is the nature of the relationship and the need it meets that determines the resultant loneliness.

If the quality of the relationship was good, it often met a major portion of the older person's needs to give and receive caring. Even when a relationship with a mate or housemate left something to be desired, it set the pattern for activities and demands of daily living. Thus the loss represents a major gap in the survivor's pattern of daily living as well as a loss of source of human intimacy.

In a mobile society, there is a high risk of another source of loss. This occurs when important individuals, family groups, or members move away from the vicinity of the older person. Frequent phone calls, personal visits, and shared social occasions are replaced with shortened, less frequent, long distance calls or with letters that consume less time and offer less opportunities for intimacy. The relationships lose anticipation of a contact, personal presence, touch, and other significant nonverbal forms of communication.

The nurse may approach this area of loneliness by listening for reports of deaths of others or moves by children or important others, or, upon noting signs or symptoms of loneliness, inquiring as to whether such events have occurred.

Urban Residence

Increased risk of loneliness has been associated with urban living, as contrasted with rural settings. It is also increased when individuals live in high risk neighborhoods where it is dangerous to venture out, even in the daylight hours. Individuals who live alone in private housing, including apartments (as contrasted to retirement communities or residences), in the city have been found to have greater risks of loneliness than those in more communal settings, although retirement residences and shared recreational facilities offer no guarantee against loneliness.

HOUSEBOUND ELDERLY. Older housebound persons, for whatever reason, are more likely to be lonely than those who are able to get out. The nurse should be alert for any factor within the environment or within the individual that restricts the ability to get out. It is a red flag predicting increased loneliness.

Change in Living Arrangements

Any change in locale or type of living for the older individual tends to disrupt established patterns of interaction and contact and, thus, presents risks of loneliness. Even when parents or grandparents *move in with the children,* there is the risk of relationships being incongruent with remembered or desired patterns of intimacy. It is quite possible for the older person to feel even more lonely in the midst of the family. Other priorities and interests or conflicting values between younger persons and the older person may result in interaction that is only a superficial facade of previous genuine intimacy—tantalizing by its possibility but frustrating in its failure. Data on these frustrations may be difficult to gather because of family loyalties and fear of losing a home, and yet the actual problems need to be specifically delineated if any effective intervention is to take place.

Moving into a nursing home or long term care facility where the majority of the residents have advanced mental and physical disability so that there is little possibility for developing satisfying relationships can also generate serious loneliness. Where these facilities are *located in isolated, outlying areas* with poor public transportation or where the individual is physically incapable of getting about, the restrictions and the change can be particularly devastating. Residents in retirement homes, even in the midst of the city, have complained also of a lack of contact with younger generations, another form of loneliness.

Change in Transportation

Any change in transportation tends to influence the pattern of human contacts; therefore, it can be a factor in producing loneliness.

LIMITATIONS ON DRIVING. Individuals who have been accustomed to driving may experience changes to which the nurse should be alert. Night blindness may interfere with the ability to drive after dark; therefore, participation is limited in social events scheduled in the evenings where younger people might normally be available. This, then, may restrict the older person to relationships with other older people who also must schedule activities during daytime hours. Evening hours, particularly dark evening hours in the winter, become lonely times.

LOSS OF CAR AS TRANSPORTATION. An absolute loss is that of loss of the car as a means of transportation. This makes the driver dependent on others or on public conveyances for transportation, often for the first time in many decades. If persons are in their late 70s or early 80s when this happens it can be quite devastating not only for the former driver but also for the mate if that individual does not drive. Certainly the anxiety over this potential loss each time the driver's license comes up for renewal is very real and recurrent.

PUBLIC TRANSPORTATION. Even individuals who have used public transportation regularly may experience problems as changes occurring with age limit their use of the system. Sometimes a change in housing makes the bus stop too far for walking, or there is an incline that is too difficult to maneuver. Changes in vision or memory prevent others from getting around.

> One older person says, "I'd get outside the store and forget which way the bus stop was, so I'd ask. But by the time I'd gotten a bit farther I would have forgotten again. It just isn't worth it, so I stay home now. You do what you have to, but it sure makes the days longer."

Change in Phone or Correspondence Patterns

The telephone and correspondence is used by both homebound and mobile older persons to maintain human contacts. The risk of loneliness increases when either of these resources changes. Loss of use of the phone may occur because of financial reasons or memory failure.

> An 83-year-old man, who had been an independent bachelor all his life and is in a nursing home following surgery complains bitterly, "I can't write my own letters; I forget how to end the sentences I start. I can't even call my friends on the phone. I have the number written down but I can't remember which numbers I've dialed . . ." He weeps in anger and frustration.

Loss of ability to write or failure of others to respond to letters creates more loneliness and a sense of abandonment. Special occasions such as birthdays, anniversaries, and holidays are times when there is high risk of feeling neglected and unloved.

Illness and Incapacity

Actual illness and disability, or even a negative view of one's health, have been found to increase the risk of loneliness. Thus, with an increase in signs and symptoms, or when the patient complains of poorer health, the nurse needs to be alert to loneliness even though relationships with others have not outwardly changed. It is as if there is an increased awareness that an individual must ultimately experience pain and disability alone (see Chapter 27, Pain).

Time

Loneliness tends to occur or increase at particular times of the day, or week, or year. Of elderly subjects who were interviewed about their experiences with loneliness, 45 percent were most lonely at a certain time of the day, 25 percent on a certain day of the week, and 27 percent at a certain time of the year. Evenings, Sundays, and Christmas were most consistently mentioned (Hood, 1974). The elderly offered several reasons for being lonely; most reasons involved changing relationships.

I miss the people at work.

The dinner hour is the worst when no one comes home to eat with me.

. . . . . when my friend used to visit.

. . . . . when I used to get up and get tea for my wife.

Wintertime when the nights are long and I can't get out. The days are grey and everything is depressing.

Christmas morning when we used to have a potluck breakfast and swap presents.

Sundays when I used to be able to go to church, and I think of the family dinners we always had afterwards.

Nurses who are aware of peak periods of loneliness or who can anticipate times of higher risk should plan with the individual, the family, or others to try to develop some resources or strategies to cope with the specific problem.

Other Factors

Several additional etiologic factors have been found to be associated with loneliness. Women are found to be more socially isolated and lonely than men (Tunstall, 1966; Palmore, 1971). There are conflicting data on whether loneliness increases with *age.* Maddox found it did while Hood's respondents said it didn't (Maddox, 1973; Hood, 1974). Older persons who *live alone* were reported in one study to be four times more likely to be lonely than those who lived with others (Tunstall, 1966). Moving from an adequate to an *inadequate income* brings greater risks of loneliness, as does a pattern of being *easily bored. Chronic alcoholism* also produces intense loneliness (see Chapter 11).

Dynamics

The need for human intimacy exists in human beings from cradle to grave. It is a basic need that ranks just above physiologic and safety needs in Maslow's hierarchy (1943); and it forms the foundation for the two higher level needs associated with accomplishing the developmental tasks (self-esteem and self-actualization). Since developmental tasks continue throughout life, the importance of satisfying needs to give and receive love do not abate with added years. It is as important after 70 as it was at 7.

Intimacy

Intimacy is a concept that characterizes a type of human relationships. The dictionary suggests such synonyms as "familiar, close, very dear, confidential, homelike, deepseated, confident, special." Verwoerdt identifies five qualities of an intimate relationship that may serve as a useful guide to nurses and other health providers when they attempt to help patients or their families meet needs for intimacy. According to Verwoerdt (1976, p. 256), a relationship that is to adequately fulfill a human's need for intimacy must meet the following criteria:

A sense of belonging	I to you, you to me, we belong to each other. There is a sense of fit and harmony.
Familiarity	Nothing new is intimate.
Repetition	It is a repetition of previous experiences and a desire for ongoing or future repetitions, not a brief encounter.
Sameness	A sense of flowing unchanged through time, binding past to present to future. It has no clock or calendar.
Sharing	Of material, time, space, and each other.

All of this suggests a quality of constancy. Continued replacement of sources of interaction, even caring interaction, does not constitute an intimate relationship, even though it may be the best one can do. This concept gives a rationale for maintaining as much stability, continuity, and predictability as possible to relationships, even those of health care providers.

Loneliness

Loneliness, the experience of deprivation of desired and needed human intimacy, can affect the elderly in at least two major directions. It causes personal suffering in the loss or absence of someone to care for and from whom caring can be received. Second, failure to have the foundation of love means that energy must be directed to meeting this more basic need or coping with the deficit rather than in accomplishing the developmental tasks of the later years.

QUALITATIVE. Loneliness involves both qualitative and quantitative elements. If available relationships fail to satisfy the recipient, there is a qualitative deficit. Thus an older person may be acutely lonely in the midst of a family gathering or with others who presumably could offer caring personal encounters. This includes nursing personnel.

> Upon returning from a vacation, the nursing director of a nursing home made rounds among the residents as early in the day of her return as they were awake and fed. Each resident was warmly greeted—some were hugged, others just touched. There was a sharing of experiences each had during the interval since they were last together—questions and answers—animated conversation where the residents could speak but, none the less, natural where they could not. The director was asked about each of her relatives, the wedding, the reunion-picnic—all the events she had told them about before she left. She, in turn, asked about the people and events in their lives. Later she told a nurse who was visiting, "I'm a part, sometimes all, of their family. Most of these people will be here the rest of their lives. They need someone to love who loves them."

QUANTITATIVE. Deprivation may also have a quantitative dimension. Contacts, when they occur, may be most satisfying, but may be so infrequent as to cause long periods of loneliness between. When both elements of deprivation—quantitative and qualitative—are present, the older person is truly lonely.

TIME ELEMENT. There is an element of time in loneliness—the past, the present, the future. The discomfort of loneliness may be generated by a *current situation*—recent losses, present unsatisfactory relationships, absences of sources of genuine intimacy. It also can be a flashback phenomenon when *recall of earlier lonely times* causes anew the signs and symptoms. Anniversaries of events—marriages, births, deaths, family celebrations, retirement—and holidays are times of high risk of loneliness generated by recall, particularly for individuals who have been married and have had children or close relations with a family.

Fear of future loneliness produces threat and anxiety. Illness in a cherished person, attending funerals of friends' mates or relatives, and reading the obituaries can trigger anxiety over future losses and attendant loneliness. How many individuals atend a funeral and weep, not for the loss of the deceased person, but for the thought of their own potential losses? The mere fact of aging brings all realistically closer to death and threats of separation. With reduced sources and opportunities for intimacy, any threat of loss is truly anxiety producing.

CONTAGION. Since everyone needs some degree of human intimacy, all are vulnerable. Thus the suffering of loneliness is contagious. It is a threat and it is anxiety producing; therefore it is alienating. *No one is safe from the threat of loneliness.* Encounters with acutely lonely people, either directly or vicariously through books, poetry, drama, music, movies, or television can create anxiety as the awareness of personal vulnerability occurs. Widows can attest to the fact that they are not as genuinely welcome in social gatherings with their married friends as they were when they were wives, even though these same people obviously still care for them.

This contagious feature of loneliness, produced by contacting lonely persons or even knowing of their loneliness, is an inhibiting force in bringing relief. Persons who might be a source of comfort may engage in distancing maneuvers during encounters in order to avoid being swept up themselves in the other person's loneliness. They may keep busy with other things, behave in a neutral or professional manner, maintain physical distances (avoiding touch or eye contact), or carry on a hearty superficial conversation that only mimics caring and blocks deeper contacts. Beyond this superficial charade, people may decrease or avoid altogether personal contacts. Even phone calls may become fewer. It is easy to deny or rationalize distancing behavior—for professionals particularly. But it does not do much to help the lonely patient deal with his problem.

DENIAL. Because of its threatening and alienating features, loneliness may evoke a denial response. People who experience it acutely are unable to talk about it during the episode or even afterward. Sullivan (1953) indicated that loneliness is so dreaded and so painful that it is avoided, disguised, or goes unnoticed. Therefore, one might predict that the direct complaints of loneliness are in inverse relationship to the suffering being experienced—the greater the suffering the more obscure and disguised the complaints. It takes astute observation of subtle cues to diagnose the problem. The same relationship holds true for the families or friends of the lonely person, and health professionals; all may deny a person's loneliness in order to protect themselves from the pain of the victim or to avoid appearing to be calloused toward a need they may feel unable or unwilling to meet.

Summary

Loneliness, then, is a deficiency syndrome, a deficit in desired and needed human intimacy for which there is no compensation. It may be related to past, present, or future deprivations. It may generate anxiety in others because of their vulnerability and, thus, prevent the kind of helpful encounters needed to alleviate the victim's suffering. Denial and dissociation are strong features that may mark or distort identifying cues.

Differential Diagnosis

Loneliness needs to be differentiated from two similar conditions—aloneness (or solitude) and lonesomeness.

ALONENESS. Aloneness exists when one is without company. It may be a mental or emotional separation, e.g., making a personal decision alone. Or, it may be a physical separation from others on a temporary or long term basis. Often the status is a chosen one, deliberately sought in order to increase concentration and productivity (Peplau, 1955). Persons who have experienced sensory overload may seek respite in aloneness. Discomfort at being without company, if any, is mild. Some individuals are comfortably solitary in nature.

LONESOMENESS. Lonesomeness is a status in which one is without the company of others, as in aloneness. The differentiating feature is that the individual recognizes a wish to be with others. Lonesomeness may occur when one is alone or with others. It reflects a desire to be closer to others. Because the discomfort usually is mild to moderate, it is a recognizable, acceptable status and,therefore, can be reported directly. Usually the individual is capable of resolving the situation and creating more desirable conditions.

Signs and Symptoms

Loneliness as a subjective state must be diagnosed either on the basis of the person's report or on associated indirect behavior. As suggested earlier,

the lonely person and significant others may avoid awareness of loneliness or be too frightened to approach it directly. Therefore, the nurse needs to be alert to those factors in the presenting situation that suggest high risk (see etiologic factors) in addition to being alert to subtle, indirect cues.

Time Oriented Complaints

The lonely person may give cues such as he is only enduring the present, time hangs heavy on his hands, or he is waiting for a change. The nurse may hear comments such as:

The days are so long now. Why, I can remember when I didn't have enough hours.

I just put in my days.

Sundays are hard days for me.

I don't sleep well and the nights are long.

The winters seem longer than they used to be.

I'm just putting in my time until I can go too.

Abandonment

The sense of abandonment can be related to the death of someone close or to a lack of attention from those with whom he wishes a closer relationship.

John left me (died) just a year ago today.

I don't see the children very often. They're so busy, you know.

People don't care for old people the way they used to. We're put on the shelf.

They are doing the best they can. They mean well, but they're so busy with . . . . .

I never get any letters any more. People have forgotten me.

. . . . . they never even phone me.

Signs

Beyond the reports indicating the enduring of time and the sense of being abandoned, there are signs that, taken together, should suggest a diagnosis of loneliness. Patients or others may report:

- A deviation from the usual approaches in activities or pace of activities. They may become frantically busy or sit back and do nothing, avoiding usual, even routine, activities of daily living.
- Increased talkativeness or unusual silences and lack of attention to input from others.
- Becoming ill as contrasting to previous good health.
- Greater intensity in previous symptoms reported or the reporting itself may become more insistent.
- Inability to concentrate or to stay with a task or activity—flitting from one activity to another without getting much done; restlessness.
- Increased irritability.
- Reporting of a sense of unreality or depersonalization.
- Postponement or avoidance of necessary decisions.
- Increased requests for clinic visits/efforts to prolong visits.

Roberts in her book on care of the critically ill (1976) speaks of "curling up" physically or, when this is impossible, psychologically in the face of extreme loneliness, as if to close out the people and the environment that seem to have closed them out.

Manifestations of Associated Problems

The problem of loneliness can in turn generate other problems or responses. Anxiety, depression, and anger, or a combination of these may be seen.

Anxiety

The symptoms of anxiety may range from mild to a near state of panic. Peplau (1955) associated the following cluster of manifestations with the four levels.

With *mild anxiety* the individual is more alert than normally. Learning ability is increased. Concentration and problem-solving ability are heightened. The individual is restless but there is no interference with motor skills.

Moderate anxiety is accompanied by a decrease in field of perception with concentration on specific areas; however, attention can be diverted to another area. Learning ability is less, but the individual can

still engage in problem solving to handle the anxiety. There may be complaints of butterflies in the stomach, headache, increased muscle tension, more perspiration, and insomnia, particularly in the earlier part of the night.

In *severe anxiety* there is further narrowing of perception with attention focused on a few specific details or on scattered details. In the area of problem solving, the person is unable to relate specifics to the whole. He may experience dread, awe, or horror. Physically, he may have headaches, dizziness, nausea, and heavy perspiration.

The most severe form is *panic*. In this state of anxiety there is not only very narrowed perceptual ability but also possible distortion. The individual may be unable to communicate verbally and may appear immobilized or engage in random movements.

Anxiety in loneliness is most often associated with anticipated bereavement or loss as well as early stages of loneliness. As the situation becomes more prolonged, the mood may shift toward a predominant one of depression.

Depression

Depression may be both a cause of and a response to loneliness. It is characterized by clusters of the following signs and symptoms:

1. Sadness, brooding; fatigue inappropriate to activity; inability to concentrate.
2. Loss of interest in formerly pleasurable activities, e.g., "I don't care much about that any more." (Family and friends may notice this before the patient does.)
3. Anorexia—food becomes tasteless "like brown cardboard," weight loss.
4. Headaches, particularly in the occipital region.
5. Insomnia characterized by waking in the early hours. (Insomnia of this type is characteristic for about two thirds of the depressed persons; hypersomnia may be present in others.)
6. Feeling worse in the morning.
7. "Shut down" in terms of activities and decision making.

(For more extensive discussion of differential diagnosis and management of depression from a generalist clinician's perspective see both Talley and

Diamon in the March 1977 issue of *Patient Care.* The articles include flow charts for decision making in diagnosing and treating depression.)

Anger

Another response to loneliness is anger—depression turned outward. When an individual feels himself powerless to alleviate his loneliness, he may move from depression to anger. It may be seen as behavior aimed at hurting or humiliating others verbally or physically. This may take the form of complaining, needling, sarcasm, making demands, scolding, or more physical behavior. Sometimes it is directed at a scapegoat and, at times, that scapegoat may be the nurse.

Anger carries some risk for the lonely person because it may further alienate persons who might be a means of reducing his discomfort. Nurses need to be particularly aware of the scapegoat phenomenon and deal with the behavior as a symptom of the problem rather than perceive it as a personal assault and reject the lonely, angry person, thus causing further alienation.

Prognosis

The prognosis of the lonely person is formulated on the basis of risk factors, much as cardiac disease. *Poor prognosis* is associated with being in ill health or having a negative view of one's health; being housebound; living alone; having inadequate money; having been happily married; and having a history of being easily bored.

Good prognosis of being able to cope with loneliness is associated with being in reasonably good health or having a positive view of one's health even if it is not good; being able to get out of the house; having an adequate income; having been single; being a male; having meaningful time-occupying activities, i.e., asking others to stop by, calling others, writing letters, or saying you are lonely; having a pet; living in a low risk neighborhood with adequate transportation; and sharing housing.

Feeling busy, having interests one can engage in, having the opportunity, ability, and resources to develop a satisfying relationship with at least one person or person surrogate (e.g., pet) seems to be a positive factor in a prognosis for recovery from loneliness.

Nursing Management

Prevention

The nurse should identify risk factors, discuss sources of strength and coping patterns, and work on change within resources. Prevent it—you have been given clues as to high risk—and intervene early.

With loneliness, a condition that so frequently generates denial, it is not surprising that older persons have few ideas as to how lonely persons can be helped by others. Almost two thirds of Hood's respondents (1974) said either that they did not know how one could help or that no one could help. This suggests that, if help is to be given, the initiative must come from an external source rather than to anticipate recognition of the problem or delineation of types of assistance coming from the lonely older person.

Nursing management of loneliness should never take a shotgun approach. Loneliness is a concept, but problems that individuals have with loneliness are specific; therefore, any intervention needs to be based on a validated diagnosis of the presence of loneliness plus:

1. Designation of the nature of the deficit in human intimacy in this presenting situation, e.g., loss of a major source, relationships with specific significant individuals that are not satisfying, barriers to desired social contacts.
2. Times of greatest discomfort or risk.
3. Goals the person has for human intimacy.
4. Current coping behaviors.
5. Usable support systems.

When data in these areas have been organized the patient's problem with loneliness should be pretty specifically defined and the desired goal and the patient's current management or degree of lack of it should be noted. Then the nurse and the patient (when he is capable of participating) can develop realistic goals and options for action.

Some of the areas of intervention the nurse may be expected to address are delineated in the following sections, together with some options that may be considered.

Time

Data on the hours and days of greatest vulnerability are needed to develop the timing for intervention. For example, many communities have "Friendly Phoner or Visitor" programs, and the nurse's input on timing may enable these agencies to either get or use data of this nature to encourage volunteers to make contact at the times of greatest risk. Relatives, too, may be made aware of times of greatest risk when the need for human contact is the greatest.

For older persons who are able to engage in activities or get about, "keeping busy" at times of high risk of loneliness has been a defense strategy that some older persons reportedly have found helpful (Lopata, 1971; Hood, 1974). Some of the activities cited include:

- busyness with "work" (housework, cooking, gardening, etc.)
- hobbies
- sports
- walking
- shopping (buying only one thing so there will be an excuse to go again)
- initiating a contact with someone else by phone or letter
- reading
- playing cards (solitaire)
- doing jigsaw or crossword puzzles
- watching television
- praying, meditating
- planning a future event or reminiscing on a past happy event.

A small number in these studies withdrew from the discomfort of loneliness by sleeping, eating, or drinking alcohol.

In order to defend against a bad experience in the matter of particular holidays or anniversary days, it is important to be aware of how these days were formerly observed. For instance, a general Christmas party may do nothing for the individual who never commemorated it that way.

The nurse, given the demands of time, may not be able to participate in the events, or even the specific planning, but may help the individual himself cope more effectively or may involve other support systems of family and community.

Transportation

Here, too, the specific coping deficit must be delineated. The acquisition of a transit pass may help a mobile lonely person without funds, but it won't help the person who needs escort service to and from a bus stop or the grocery store because of the high risk neighborhood. If external escort service is not available, some suggestions for buddies or carpools may help in some circumstances.

Where the long term car owner/driver loses the right to a driver's license because of physical condition or loses the car because of expense or giving in to the children's insistence, the nurse needs to determine what needs the individual is experiencing in learning to use public transportation (building new habits, vision, geography of bus routes, location of stops, and so forth). Strategies for coping with shopping and getting to appointments and social events are important also. The reversal of role from offering transportation to asking for it may require some discussion or role playing to work through problems. The "independents" and the givers are not always good in dependent or receiving roles.

If the community, church, or volunteer groups provide rides, linkage with these support systems may be made. If there are options in long term care facilities or retirement apartments, consideration of transportation to family, friends, or an acceptable diversion source should be considered. There are groups who provide volunteer drivers, a carpool with a driver and his regular passengers, paid by Medicaid not Medicare.

Bereavement

Giving the individual support in the work of grieving, helping him bridge the gap, and later repeopling his world are three aspects of nursing management when a major source of human intimacy has been lost. In some communities there are "solo" rap groups for widows, widowers, and newly-single persons. Here, because others understand and share the experience through their own loss, mutual help emerges. Nurses often have been involved in organizing such groups. Or, knowing of them, they help the bereaved person move into them.

Where these support systems do not exist, the individual may be linked with another person whom he may call when things get bad. Although it doesn't relieve the suffering, helping the person and his family understand the nature and work of grieving, does lend perspective and a sense of its normality and necessity. When the work of grieving is not completed initially, it tends to reappear. As difficult as it is, grieving should not be avoided. Anywhere from three weeks to three months has been cited as a normal time period for working through bereavement.

Lonely Meals

In studies of nutrition among the elderly, the problem often has been found to be loneliness rather than food or money. Women who have always cooked for husbands, families, or housemates are highly vulnerable to loneliness at meal times. The person whose mate, or sibling, always ate meals with him, and faced him across the table, feels his loneliness with an empty chair facing him.

Nurses in retirement complexes have been facilitators of setting up systems where individuals trade off providing meals and form groups for eating together. Some widows in church groups, for whom Sunday dinners and the afternoon are particularly lonely, have begun rotating this meal at their various residences.

The nurse's role is in gathering the data on significant meals and possible resources or support systems, and then, working through the individual family, or others, testing alternative plans. Some schools and churches sponsor group meals (see Chapter 9, Nutrition).

Repeopling Their World

Older persons have been found to be most often lonely for someone who is deceased. Helping them to "repeople" their world and to develop new roles and relationships is one form of management. Day care centers, senior centers, rap groups, senior citizens groups in churches, and classes open to older persons on college campuses are some means of making new contacts.

Companions of the same age seem to be as important to older persons as to younger people. Single persons living with siblings have been found to be less lonely than those whose siblings are not alive or near. In some studies, living children were able to lessen loneliness (Shanas, 1973; Tunstall, 1966), while in another this was not significantly related to the amount of loneliness reported (Hood, 1974). Females tend to find relief with their families; males more with friends. However, for either sex, living alone has been found to increase the likelihood of loneliness.

Retirement communities offer one option for repeopling one's life; sharing housing with someone is another form. Some older folks are trying a communal form of living to provide companionship, safety, and reduced expenses. The nurse can help in brainstorming options, examining pros and cons, and implementing decisions.

Nursing personnel who work in long term care settings have an opportunity to offer a dependable and predictable caring presence to patients—if they can maintain their own well springs in the process. Nurses who have "charge" responsibilities in these settings have the task of serving as the role model and of helping young unskilled persons understand that care for these older persons involves treatment of their loneliness while they are ambulating, turning, changing, feeding, and cleaning. Staff development sessions to enable them to participate effectively in this activity may be supportive.

The same role may be possible in a more episodic fashion with the nurse who functions in ambulatory and home health care settings where she is helping the patient to manage his health problems and activities of daily living on the phone or in a visit.

People Substitutes

Pets sometimes serve as surrogates for human intimacy, although they can be a bother too. They are available as a source of comfort during the high risk evening and night hours or the Sunday afternoons when others are busy. Where human contacts are limited and where the person's lifestyle and finances could accommodate a pet, this may be an effective way to offer a dependable living presence and help the person occupy his time. The pet owner can feel needed, and often there is a source of dependable affection. Some humane societies donate pets to persons over 65. If pets are given as a gift, be certain of the person's preference. Don't give a cat to a dog lover.

Reducing Distancing Behavior

A nurse may make a major contribution to solving the patient's problem of loneliness by diagnosing distancing maneuvers in herself and others as they relate to the lonely person. Being aware of the dynamics of each person's vulnerability to the threat of loneliness as a basis for a natural desire to avoid contact can help a person understand the basis for the behavior. It may also reduce the guilt that further alienates family members and health care providers. Then it is possible to explore ways of reducing the need to distance oneself.

In the same vein, the anger response of the lonely person needs to be interpreted as a symptom of frustration and powerlessness in his efforts to deal with the cause of the loneliness. Individuals also need to understand how it may be disguised or applied to scapegoats. Often, when recipients of the angry behavior understand that it is a response to feeling helpless, they are more willing to respond in a caring rather than retaliatory manner, thus moving toward rather than away from the lonely person. There are times when a person needs another individual with whom it is safe to be angry. Where there is anger, at least it shows the individual is still in there working—not giving up.

Depression

Current thinking on the management of reactive depression (grieving over loss) is that interpersonal support is the preferred form of therapy. Antidepressives are not seen as therapeutic and may only cause a delayed response.

Where a diagnosis is made of endogenous depression (deficiency in neurotransmitters that facilitate conduction of nerve impulses across synapses), pharmacologic management using tricyclic antidepressants is seen as therapy of choice. Endogenous depression may occur with loneliness or may be a cause of loneliness as others avoid the depressed person. The following symptoms occurring in clusters should alert a health care provider to consider endogenous depression in addition to whatever other presenting complaints may be present:

1. Sleep disturbances characterized by early awakening.
2. Generalized headache in the occipital region.
3. Chronic pain (depressive equivalent).
4. No energy—fatigue unrelated to work and unrelieved by rest.
5. Weight loss.
6. Emotional state of sadness—hopelessness.
7. Psychomotor slowing usually associated with depression.

Tricyclic antidepressants cause significant common side effects. The side effects include dry mouth, urinary hesitancy (especially among the elderly), transient mild dissociation, constipation, postural hypotension, ejaculation or other potency disturbances, sweating, tachycardia, flushing, drowsiness, muscular twitching tremor, paresthesia, weakness,

fatigue, headache, nausea, and heartburn. Since tricyclic drugs present major side effects in the first weeks of treatment, while usually failing to show desired effects until the third week, patients need to be alerted to both the expected symptoms and the need to be patient and continue taking the drug despite lack of relief. Practitioners have found it helpful to tell patients that a few lucky people will begin to feel better in a week or two but the majority do not get results for about three weeks. This regimen often is a long term one; thus patients also need to know that the medication replaces a chemical deficiency and, therefore, is nonaddictive.

Complications

The signs and symptoms of loneliness may result in a positive feedback cycle whereby those who might relate to the person become so uneasy that they reduce contact, and so the person is more deprived of human intimacy than before. Multiple losses and changes associated with them have been associated with near-future illness likelihood (Rahe, 1972).

Suicide, fast or slow, is another complication that cannot be ignored. Sometimes those patients who are so lonely they "wish they could die" will attempt to accomplish this in an acute or chronic fashion.

Evaluation

Response to intervention (or nonintervention) may be evaluated in terms of abatement or continuation of the manifestations. When persons begin to regain their previous affect and lifestyle and when they report being happier, having more enjoyable encounters with others, being busier, and being able to get more done and concentrate more easily, then improvement is being made. They may have fewer complaints that days or evenings are too long. They may report sleeping better, eating better, gaining weight, being less tired, or having fewer headaches. They may make fewer demands on the health care system and be less intense in reporting their symptoms.

Significant others may report enjoying the persons more, wanting to be with them more, or, at least, finding it easier to be with them. One might hear comments that they are "more like their old selves."

Where signs and symptoms of loneliness persist

or increase, the intervention is not succeeding or the loneliness is not going away by itself.

BIBLIOGRAPHY

Bacon, M. H.: Why the old are getting mad. Saturday Rev. of Society 1:4, 1973.

Berblinger, K.: A psychiatrist looks at loneliness. Psychosomatics 9:96–102, 1968.

Bowman, C.: Loneliness and social change. Am. J. Psychiatry 112:194–198, 1955.

Buhler, C.: Loneliness in maturity. J. Humanistic Psychol. Fall 1969.

Diamond, S., et al.: 9 experts review an FP's (Family Practitioner) depression regimen. Patient Care 11:20–41, 42–77, 1977.

Frankl, V. E.: Man's Search for Meaning. Boston: Beacon Press, 1963.

Fromm, E.: The Art of Loving. New York: Harper & Row, 1972.

Fromm-Reichmann, F.: Loneliness. Psychiatry 22:1–16, 1959.

Goldman, G. D.: The lonely person. Group Psychotherapy 8:247–253, 1955.

Gorer, G.: The American People. New York: W. W. Norton, 1948, p. 130. As cited by F. Fromn-Reichmann in Loneliness. Psychiatry 22:1–16, 1959.

Greer, I. M.: Roots of loneliness. Pastoral Psychology 4, 1953.

Guptan, M.: An interruption in loneliness: The use of concrete objects in promotion of human relations. J. Psychiatr. Med. 9:23, 1971.

Holmes, T., et al.: Experimental study of prognosis. J. Psychosom. Res. 5:235–252, 1961.

Hood, P. H.: Perceived Loneliness Among the Aged and Associated Factors. Unpublished Master's Thesis, University of Washington, Seattle, 1974.

Howell, A., and Loeb, M. B.: Nutrition and aging. A monograph for practitioners. Gerontologist, Part II, 9:3, 1969.

Hurlbut, K.: The loneliness of suffering. Can. Nurse 61:299, 1965.

Knight, T.: Loneliness: A clinical nursing problem. In Maloney, E. (ed): Interpersonal Relations. Dubuque IA: William C. Brown Co., 1966.

Lopata, H. Z.: Widowhood in an American city. Cambridge, Mass.: Shenkinan Publishing Co., 1973.

Lopata, H. Z.: Loneliness: Forms and components. Family 35:2, 1971.

Maddox, G. L.: Themes and issues in sociological theories of human aging. In Brantl, V. M., and Brown, Sister M. R.: Readings in Gerontology. Saint Louis: C. V. Mosby, 1973.

Maslow, A.: A theory of human motivation. Psychologic Rev. 50:370–396, 1943.

Moustakas, C.: Loneliness. Englewood Cliffs, NJ: Prentice-Hall, 1971.

Munnicks, J.: Loneliness, isolation and social relations in old age. Vita Humana 7:228–238, 1964.

Palmore, E.: Variables related to needs among the aged poor. J. Gerontol. 26(4):524–531, 1971.

Paul, H., et al.: Rx for loneliness: A plan for establishing a social network of individualized caring through caring. Crisis Intervention, 4(3):63–83, 1972.

Peplau, H.: Loneliness. Am. J. Nurs. 55:1476, 1955.

Rahe, R. H.: Subjects' recent life changes and their near-future illness reports. Ann. Clin. Res. 4:250–265, 1972.

Reisman, D.: The Lonely Crowd. New Haven: Yale University Press, 1950.

Roberts S.: Loneliness. In Behavioral Concepts and Nursing Throughout the Life Span. Englewood Cliffs, NJ: Prentice-Hall, 1977.

Roberts, S.: Behavioral Concepts and the Critically Ill Patient. Englewood Cliffs, NJ: Prentice-Hall, 1976.

Shanas, E.: Family-kin networks and aging in cross-cultural perspective. J. Marriage Family 35(3): 505–511, 1973.

Steig, W.: The Lonely Ones. New York: Duel Sloan and Pearce, 1942.

Sullivan, H. S.: The Interpersonal Theory of Psychiatry. New York: W. W. Norton, 1953.

Talley, J.: Treat depression as the curable disease it is. Patient Care 11:20–41, 42–47, 1977.

Tanner, I.: The aloneness and loneliness of the aged. In Fear of Love. New York: Harper Row, 1973.

Tunstall, J.: Old and Alone: A Sociological Study of Old People. London: Routledge and Kegan Paul, 1966.

Van Slambrook, M.: Boredom and loneliness in growing old. Geriatric Nursing April, 1968. pp. 3–4.

Van Zonneveld, R. J.: The Health of the Aged. Assen, Netherlands: Van Gorcum and Company, Ltd., 1961.

Verwoerdt, A.: Clinical Geropsychiatry. Baltimore: Williams and Wilkins, 1976.

Von Witzleben, H.: On loneliness. Psychiatry 21: 37–43, 1958.

Weigert, E.: Loneliness and trust—Basic factors of human existence. Psychiatry 23, 1960.

Zilboorg, G.: Loneliness. Atlantic Monthly, 45–54, 1938.

26

Losses of Aging

Caroline Preston

QUICK REVIEW

LOSSES OF AGING

DESCRIPTION	The older individual is deprived of valued attributes, relationships, and property at an increasing rate and intensity; this threatens or overwhelms the ability to adapt and reintegrate.
ETIOLOGIC FACTORS	Threat of or actual decrements of energy, functional capacity, status, roles, financial resources, mobility, beauty, opportunities, control, and so forth disrupt the older person's well-being.
HIGH RISK	Increased frequency and intensity of losses adds to risk of inability to make adjustments. Vulnerability in losses is increased if individual lacks skills, interests, and resources for making friends; adequate financial resources; or a positive perception of health.
DYNAMICS	Loss is based on deprivation in present as compared to past. Intensity of loss is based on the value the individual placed on that which is lost. Time and energy required for grieving and reintegration are not available for other tasks of ADL. Where intensity and frequency of losses overwhelm coping resources, disintegration of coping and lifestyle occurs.
SIGNS AND SYMPTOMS	Alluding to or reporting of losses (may be indirect or covert). Denying losses or using overcompensating behavior. Anger at persons, system, self. Depression, withdrawal, apathy, anorexia, fatigue in conjunction with data on actual or suspected losses.
COMPLICATIONS	Depression, sensory deprivation, feelings of worthlessness, fatigue, suicide.
PROGNOSIS	Dependent on intensity and frequency of losses, previous ability to "make do," perceived health status, financial status, and ability and resources for repeopling his world.
MANAGEMENT	Support productive patterns of delaying losses or dealing with them—denial, acknowledging but ignoring them, making do, finding substitutes. Encourage and participate in reminiscing. Accept and help person and family understand the losses the person is experiencing (if denial is not being used or is used ineffectively). Help person and family understand the time needed for grief work (for intrapersonal losses as well as interpersonal) and its impact on affect, energy, and decision making. Develop ADL plans that take grief work into account.

Continued on next page.

EVALUATION	Individual and family behavior that delays or defends against losses or compensates for them. Individual and family adjustments in lifestyle to accommodate to the grief work. Acceptance of older individual's grief associated with intrapersonal losses as legitimate. Effective utilization of personal, environmental support systems. Evidence of reintegration and restitution.

Although losses are not unique to old age, a fact of the human condition is that losses not only occur with greater frequency and greater intensity as one ages but also can compound disastrously. Avoiding losses, delaying them, adapting to them and making restitution for them can be demanding, and sometimes overwhelming. Yet coping with loss remains the salient developmental task in the aging process. This task includes coping with the increasingly imminent and crucial loss of the self in death. (Since Chapters 25 and 28 on loneliness and powerlessness deal with interpersonal losses, the focus of this chapter is *intrapersonal* losses.)

Loss can be defined as giving up or having something of value taken from one. Intrapersonal losses in aging include energy, functional capacity, status, material wealth, the richness of one's sensory environment, beauty, roles, opportunities, control, a variety of other areas of possession, and, as stated previously, the loss of self in death.

In helping older persons live with actual losses or the threat of them, nurses are concerned with:

- The person's definition of the loss
- The person's concern regarding potential losses
- Objective data indicating loss or risk of loss
- The significance of loss to the person
- The impact it has on his daily living and lifestyle
- The response in coping with losses, both past and present

The value the person attaches to the area within which the loss occurs will determine in part the intensity of the deprivation experienced and will be a factor in the response to and evaluation of the effectiveness of nursing intervention.

Areas of High Risk

Losses of an intrapersonal nature are those associated with being an aging person in a technologic society in which people not only age, but obsolesce in deteriorating bodies and in vague rolelessness. The physical losses and the consequent decreases in independence make for an ever-dwindling array of choices and control over one's life. (See Powerlessness, Chapter 28.) The following vignettes, in the words of the elderly themselves, illustrate areas at high risk of loss in the elderly.

Loss of Mobility

As discussed in Chapter 25, loss of mobility is common in the elderly, whether it pertains to transportation or to physical deterioration which inhibits mobility.

A woman with glaucoma remarks: "Even if I could see to drive, I don't have the strength to carry in the groceries. If I try to, I tremble so with fatigue, it takes me hours to get enough strength to prepare a meal."

A woman has this to say about traveling: "When you are in your 60s, the first freedom of retirement is great. But, by the time you get to the mid-70s, you begin to lose courage. What if you are far from home and get sick, leave your purse somewhere, have your passport stolen. You begin to wonder if you are sharp enough for decisions or emergencies. Or, if you do go on traveling, you begin to feel like that poor Flying Dutchman who can't ever go home until he finds someone to love him."

Loss of Diversion

Many lonely hours are spent when there is not a variety of things to do, especially if the person led an active, diversified life.

> Another woman who had always delighted in her fine handiwork, says, "How can I fill the hours of the day now that my sight is going? What is there to do beside sit in front of the television and doze the days away. Then all night I have nightmares—I don't need the sleep—I have had enough already."

Loss of Communication

The loss of the ability to reach out to others, or communicate with them, is frightening and depressing, and many times that loss increases with age.

> A man says of his hearing loss and the aid he wears unhappily, "I used to think people were mumbling to keep me from knowing the bad things they were saying about me. Now, when I turn up my aid I can hear voices, but I also hear all the other sounds and scratches. These are painful to my ears."

Loss of Resistance to Disease and Trauma

Increasing bouts of illness and days in bed or the hospital, further sap waning vigor.

> An 80-year-old person laments, "You catch things so much more easily and get over them more slowly. But the longer you are inactive, the more your strength goes and your appetite. It's a vicious circle of greater and greater vulnerability. In the flu season, you're afraid to leave your apartment for fear of catching something—crowded elevators are especially frightening."

> A woman in her mid-70s comments, "Going down steps, especially without railings, I avoid as much as I can. They say you don't fall and break your hip—rather, your hip breaks and that's why you fall. If you are also unsteady on your feet or dizzy in your head, or the light isn't very good, even a cane isn't much comfort."

Loss of Beauty in Face and Body

Contemporary advertising and television compound the problem of beauty loss with their accent on youth, beauty, and virility. The inevitability of having to exist in an increasing alien, infirm body with sagging, wrinkled skin, is a parody of youthful appearance.

> Of these narcissistic insults, a formerly beautiful 75-year-old woman claims, "When I look in the mirror, there is not the vestige of me left, but I don't really feel as old as I look. That me is still there, somewhere, but it's no longer in my face."

> A sexually-active 80-year-old woman, whose partners tend to be much younger, stated, "I don't like my lovers to see my fat old body. I turn the lights off and get into bed in the dark. I don't think it is so bad for them to feel me but I don't want them to see me."

> A vigorous old man in his 70s remarks, "When I look in the mirror, I am reminded of a cross between a turkey and a bloodhound with my baggy, bloodshot eyes and my chin and neck with flesh folds like wattles. I think about plastic surgery, but who my age could afford it?"

Loss of Sexual Urgency and Orgasmic Capacity

Few old people in the current generation, especially women, are able to discuss losses in the area of sexual function. This is understandable in light of prevailing sexual mores to which they were exposed in their formative years. One wonders, however, if the paucity of material about sexual functioning among the aged may be due to the fact that they are rarely asked to discuss this facet of their existence.

We are mainly indebted to Masters and Johnson's study of the sexual response among the few old subjects included in their sample for information concerning age-associated changes in orgasmic reactions. Masters and Johnson discuss the slower erections, longer refractory phases between copulations, and decreased pressure to ejaculate experienced by men as they age. Women often experience thinning of the vaginal tissue, making intercourse painful. They may also lose the capacity for pleasurable orgasms, and these may even be associated with sudden, severe abdominal pain (Masters and Johnson, p. 197, 241).

> Of his sexuality, one man in his 70s remarks, "After my prostate gland examination, the doctor said I was okay. I wanted to ask how I could keep things okay, keep having the capacity for erections. But I never had a chance to ask."

Loss of Confidence in Cognitive Functions

There are several well-documented changes in problem-solving and learning skills associated with age. The degree to which decrements in these functions are physiologic in origin, or functional, i.e., stem from motivational defects related to anxiety and loss of confidence, is much less clear.

> One older person observed, "I live in a retirement community. Everyday I see people going down hill—being more forgetful, getting lost, not recognizing me. It scares me. When I lose my glasses, lock the keys in the car, forget an appointment—things I have done all my life at one time or another—this is different now. I tell myself, 'Here it comes; here it is' —senility, not creeping up on me but jumping out on me like a beast in the jungle."

> Another elderly person says of efforts to learn a new language, "I enrolled in a Spanish class. Most of the students were decades younger than me. They had no trouble learning about 10 new words each day; I found I couldn't keep up. Finally I gave up and dropped out."

Often couples differ not only in vigor but in the maintenance of cognitive skills.

> One woman, with an older husband, scrutinizes her relationship with him, "I am still eager for new adventures, to acquire new skills—but not my husband. He feels he can't keep up, resents my activities, my leaving him alone. What am I supposed to do? Resign myself to being his nursemaid for the rest of our lives together?"

Loss of First Class Citizenship

Another area of loss is that of being a member of the adult majority. Older persons experience being patronized, ignored, or treated in a "special" way. Many have never experienced being a member of a minority group while others experience being a double minority.

> "When I go to the theater, or to the zoo, or any number of other places and see seniors and children, *half price,* I am ashamed to ask for the bargain. To make it worse, sometimes I am given it without even asking—just one look at my face. Children and seniors—the disfranchised!"

High Risk Populations

While every person experiences losses in the process of aging, the more vulnerable elderly are those who cannot live effectively, comfortably, or stoically with their losses. Individuals at high risk of suffering seriously and making ineffective adjustments, show the following characteristics:

1. Lack skills, interests, and resources for continuing to make friends.
2. Lack adequate economic resources for their usual lifestyle.
3. See themselves as being in poor health.

A lifelong pattern of "making the best of things" seems to foster the weathering of aging losses more effectively.

Manifestations

Loss can be inferred from an unpropitious *change* in the present from circumstances or conditions of the past. Therefore, history is very important in determining the existence and nature of losses. An individual must feel the possession of something valued at one time in order for a significant loss-experience to occur. What is loss to one is not to another. When losses occur or threaten to occur, indicators that the individual is suffering because of them often emerge. Thus the nurse should gather data in the areas known for high risk of losses in aging, or observe cues that indicate suffering associated with loss or threat of loss in assessing the presenting situation.

Subjective Data

The reporting of concerns over losses or concern for potential or imminent losses may be overt. An example is the individual with failing eyesight who is worried about driver's license renewal tests. On the other hand, a loss may be alluded to only in a indirect and obscure manner: "I used to be so active in my garden." "I can't keep up the house the way I did— sad to see it go down hill, but. . . ." "I was head of the fire brigade in this town, during the early years." "I once was able to give the children and grandchildren nice things at Christmas; now I don't even bother with a tree." Some of the losses most personally devastating or demoralizing, however, may be the most difficult to share.

The gathering of subjective data on losses is to touch on sensitive areas; it should be approached carefully by the nurse. Time is needed to learn what is or was of value to the individual. People, including the elderly, do not readily open up and share this kind of information until trust has been built—unless they are desperate. If the nurse confronts the older person with a statement about a loss that has been perceived, even though the observation can be valid, the individual may find it necessary to deny the loss. To acknowledge it at that time may be too painful or devastating. The person's coping resources may not be sufficient at this point. Gathering data on losses requires both patience and sensitivity—a sense of when confronting a loss will be helpful and when it will not.

Objective Data

Objective data also suggests areas of loss, validates losses described in the subjective data, or helps to identify patient reactions to losses. One should note the richness or barrenness of the sensory environment, the contrast between beauty and form in old photographs and present appearance, the roles the individual occupies (or lack of them), and the condition of the immediate environment, activity, mobility, cognitive ability, and finances. All of these circumstances yield concrete data to help determine loss and response to it, if assessed in the context of the individual's earlier life to determine whether a loss in truth exists and what its nature is.

Prognosis

Prognosis is based on the frequency and intensity of losses and their cumulative effect, when new significant losses occur before restitution and adjustment have been accomplished for earlier ones. In addition to the incidence of losses, prognosis is related to resources and past coping styles. Prognosis is improved if at least two of the following three resources are available:

1. Ongoing capacity for making friends and maintaining relationships.
2. Financial status seen as adequate by the person.
3. Physical status viewed as "healthy" or positive by the individual.

Successful aging, including coping with losses, is related to retaining some sense of control—feeling able to "make do" rather than being victimized by events or fate. Careful assessment of just *how much* adaptive change is being required and the resources that are available is essential in predicting prognosis.

Complications

Depression among the aged is serious. Often it is not manifested by the usual symptoms of sadness but, rather, masked by complaints of fatigue, general sense of malaise, sometimes simulating the symptoms of senility, i.e., disorientation, confusion, and memory defects. The depression may result in suicides or suicidal attempts, alcoholism, or poor nutrition. Symptoms of senility often disappear if people are helped to overcome their depression.

Treating chronic illness is not the most rewarding enterprise. Many professionals are reluctant to get involved with the elderly. This is especially true among those professionals who cannot overcome their "rescue fantasies," i.e., those who tend to avoid those they cannot cure because they regard both the patients and themselves as failures if a cure is not established. Mutual discouragement can be hard to avoid and may result in spiraling complaints and/or "shopping" for miracles. Nurses and the elderly persons they serve must be content with small increments of improvement and gain, and must often settle for comfort instead of cure.

Nurses must be alert to the possibility that so much of the patient's energy is or must be invested in the work of mourning that little is available for sustaining most or all of the activities of daily living. The consequences may be anorexia, insomnia, and severely curtailed patterns of activity. A vicious cycle is created that involves increasing sensory deprivation so that cognitive function is in disarray or disuse, which causes inevitable cognitive deterioration.

Prevention and Management

Prevention

Since most intrapersonal losses are part of the aging process, perhaps the only bulwark anyone can erect against devastation or disintegration in the face of such losses is a lifelong effort to develop constructive habits of coping with losses. Denial is seen frequently among the aged, and for some this proves an effective defense. For others the work of mourning can only be postponed but must eventually be performed before reintegration of coping patterns can occur.

Another mechanism for avoiding a painful or empty-from-losses present is reminiscing—recalling times when one had more self-worth and life was more rewarding and pleasant. The repetitiousness of the elderly is not the idle, attention-getting device it appears to be. Repeating stories of one's lifetime is one of the ways in which one confronts the fact that life is nearly over and cannot be relived. Sometimes, in reviewing their lives, older persons are able to re-structure their histories through stories that help to view life from the perspective of many years. Further, it offers the person and others a basis for interaction in terms of earlier successes and roles. In a study of older persons discharged from a hospital in New York, those who seemed to find comfort by liv-ing in the past when the present and future were undeniably bleak tended to survive longer with fewer hospital readmissions than those who focused on the problems of the present and the uncertainties of the future.

Nurses can participate therapeutically not only by fostering reminiscing but also by learning of the individual's earlier achievements and giving recogni-tion for them. Recognizing the function of reminisc-ing and the describing of earlier roles should not be merely tolerated, but actively encouraged as legiti-mate and helpful methods of dealing with a painful present and uncertain future.

Management

The same principles of management outlined in loneliness through interpersonal losses apply to the management of intrapersonal losses. Recognition of the need for time to grieve is essential; expecting normal function or affect during this process is neither helpful nor supportive. The duration of a grief reaction is variable but may extend for months. Acknowledging necessity of mourning and sharing it (rather than engaging in distancing maneuvers) can be helpful.

As soon as the energy to engage in ego-suppor-tive activities begins to re-emerge, people can then begin the process of educating themselves to make restitution for losses. Many older people can be ob-served to initiate such programs for themselves with the encouragement of understanding families and friends. Some may need the intervention of more pro-fessional help in individual or group counseling.

In dealing with the older person who has had exposure to intrapersonal losses, the practitioner or counselor needs to assess available assets and sup-ports. The person can be encouraged to keep a log of daily activities. Such a log can then be useful in assessing current levels of engagement, in pointing up deficiencies in such levels, and in suggesting areas for potential increases in activities and engage-ments with the goal of a gradually expanding pattern of both.

The evidence from longitudinal studies of cogni-tion and the aging process reveals that people who continue to exercise learning skills show few signifi-cant deficits in their learning capacities. The key to the process of making restitution for losses lies in this fact, that people can and do learn new and different coping mechanisms and interest patterns.

Many potential methods of helping people exer-cise their learning capacities are available. First of all, people should be encouraged in every possible way to heighten their involvement in enriching their own lives and those of others. Old age can be con-strued as a time of enormous potential growth and development if the individual embarks on and main-tains intense investment in being alive and free of the responsibility of job and career. One man in his 80s maintains, "if you are willing to put your shoulder to the wheel of the better life for everyone, you can be involved 24 hours a day." The militant Gray Panther, Maggie Kuehn, is exemplary. She mounts the barri-cades in the interests of all humanity, not just the old. The old are the most free to rebel against the status quo; this is not the least of the new careers open to them. Victims of ageism themselves, they can well recognize the work to be done to overcome these stereotypes and achieve full class citizenship status.

For the health professional, the first principle is to recognize the potential strengths in all older peo-ple. They may need guidance in a program of con-sistent physical exercises and in adequate nutrition. The importance of maintaining viable friendships and actively seeking new contacts must be empha-sized. As the SAGE (Clare Luce) program has demon-strated, the old can use all the techniques in our armamentarium toward increased self-esteem and well-being: consciousness raising groups, assertive-ness training, and practice in exercises of being graceful givers and generous receivers and in manag-ing increasing dependency and interdependency needs. Oldsters can learn massage, yoga, breathing exercises, meditation, and relaxation techniques, which appear effective at any age as countermeasures for depression and anxiety.

A noted gerontologist stated, "there is not a sin-gle program geared to improving the mental health of the elderly in the country that has not been a smash-ing success." (Eisdorfer, personal communication.) (See Chapter 29 for program ideas.) The mental health practitioner does well to keep his encouraging outlook for work with the aged in the forefront of his or her interventional programs. The older person must not be written off with the contemptuous dismissal that disheartens so many, "at your age, what can you expect?" The elderly must learn to answer this question, as women have: "everything."

Evaluation

As with the resolution of interpersonal losses, so too with intrapersonal loss, one must depend on observation of what people who experience losses are able to say and do. Alertness to the ebbing of sadness and reawakening of interest and involvement is critical to these developments which must be encouraged and supported. Activity patterns in general, but especially those connected with the activities of daily living, and reinvolvement in the lives of others are probably the most reliable indices of loss-coping behavior. Even people who may be unable to verbalize feelings of devastation or discouragment can begin to engage in behavior that reflects the regaining of a firmer grasp on one's bootstraps. As they begin to experience this control, some people can be openly verbal about an increase in feelings of well-being. It is helpful to give reassurance that it is normal to have setbacks in progress. Resources in the community for the support of older people are one of the most significant consequence of recent social policy and planning. Professionals should be well informed of these developments and encourage older people to take full advantage of the emerging fact that our society no longer tolerates the abandonment and neglect of our older citizens.

REFERENCES

Masters, W. H., and Johnson, V. E.: Human Sexual Response. Boston: Little Brown, 1966.

27

Pain

Dorothy Crowley

QUICK REVIEW

PAIN

DEFINITION	A concept of personal and private sensation of hurt, a set of responses, a signal of harm or potential harm to tissue.
HIGH RISK	Aged persons with multiple moderately severe pathologies or those whose adaptive capacities are already severely taxed.
DIFFERENTIAL DIAGNOSIS	Absence of pain in acute conditions that are normally characterized by pain; depression.
MANIFESTATIONS	Cultural values shape pain behavior and influence attitudes toward pain and the appropriate management of pain.
PROGNOSIS	Prognosis tends to be better if (1) person has confidence in care provider and in mode of management; (2) pain is of short duration; (3) secondary gains from pain are less than the gains of being pain-free; (4) person can become *actively involved* in control of the pain; (5) person can find meaning in the pain.
PREVENTIVE MANAGEMENT	Reduce anxiety and fear; help the person achieve control over the pain and maintain meaningful relations to self, others, environment; support person's strengths and coping abilities; interpose activities incompatible with pain or anxiety responses. In management of recurrent pain, administering medication *before* the pain recurs will reduce anxiety and the amount of analgesic required to control pain.
EVALUATION	Patient's subjective report of decrease in pain intensity; reduction in analgesic intake; increase in activity; evidence of interest in things other than self and pain.

Complaints of pain appear to increase with advancing age. Part of the reason for this is the fact that the incidence of chronic ailments, many of which are associated with pain, is higher. "Body monitoring," a concern with the care of one's body and its functioning, is a common feature of old age (Butler, 1973, p. 34). It serves to make one more aware of aches and pains that might either have gone unnoticed or been dismissed as of no consequence at an earlier stage of life. At the same time, pain imposes an additional strain that may severely tax the ability to cope with it at a stage in life when the person's adaptive capabilities may already be heavily burdened by adjustments required in other aspects of living.

Definition

Although many attempts have been made to define pain, no definition is completely satisfactory, even as we define it for ourselves. Through life experiences, we build up an idea of what it means to hurt, how it feels, how we think others feel when they say, "I hurt," and we observe how we and others behave when hurt. If one is of a reflective bent, one may have been puzzled by the experience of pain—why toothaches hurt worse in the middle of the night; why an injured ankle didn't hurt when one was engrossed in an exciting game; why a child's bump is soothed by mother's kiss; why pain may not seem as severe when another person is present; why similar amounts of trauma may hurt worse in some situations than in others.

In attempting to understand this complex and seemingly paradoxic phenomenon, it may be tempting and, at times, even necessary to think of pain simplistically as a response to a noxious stimulus. One steps on a tack, and it hurts; remove the tack and it feels better. Much of one's experience with pain can be understood within this framework of thought. However, much of what one observes clinically does not fit into this simplistic model.

Sometimes patients fail to complain of pain in the presence of organic pathology or, conversely, complain of pain in the absence of identifiable pathology. Often one can observe very little relationship between the intensity of the stimulation and the intensity of the pain. Patients report relief from pain through use of agents with no known pharmaceutic action; and yet, they may fail to experience relief with drugs of demonstrable pharmaceutic action.

With some of these types of problems in mind, Sternbach has suggested that pain can be considered as ". . . an abstract concept which refers to 1) a personal, private sensation of hurt; 2) a harmful stimulus which signals current or impending tissue damage; 3) a pattern of responses which operate to protect the organism from harm." (Sternbach, 1968, p. 12). Such a definition has the advantage of providing a more comprehensive view of pain, and, hopefully, a view that makes it possible to appreciate some of the clinical manifestations of pain which are difficult to accommodate in a more simplistic stimulus-response model.

As an abstract concept of a personal and private sensation of hurt, pain can be considered as a product of consciousness derived from the processing of sensory data within the central nervous system. To develop such a concept of pain, it is essential that the person (1) has had exposure to noxious stimuli at some time and (2) has a nervous system capable of processing such stimuli. Most persons have repeated exposure to such stimuli in the normal course of living and, over time, develop ways to process the data derived from these experiences so as to provide protection from harm.

As a hurt that is felt, "pain is a single, unified concept." It is neither mental nor physical, nor is it the interaction of the mental and physical, although our attempts to explain or describe the experience resort to the terms of the various disciplines that have been concerned with trying to understand pain (Sternbach, 1968, p. 4).

A part of the concept of pain is the idea of a harmful stimulus that signals tissue damage. The ability to experience pain is an important protective mechanism. Without the ability to perceive pain, one would be in constant jeopardy from one's environment. Nevertheless, even with an intact nervous system, tissue damage can occur without pain, and pain can occur in the absence of tissue damage.

In spite of the fact that nervous pathways that subserve pain have been identified, pain cannot be understood simply as a sequence of tissue damage, stimulation of an end-receptor, and transmission of impulses through certain pathways in the central nervous system.

The concept of pain also encompasses the notion that there is a pattern of responses, which involve the whole organism, to that which is harming or threatens to harm the person. This pattern of responses is influenced not only by the nature of the stimulation but also by the meaning of the stimulation, the context of the situation in which it occurs, and past experiences and associations with pain and the learning that has accompanied these experiences (Benoliel and Crowley, 1973, p. 72).

High Risk Populations or Situations

Aged persons are at risk for the development of chronic pain problems for the following reasons:

1. The years already lived have increased the chances of developing a pathologic condition through disease or trauma that may cause pain.
2. The presence simultaneously of several moderately or mildly painful conditions, any one of which if present singly might be ignored, may lower the persons's threshold for pain.
3. Adaptive capabilities, already taxed by the adjustments imposed by aging, may lower the tolerance of the aged person for pain.

Such factors may serve singly or in unison to make the aged person more vulnerable to the development of pain problems.

On the other hand, some persons as they grow older, seem to cope successfully in spite of increased vulnerability. A recent comment by one octogenarian reflects her views on this point, "I don't know that pain is any different than when I was younger; it feels the same to me. One seems to have more aches and pains, but I notice among some of the older women (that lady you met at the elevator is 95)—they just keep going and don't let it bother them."

Dynamics

Although the aging process affects the experience of pain, so many factors influence pain and the variations between individuals is so great that it is difficult to determine precisely how pain is affected. Degenerative changes related to aging which occur in the skin and peripheral nervous system may affect sensitivity to pain (Schludermann and Zubek, 1962, p. 300). It is also possible that changes in the central nervous system associated with age may exert an influence on the processing of sensory data relevant to pain.

Findings from experimental studies on the relationship of age and the pain threshold, while by no means in complete agreement, tend to suggest that subjects over the age of 60 report noxious stimuli as painful at a higher level than patients less than 60. Whether this finding is related to a decrease in pain

sensitivity related to age (Schludermann and Zubek, 1962) or whether it is related to a tendency of older subjects to want to be more sure about what they are reporting is not clear.

Lower pain tolerance levels related to age have been reported by Procacci (1975). However, reports indicate that when a distinction is made between tolerance for cutaneous pain, as measured by radiant heat, and tolerance for deep pain, as measured by pressure on the Achilles tendon, older subjects have higher tolerance for cutaneous pain and lower tolerance for deep pain (Woodrow, et al., 1972). Again, the picture may be confounded by differences in attitudes toward tolerating pain between older and younger subjects. Reports of clinical observations, tend to support the view that, even recognizing variations between individuals, there is some decrement in the perception of pain associated with aging.

Unfortunately, some of the important consequences of pain for the person aggravate, and are aggravated by, aging. First of all, pain weakens one's relatedness to one's self as a whole person, to other people, and to one's environment, time, and space. Second, it generates negative affect, especially anxiety and fear. These, in turn, increase the severity of pain. Third, it is apt to seem meaningless; it is very difficult to understand why pain exists or why we need to try to live with it. Fourth, it promotes a sense of helplessness.

Manifestations

Since the experience of pain is personal and private, what one knows of another's experience depends upon what the person in pain communicates overtly and covertly. Based on the message received, we tend to assess it in terms of our own experience, knowledge, beliefs, and attitudes about pain and make inferences about what the other's pain is like. Because pain plays such a critical role in testing reality, we tend to place trust in our own experience of pain as true and accurate, and discount the accuracy of evidence that is contrary (or apparently contrary) to our own internal standards. Therefore, it is difficult to accept the fact that individuals exposed to identical intensities of noxious stimulation may have quite different pain experiences or that one individual exposed to equal amounts of noxious stimulation in two different situations may experience severe pain in one situation and little or no pain in the other.

Anthropologists, missionaries, adventurers, and others who have had an opportunity to observe persons in other cultures have been puzzled by the evidence that people in different cultures often seem to experience and handle situations such as childbirth, physical injury, and illness very differently. That cultural orientation is an important influence on how persons deal with noxious stimuli is generally recognized. Precisely how differences in cultural orientations manifest themselves clinically is not well understood.

Zborowski (1969) in a study of patients of "Old American," Irish, Italian, and Jewish ethnic orientation was able to identify patterns of pain behavior commonly observed in each of these ethnic groups. Within each group, he found that, while a modal pattern could be delineated, there were wide variations from this pattern by individuals in the group. One of the most important findings in this study was that, while the pattern of modal behavior of persons in two ethnic groups might be similar, the cultural values expressed by these patterns of behavior might be very different.

Cultural values influence how persons in a given society think and feel about what should be done about pain and how others should respond to them when in pain. In the United States, science, technology, specialization, and activity tend to be highly valued; we tend, as a people, to favor the elimination of pain at almost any cost rather than to accept it as a part of the human condition. This orientation is neither "right" nor "wrong," nor can it be defined as "good" or "bad." The facts remain, however, that pain is part of the human condition, not all pain can be eliminated, and the price for eliminating some pain may be higher than the person in pain wishes to pay.

In considering the role that cultural beliefs and values play in the shaping of pain behavior, it is essential for clinicians to recognize that they, as well as their patients or clients, are a product of their society. Knowledge of one's own views and attitudes about pain, and sensitivity to how these views and attitudes affect one's behavior in responding to persons in pain, make it possible for clinicians to become more open to listening and understanding the person in pain.

In working with older persons in pain, it is particularly important to listen for cues as to how they believe that age itself affects pain and what prerogatives, if any, age may bring. Deeply felt cultural values may be significant elements in shaping these views. For example, some aged persons believe that one must expect to have pain and that the best way of handling pain is to "try to ignore it." Some persons may be disturbed by treatment that makes them less aware, lethargic, or confused, preferring to live with at least mild and moderate pain rather than risk loss of awareness. Others feel that, as older persons, they have earned the right to relief from pain and believe that they should not have to live with any pain that can be eliminated.

Differential Diagnosis

One of the most difficult problems in respect to differential diagnosis is the absence of pain in certain acute chest or abdominal conditions in which severe pain is typically a cardinal symptom. In an excellent analysis of myocardial infarctions in aged persons, Pathy (1967) found chest pain reported in only 19 percent of cases. Pain may be absent or minimal in other acute inflammatory conditions of the chest or abdomen, such as perforated appendix, perforated ulcer, mesenteric infarction, acute pericarditis, and pleurisy. On the other hand, chest pain is often reported in conditions involving the esophagus or diaphragm, such as hiatal hernia. Thus, reliance upon pain as a diagnostic indicator in acute abdominal and chest conditions in aged persons becomes problematic.

A second aspect of pain which, while not necessarily more prominent in aged persons, confounds differential diagnosis is that pain may mask a severe depression. Clinically, depression and chronic pain are often associated. It has been observed that relief of depression either through antidepressant drugs or other treatment often relieves chronic pain. On the other hand, acute depression in a patient with chronic pain may be precipitated by the relief of pain. The precise nature of the relationship between depression and chronic pain is not well understood. Although it is possible that some instances of depression accompanying chronic pain are a reaction to the problem of coping with this pain over a long period of time, it is less clear how that pain may appear to be interchangeable or a substitute for depression in some persons (Sternbach, 1974, pp. 40–51). There has been speculation that the key to understanding this puzzling association may be related to biochemical changes occurring in the central nervous system. Such speculation is based on the recent discovery of natural morphine-like substances in the brain that are believed to exert a modulating effect not only on pain but also on mood.

Complications

Depression and undesired reactions to drugs are important complicating factors in the management of pain in the elderly. Either severe acute pain or moderately severe chronic pain constitutes a significant source of stress which may tax the adaptive capacities of the older person to the point where depression ensues. The overlying depression further complicates the problem of effective management of the pain.

Undesired drug reactions not only are more common in persons in older age categories but also are apt to be more severe and more difficult to reverse if they do occur. Of particular importance in the reactions to drugs used to combat pain are confusion, disorientation, and impairment of the sense of equilibrium which may contribute to falls; profound depression of the central nervous system functions resulting in lethargy, immobility, and pulmonary congestion; and disturbances of gastrointestinal function resulting in anorexia, constipation, and/or gastric hemorrhage.

The frequent occurrence of adverse drug reactions in the aged has been attributed to (1) reduction in metabolic turnover which may make it possible to achieve a therapeutic level of drug concentration with a relatively low drug dosage; (2) changes in the central nervous system which make the person more susceptible to confusion and disorientation; (3) impaired homeostatic mechanisms; (4) impaired renal and hepatic function which may slow the rate at which drugs are eliminated; and (5) the high variability in response to drugs among aged individuals owing to variations in the effects of aging, disease, and/or trauma on various organs (Exton-Smith and Windsor, 1971, pp. 369–371).

Close supervision and skilled management of medication for relief of pain is of particular importance not only in minimizing adverse reactions to drugs and the possibility of overdosage but also in avoiding the possibility of failing to provide relief by inadequate dosage. Adequate medical management of pain is sometimes denied the older person because of a mistaken belief that nothing can be done because of the patient's advanced years.

Prognosis

Fortunately, many of the conditions that give rise to pain either are self-limiting or can be effectively managed if associated anxiety, fear, and depression can be relieved. Fears that pain may signal crippling or increased dependency or that the pain may reach an intensity that cannot be coped with are particularly troubling, particularly in the elderly. Anxiety and intensity of pain can be reduced markedly if reassurance can be given that crippling and dependency will not necessarily be increased. The most convincing way to reduce fears associated with successful coping with future pain is to demonstrate the ability to successfully manage the patient's present pain.

The prognosis for successful management of pain is better if the person has confidence in the persons who are responsible for care and treatment and in the particular approach employed in pain management. Prognosis is good if the pain has been of relatively short duration, if the secondary gains from having the pain do not exceed the advantages of being pain-free, and if the person can become actively involved in control of the pain.

The prognosis is less optimistic if any of these factors are lacking; however, since so much of the successful management of pain is dependent upon the relationship with the patient and the context within which care and treatment is given, pain is rarely, if ever, completely intractable.

Prevention and Management

Unfortunately, there are no easy solutions to the prevention and/or management of pain. Pain is influenced by a wide variety of factors, some of which are intrinsic to the individual, and others that impinge on the individual from the environment or the context in which noxious stimulation and/or treatment of pain occurs. Insofar as clinical pain is concerned, there are wide variations among persons in respect to sensitivity to pain, ability to tolerate pain, the meaning of pain, beliefs about appropriate pain behavior, and even the propensity to develop pain problems (Engel, 1959, p. 9). Nevertheless, there are general principles or guidelines that can be suggested.

1. Measures that reduce negative affects, particularly anxiety, fear, and depression, usually reduce both pain behavior and the intensity of pain experienced. Since anxiety potentiates the pain response, measures taken to reduce anxiety may either eliminate or dramatically reduce the experience of pain. Such measures may take a variety of

forms, such as (1) understanding the nature of the pain mechanism, (2) learning to work with the body's own potentials for coping with pain, and (3) learning to interpose activity incompatible with anxiety or pain response and/or to utilize the environment to support the person's coping strategies. When pain is constant or when it can be predicted to occur at regular intervals, administering analgesic medication at short regularly-spaced intervals is generally regarded as preferable to waiting for the pain to recur, anxiety to build up, and associating pain relief with the taking of pain medication.

2. It is important to demonstrate to the patient that the pain that is being experienced can be controlled and he or she has a part to play in that control. Introducing the patient to techniques to head off anxiety, to prevent pain, or to engage in behavior incompatible with pain are means of assisting patients to gain a feeling of control over the pain. Patients can also enter into the process of decision making in relation to such things as the reduction of dosage of analgesic required to control pain, the evaluation of therapeutic outcomes, and the choice between given alternatives of intervention (Moss and Meyer, 1966).

3. Measures that provide a means for the person in pain to reestablish his relatedness to the environment, to other people, and to himself as a person are important to combat the feeling of isolation that accompanies severe pain and/or long term pain. Patients with pain need to know that they have been heard and that what they have said about their pain is understood and taken into account.

Once relief is obtained, even if it is temporary, the individual who has chronic or recurrent pain needs to learn to focus attention outside himself on interests other than his pain problem. Activity that is of interest and meaningful to the person is important. Keeping a record of such activity is useful as a means of obtaining visual feedback of progress being made. It is also important to find ways to keep one's self related in time and space in ways that are meaningful outside of pain and pain medication.

4. Persons with pain need to find meaning in their pain—something that makes sense to them. Since this is very personal helping the patient explore the pain experience (i.e., what the pain is like, what worries him about it, how it interferes with normal activities of daily living, ways of coping that have been found successful in the past) not only provides data for assessment but also can be helpful in individualizing the plan of care with the patient (McCaffery, 1972, pp. 88–92).

Evaluation

It is difficult to judge precisely the effectivensss of any given measure taken to relieve pain because (1) there is no completely satisfactory way to quantitatively measure the intensity of pain in a given individual, and (2) the context within which pain occurs and management is undertaken can and do affect the outcomes of intervention. On the other hand, well-oriented, cooperative persons are able to reliably rate their subjective assessment of the intensity of pain at a given point and, also, to indicate the amount of relief obtained.

A number of techniques may be used to elicit the patient's rating of the intensity of pain. One way is to ask the patient to rate the intensity of current pain on a scale from zero to ten, with zero representing no pain and ten representing the most intense pain the person has ever experienced. This is considered a reasonably reliable measure of the person's subjective assessment of intensity. To determine the relief obtained after a measure with therapeutic intent has been completed, the person may be asked to indicate at intervals of a half hour, one hour, and two hours whether the pain is one-quarter, one-third, one-half, two-thirds, or completely gone. Such ratings yield data to judge the intensity of pain in this person's experience and also the amount of relief experienced. It does not yield data to judge intensity of pain across subjects, nor does it necessarily indicate that relief is due to the intervention taken.

When pain has persisted over a prolonged period of time, asking the patient to keep a diary of activity, pain medication, and pain severity for seven to ten days prior to initiation of treatment provides invaluable baseline data for evaluating the subsequent progress. If it is impossible to obtain such data prior to initiating treatment, keeping such a diary immediately after the initiation of treatment and at intervals in the succeeding weeks may also be useful. An increase in activity, a decrease in analgesic intake, and the patient's subjective judgment that pain is less severe are all indicators of pain relief.

BIBLIOGRAPHY

Agate, J.: The natural history of disease in later life. In Rossman, I. (ed.): Clinical Geriatrics. Philadelphia, J. B. Lippincott, 1975.

Benoliel, J., and Crowley, D.: The patient in pain. Proceedings of the National Conference on Cancer Nursing, American Cancer Society, 1973.

Butler, R.: Aging and Mental Health. St. Louis: C. V. Mosby, 1973.

Engle, G.: Psychogenic pain and the pain-prone patient. Am. J. Med. 26:899–918, 1959.

Exton-Smith, A. N., and Windsor, A. C.: Principles of drug treatment in the aged. In Rossman, I. (ed.): Clinical Geriatrics. Philadelphia: J. B. Lippincott, 1971.

Kenshalo, D. R.: Age changes in touch vibration, temperature, kinesthesis and pain sensitivity. In Birren, J., and Schaie, K. W. (eds.): Handbook of the Psychology of Aging, 1977.

McCaffery, M.: Nursing Management of the Patient in Pain. Philadelphia: J. B. Lippincott, 1972.

Moss, F., and Meyer, B.: The effects of nursing interaction upon pain relief in patients. Nursing Research 15:303–306, 1966.

Pathy, M. S.: Clinical presentation of myocardial infarction in the elderly. Brit. Heart J. 29:190, 1967.

Procacci, P., et al.: The cutaneous pricking pain threshold in old age. In Weisenberg, M. (ed.): Pain: Clinical and Experimental Perspectives. St. Louis: C. V. Mosby, 1975.

Riley, M., and Foner, A.: Aging and Society, Vol. I. New York: Russell Sage Foundation, 1968, pp. 248–249.

Schludermann, E., and Zubek, J. P.: Effect of age on pain sensitivity. Perceptual Motor Skills 14:295–301, 1962.

Sternbach, R.: Pain Patients: Traits and Treatment. San Francisco: Academic Press, 1974.

Sternbach, R.: Pain: A Psychophysiological Analysis. New York: Academic Press, 1968.

Woodrow, K. M., et al.: Pain tolerance: Differences according to age, sex and race. Psychosom. Med. 34:548–556, 1972.

Zborowski, M.: People in Pain. San Francisco: Jossey-Bass, Inc., 1969.

28

Powerlessness

Tom Hickey

QUICK REVIEW

POWERLESSNESS

DEFINITION	Expectancy that one cannot determine the outcome of one's behavior.
ETIOLOGIC FACTORS, HIGH RISK	A developmental phenomenon. Decline in physical vigor and body capability—chronic disease. Societal induced—removal of persons from the power structure. Socialization into the role of being old and powerless. Loss of determinates of power: property, independence, finances, belongings, useful knowledge, productivity. Relocation, institutionalization. High level anxiety.
DYNAMICS	A deficiency, based on what is "important" to the older person.
SIGNS AND SYMPTOMS	Reminiscence without reintegration. Turning into one's self. Expressed fear of being overwhelmed by external forces.
MANAGEMENT	Encourage freedom of expression of personal fears and concerns. Accept initial dependent behavior with new power loss situations. Foster positive assertive responses. Do not negate aggressive, narcissistic, demanding behavior; since it is an indicator of attempts to retain control and power. Locate and help person to see realistic areas of control and areas for future control (goals). Set up encounters with others who lost power and then were able to regain control. Encourage reminiscence and integration. Identify for areas where control realistically can be exerted.
EVALUATION	Observe pattern of participation in decision making and control activities. Determine areas of satisfaction and/or continuing frustration.

Granted that physical vigor is lost in old age: no one expects physical vigor of the old. That is why, both by law and by custom, men of my age are excused from responsibilities which cannot be carried on without physical exertion, and the end result is that we are not only not required to do more than we can, but not even as much as we could.

(Cicero: On Old Age)

For Cicero and many writers since then, powerlessness is in the eyes of the beholder. In its most literal sense, it is the perception of loss of power. When identified with old age and the elderly, this powerlessness is both a self-perception and a societal stereotype, i.e., the perception of others of the generalized role and functions of old people. It is a form of alienation. It can also become a self-fulfilling prophecy, especially when viewed in the context of earlier life roles and functions. To nurses and other health care practitioners, the powerless behavior of elderly patients frequently is detrimental to good health care; it usually creates an atmosphere of higher dependency on the health care system and more work for care personnel. To understand this phenomenon it is important to define initially the psychologic and social determinants of powerlessness.

Definition

On a philosophic level, the concept of powerlessness is inherent in the theoretic literature that deals with alienation. In Marx's theory of alienation, a central issue is the chance an individual has of "controlling his social and natural environment rather than being a victim of uncontrollable forces" (Israel, 1971, p. 5). The social role of man—central to Marxian philosophy—is also a key to understanding the sense of powerlessness and alienation experienced by older people in their social environments. Seeman (1961) defines alienation in terms of five states: powerlessness, meaninglessness, normlessness, isolation, and self-estrangement. These states suggest that, for the most part, socioeconomic concepts and contemporary kinship structures—that is, our current social structure—cast the elderly in a role of alienation and powerlessness. On a psychologic level, on the other hand, the older individual's self-perceptions in the larger societal context will determine the extent to which powerlessness has become personal-

ized. The geriatric health practitioner must understand the social structure, and attempt to determine and define psychologic states on an individual level in order to better work with the older patient.

In his nationally acclaimed documentary on being old in America, Dr. Robert Butler summarized it slightly differently: "Powerlessness is a condition considered by many to be synonomous with old age in America. All too many people have been brainwashed and pacified into believing they are powerless." (Butler, 1975, pp. 321–322).

Both the early observations of Cicero and these contemporary comments by Butler suggest something of additional importance beyond what could be termed the "condition" of powerlessness in the aging. There is the clear implication that social and psychologic states of powerlessness may differ. In other words, the social structure (and resulting stereotypes) frequently encourage us to carry the concept of powerlessness too far with the elderly—to ignore, to expect nothing, to cast aside. Similarly, many old people convince themselves and others around them upon whom they are dependent (e.g., family, nurses, other service providers) that they are totally powerless. Little is expected or demanded because that has become the generalized perception within the individual and in his immediate relationships.

Looking again at the literature on alienation theory, we find both the psychologic and social concepts of powerlessness closely linked. Perhaps both perspectives are best summarized in the writings of Seeman where powerlessness is the individual's *expectancy* that he cannot determine the outcome of his behavior, i.e., that his behavior is not instrumental in his goal attainment which is determined largely by powers outside of himself. The key term here is "expectancy." For the geriatric practitioner it becomes as critically important to assist the elderly in defining realistic individual expectancies for themselves as it does to modify the expectations of nurses and important others in that individual's immediate surroundings.

Etiologic Factors

As implied in the preceding section, the etiologic factors of powerlessness are twofold. On the one hand, it is a *developmental* phenomenon, related to the decline of physical vigor and the bodily systems generally. Although this is largely an age-related phenomenon, there is wide variation in individual conditions, with notable genetic and sex differences apart from age. Moreover, an individual's level of acceptance of loss of power and his or her ability to compensate, adapt, or otherwise cope with this phenomenon tend to vary greatly as a function of lifelong personality styles, adaptation to previous life events and crises, and the like.

On the other hand, powerlessness is a *societal-induced* phenomenon. As previously discussed, there is a somewhat generalized expectation that old people are withdrawn from the power structure of society. In the framework of disengagement theory (Cumming and Henry, 1961), either the individual withdraws or society withdraws from the individual. There have been ongoing debates about whether such a process is universal, and this chapter will not attempt to continue such discussions. Nevertheless, there is a somewhat generalized expectation—both by society and by the individual—that regardless of the older person's level of activity (along a continuum of engagement-disengagement), the personal and societal stereotype of old people is one of lack of power and status. Although this phenomenon is also an age-related one, there is a great deal of variation in the acceptance of this perception or belief. Nevertheless, we have generally tended to marvel and praise as extraordinary, the intellectual, physical, or other creative accomplishments by the very old (e.g., Adenauer, Pope John XXIII, Grandma Moses, Picasso, and so forth).

One of the better perspectives for analyzing this dual etiology of powerlessness emerges from the behavioral sciences. Behavioral scientists frequently view age-related changes from the context of life-long socialization. Most people are socialized to new roles throughout their lives, e.g., first entry into school, adolescence, entry into the labor force, marriage, parenthood, separation and return to a single role caused by divorce or widowhood, retirement, and perhaps institutionalization. Regardless of an individual's expectations or preparations, these new roles have different obligations, right, standards, and norms of behavior. Whether the individual is formally trained or initiated into the new standards and expectations, there is at least an informal change of some significance. As Rosow has pointed out, "In various ways he is instructed in his new obligations and rights, in the norms that are supposed to guide his conduct and relations with others, in what they can expect of him and he of them. This induction is the process of socialization" (1974, p. xii).

Despite the similarity of the process as it affects the individual at various stages in life, there does not seem to be an effective socialization process to many of the important life events found in old age—beginning, perhaps, with retirement. One can speculate that this is changing in a positive way as new cohorts reach their post-retirement years, with the emerging emphasis on old age as a distinct period of American life. The newly old people are moving into a period which now has more visibility, and they are doing so with greater personal resources and independence, including better health. However, this possible change represents the future, not the present cohort of very old people who are the current participants in the health care system. The phenomenon of powerlessness, related to what is, at best, an ambiguous socialization process to old age, is still quite present to nurses and other health providers as they work with their patients in the geriatric care context.

Loss of Determinates of Power

The loss of power by the elderly cannot be defined simply in terms of an inability to socialize or be socialized into old age. More specifically, it is the loss of the determinates of power as earlier defined in adulthood, combined with the inability to define, accept, or adapt to different expectations which accompany old age. Rosow (1974) relates power to status, defining several factors that determine adult status in our society. Some of these are briefly defined here in terms of both their social and health-related dependency implications.

PROPERTY OWNERSHIP. Property ownership traditionally has been an important criterion for power, independence, and security. Moreover, older people have been able to command a certain amount of deference and respect from the young until property is passed on to the latter, frequently not until after the elder's death. This phenomenon has gradually changed in American society to the extent that the deferential relationship has eroded. The obvious residual status of property ownership is the independence it provides. Thus, it is a very real fear which older people have about the loss of independence (power) which might result from a catastrophic illness and/or institutionalization. On the one hand, the caution, suspicion, or apprehension with which many older people approach the health care system is frequently based on a realistic fear that there may be no cure or relief for their illness. On the other hand, there is an equally realistic fear that the cost of health care will erode their financial security including the irrevocable loss of their property and its incumbent status.

INSTITUTIONALIZATION. On somewhat of a micro level, we see similar concerns and behaviors in the institutionalization process—which may take place much after the loss of real property. There is a real sense of loss and powerlessness inherent in becoming housed in a building and a room that contain few, if any, material and tangible personal properties. A few family pictures and letters among a handful of other personal items in a bedside drawer may represent the last vestiges of an individual's personal relationship to his surrounding world. It is not surprising then that institutionalized older people behave in a way that reflects a high degree of apathy, dependency, and powerlessness. This is their perception— one which is frequently reinforced by the institution and the health practitioner. In any event, whether we are dealing with the institutionalized older patient or an older person at the outset of a diagnostic and treatment phase, it is unfortunate that more attention is not given to this basic fear. It is a real fear of loss of control and power in one's life, of being stripped, so to speak, and of losing the relationship to an immediate environment which is inherent in the possession of property.

KNOWLEDGE. Knowledge has always been a determinate of status and power. Traditionally, this has been linked with age, experience, and wisdom. The aged were typically viewed as authorities, teachers, and models for the young because of their possession of vast amounts of important knowledge. As Toffler (1970), Rosow (1974), and others have noted, the rapid rate of societal change, the speed with which new knowledge becomes strategic and old knowledge obsolete, have minimized the importance and value of the knowledge possessed by older people. The newly powerful are the recently trained and the discoverers or technicians of new uses of knowledge. Thus, knowledge still is an important determinant of power and status. Given this context, the all-too-frequent perception of society and of older people themselves is that the elderly generally possess little or nothing in the way of useful and important knowledge and experience.

This appears to be a much-too-generalized perception. For example, there is a returning interest among many young people in the cultivation of plants, herbs, and vegetables, in such artisan crafts as pottery and needlework, and so forth. Much of the expertise for these and other activities resides with the current generation of old people. Thus, while the power traditionally inherent in knowledge has

changed to favor the young, the versatile, the technicians, and the futurists, this should not result in a sense of total powerlessness by the aged. In the health care setting, for example, Maddox and Douglass (1973) demonstrated that older people were frequently more "knowledgeable" about predicting and diagnosing their own health status than was the health care profession.

PRODUCTIVITY. Productivity is another determinant of status in Rosow's framework. In a strict socioeconomic sense, older Americans are relatively powerless. With the exception of various professions and some highly selective and self-reliant occupations, older people are expected to retire, and are perceived as not productive in relation to the national economy. Many old people are able to redefine productivity in terms of other activity. Such retirement activity can frequently take on more personal meaning and value for the individual than the productive values of a previous career. If we were to expand our economic definition of productivity to include broader social concerns, then the status of many of the elderly—and their retirement activities—would increase significantly. This writer and others (e.g., Cowgill, 1974) have suggested that such a change in society's views of productivity may gradually be taking place, at least among the younger adult cohorts. In any event, the significant issue for nurse and practitioner is that the current cohort of older people have been socialized in a society which values productivity. The loss of such is perceived as a real loss of power and status.

PERSONAL INDEPENDENCE. Another valued outcome of our American system is personal independence, which is a high degree of status and power. Thus, a very ambiguous socialization faces older people with increasing dependences. As Rosow has well-stated: "Thus, prosperity and autonomy have weakened the informal mutual aid networks that have traditionally been the most important mechanisms for meeting the needs of older people. In a mass society, responsibility for them is becoming increasingly formalized, ritualized, and depersonalized as a public problem" (1974, p. 5).

The powerless behavior and response of the institutionalized elderly seems to be: "Why am I here among people I do not know? Where are my family and friends? This is not my home." This is the ultimate loss of power—the life event for which there is the least amount of anticipatory socialization. It is no wonder that old people fear the onset of any illness and the generalized loss of power. Clinical interviews have shown that these fears are most frequently related to an ultimate and deeply rooted fear of institutionalization and its implied loss of personal independence.

SENSE OF COMMUNITY. Related to independence is the whole structure of kinship and community. The smaller nuclear family and its mobility have greatly reduced the ties that traditionally bound families together, both vertically between several generations and laterally across siblings and their families in the same community. The binding ties are now fewer and typically characterized by geographical separation. Thus, as dependencies increase with age, older people sense a powerlessness in being forced to seek help locally among strangers—unable to rely on significant others for the assistance they need.

Consequences of Loss

The major consequence of losing the trappings of status is the pervading sense of powerlessness. Rosow's (1974) negative perspective on the lack of effective socialization to old age concludes that (1) older people are generally devalued by younger people as determined from the latter's rejection behavior and negative attitudes; (2) the aged are viewed as stereotypes (much like other minorities) rather than as people; and (3) they are excluded from society—largely owing to role loss and the ambiguous identity which results from the previously described negative status changes.

The foregoing discussion suggests that the concept of power(lessness) is very deeply rooted in both our social structure and individual development throughout adulthood. It is both a social and a psychologic phenomenon. Rosow's socialization framework suggests that we are "just not ready" for old age when we reach it. In fact, when we view this from a life-span perspective, many of the previously described losses are contradictory. Power is the ultimate result of mastery of basic human goals inherent in all child development theories, e.g., independence, autonomy, integrity, actualization. Human development seems to occur gradually and somewhat systematically, whereas physical and psychologic decline seem to come more rapidly and erratically. It is not surprising that we are not ready for it.

Dynamics

In many ways powerlessness is not a problem until it is perceived as such. It begins to operate as a dynamic in other behaviors—including the illness role—when the cumulative experiences of past losses and the probability of immediate future losses are real and imminent to the older person. Moreover, physical powerlessness of the body, especially either visual or ambulatory deficiencies, reinforces a generalized sense of powerlessness throughout the system.

Much like loneliness, which is described in Chapter 25, powerlessness is analogous to a deficiency disease. Elderly people are deficient in something significant to bodily and system functioning and/or perceive themselves to be significantly deficient, and are treated as such. It is most likely that the extent to which the perception of deficiency is overgeneralized by the older individual will determine, in large part, the degree to which the individual is treated as deficient by the nurse. The depth and extent of the symptomatology will vary as a function of expectancies and perceived reinforcements. Beyond defining the "real loss" or deficiency, the nurse needs to determine what is most important in the loss from the individual's standpoint. In the patient's view, part of the perception of deficiency is related to the probability of reversing the problem or at least obtaining compensatory mechanisms as substitutions. Should such opportunities or alternatives exist, the generalized sense of deficiency and overall powerlessness may shrink considerably. The nurse is undoubtedly in a more enlightened position to suggest viable compensatory mechanisms or alternatives to meet an important need or to minimize the personal concerns surrounding a deficiency. A frequent reaction to a depressed or recalcitrant patient is that "there is nothing we can do." However, the real problem here may be that the appropriate lever has not been found. Many people can tolerate all kinds of chronic problems *if* there were some mechanism to compensate for one of their deficiencies which has assumed maximal personal significance.

An important starting point then is to deal effectively with perceptions and expectancies. On another level, the dynamics of powerlessness suggest that physical and psychologic manifestations be differentiated in the diagnosis of problems. It is not uncommon, for example, for some of the psychologic problems to diminish somewhat during treatment of physical problems, only to reappear later. As attention is focused on the older person and a specific physical problem, a sense of renewed self-importance may develop. Control and power may return as patient demands are met. However, as the patient recovers and attention declines, the feeling of importance and control may subside and lead to depression. The physical and psychologic manifestations of powerlessness must be treated separately.

Problem Manifestations

The aged population is generally at risk to the deficiency problems related to powerlessness. There are a number of specific situations and high risk areas to be considered by the health practitioner. Before discussing these, however, it might be useful to describe the more general health context of older people and some of the normal aging phenomena. This is undoubtedly a restatement of what appears in other sections of this book; however, full knowledge of the health status of older people and about the normal aging process is of great importance to our understanding of powerlessness.

Health Care Service

The most obvious issue facing the health practitioner is the disproportionate number of older people among the population requiring health care and services. Although they represent approximately 10 percent of the general population, people over the age of 65 account for nearly one third of the costs of health care in this country. Moreover, data of the National Center for Health Statistics (1974) provide the following additional information. Hospital discharge rates for age 65 and over are 346 per 1000 persons— more than double the rate for the general population. The average length of hospital stay for the elderly is approximately 12 days, almost five days longer than the average for all ages. Hospitalization for older people is most frequently caused by diseases of the circulatory system (105 discharges per 1000 persons), diseases of the digestive system (45 discharges per 1000 persons), and neoplasms (38 per 1000 persons).

Thus, the problems most frequently being treated are chronic diseases, including heart disease, arthritis, various orthopedic conditions, and problems related to vision and hearing impairments. Chronic diseases lead to impairment in function which in turn leads to a sense of powerlessness. In fact, more than two out of every five older persons report some form of limitation of important activities caused by chronic conditions. This is four times the rate for the general population. Thus, in contrast with more generalized acute care settings, the geriatric nurse is dealing with an older population of sick people who come more often to seek health care and treatment,

who stay longer, and who are rarely cured or completely well.

Physiologic Changes

There are a number of physiologic changes associated with the normal aging process which can lead to system deficiencies and a generalized sense of powerlessness and to chronic illnesses and related dependencies. These changes vary with individuals according to chronologic age, genetic makeup, and other degrees of impairment. The overall effect of these changes is a decreased capacity for homeostasis, or the ability of the bodily system to cope with new stimuli and return to normal state. There are changes in some organ systems that are due to aging while other organ systems remain relatively stable throughout life.

NERVOUS SYSTEM. The nervous system of an individual gradually loses its efficiency as a result of a decreased number of cerebral neurons and a slowing of the passage of impulses along the neural tracts. This results in a slowing of reflexes, muscle responses, and sensory efficiency. The senses of smell and taste diminish as do the visual and hearing abilities of older persons. Presbycusis is a hearing condition that is the loss of ability to hear high-pitched sounds. Vision generally declines slowly, although some individuals do experience the development of cataracts or glaucoma. All sensory losses decrease the ability of the individual to relate effectively to his environment and to control his life situations.

CARDIOVASCULAR SYSTEM. The cardiovascular system continues to function well unless a disease state such as arteriosclerotic heart disease or hypertensive disease is present. There is an increase in blood pressure with increasing age because of reduced elasticity of arteries. Usually the heart does not increase in size but does decrease in ability to provide functioning response to excessive exercise or stress.

SKELETAL SYSTEM. The skeletal system very often suffers the effects of decreased joint mobility as fluids harden and tendons stiffen and shorten. A condition known as osteoporosis alters the structure of some bones and the ability of the body to withstand stress. An effect of this is seen in the frequent hip fractures experienced by older persons, a condition that severely limits mobility and frequently results in a fairly long hospitalization for the individual.

GASTROINTESTINAL SYSTEM. The gastrointestinal

tract is a system that can remain relatively efficient throughout life because the cells reproduce themselves. Yet the decreased taste sensations and the problem of decayed or missing teeth contribute to poor nutritional intake. Often, owing to lack of sufficient funds, the aged person is not eating a balanced diet and either gains excessive weight or suffers from malnutrition. Also, decreased muscle tone contributes to decreased peristalsis and constipation.

Physiologic Coping Mechanisms

The elderly person is susceptible to the deleterious effect of any disease state. Because of the many physiologic changes that occur, he has a decreased ability to respond to an onslaught to any system. His physiologic coping mechanisms are deficient to respond to infection, dehydration, electrolyte imbalance, anemia, or any other disease process. One of the first systems that is affected by these are the cerebral neurons. The brain requires 20 percent of the total oxygen of arterial blood. The need is increased by an increased body temperature or increased body demands. The brain has no capacity for storing oxygen, and a deficiency interferes with the production and function of neurohormones and cerebral metabolites, thereby causing an inhibition of impulses through anatomic pathways, affecting motor and sensory impulses and emotional and intellectual aspects of consciousness. Dehydration and inadequate renal function secondary to poor cardiac output cause sodium retention and cellular dehydration. Insufficient glucose intake combined with hypoxia leads to energy deprivation. Poor vitamin intake leads to inactivation of cellular activity. All of these cellular changes are the physiologic causes of confusion that are so often a manifestation of illness by an aged person. Confusion which does not allow the person to be fully aware of his surroundings contributes to his feeling of powerlessness.

Psychologic and Emotional Processes

In addition to physiologic processes that contribute to a feeling of powerlessness in the older person, there are numerous psychologic and emotional needs and processes that function to promote health or disease. Initially, it will be beneficial to focus on the personality of the individual. For any individual throughout his lifespan, there is an attempt to develop a sense of self, an identity. There is a searching for a balance between how one perceives himself and how others perceive him. There is a searching for an answer to the question "Who am I?" that tries to find the balance between the ideal self (the way we wish we were) and the real self (the way we are). Knowledge and acceptance of self is necessary for growing older successfully.

REMINISCENCE. One of the processes through which an aging person begins to accept decline is reminiscence. This is characterized as the progressive return to consciousness of past experiences and an attempt to integrate these into the self in a meaningful way and to resolve past conflicts. If this reintegration can be achieved, there is new meaning to a person's life and even a preparation for death. If reintegration does not occur, depression and anxiety can be the result (Butler, 1963). Illness can deter this reintegration because it requires the elderly person's energy be directed towards coping with the illness. Hospitalization can prevent this reminiscence because no one person will take the time to listen to the person; instead, by his return to previous life, he is labeled as "senile." If one does not know the therapeutic value of this reminiscence, one cannot support this behavior.

INTERIORITY. Another aspect of "turning into one's self" is a fairly normal developmental change. There seems to be a subconscious force at work that begins developing in middle age. This is known as "interiority." A person shifts from active to passive modes of mastery. He often sees the world as complex and threatening, and sees himself as being unable to cope (Huyck, 1974). This shift into self and the fear of becoming overwhelmed by external forces are frequently a cause for a patient's reaction to the technical orientation of a modern hospital. He feels he cannot cope with the equipment and procedures which are designed to help him recover but which are frequently painful, tiring, and incomprehensible in purpose.

Sensory Loss

The interaction between sensory loss and a person's self-concept is another prominent feature in the overall reaction of an elderly person to hospitalization. An elderly person who has a hearing or vision loss, who is placed in a new environment and subjected to either a sensory deprivation or sensory overload, cannot adequately order his environment. If he attempts to communicate but cannot hear, a nurse may not effectively explain his surroundings. Often she does not take the time, but she may also fear disturbing other patients in the immediate area. If a patient cannot see, he may be unable to experience his surroundings or anticipate intrusion into his personal space. Anxiety and anger may be the result. Even normal human subjects, who are subjected to deprivation of sensory stimulation, lose their powers of awareness and perception. An elderly person who is confined to bed by siderails, handicapped by various tubes and equipment, and suffering from pain and weakness will soon become disoriented and confused. If he then attempts to remove himself from his bed, he is very often restricted to the bed by use of body or limb restraints. These increase his sensory deprivation and his ultimate confusion.

Other Processes

This section has been describing the elderly in general and the normal aging process as the risk factors in the powerlessness syndrome. What other phenomena or specific situations would suggest a higher than normal risk? On the psychosocial level there are a number of fairly obvious life events that would increase the potential for powerless behavior. Retirement, widowhood, relocation, or institutionalization are primary examples. The recency of their occurrence and the patient's adaptation to them should be explored by the health care practitioner as important components of any illness diagnosis.

On the psychophysiologic level, high risk patients are those who exhibit high levels of anxiety. Coping with normal aging phenomena can easily lead to a continuing state of anxiety which tends to reduce the effectiveness of various treatment interventions. It should be kept in mind, however, that mild anxiety can serve as a motivating force and set the stage for learning new adaptive behaviors and developing compensations for other losses. On the other hand, severe anxiety reduces focus and concentration along with the patient's involvement in his or her immediate environment. It becomes more difficult to work with this patient, and other symptoms and problems will compound this general deficiency. An anxiety neurosis, or chronic anxiety state typically leads to some form of chronic depression. It is a tremendous challenge to deal with these patients either diagnostically or therapeutically. In fact many are routinely dismissed as "senile." Thus, the onset of a recurring level of mild anxiety is the point at which there is both highest risk of rapid decline and greatest potential for successful treatment intervention.

Treatment and Assessment Issues

This chapter has intentionally not addressed issues of prevention. The proper treatment of deficiencies and actions taken by both patient and practitioner to avoid the generalization of a deficiency to an overall powerlessness syndrome are the most effective ways to prevent further decline in this area. There is unquestionably no way to prevent some semblance of a self and body perception as powerless by the patient, nor any way to prevent the societal role and status structure which sets the stage for such perceptions.

The basic issue here seems to be that of treating problems, not concepts, and treating them in their order of importance. Since the elderly and the chronically ill frequently present themselves for health care with multiple symptoms, problem identification and definition and the hierarchical ordering of problems is critical for successful treatment. Once these are identified, the nurse is in a good position to suggest useful support systems, to assist with the use of compensatory mechanisms and to reinforce good coping behavior. The effectiveness of treatment is to be found in the increase of behaviors that counteract generalized powerlessness and exhibit a realistic autonomy in the context of objective limitations and deficiencies.

In their extensive research on institutional patients who experience transfer or relocation, Lieberman (1975) and his colleagues reported that positive and assertive behaviors were more often predictors of better adjustment. Patients who were aggressive, irritating, narcissistic, and demanding were typically better off in the crisis situation. This is an important dimension to consider when evaluating treatment effectiveness and behavioral change. It is frequently thought that the quiet, passive, and likable elderly patient is the best. In fact, this may be the patient who is regressing, withdrawing, and perhaps giving in to the deficiencies he is experiencing.

Finally, this chapter concludes with some of the treatment procedures suggested by Rudd and Margolin (1968) for dealing with dependent behaviors and anxieties which so frequently result from the onset of the sick role in old age.

First, the staff must be prepared to accept this initial dependent behavior and communicate to the patient that dependency resulting from illness does not mean lowered esteem in their eyes. Then the patient should be helped to see that he has a measure of control over his destiny and what is being done to him, and that he can and should participate in his care. He can be helped to see that other people have been in the same circumstances and have recovered. Before a person can accept these motivational concepts, he must first feel free to express his personal fears and concerns. If the expression of these fears and concerns meets with understanding and acceptance, he can then begin to express a tentative control over his environment.

The art of communicating with an older person often requires short, simple communication. Sometimes the initial interaction will be stimulated by questions regarding his past life and accomplishments. A nurse can build on this interaction to begin a program to build a sense of self-awareness and confidence in the person's own ability. From there, a patient can be helped to realize that, if he participates in care, he will be exercising control over his own life and helping himself to achieve the fullest possible return to health.

These are but a few of the approaches that the innovative nurse will use to meet the needs of this ever-increasing segment of our population. The evaluation of these measures will be possible in the future as nurses become aware of the growing need for quality assurance in providing care. As nurses become aware of the methods of developing and using evaluation tools, they will be able to assess their efforts and plan further measures to improve care. At the present time, a nurse can and does evaluate an elder's response to care in the same measure she evaluates any other age group. Further research into nursing measures and outcome criteria must be carried out if progress is to be expected in this area of geriatric nursing.

REFERENCES

Butler, R. N.: Why Survive? Being Old in America. New York: Harper & Row, 1975.

Butler, R. N.: The life review: An interpretation of reminiscence in the aged. Psychiatry 26:65–76, 1963.

Cicero, M. T., (Copley, F. O., tr.): On Old Age. Ann Arbor: University of Michigan Press, 1971.

Cowgill, D. O.: The aging of population and societies. In Eisele, F. R. (ed.): Political consequences of aging. Ann. Amer. Academy of Pol. Soc. Sci. Philadelphia: American Academy of Political and Social Science, 1974, pp. 1–18.

Cumming, E., and Henry, W.: Growing Old: The Process of Disengagement. New York: Basic Books, 1961.

Huyck, M. H.: Growing Older. Englewood Cliffs, N.J.: Prentice-Hall, 1974.

Israel, I.: Alienation From Marx to Modern Sociology. Boston: Allyn & Bacon, 1971.

Lieberman, M. A.: Adaptive processes in late life. In Datan, N., and Ginsberg, L. H. (eds.): Life-Span Developmental Psychology: Normative Life Crises. New York: Academic Press, 1975, pp. 135–159.

Maddox, G. L., and Douglass, E. B.: Self-assessment of health: A longitudinal study of elderly subjects. J. Health Soc. Behavior 14:87–93, 1973.

National Center for Health Statistics, 1974, Utilization of Short-Stay Hospitals: Annual summary for the United States. USDHEW, Public Health Series 13, No. 26, Washington, D.C.

Rosow, I.: Socialization to Old Age. Berkeley: University of California Press, 1974.

Rudd, J. L., and Margolin, R. I.: Maintenance Therapy for the Geriatric Patient. Springfield, Ill.: Charles C Thomas, 1968.

Seeman, M.: On the meaning of alienation. Amer. Sociolog. Rev. 26:753–758, 1961.

Toffler, A.: Future Shock. New York: Random House, 1970.

Part 5

A Look to the Future

29

Encouraging Continued Growth
in the Elderly

Richard L. Grossman and Robert B. Greifinger

The woman sitting in front of us is an erect, cheerful, clear-eyed person with obvious energy and a ready smile. She enjoys talking to other people, but not just about herself. There is curiosity in her twinkling blue eyes. She says to us, "I'm 71, and I've been living in St. Petersburg for 11 years. I've had arthritis for a long time—even before I moved down here." Then she tells us with a chuckle, "I just know that when I get up in the morning I'm going to feel stiff all over, so I kind of limber myself up by walking around my bed and bending several times as a kind of exercise." Physical examination discloses that Mrs. B has mild degenerative joint disease but, in every other respect, is a strong person physically. Further interview reveals that she continues to be an active gardener and she goes sailing with some younger friends in St. Petersburg. When we ask her how she deals with her arthritis when she is busy she says, "Well, you know, when you're doing something you like, you tend to forget what's bothering you. Of course, there are some things I can't do—I have someone else do the heavy digging in the garden, for example, and I'm afraid I'm no longer a perfect crew member when we go sailing." As we continue to talk, a feeling of mutual respect and trust develops. Mrs. B tells us quite forthrightly but in a lowered voice, "The thing is that I still live alone, you know. I don't have any family any more. What concerns me is that I know I should be preparing somehow for what they used to call 'the visit of the grim reaper' and I feel that I don't know how to do this. I don't think I'm afraid of death, but I'm wondering if there isn't something I can do to make more of this last chapter of my life."

In the past it was thought that the chief contribution a nurse could make to the older patient consisted in providing "Tender Loving Care." We propose that the latter day successor to "TLC" is a more specific technique: dealing with the inevitable *thrust toward growth* which continues even though the older person often perceives his life to be in a continuing decline. As Doctor Gay Luce, the developer of the Senior Actualization and Growth Exploration group in Berkeley, California says, "People can grow as much at 75 as at 25, if they are given the same conditions that inspire growth in the young—nurturing, support, challenge, freedom, and continued activity." Doctor Luce's philosophy is one more aspect of the evolving definition of human health, namely, that *health is not the condition in which a human being finds himself, but is rather the process by which he becomes the whole person of which he is capable.* In the United States the older person is too often considered (by himself and by those around him) to have already completed this process of becoming, and to be in a state of decline simply because there is a loss of elasticity in the connective tissue of his body. The acceptance of this image of the older person contributes to behavior patterns that (1) discourage the full use of the body, (2) disregard healthful diet, and (3) lead to loss of hope, faith, and laughter. The older person simply ceases to believe in a meaningful future.

If health, however, is seen as more than merely the functional capacity of the human body, the role of health practitioners is to work with the endowments, behaviors, and skills that the older person has accumulated in his lifetime. These are the health attributes of the elderly, their subliminal resources, their extant strengths.

How can the nurse help to uncover these positive attributes? How can the nurse feed back these qualities to the patient? How can the nurse develop an alliance with the older person that will direct the use of these resources toward his continuing healthful movement?

> Mrs. B from St. Petersburg continues, "I'm more and more preoccupied with dying. I don't want to end up in one of those homes, lying helpless in my bed, just a burden to everybody. I think about how my own mother died, just as dependent as a baby. It was terrible."

This sort of fear and preoccupation does not seem very promising as a "health attribute." But the first step in achieving a positive orientation in dealing with the old person is to trust and respect the patient *exactly as he presents himself*. We go toward the positive by working first with the articulation of subjective feelings and ideas matched with our objective appraisal. In the case of Mrs. B, for example, we have already observed in her the following positive health attributes which we might use to work with her on the subject of planning her so-called last chapter:

1. She is alert and curious.
2. She has a health-seeking attitude. ("I want to make more of my life")
3. She has an active, committed, physical life, including exercise, gardening, and sailing.
4. She is not afraid of talking about her death.
5. She has integrated the disability of her arthritis into her life.
6. She lives independently.
7. She looks forward to a future—even a future death—that she considers to be better than her mother's.
8. She has friendships and activities involving people of other generations.

These eight attributes are only the *obvious* positive resources Mrs. B exhibits. Against them we have the evidence of her real—and not inappropriate—distress about preparing for her death. Clearly these two kinds of data cannot be neatly separated. We owe Mrs. B a working response to the issue that brought her to us, but we also have the opportunity to introduce her to ways of exploring her potentials for growth that are implied by her evident strengths. Doing both these things is the most humanistic strategy available to us.

What do we do for Mrs. B? What do health care workers do for elderly persons at large, who are universally characterized by possessing untapped, unused health attributes at the same time they are experiencing stress or disability?

GROUP APPROACHES AND ACTIVITIES

The key themes of a positive-oriented approach to older people were stated by Doctor Luce when she said the requirements for growth are "nurturing, support, challenge, freedom, and continued activity." The nurse's role is central in creating the environment in which those themes can be made real. The remainder of this section deals with guidelines that might be used in working with the health attributes of the elderly.

We're All in the Same Boat

The nurse can take responsibility for organizing groups of older persons to meet on a regular basis. Experience has demonstrated that the setting for such a group is of great importance. It should be an area as large as possible, a space comfortable for sitting and lying on the floor, and spacious enough to permit exercises involving dance movements, walking, and stretching. The members of the group should sit either on the floor or on pillows rather than on chairs. The nurse-leader might consider burning a mild incense at each meeting, or using background music for some of the exercises. Ideally, this room should have access to the outdoors so that in good weather some of the activities could be extended beyond the room itself.

The strength of peer groups is obvious and well established. In the case of older persons it is particularly important and enriching for them to be able to meet people who have many of the same concerns they do. They are often quite surprised that there are *many mutual concerns and fears*. A mixed group of men and women is desirable. The role of the nurse-leader should emphasize her facilitative qualities; the style of leading the group should be patient-centered, that is, not directive or didactic. The atmosphere should at all times be kept as informal and friendly as possible, with the members of the group sitting as close together as is comfortable. They should be encouraged to speak to each other directly. At the first session the leader would be well advised to emphasize that the group is not "therapeutic." There should be some discussion of the fact that *old age is not illness* and that, although the nurse is highly qualified to cope with the emergencies and distress of all people, in this setting her role is to help the group elicit its individual and communal strength in order to make this period of life richer, more vital, and more active.

The group should have a specific time for meeting, preferably no less than once a week. Each session should run from one to two hours, with the understanding that any member may leave the group at any time without explanation, but that regular attendance will be beneficial to all. In addition, the ground rules for the group should include the understanding that any issues that come up for discussion, such as sexual activity, death, financial problems, and other similarly confidential and extremely personal information, are on a purely voluntary basis. No member should be made to feel that by belonging to the group he is under any obligation to deal with any personal matters that might be embarrassing.

On the other hand, the main theme of the first few sessions of the group will be on developing trust and respect for all group members and understanding that the group is an unusual and privileged opportunity to deal with matters that group members may not have been able to discuss with anyone before the group was formed. The theme, therefore, is total honesty, confidentiality, mutual respect, and equal consideration for the privacy of all group members.

It Feels Good to Talk

All sessions, but particularly the first two or three, should emphasize the freedom of everyone present to talk about anything that concerns him. It is important that the leader be gentle in guiding the discussions and in reminding members about the ground rules they have adopted for their discussions. The nurse should feel free to discuss her personal experiences as well, thereby encouraging candor and detail. The group leader should be especially sensitive to the common problem of loss; the *loss of other people in his life* to death and the *loss of experiences in the workplace and family setting.* These are experiences that have extended over many years and have suddenly been truncated. Continuing loss generates unique fears in the mind of the older person. Ventilating the feelings that accompany those fears with others who are in comparable positions is the fundamental vehicle for creating trust and love within the group.

Touching Is Believing

One of the most important commonplace experiences that disappears from the life of the elderly person is the repeated touching of others and the touching of himself. In many older people, this leads to a fear of being touched, often accompanied by a belief that anyone who approaches is likely to touch in a hostile fashion. This situation emphasizes the *isolation, loneliness,* and *"ghetto"* circumstances of the older person. This can begin to be remedied in group work, especially by the teaching of full abdominal breathing exercises. These exercises will form the essential vehicle for learning many deep body relaxation techniques, and for employing techniques of visualization, imagery, and fantasy. Because the breathing exercise is so important, it should be a standard part of every group meeting and should be repeated at each session. The best way to learn the breathing technique is in pairs. Learning this technique offers a comfortable and nonthreatening opportunity for older persons to once again touch each other.

One member of each pair should lie comfortably on the floor with his partner on his knees next to him. The helping partner places one hand on the person's chest and his other on the abdomen. The person in the breathing position (recumbent) places his hands on top of the helper's hands. The helper asks his partner to take slow and rhythmic breaths, introducing the concept of *rolling breathing* by asking his partner at the beginning of inspiration to fill the abdomen and place pressure against the hand covering the abdomen. With each inspiration they should concentrate first on lowering the diaphragm and expanding the abdomen. After the abdomen has been expanded and pushed against the hands, energy should be directed toward filling the chest with air, raising the anterior ribs until the breath is felt to lift the clavicles. Expiration is simply the reverse of this process. The breather should allow expiration first to leave the collarbones, then to deflate the chest, and finally to relax and empty the abdomen. This completes the breath cycle.

With patience and concentration, first expanding the abdomen and then the chest, the helper can encourage a rhythmic, rolling, relaxed breath, which will be perceived as a wave beginning in the abdomen, moving up toward the chest, relaxing in the chest, and then returning to the abdomen.

It will not be unusual for people to have difficulty at first with rolling breathing, as it is culturally established for us to breathe solely with the chest. However, encouragement of deep abdominal breathing, with its complete filling of the lungs, can be learned without much difficulty. For those who have trouble expanding the abdomen, the group leader may ask them to place their hands behind their necks with their elbows extended as high as possible away from the shoulders. This, in effect, cancels the possibility of using the accessory muscles of respiration, and focuses the respiratory effort solely on the diaphragm. The diaphragm has a natural movement to expand the lungs toward the abdomen, giving the sensation that the abdomen is being expanded.

Rolling, rhythmic breathing should be continued for approximately five minutes. It is often helpful to encourage participants to close their eyes and, after breathing is begun in a rhythmic way, to concentrate on relaxing the muscles and letting energy flow through the body. The touch of the helper is extremely important in creating a secure environment for relaxation. Having learned this technique, older people should be urged to add rhythmic deep breathing to their daily routine. This is helpful for encouraging general relaxation, promoting restful sleep, and dissipating pent-up energy from anxiety or inactivity.

Another technique that involves touching between the members of the group is a *basic massage*. The technique of *self-massage* should be taught first. This introductory massage for the head and shoulders is something every member of the group can do for himself. After it becomes a familiar routine, it is an appealing introductory exercise to massaging another person's head and shoulders.

After the technique of self-massage is practiced at a number of sessions, members of the group should be encouraged to try massaging each other. A good way to do this is to have each person lie on the floor and have a partner on his or her knees at the head of the person lying down. A gentle massage of the head, face, ears, and neck will be easy for the person to do since he has now had daily experience in his own self-massage. As in the case of the breathing exercises, the partners should then alternate so that each gets the experience of both touching and being touched by another in a supportive fashion.

Motion Is Movement

A characteristic of the elderly is tentativeness in moving and walking. This is due partly to a lack of confidence in the body's ability to avoid difficult situations, or to move rapidly. Some of it is due to a fear of mingling with crowds of people (usually younger) who are moving so rapidly that the older person feels threatened. Walking in particular is experienced by many as a difficult task, one which reminds them of their declining strength and autonomy. For these reasons, exercises involving use of the body in motion are of immense consequence to the older person. The group should not be lectured about its abilities but, rather, should be invited to participate in experiential exercises that *confirm* for them their ability to maintain balance and control over parts of their bodies.

For example, while sitting on their pillows in the circle, an exercise of "slow motion" can be used. Tak-

---

INSTRUCTIONS FOR SELF-MASSAGE

1. Begin by tapping the top of your head gently with your fingertips. Let your fingers dance around all over your skull.
2. With the tips of your fingers, begin to massage your ears starting with the top rim and circling your entire ear.
3. When your fingers approach your ear lobes, massage gently in a circular way. Let your fingers move to the indentations right behind your ear. Do a slow circular massage on these indentations.
4. Gently rub your neck muscles from the base of your skull downward.
5. Move your hands around to your face. Pull your forehead horizontally from the midline to the side, running your hands along your forehead in a gentle movement from side to side.
6. Massage around the sinuses and the bony orbit of your eyes (be sure not to massage your eyeballs).
7. Use your fingertips to massage the sides of the tip of your nose.
8. Move your fingers in a circular motion on your jawbones, coming forward slowly from your ears down to your chin.
9. When you come to the tip of your chin, use your hands to pull downward gently on the front of your neck.
10. Crossing your left hand over your body, massage your right shoulder muscles vigorously, keeping the other arm and hand tucked behind you to support your back. Do the same for your left shoulder with your right hand. Knead your shoulders, particularly in back and toward the neck.
11. Throughout this massage, close your eyes and concentrate on the feeling in your fingers, skin, and body. Relax. Breathe deeply and slowly.

ing partners but remaining seated facing the center of the circle, the participants practice turning their bodies toward their partners by rotating their pelvis in an exaggeratedly slow manner. They should be encouraged to make their ordinary movements as slowly as possible. They then reach out their right hands for the purpose of shaking hands, again exaggerating as much as possible the slowness of the movement toward the other person. Together they shake their arms up and down as slowly as possible and feel the rhythm of their own reduction of movements to an exceedingly slow pace.

For their exercises at home, they can be encouraged to dress in slow motion or pour a glass of water in slow motion. The object of these exercises is to give each person a sense of the way in which his body moves, and an equal sense of the manner in which he controls that movement. The beneficial side effect of slow motion exercises is that it encourages a feeling of calm and tranquility.

Another movement exercise (which emphasizes that the older person can practice controlling his body at any time in an ordinary setting) is a stretching technique that has been called "picking grapes." In this exercise, each member of the group is standing with his feet separated about the width of his shoulders. He is encouraged to stand for a few moments with knees unlocked and the body in as relaxed a state as possible. For the first few moments, participants are encouraged simply to do deep breathing until they feel they are totally relaxed. The exercise begins by permitting the body to fall forward from the waist, without any attempt to touch the ground but extending the arms and allowing them to fall, fingers outstretched toward the ground, again in as relaxed a manner as possible. Then, slowly and rhythmically, each person rises from the bent position, allowing his upper torso to follow the lead of his arms as they ascend and eventually reach toward the sky. At the point when his arms are extended as far as possible, he stands on tiptoe and wiggles his fingers, reaching toward an imaginary grape arbor as if picking the fruit of the vine. The main sense that each person should feel is that the spine and back are being gently arched and stretched, and that the hips are rolled back, with the face looking upward as the fingers pluck "the grapes." After several moments in this outstretched position, he slowly permits his upper torso once again to fall forward with his hands, head, and shoulders descending toward the floor. After a few moments of remaining in the best position, he repeats the "picking of the grapes" sequence.

Both the rising and falling segments of the exercise should be repeated five to ten times after the group members have been introduced to the exercise.

Persons should be encouraged to move around during the exercise if that is comfortable for keeping balance. It is important to stress that this is not a calisthenic exercise in which a person should be straining to touch the floor or his toes; rather it is an exercise requiring relaxed movements.

The Age of the Higher Self

The elderly, in many cultures, are expected to devote their energy to spiritual matters and to acting as a resource of wisdom for younger people. Our culture has no tradition for this special privilege; nevertheless, there are ways in which the older person can devote himself to matters of the spirit and be personally rewarded in the process. One way this can occur is in the person's learning new ways to be serene and quiet, and to contemplate one idea or feeling at a time. This can be accomplished by an informal exercise in *mindfulness*, or concentration, in which the communication is internal rather than directed to the outer world. A good group technique in doing this is to place a large, lighted candle in the center of the circle. After determining that the members of the group are seated in a comfortable and relaxed position and have gone into the rhythm of their, by now familiar, deep breathing, ask them to concentrate quietly on the flame of the candle until such time as they might wish to close their eyes and direct their concentration inward. This exercise can be accompanied by quiet music, such as one of the baroque canons, or other sounds that are conducive to tranquil contemplation.

There is an exercise that has no immediate application to ordinary daily living but can be very rewarding to group members in reinforcing their sense of community and membership in the human race. It is to form a living *mandala,* a mandala being a Hindu or Buddhist symbol of the universe. In this exercise, members of the group lie in a circle with their heads forming the hub of the circle; they hold hands with the persons on either side of them. With a background of quiet music, or in total silence, the group performs regular, rolling, deep breathing. With his eyes closed, each person concentrates on images of all the members of the group and of himself. He directs his conscious attention to his membership in the group and to his relationship with the people he has grown to know and trust. This exercise may be used as a finale to individual group sessions, or a special 10- to 15-minute period may be set aside at sessions for the experience. The leader should remember that, in the case of both the candle contemplation and the living mandala, members of the group may first exhibit some self-consciousness over doing things that are not customary. Likewise, at the end of such exercises, they may wish to discuss with each other some of the thoughts and feelings that accompany the experience. The leader should encourage this kind of exchange and, with respect to any feelings of intimidation, should urge the person to do only that with which he is totally comfortable. (Incidentally, in all these exercises, the leader should participate as a full member.)

One device that seems to alleviate feelings of self-consciousness and makes the experience more readily available to group members is to close the eyes while doing the exercise, emphasizing the feeling of privacy and individuality.

The Gift of the Senses

For the most part, the resources of the five senses remain available to the older person, and can be stimulated for the purpose of creating immediate and meaningful rewards. A large literature and documentation of "sensory awareness" techniques now exists, and many of the principles established by innovative developers of these systems can be adapted to the special growth needs of the older person.

For example, if the weather and the outdoor setting permits, one particularly meaningful exercise that might be employed is the "the blind walk." Group members are encouraged to form two-person partnerships. One member of the partnership is blindfolded and entrusts himself to the other for being led through an outdoor walk. They join hands and the responsible, leading partner guides the other person on a gentle exploration of the surroundings. From time to time the leading partner stops and picks up objects that might be smelled (flowers, leaves, berries) or an object that might be explored by the touch (stones, bark from a tree, clumps of grass, twigs). In each instance, the leading partner pauses long enough to allow the blindfolded person to use his smell or touch to explore all the qualities of the objects: the texture, the odor, the shape, the size, things on which we do not normally concentrate. As in other partnership exercises, the roles are reversed so that the leading partner may also have the blindfold experience.

This exercise could well be followed by a discussion of some of the unusual ways in which the senses record an experience for the older person that he had long since thought of as matter-of-fact and ordinary.

In the event that the setting or the weather does not favor the blind walk, an indoor adaptation of the exercise is the "tangerine peel." In this exercise, everyone in the room is given either a tangerine or an orange and, again in partnership, one person is blindfolded (or closes his eyes) and peels, smells, explores with his fingertips, tastes, chews, and swallows the fruit. Once more, the highlight of the exercise is the exchange of the experience of each person. The principle of the tangerine peel is to emphasize that even though, in the case of older persons, some of the senses may be weakened as a result of physiologic changes, the reserve capacity of all the senses is still reachable, and the "peel" becomes an immensely rewarding experience for those who consciously set out to explore its richness. The object of all sensory awareness exercises is to emphasize *autonomous control* of the five senses, whether they are being used retrospectively or actively.

The Rhythms of Life

The changes that occur in the body of the older person are sometimes subtle, sometimes dramatic. In addition to specific organic change and to changes in the appearance and parts of the body, many of the processes that we call "normal" operate with different rhythms as people grow older. These changes occur in sleeping patterns, digestion and evacuation, sexual appetite, and, of course, mood and outlook.

These changes can often be frightening and threatening for the older person. One way to defuse these alterations of their intimidating quality is to keep a regular record of them over a considerable period of time. For that reason, one of the most constructive things that the nurse can do in dealing with older people is to encourage them to keep a *Body Rhythm Diary* (see Appendix 29-1). This form should not be construed as being rigid, and the nurse may wish to revise some details of it, depending on the group with which she is working. Its general outlines give the older person an opportunity to understand consciously more of the things that are going on in his physical life.

The nurse can take the responsibility of conducting discussions of the diary entries of various group members (or of an individual if she happens to be working private with someone) and take account of some of the data that is acquired as a result of posting the entry into the daily diary. For example, it is particularly useful for older people to become aware of which hours of the day are those in which they feel they have the highest energy available to them. By keeping the diary and plotting its information on a simple graph it becomes quite clear, for instance, that someone who wishes to pursue a particularly active schedule of dancing, woodworking, or teaching has an optimal period in each day in which to do these activities.

The concept that the person can responsibly choose which hours to work in order to take advantage of that high energy will reinforce the feeling of *independence* that many older people feel they are losing as the aging process takes place. Likewise, the regular maintaining of the Body Rhythm Diary will give the individual precise, subjective feedback about his own experience, and add to the realization that there are some things he can take control of, or adapt to, which prior to the diary might have been experienced as inevitable disabilities.

Another form of diary keeping that can be especially rewarding to the older person is the keeping of a *Dream Journal*. Again the support of the group is useful in encouraging people to maintain, examine, and discuss their dream life, and to act on any messages in those dreams that seem particularly appropriate to them. We know of a number of cases, for example, in which older people were reunited with members of their own families or with old friends, from whom they had had previous angry separations. Having dreamed of such a reunion, they were supported in their efforts to make that dream become reality. The emphasis on using dreams in this way is to accept as valid any subjective or personal interpretation of the dream of the person in the group, rather than try to submit it to definition by some fixed psychologic system. The use of dream journals calls for the nurse to be particularly sensitive to the animation that members of her group exhibit in discussing dreams and to support those acts in waking life which the person feels are deeply motivated.

Balance is All

There is a sequence of feelings and experiences which cause a great many older persons to feel particularly insecure physically as they move through daily life with other people. As mentioned previously, the aging process often causes people to feel they do not have "normal" stability in walking, or in

boarding busses, or in getting in and out of automobiles. As a result they adopt a tentative, and defensive, style of moving; they attach an inordinate amount of consciousness and mental attention to a process usually accomplished almost semiconsciously. The result is that most of the consciousness of the older person in walking becomes, in such situations, so attached to his head that the rest of his body is almost dangling from his preoccupied skull. Therefore, it is useful to help older persons reestablish a firm connection with the earth over which they walk. The best way to do this is to reinforce their consciousness of their pelvis and of its connection as the major link between the legs and the upper torso. One exercise that is particularly useful for this, sometimes called "Bozo the Clown," is described here.

In this exercise, members of the group sit on a floor in as comfortable a position as possible, preferably cross-legged. They begin by breathing deeply with their eyes closed, imagining the breath coming in from the anterior base of the spine. For women, conceptually, this is like breathing in through the area of the vagina and taking the air up the front of the spine. Then they imagine exhaling the air down the back of the spine, and feeling a floating sensation with each exhalation.

The head sits on the center of the spine. One way to emphasize this is to move the head several times, nodding "yes" (forward and back), "no" (turning the head from side to side), and "maybe" (tilting the head from one shoulder to the other). Another way to get the sensation of the head being centered on the spine is to move the head back while inhaling deeply, moving it forward while exhaling deeply, concentrating on the balance of the head.

Once the group members feel comfortable with their heads "centered" and their hands folded in their laps, they should be encouraged to try to feel as bottom heavy as possible. "Try to imagine that in the pelvic area there is a heavy weight, like a medicine ball running from hip to hip. Try to feel that a large weight just below the navel is weighing you down." "Now lean forward slowly, and rock forward, continuing to feel that centered weight." "Then lean to the right, emphasizing again the feeling of weight just below the navel." "Now lean to the left, again imagining the weight in the pelvic area."

The nurse can go around the room and gently tap people on the shoulder, urging them to react as "Bozo the Clown" might (the weighted top that children hit and which returns to an upright position because it is weighted on the bottom). All the members should be encouraged to let their bodies move in whatever direction they have been tapped by the nurse, and then return to the centered position. The entire exercise should continue for at least 15 minutes, with all group members practicing the leaning forward and backward, leaning to the right and left, and leaning around in a circle, breathing into the stomach, and feeling that a special weight is keeping them balanced.

The next phase of the exercise is to have everyone stand, close his eyes, and imagine once again the feeling he had while leaning and rocking on the floor. This exercise attempts to encourage the subjective feeling that the center of gravity is actually low in the body, just above the genitals, and not as most of us believe, mentally held in the head, chest, or throat. After a few moments of deep breathing and recollection of the weighted feeling in the pelvis, group members should be urged to walk very slowly back and forth, and around the room. The nurse should encourage all group members to breathe deeply and concentrate on the feeling of centeredness in the hip area. After this exercise, as with all exercises, a discussion of the subjective experiences of the group members usually is helpful, and the consensus of the group may well be that they would like to repeat the exercise after exchanging their impressions.

Again, the objective of this exercise, while it has specific effects on the way people use their physical bodies, is also to encourage them to believe in their own ability to control the way they move, even though advancing age may have slowed them down or caused them to have to compensate for some specific disability in their bodies. It might be described as an attempt to show older people how to use their bodies in a healthy way, even though those bodies may be smaller and weaker than they used to be.

SPECIAL TIPS ON WORKING WITH THE HEALTH ATTRIBUTES OF THE ELDERLY

1. The nurse is highly trained to cope with the needs of the older person as those needs relate to distress and disability. However, in working with the positive but unused endowments, behaviors, and skills of the older person the nurse clinician is not a therapist, but a facilitator. In this role, her goal is to educe what is already *present* as a potential strength in the older person, rather than treat that person as someone who is ill or distressed.

2. The main objective of all work with the health attributes of the elderly is to emphasize the potential for *autonomous self-governance*. All the exercises are designed specifically to give the older person a small but profound insight into his ability to increase his own amount of self-sufficiency. The nurse, therefore, plays the part of a gardener of older trees, attending to their continuing growth without attempting to force that growth.

3. There is a growing body of literature about the aging process in all its aspects and also about death and dying. Nurses should familiarize themselves as much as possible with this work and share it whenever they can with the older persons with whom they work.

4. The chief criteria for the successful nurse in working with the growth potentials of older persons are sensitivity, patience, and the ability to be self-aware.

5. Much of the nonmedical assistance directed toward older persons casts those people in the role of audience. Music, games, entertainment, religion, and other performances are brought to older people, who become passive consumers of other people's work. The key to working with the health attributes of the elderly is to find ways to make them active, talking, experiencing participants in the process of individual growth.

6. The elderly among us are not merely our fathers and mothers, our grandfathers and grandmothers—they are the future incarnations of ourselves, reminders that we, too, are involved in the continuous aging process even though we may still be chronologically young. The respect and regard we hold for ourselves and for our own possibilities and hopes are the same feelings we owe to the elderly. We are members of the same society that has promoted the idolization of youth and the deploring of old age. The only way to redress that obvious imbalance is to respect and regard the abilities of older persons to continue to grow within themselves even though that growth may not be of the same kind that we associate with younger people whom we describe as "successful," "productive," or "high achievers." The older person grows in different ways, and perhaps even in a less active setting; he, nevertheless, is entitled to the richness of that experience. No one is in a better position to nurture and support that process than the geriatric nurse. Believing in the possibilities of continued growth and loving the people who are trying to explore those possibilities are the necessary conditions for making them come true.

APPENDIX 29-1

BODY RHYTHMS DIARY

Date: _____

Day of week: _____

AWAKENING DIARY:

1. *Time:* _____
2. *Pulse rate:* _____/minute
3. *Awakening mood:*   positive, good spirits   5   4   3   2   1   low, depressed
4. *Feeling of energy:*   energetic, fresh   5   4   3   2   1   fatigued, sluggish
5. *Expectation for today:*   interesting, hopeful   5   4   3   2   1   fearful, stressful
6. *Quality of sleep:*   refreshing, deep   5   4   3   2   1   fitful, restless
7. *Amount of dream activity:*   more than usual   5   4   3   2   1   less than usual
8. *Character of dreams (positive, fearful, tranquil, etc.):* _____
_____
9. *Sleep duration:* _____ hours
10. *Awakening temperature:* _____°F
11. *Body weight:* _____ lb.

BEDTIME DIARY:

12. *Time:* _____
13. *Moods and feelings today:*
   a) *Desire to be with others:*   extroverted   5   4   3   2   1   introverted
   b) *Feelings of freedom:*   free   5   4   3   2   1   restricted, trapped
   c) *Feelings of happiness:*   joyful   5   4   3   2   1   sad, gloomy
   d) *Feelings of emotional satisfaction:*   fulfilled   5   4   3   2   1   empty
   e) *How others felt about you:*   admired, respected   5   4   3   2   1   disliked
   f) *Feelings of calmness:*   peaceful, centered   5   4   3   2   1   anxious, insecure
   g) *Feelings of energy:*   tremendous energy   5   4   3   2   1   exhausted, worn-out
   h) *Feelings of self-confidence:*   self-assured   5   4   3   2   1   inadequate
14. *Did you laugh today?* _____ cry? _____
15. *Interest in sexual matters:*   very interested   5   4   3   2   1   couldn't care less
16. *Amount of sexual activity:*   more than usual   5   4   3   2   1   less than usual
17. *How fast did time go by today?*   very fast   5   4   3   2   1   dragged slowly
18. *Were you "on time" and punctual today?*   usually   5   4   3   2   1   rarely
19. *Did you fantasize or daydream today?*   a lot   5   4   3   2   1   very little
20. *Intellectual functioning:*   very sharp   5   4   3   2   1   dull, slow
21. *Attention span:*   very concentrated   5   4   3   2   1   easily distracted
22. *How was your memory today?*   excellent   5   4   3   2   1   frequent lapses
23. *Motor coordination today:*   adroit   5   4   3   2   1   clumsy
24. *Physical exercise today:*   overexerted myself   5   4   3   2   1   less than usual
25. *How much stress was there in your day?*   very stressful   5   4   3   2   1   little stress
26. *Did anything unusual happen to you or your family today?*
   (accident, marriage, death, birth, new job, crisis, etc.) _____
_____
27. *What was the weather like today?* _____
28. *Were you particularly aware of any of your senses today?*
   touch _____ taste _____ smell _____ hearing _____ sight _____
29. *Appetite today:*   insatiable hunger   5   4   3   2   1   no hunger
30. *Food today:*   regular, well-balanced meals   5   4   3   2   1   irregular eating
   Any comments on food eaten today? _____

31. *Bowel movements today:*   number _____
    time of day _____ character _____
32. *Amount of liquid consumption:*   more than usual   5 4 3 2 1   less than usual
33. *Frequency of urination:*   more than usual   5 4 3 2 1   less than usual
    color of urine _____
34. *General state of your skin?*   (clear, pale, pimply, dry, oily) _____
35. *Feelings of health today:*   very healthy   5 4 3 2 1   poor health
36. *Did you have any unusual symptoms today? If so, when?*

    anxiety _____   breathing difficulty _____   sore throat _____
    allergies _____   sinus problems _____   fatigue _____
    skin rashes _____   itchiness _____   nausea _____
    headache _____   stomach ache _____   fever _____
    body pains _____   constipation _____   other _____
    eye troubles _____   diarrhea _____

37. *Did you use any drugs or medication today? If so, what?* _____
    _____

38. *What part of the day* (morning, afternoon, evening, night) *were you most:*

    productive _____   sensitive _____   happy _____
    energetic _____   depressed _____   tired _____
                                                                              irritated _____

39. *What is your overall feeling about today?*   one of my best days   5 4 3 2 1   one of my worst days
40. *Any further comments:* _____
    _____
    _____
    _____
    _____
    _____

Reprinted from Sobel, D. S., and Hornbacher, F. L.: An Everyday Guide to Your Health. New York: Grossman Publishers, 1973. With permission.

30

The Challenge for Nursing

Maxine Patrick and Doris Carnevali

A reality of professional life for most nurses is that they are going to be involved in some aspect of health care for the elderly during their nursing careers. In fact, older persons may represent an increasing proportion of nurses' case loads as more individuals live longer and health care patterns and payment systems change. This suggests that not only nurses specializing in the care of the elderly but also any nurse who provides services to older persons needs working knowledge of age-related changes and their impact on health, illness, and management of daily living.

Nowhere in health care is there as great an opportunity for nurses to do what they say they want to do as in the care of older people. They can examine, treat, work with families, be accountable, serve as advocates, plan and institute care, and collaborate with others, because, as yet, no other professions are doing it. But the time may not be far distant when others will step in and do what nurses have not done. Medicine is awakening. More medical schools have geriatrics courses now than do nursing schools. And, a recent conference devoted its agenda to the need for medical education in geriatrics and ways to develop such curricula. The Veterans Administration is training some physicians but not nurses in the care of the elderly. At present and in the past there has not been competition for the care of the elderly sick. This picture may be changing. Nurses need to be alert to what could happen and become involved initially rather than complain when others take over.

Few nurses graduate from schools in which nurs-

ing care of the elderly has been taught as an area requiring special knowledge and expertise—comparable, for example, to pediatrics. Nor do licensure examinations give attention to the older age group with special segments as they do to the very young. It is as if knowledge of growth and development (which tends to focus on the first third of life in most courses) and medical-surgical nursing (which tends to focus on pathophysiology and treatment of "adults") automatically makes a nurse ready to care for the elderly. Thus, most nurses graduate from basic programs with little emphasis in their background on age-related changes in the elderly and the implications for nursing management. The very absence of this attention to the elderly communicates a message to nursing students.

Beyond the basic preparation of nurses, clinical specialization in practice gives only token recognition to age-related factors and implications for practice. In many clinical specialty areas the emphasis has been directed almost totally to body systems and phenomena encompassed by the clinical specialty, as in orthopedic specialization which treats diseases of the musculoskeletal system; or the focus may be on the pathologic process as it affects body systems, as in oncology. For other nurses and some physicians the specialization may be related to the acuteness of the presenting situation rather than the system or the disease process, as in intensive care nursing or in emergency room or recovery room specialization. The fact is that, aside from maternal-child nursing, a nurse in any specialty area, regardless of its focus, is going to provide care to the elderly. The nurse specializing in orthopedics is probably going to see more elderly persons with fractured hips and degenerative joint disease than youngsters with broken arms or ski injuries. Certainly cardiac disease, except for congenital anomalies, is one of middle and old age, as are strokes and peripheral vascular disease. Cancer has a higher incidence in the elderly. So does diabetes. Nurses in emergency and intensive care units treat the elderly at least as often as other age groups.

Further, more than 90 percent of people over 65 are not in institutions specializing in health care for the elderly. They are receiving health care in ambulatory health care settings, general hospitals, their own homes, classes and clinics in senior citizen centers, or retirement homes.

One of the challenges for the practicing nurse and the nursing profession is to recognize the deficit in basic education for today's practice. Individual nurses whose basic or advanced education omitted the knowledge and expertise necessary to safely and effectively nurse the elderly need to remedy the situation through reading, continuing education or advanced formal education, and more critical evaluation of their ongoing practice as it involves older persons. The profession and the educational systems that prepare practitioners need to examine priorities that devote entire quarters to, and special segments of a licensure to, the particular knowledge and expertise associated with the very young and neglect the same areas in the very old. And this despite the fact that the majority of practitioners will be delivering care to the old—not the very young. It is a challenge.

Beyond knowledge and expertise is the very real issue of values of the profession and the way in which students and beginning clinicians are socialized into their professional roles. Students and clinicians are still being taught in multiple ways that participating in the curing process is the way to go for professional "success." Knowledge related to pathology and treatment for survival and curing is emphasized; role expectations tend to be related to cure-oriented activities; role modelling tends to highlight cure related attitudes, values, and activities; and critical thinking most often addresses diagnosis and management of acute health problems. Maintenance tends to tag along as more of a compassionate intuitive component. It is often seen, but not nearly as aggressively taught or modelled. The critical thinking associated with the long term problems of main-

tenance and the difficult skill of finding the criteria for measuring response in maintenance receive less attention than do the immediate needs in acute care.

As long as there is societal and peer pressure for the best nurses to go into life-saving, curing, dramatic settings, it will be difficult to recruit a critical mass of outstanding professionals to creatively address the needs of the elderly, particularly the dependent elderly. There is the risk that lip service, but not real impetus, will be given to the care of the elderly—in continuing education, in lobbying for legislation as it involves nursing and health care for the elderly, in quality of publication about nursing the elderly, and in associated research and funding for research.

Creativity and rigor in providing *high quality nursing care* for the elderly, regardless of their presenting situation or the setting within which the care is delivered, warrants recognition and status. Students, clinicians, and scholar-researchers need the support of status but also that of critical review if nursing of the elderly is to keep abreast of professional developments in other areas of the discipline.

THE CHALLENGE TO THE INDIVIDUAL CLINICIAN

Nursing the elderly is going to involve nurses in two types of case loads. For some, the elderly will comprise a total case load. Geriatric nursing will be a clinical speciality for them and they may deliver care to the ill or fragile elderly in long term care settings, home care, or geriatric clinics. A future dimension of geriatric specialization should be the presence of a geriatric clinical specialist in acute care institutions who, like the stroke, mental health, or oncology clinical specialists, would serve as consultant to the entire nursing staff, from the emergency ward to the medical units to the intensive or coronary care units. Probably because of the number of people over 65 in institutions on any given day, all hospitals could gainfully employ such a person to give the staff the necessary expertise to deal with problems peculiar to the elderly.

For another group of nurses working in hospitals, clinics, offices, and perhaps home care service, the older persons will be only a part of a case load that includes other age groups.

The demands and skills in the nursing roles for each of these two groups of nurses as they care for the elderly will be different.

The Nurse with a Total Load of Elderly: The Geriatric Specialist

To nurse where patient change is slow, and eventually downhill, where measurement of change is difficult, and where the curer's nemesis, *death*, is an inevitable, foreseeable ending, requires special wisdom, satisfaction in practice, and stamina. Such nurses need to be aware of the drains on themselves and the need to maintain a vitality and fresh vision as well as expertise based on current knowledge of the state of the art. They need to recognize the wisdom of filling their own wellsprings of creativity and knowledge in order to practice with ongoing enthusiasm and skill. *Nurses need to be on the cutting edge of health care in this field where nursing is such a critical component.*

Nurses in Other Specialty Fields

Those nurses for whom the elderly are only a portion of their case load face the same challenges to remain abreast of the current state of the art of geriatrics as do the specialists in the field. However, their task is complicated by the day-to-day requirement to treat patients of different ages and retain current expertise in another specialty field. A fast moving nursing case load, whether in an institutional or ambulatory care setting, in which nurses see patients of different ages, requires them to be facile in rapidly and purposefully shifting their frame of reference according to the age differences among patients they are seeing. They need to know when to call upon a specialized knowledge base on age-related changes and responses to therapy, lifestyle, and the need for support systems. They may need to adjust their expectations, perspectives, data base, and, occasionally, style in caring for the very old. Such frequent, rapid "gear shifting" can be demanding. However, it should be done enough to become a habit.

Beyond this, nurses functioning in a particular specialized clinical field need to have current knowledge within the speciality area about the implications of age-related changes or to know when such substantiated knowledge is missing. They need to view laboratory data in terms of age-related norms or to press for such norms where they do not exist. They need to be aware of the adjustment of drug dosages in terms of changing laboratory findings and to know where manifestations of drug side effects are different for the elderly. Clinical specialists and clinicians in special fields need to alert researchers and teachers to the special problems the aged have in particular disease areas within their field and to urge that attention be given in ongoing research to develop more precise, accurate knowledge and predictably effective nursing management.

These are difficult, unsung jobs. Still, many nurses have devoted their professional lives to the care of old people and have made major contributions to the well-being of this large segment of our population. The mention of geriatrics, like rehabilitation, is not very thrilling to many nurses. Still those same nurses, given a chance to work with older people, frequently become excited and challenged by this kind of nursing. They find that it is not nearly as dull as they had imagined. There are a growing number of nurses who are tremendously enthusiastic about nursing older people. They are doing a creative professional job.

Medical advances have made it possible to add to the number of years human beings survive. *Nurses have the opportunity to contribute to the quality of life in those extra years.* Meeting the health care needs of the elderly in a holistic approach presents a particular challenge to the nursing profession, but nurses and nursing have met challenges such as this before. Given enough expert clinicians, educators, and scholars who are willing to address the broad health needs of the elderly as well as the needs of those who nurse them, we can no doubt address this one with the verve and wisdom the challenge deserves.

Index